S0-BXN-509

TUMORS OF THE SOFT TISSUES

Contributors

Robert B. Epstein, M.D.
Eason Professor of Medicine
Department of Medicine
College of Medicine
The University of Oklahoma at Oklahoma City
Health Sciences Center
Oklahoma City, Oklahoma

Edwin J. Liebner, M.D.
Professor of Radiology
Director, Radiation Therapy Section
The University of Illinois at the Medical Center
Chicago, Illinois
Consultant,
Veterans Administration West Side Hospital
Chicago, Illinois

TUMORS OF THE SOFT TISSUES

Tapas K. Das Gupta, M.D., Ph.D.

Department of Surgery
Division of Surgical Oncology
University of Illinois at Chicago
Cook County Hospital
Veterans Administration West Side Hospital
Hektoen Institute for Medical Research
Chicago, Illinois

RC280
S66
D265
1983

APPLETON-CENTURY-CROFTS/Norwalk, Connecticut

0-8385-9045-4

Notice: The authors and publisher of this volume have taken care that the information and recommendations contained herein are accurate and compatible with the standards generally accepted at the time of publication.

Copyright © 1983 by Appleton-Century-Crofts
A Publishing Division of Prentice-Hall, Inc.

All rights reserved. This book, or any parts thereof, may not be used or reproduced in any manner without written permission. For information, address Appleton-Century-Crofts, 25 Van Zant Street, East Norwalk, Connecticut 06855.

83 84 85 86 87 88 / 10 9 8 7 6 5 4 3 2 1

Prentice-Hall International, Inc., London
Prentice-Hall of Australia, Pty. Ltd., Sydney
Prentice-Hall Canada, Inc.
Prentice-Hall of India Private Limited, New Delhi
Prentice-Hall of Japan, Inc., Tokyo
Prentice-Hall of Southeast Asia (Pte.) Ltd., Singapore
Whitehall Books Ltd., Wellington, New Zealand
Editora Prentice-Hall do Brasil Ltda., Rio de Janeiro

Library of Congress Cataloging in Publication Data

Das Gupta, Tapas K., 1932–
    Tumors of the soft tissues.

    Bibliography: p.
    Includes index.
    1. Tumors.   I. Title.   [DNLM: 1. Soft tissues neoplasms.   WD 375 D229t]
RC261.D265   1983   616.99′2   82-16421
ISBN 0-8385-9045-4

PRINTED IN THE UNITED STATES OF AMERICA

In grateful appreciation
of their early guidance and encouragement
this book is dedicated to the memory of
Gordon P. McNeer and Richard D. Brasfield
of Memorial Sloan-Kettering Cancer Center.

Contents

Preface

Nothing can be learned unless man proceeds from the known to the unknown. With this thought, I have attempted to synthesize my experience in the diagnosis and treatment of soft tissue tumors with the presently available data on this fascinating group of human neoplasms.

The first section deals with the epidemiology, classification, pathology, and methods of diagnosis. The second section describes the various modalities of treatment of soft tissue tumors and the vast strides made in treatment methods. The third section is devoted to the natural history of the benign and malignant tumors arising from each individual tissue type. The last section describes the characteristics of childhood sarcomas.

I deeply appreciate all the help and encouragement I have received from my family, colleagues, and friends, and above all, my patients. My thanks to Dr. Edwin J. Liebner for contributing the chapter on Radiation Therapy and to Dr. Robert B. Epstein for the chapter on Immunology and Immunotherapy. My colleagues in the Division of Surgical Oncology, Drs. Henry A. Briele, Prabir K. Chaudhuri (presently at Loyola University Medical School, Chicago), Edward L. Felix (now practicing in Fresno, California), John A. Greager, Donald K. Wood, Carl Cohen, and Craig W. Beattie, made valuable suggestions and corrections. Dr. Olga Jonasson (Professor of Surgery and Chairman, Department of Surgery, Cook County Hospital), Dr. Robert J. Baker (Professor of Surgery and Chief of General Surgery, University of Illinois Hospital), Dr. Gerald Moss (Chief of Surgery, Michael Reese Hospital, Chicago), Dr. Ralph R. Weichselbaum (Associate Professor of Radiation Therapy, Harvard University Medical School, Head of the Peter Bent Brigham Division of the Joint Center for Radiation Therapy), and Dr. Rao Mantravadi (Assistant Professor of Radiology and Radiation Therapy, University of Illinois) have provided valuable criticisms on several chapters. Dr. John P. Waterhouse and Dr. Bina Chaudhuri reviewed the chapter on Pathology. Dr. Chaudhuri also helped in the selection of photomicrographs. Ms. Bobbie Newson is credited for producing the electron micrographs.

I am deeply indebted to Dr. Lloyd M. Nyhus, who not only had the foresight to initiate a Division of Surgical Oncology, but also to provide a milieu conducive to its growth and development. His continued encouragement is sincerely appreciated.

I would also like to express my appreciation to Dr. Samuel J. Hoffman, Director of Laboratories, Hektoen Institute for Medical Research, for his continued support and help throughout the time this book was in preparation.

Ms. Roberta Macke not only typed the manuscript, but also helped in all other details required for the production of this book.

Finally, my limitless thanks to Ms. Mary Conn for editing the entire manuscript.

TUMORS OF THE SOFT TISSUES

SECTION ONE: Principles of Classification and Diagnosis

1

Introduction

Tapas K. Das Gupta

Soft somatic tissue (connective tissue) comprises the form and substance of the human body. It accounts for about 50 percent of the body weight in adults and 25 percent in children. Height, weight, and body conformation are largely determined by its distribution. The shapes, such as facial features, are welded in a hereditary pattern by the functional equilibrium of intergrowth of these tissues. The shape, size, and contour of all mature viscera are inherently dependent on the amount, composition, and geometric configuration of the connective tissue elements.

The mesenchymal constituents of the body mass theoretically have the same risks for the development of diseases, tumors, and other morbid conditions as has the rest of the human body. In 1950, Klemperer,[1] in an initial systematized study, offered a nosologic scheme to such apparently diversified pathologic entities of the somatic tissues as rheumatic fever, rheumatoid arthritis, polyarthritis, acute lupus erythematosus, scleroderma, and a host of other diseased conditions. Since then, the subject of diseases of the connective tissue has been well investigated. It appears that, although degenerative diseases, metabolic disorders, and certain muscular afflictions are relatively common, an inverse relationship exists between this large body mass and the development of tumors and

tumorlike conditions in the soft somatic tissues. Strangely enough, this curious biologic paradox of a large body mass with a low incidence of tumors did not, for a long time, arouse sufficient interest among clinical scientists to spur a major investigative program.

Of the tumors arising from the primitive mesenchyme, the lymphomas[2] and bone tumors[3-5] have received maximum attention. In contrast, soft somatic tissue timors have been sparsely studied and, until recently, they received only cursory mention in most textbooks.

Reports on the natural history of these tumors or tumorlike conditions appeared in the medical literature in the latter part of the nineteenth century, but the focus was primarily on bone tumors. It was not until this century that interest in a systematic study of mesenchymal tumors was aroused. Ewing[6] originally generated interest in the study of primary mesenchymal tumors, but his major interest was always the tumors of the skeletal tissues.[7]

Stout[8,9] was the first investigator to provide a detailed description of tumors of the soft tissues. Largely on the basis of his original and critical studies, this group of neoplasms was histogenetically classified and their histologic criteria established. The enormous number of papers by Stout and his colleagues referred to in the body of this text is testimony to his pioneering work in the field. The fascicle on *Tumors of the Soft Tissues* by Stout and Lattes[10] still constitutes the mainstay of histologic diagnosis of these tumors.

Systematic clinical studies of soft tissue tumors were primarily initiated by Pack and his colleagues.[11] The volume of material published by Pack, and later by his associates at the Gastric and Mixed Tumor Service at Memorial Hospital in New York, is astounding. Today, most authors reporting on end result studies use the data provided by Pack and his co-workers as the historic reference point. For certain histologic types, Pack's studies are still valid and have been confirmed by more recent publications.

The contributions of Enzinger and his colleagues at the Armed Forces Institute of Pathology have helped to better understand the histology and histogenesis of these tumors. The multitude of papers by Enzinger and his co-workers, cited in various chapters of this text, testify to the fundamental nature of his group's contribution to this subject.

In recent years, histopathologists have provided us with elegant morphologic studies, making histogenetic classification easier and establishing a sound basis for the management of tumors of the soft tissues. Although a number of excellent clinicopathologic papers, cited elsewhere in this text, have recently been published, in general clinicians have not as yet synthesized and applied these morphobiologic data to the understanding of the natural history and overall management of these tumors.

With the establishment of the Division of Surgical Oncology at the University of Illinois, the author decided that accurate data on all these soft tissue tumors or tumorlike conditions would be maintained on a prospective basis. The results of our treatment program have been compared with the burgeoning new clinicopathologic findings, and we have attempted clinicomorphologic correlation of these diverse tumors.

Overall, we have managed 681 evaluative primary and 232 metastic malignant soft tissue tumors (Table 1.1). The experience derived from study of these tumors, along with their benign counterparts, constitutes the basis of this book. All patients were evaluated and managed under the supervision of the author. The tumor specimens, whenever feasible, were ultrastructurally studied in the author's laboratory, in-

TABLE 1.1. HISTOLOGIC CLASSIFICATION OF 681 MALIGNANT TUMORS OF THE SOFT SOMATIC TISSUES TREATED AT THE UNIVERSITY OF ILLINOIS

Liposarcoma		95
Dermatofibrosarcoma protuberans		28
Aggressive fibromatosis		45
Abdominal wall	9	
Extra-abdominal	36	
Fibrosarcoma		79
Malignant fibrous histiocytoma		47
Leiomyoblastoma		10
Leiomyosarcoma		57
Somatic tissue	21	
Other sites	36	
Rhabdomyosarcoma		59
Embryonal		
Orbit	8	
Other head and neck sites	23	
Trunk and extremities	21	
Genitourinary tract	7	
Pleomorphic		32
Alveolar		12
Malignant schwannoma		74
Solitary	56	
With von Recklinghausen's disease	18	
Ganglioneuroma		4
Neuroblastoma		10
Synovial cell sarcoma		34
Clear-cell sarcoma of tendon sheath		4
Epithelioid sarcoma		8
Hemangiopericytoma		19
Angiosarcoma		17
Kaposi's hemangiosarcoma		25
Lymphangiosarcoma		5
Extraskeletal osteosarcoma		5
Extraskeletal chondrosarcoma		3
Ewing's sarcoma of soft tissues		2
Malignant granular cell myoblastoma		1
Alveolar soft-part sarcoma		6
Total		**681**

dependently of the pathology department of the University of Illinois. Currently, all available tumor specimens are being stored for various biochemical, immunologic, and hormone receptor studies.[12]

The chapter on pathology is written primarily for the clinician and in no way attempts to be a major text reference for histopathology of somatic tissue tumors. Although the tumors arising from the peripheral nerve tissue are neuroectodermal in origin and are in no way similar in biologic behavior to mesenchymal tumors, because of their similarity in clinical presentation and the concomitant difficulty in management, they are included in this book. To provide a better perspective for comprehension of the natural history of these diverse mesenchymal and neuroectodermal neoplasms, tumors arising from each tissue type have been individually discussed and the pertinent literature has been summarized. The end results after various types of treatment, as found in the published reports, have been compared with those observed in the patient population treated at the University of Illinois. The operative techniques described in Chapter 6 are those performed by the author and his group in the Division of Surgical Oncology. However, we do not claim any originality or innovation in the techniques of these often-complicated operations. The chapter on chemotherapy of soft tissue sarcomas primarily describes the experience derived from cases treated in our Division of Surgical Oncology and in no way attempts to represent a summary of all the currently available publications on the subject.

The chapters on immunology and immunotherapy and on radiation therapy have been contributed by Drs. Robert Epstein and Edwin J. Liebner. However, this book primarily represents the author's experience with these types of tumors, and reflects his opinions and conclusions. In our Division of Surgical Oncology, although various in-house treatments and investigative programs are in progress, the general principles outlined in different sections of the book are routinely followed in the management of most of the common forms of soft tissue sarcomas.

It is hoped that our experience with these rare, fascinating tumors, our methods of management, and our data on their natural history and biologic behavior will be useful to all interested in the study of these tumors and tumorlike conditions.

REFERENCES

1. Klemperer P: The concept of collagen disease. Am J Path 26:505, 1950
2. Gall EA, Mallory TB: Malignant lymphoma: A clinicopathological survey of 618 cases. Am J Path 18:381, 1942
3. Bloodgood JC: The diagnosis and treatment of benign and malignant tumors of bone. J Radiology 7:147, 1920
4. Codman EA: Bone Sarcoma. New York, Paul B. Hoeber Inc, 1925
5. Coley BL: Neoplasms of Bone and Related Conditions; Their Etiology, Pathogenesis, Diagnosis, and Treatment. New York, Paul B. Hoeber Inc, 1949
6. Ewing J: Neoplastic Diseases, 4th ed. Philadelphia and London, W.B. Saunders, 1942
7. Ewing J: A review of the classification of bone tumors. Surg Gynecol Obstet 68:971, 1939
8. Stout AP: Panel on Soft-Part Tumors. Proc Nat Cancer Conf, 1949, p 206
9. Stout AP: Tumors of the Soft Tissues. Atlas of Tumor Pathology, Sect 2, Fasc 5. Washington DC, AFIP, 1953
10. Stout AP, Lattes R: Tumors of the Soft Tissues. Atlas of Tumor Pathology, Sect 2, Fasc 1. Washington DC, AFIP, 1967
11. Pack GT, Ariel IM: Tumors of the Soft Somatic Tissues. New York, Paul B. Hoeber Inc, 1958
12. Chaudhuri PK, Walker MJ, Beattie CW, Das Gupta TK: Presence of steroid receptors in human soft tissue sarcomas of diverse histologic origin. Cancer Res 40:861, 1980

2

Epidemiology and Etiology

Tapas K. Das Gupta

The factors leading to the development of human mesenchymal tumors have not yet been adequately identified. Most of the correlations are indirect, and conclusions have been derived from evaluation of clinical coincidences. Unlike the more common forms of human neoplasia, such as cancers of the breast and colon, the rarity of these tumors makes epidemiologic studies difficult. Chemically and virally induced sarcomas in experimental systems have provided a body of scientific data on the etiologic factors,[1-9] but little of this information is as yet applicable to human sarcomas. In this section, current knowledge of the genetic, racial, and environmental factors underlying the etiology and epidemiology of human sarcomas is briefly reviewed.

FAMILIAL AND GENETIC FACTORS

Only a small proportion of human malignant tumors are inherited in a mendelian pattern, indicating single gene transmission that occurs as an inherited trait or as a complication of inherited precursor lesions that are clinically recognizable (Table 2.1). Recognition of these preneoplastic hereditary syndromes would allow the early screening of family members for possible early treatment and the delineation of bio-

chemical and physiologic mechanisms linking gene defects to these neoplasms.

The familial preneoplastic and neoplastic syndromes directly related to mesenchymal tumors are rare, and each of these entities has been discussed in detail elsewhere in this book. In this section, they are briefly reviewed to provide a better perspective of the multifactorial influences on the etiology of human soft tumors.

Gardner's Syndrome

Gardner's syndrome is characterized by the appearance of multiple mesenchymal and skeletal tumors in conjunction with colonic polyposis. The extra-alimentary tumors are usually osteomas, lipomas, or epidermal cysts.[10] The close association of aggressive fibromatosis and low-grade fibrosarcomas in patients with Gardner's syndrome is well known. This syndrome is discussed in detail elsewhere (Chapter 12).

Chemodectomas

Chemodectomas are paragangliomas and can arise anywhere in the sympathochromaffin system. The most common locations are the carotid bifurcation and the nodose ganglion in the neck. These tumors sometimes produce catecholamines. Familial carotid body tumors are frequently bilateral (Chapter 14).[11]

TABLE 2.1. HEREDITARY NEOPLASTIC SYNDROMES

A. Hereditary neoplasms or sarcomalike conditions
   1. Gardner's syndrome
   2. Chemodectoma
   3. Retinoblastoma
   4. Pheochromocytoma and medullary thyroid carcinoma
B. Preneoplastic conditions (hamartomatous syndromes)
   1. Neurofibromatosis
   2. Tuberous sclerosis
   3. von Hippel-Lindau syndrome
   4. Multiple exostoses
   5. Peutz-Jeghers syndrome

Retinoblastoma

Although retinoblastoma, strictly speaking, is not a sarcoma, it is included in this chapter because its biologic behavior is akin to that of mesenchymal tumors. Retinoblastoma is an embryonic ocular tumor that occurs in young children, the incidence being about 1 in 20,000. In 5 to 10 percent, the occurrence is familial; bilateral involvement is more common in familial than in nonfamilial cases. Penetrance is 80 to 90 percent; therefore, clinically unaffected persons may occasionally transmit the tumor.[12,13] Jensen and Miller[12] suggested that deletion of the D chromosome is a frequent manifestation in retinoblastoma. Associated congenital malformations of varying degrees have been reported.[12–16] Jensen and Miller[12] found that 53 of 1,077 evaluable children with retinoblastoma had major congenital malformations. Additionally, 21 were mentally retarded, whereas four to seven cases would normally be expected. A further finding was that 30 children had a second primary cancer, osteosarcoma being the most common. One case of rhabdomyosarcoma in a child with retinoblastoma has also been reported.[17] Although radiation-induced cancers of the head and neck region are well recognized, the osteosarcomas and fibrosarcomas reviewed by Jensen and Miller[12] were distant from the irradiated area.

Pheochromocytoma and Medullary Thyroid Carcinoma

These tumors occur either singly or together.[18–20] The reported penetrance is 85 percent; a higher rate may be found upon careful screening of the patient's family for increased production of catecholamines and calcitonin by otherwise silent tumors. These tumors are usually diagnosed after the second decade of life and tend to arise bilaterally or at multiple foci in the adrenal medulla and the thyroid. The syndrome occasionally includes parathyroid hyperplasia and neoplasia, which may be a complication of hypercalcemia resulting from increased circulating levels of calcitonin.

Preneoplastic Conditions or Hamartomatous Syndromes

Structural defects in several organ systems can be identified in these conditions. Usually they are defects in development, with incorrect differentiation and random mixing of all the component tissues. One or more of these tissues may proliferate as a localized growth (hamartoma). The hamartomas are classified primarily as malformations, as opposed to true benign neoplasms (Chapter 4).[21] As with hereditary neoplasms, autosomal dominant inheritance is indicated in these syndromes, and there is no evidence that environmental factors contribute to the development of these neoplasms.

Neurofibromatosis

Neurofibromatosis, or von Recklinghausen's disease, occurs in about 1 in 3,000 live births and is characterized by multiple café-au-lait spots and multiple neurofibromas. Frequently, it is associated with lipomas, lymphangiomas, and hemangiomas. A detailed discussion of this syndrome and variations thereof can be found in Chapter 14.

Although central or peripheral nervous system tumors not associated with von Recklinghausen's disease usually do not appear to be familial, Young, Eldridge, and Gardner[22] described bilateral acoustic neuromas in a large kindred. They concluded (1) that if a patient with a unilateral acoustic neuroma is young, or if there is a family history of acoustic neuroma, the possibility of eventual bilateral disease is great; (2) if a diagnosis of bilateral acoustic neuroma is established, the patient should be carefully watched for development of other central nervous system tumors and his or her relatives should be screened for acoustic neuroma; and (3) that the tumors that occur both unilaterally and bilaterally, such as acoustic neuroma, neuroblastoma, retinoblastoma, pheochromocytoma, and chemodectoma, are generally sporadic and nonfamilial when unilateral, but when bilateral are frequently genetically determined and transmitted as an autosomal dominant trait. Lee and Abbott[23] confirmed the observations of Young and co-workers[22] from a study of their own clinical material.

Tuberous Sclerosis
Tuberous sclerosis is associated with the clinical triad of adenoma sebaceum, epilepsy, and mental retardation. Characteristic hamartomas occur in the brain, retina, heart, lungs, and kidneys. Giant cell astrocytomas of the brain develop in about one to three percent of these patients.[18]

von Hippel-Lindau Syndrome
This syndrome features angiomatosis of the retina and cerebellum and often is associated with cysts and angiomas of the viscera and of the cutaneous and subcutaneous tissues. Patients with this syndrome show a predisposition to associated hypernephromas, pheochromocytomas, and ependymomas. Table 2.2 shows the hereditary neurologic disorders associated with cutaneous and subcutaneous angiomas.

Multiple Exostosis (Diaphyseal Aclasis)
Multiple exostoses are osteomas occurring at surfaces of growing bones. Severe deformities often result and transformation to chondrosarcoma is reported in 5 to 10 percent of cases.[18,24]

Peutz-Jeghers Syndrome
In Peutz-Jeghers syndrome, hamartomatous gastrointestinal polyps are associated with melanin pigmentation of the buccal mucosa and lips. These polyps are usually in the small intestine and rarely become malignant.[18,25]

CANCER FAMILIES

The concept of "cancer families" has recently been broadened to include familial neoplasms of dissimilar cell types.[18,26] In a study of childhood rhabdomyosarcoma, a tendency for the cancer to aggregate in siblings was associated with a high frequency of various other cancers in parents and other relatives, especially in the female breast.[27] Sarcomas in children are also found in association with adrenocortical carcinoma, brain tumors, and other childhood tumors, as second primaries.[28,29] Miller [30] found that siblings of children who died of brain tumors were at excessive risk of sarcomas of the muscles and bones. Adenomatous polyps of the colon (familial polyposis) may be associated with familial adenocarcinoma[26] and, in familial aggregations, with brain tumors[31] and various sarcomas.[28]

RACIAL VARIATIONS

Genetic factors, environmental exposures, or both, may account for the substantial racial and ethnic differences that appear in the distribution of certain cancers. In the spectrum of sarcomas, this is particularly apparent in the incidence of Kaposi's hemangiosarcoma, a disease that predominantly affects elderly persons of Eastern European descent. In contrast, Kaposi's sarcoma is a common form of childhood cancer in equatorial Africa (Chapter 16). Ewing's sarcoma in children is less common in blacks than in whites in the United States. An adequate explanation of this racial or ethnic variance in the incidence of certain sarcomas has not been advanced.

CONGENITAL DEFECTS AND SARCOMAS

It has long been known that certain childhood sarcomas are associated with congenital anomalies.[32,33] Miller[32] found that among children with Wilms' tumor[33] and neuroblastoma[34] the peak mortality is at about 4 years of age. A similar mortality pattern was found in patients with primary liver cancer[35] and adrenocortical neoplasia.[36] In general, the following congenital defects occur sporadically and may be due to fresh mutation of genes:[18] sporadic aniridia with Wilms' tumor; congenital hemihypertrophy or visceral cytomegaly with Wilms' tumor; adrenocortical tumor or hepatoblastoma; enchondromatosis or enchondromas and hemangiomas with chondrosarcoma; and gonadal dysgenesis with gonadoblastoma.

TABLE 2.2. HEREDITARY NEUROLOGIC SYNDROMES ASSOCIATED WITH CUTANEOUS AND SUBCUTANEOUS ANGIOMAS

Syndrome	Inheritance	Sex	Onset	Skin Lesions	Central Nervous System Findings
Ataxia, telangiectasia	Autosomal recessive	Equal	Childhood	Telangiectasia increased by sun exposure	Cerebellar ataxia; ocular telangiectasia; nystagmus; mental retardation; dysarthria
Fabry's disease	Sex-linked	Males show full syndrome	Childhood	Angiokeratomas in clusters	Cerebrovascular accident; neuronal glycolipid deposition (peripheral neuritis)
von Hippel-Lindau	Autosomal dominant	Equal	Adulthood	Port-wine stain or no lesion; café-au-lait spots	Cerebellar hemangioblastoma and cyst; spinal hemangioblastoma (rarely)
Osler-Weber-Rendu's disease	Autosomal dominant	Equal	Childhood	Telangiectasia of skin, mucous membrane	Angiomas in brain or spinal cord, with signs of local tumor
Sturge-Weber	Autosomal dominant or not familial	Equal	Birth (in two-thirds of patients)	Port-wine stain in distribution of 5th cranial nerve	Angioma of meninges, intracranial calcifications; mental retardation; epilepsy; hemiparesis; visual impairment

VIRAL, CHEMICAL, AND PHYSICAL FACTORS

Viral Factors

Although type C viral particles have been isolated in several animal sarcomas,[1,2] there has been no confirmed isolation of infectious type C virus from normal or transformed human tissues. Recently, however, several groups have reported the identification in human tumor tissue of nucleic acid sequences or reverse transcriptase from the known well-characterized mammalian type C viruses. Kufe and associates[1] demonstrated that RNA sequences homologous to certain sequences of Rauscher mouse leukemia virus can be detected in human sarcomas. Although these or similar data[2-8] are of intense interest, direct correlation of a possible association between type C viruses and human neoplasia must await the isolation of infectious type C virus from human tissues, or at least the identification of a human cell culture that releases human type C virus in high titers.

Chemical Factors

Sarcomatous transformation induced by chemical carcinogens in experimental animals has long been described.[9] But, although polycyclic hydrocarbons produce sarcoma in rats, mice, and guinea pigs, and express a diversity of neoantigens, no direct evidence exists that any of the known carcinogens induce human sarcoma, with one exception: epidemiologic studies have shown that polyvinyl chloride exposure is linked with the development of hepatic angiosarcoma (Chapter 16).

Physical Factors

Foreign Body. The linkage of foreign-body-induced sarcomas in animals and man is much better substantiated.[37-44] Although the evidence in man is based on isolated case reports, the fact that such instances are documented should arouse considerable interest among clinical oncologists.

Tumors associated with foreign bodies have been reported intermittently since 1880.[45] Around the 1940s, several investigators[38,40,41] found that rats may develop sarcomas after plastic material is implanted in different body sites. This observation was further explored by Oppenheimer and co-workers,[46-48] Nothdurft,[49-52] Zollinger,[53] and Alexander.[37] These elegant studies established the etiologic role of foreign bodies in the induction of sarcomas in experimental animals. By excluding the chemical factors, the conclusion was reached that the physical presence and nature of the foreign body were singularly responsible for sarcomogenesis. Since artificial implants of various kinds are increasingly used by surgeons for anatomic, functional, or cosmetic reasons, extensive investigation of the biocompatibility of these agents has recently begun.[41,48,54-59]

Considering the increased frequency of foreign-body implantations in humans during the past two decades, the actual number of induced sarcomas is surprisingly small, compared with the number induced in mice and rats.[46-53] No sarcomas were reported by Rubin and co-workers[60] among 281 patients with facial prostheses, nor by deCholnoky[61] among 11,000 women who underwent augmentation mammoplasty. Similar negative reports have been published by other investigators.[43, 62-64] The differences in sarcoma incidence between human and murine species may relate, at least in part, to the differences in average tumor latency, which in mice is usually between 6 and 24 months, and in man, several years. Artificial implants frequently are performed in older patients, and the tumor latency might exceed the normal life expectancy of a large number of these patients; however, such is not the case with augmentation mammoplasty. Burns and associates[42] reported the development of a sarcoma 10 years after arterial repair by a Teflon-Dacron prosthesis. In another instance, a chondrosarcoma developed 18 years after implantation of Lucite spheres in the pleural cavity.[65] In 1970, Ott[45] collected all cases of foreign-body-induced sarcomas up to 1966 and found that in some instances the latency period was 40 years or more. The foreign bodies included metal implants, bullets, shrapnel pieces, and homotransplants. Human sarcomas associated with implanted plastic material have also been reported by Bischoff.[39]

A conspicuous characteristic of foreign-body sarcomas is that they appear in a great variety of histologic types. In man, these include fibrosarcoma,[42] chondrosarcoma,[65] and meningioma,[39] as well as asbestos-induced mesothelioma.[66-68] The findings in experimental animals are similar.[38,44,46,55,69] The histologic features of foreign-body-induced sarcomas have been grouped according to the degree of anaplasia, and four grades have been developed.[59] The majority of the tumors were found to be grades 3 and 4 by Johnson and co-workers.[70–73]

Foreign-body-induced sarcomas in experimental systems have been extensively investigated as to morphology, growth characteristics, antigenicity, karyologic aberrations, factors determining the preneoplastic conditions, tumor incidence, and latency.[59] Various hypotheses have been proposed for the mechanisms of induction of sarcoma by a foreign body.[59] Even viral particles have been isolated from some of these experimentally induced sarcomas,[51,71,72] but the mechanisms involved are still unknown.

Despite the apparent rarity of foreign-body-induced sarcoma in man, it would be unwise to be complacent. Several measures should be undertaken to minimize the incidence.[59] They include (1) a restrictive approach to artificial implantations, especially of medically unnecessary cosmetic procedures; (2) reexamination of implant carriers at frequent intervals; and (3) a centralized registry for gathering information on instances of foreign-body-induced neoplasia.

RADIATION FACTORS

Ionizing radiation in sufficiently high doses acts as a complete carcinogen, serving as both a tumor initiator and a promoter. Malignant transformation can be initiated in nearly any tissue or organ of man or of experimental animals by the proper choice of radiation dose and exposure schedule. The principal interest in radiation as an environmental carcinogen is not at high dosage levels. Relatively few patients receive such high dosage, and in most cases in which they do, the radiation is given as a localized treatment for a malignant tumor.

From an environmental standpoint, radiation exposure has not yet been linked with the development of soft tissue sarcomas. The induction of bone tumors by radiation was first observed in clock dial painters after accidental ingestion of radium while painting the luminous dials.[74,75] In addition to osteosarcomas, such victims showed an excessive incidence of fibrosarcomas and carcinomas of the paranasal and mastoid sinuses.[76,77] The latent period for induction of the tumors varied inversely with the radium content of the skeleton, being as short as 10 years in persons with 5 to 6 μg of radium and more than 25 years in those with smaller radium burdens.[78] The incidence of bone tumors has been interpreted to vary roughly as the square of the terminal concentration of radium in the skeleton, exceeding 20 percent at levels of 5 μCi or more, but with no evidence of tumor induction at levels of less than 0.5 μCi.[79]

Induction of both skeletal and extraskeletal sarcomas has been documented after therapeutic radiation.[80] Osteosarcomas have been noted following external radiation therapy with doses ranging from 3,000 to 15,000 rads.[80] The latent period in such tumors has been an average of nine years. At the University of Illinois, we found one incidence of chondrosarcoma of the chest wall seven years after therapeutic irradiation of the anterior chest wall for carcinoma of the breast (Fig. 2.1A and 2.1B). Fibrosarcomas are also known to occur after therapeutic radiation. A detailed analysis of postirradiation fibrosarcomas will be found in Chapter 12. It is generally recognized that curative doses of all therapeutic radiation might result in some form of sarcoma. Radiation-induced malignant mesenchymal tumors have provided the cancer biologist with a myriad of valuable data;[81,82] however, the only conclusion of any practical importance is that neoplasms of virtually any type can be induced, given appropriate conditions of irradiation and a suitably susceptible host.

TRAUMA

Although the clinician is frequently faced with a patient who historically links a sarcoma to an antecedent episode of trauma, there is no evidence to suggest that trauma plays any role in the induction of human mesenchymal malignant tumors.

IMMUNE DEFICIENCY STATES AND SARCOMAS

The incidence of malignancy in patients with primary immune deficiencies is roughly 10,000 times that in the general age-matched popula-

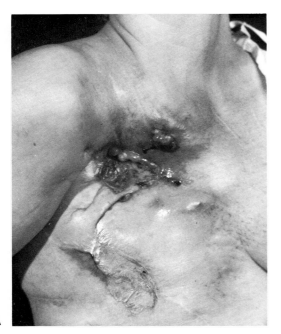
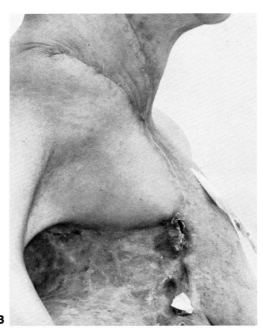

Figure 2.1. **(A)** This 51-year-old woman had radiation therapy to the anterior chest wall following a radical mastectomy for carcinoma of the breast. She was seen in our clinic for a chondrosarcoma, radiation necrosis, and a pleurocutaneous fistula. The tumor extended to the root of the neck and arm. At operation it was found that the intrathoracic extension consisted of involvement of the pulmonary parenchyma. She underwent a neck dissection, forequarter amputation, chest wall resection, and pneumonectomy. **(B)** Appearance three months postoperatively. She died four years later of an apparent coronary infarction. No autopsy was obtained.

tion.[83] In most instances, the malignant disease associated with immune deficiency states is lymphoma. Of the 55 cases reported by Melif and Schwartz,[83] only 11 (20 percent) were of the nonlymphoreticular variety. Six of the 11 were adenocarcinomas of the stomach, and there was one each of astrocytoma, glioma, cerebellar medulloblastoma, ovarian dysgerminoma, and basal cell carcinoma. No evidence of sarcoma in association with primary immune deficiency disease was observed.[83]

Similar malignant neoplasms are encountered in post-transplant patients receiving immunosuppressive therapy.[83] A registry of 5,170 recipients, consisting of 5,000 with kidney and 170 with heart allografts, was compiled by Schenk and Penn.[84] In 52 (1 percent) of the patients a neoplasm developed: 28 were of epithelial origin (skin, cervix, and tongue), 22 were lym-

phomas, and 2 were leiomyosarcomas. Although there is no doubt of the malignant nature of most of these neoplasms, there is some confusion as to the mechanism of their development in supposedly immunosuppressed patients.[84,85] Therefore, while there may be a risk of soft tissue sarcoma developing in immune deficiency states, only rarely does this occur.[86]

REFERENCES

1. Kufe D, Hehlmann R, Spiegelman S: Human sarcomas contain RNA related to the RNA of a mouse leukemia virus. Science 175:182, 1972
2. Lieber MM, Todaro GJ: Mammalian type C RNA viruses. In Becker FF (ed): Cancer: A Compre-

hensive Treatise, vol 2. New York, Plenum Press, 1975

3. Rauscher FJ, O'Conner TE: Virology. In Holland JF, Frei E III (eds): Cancer Medicine. Philadelphia, Lea & Febiger, 1973, p 15

4. Bernhard W: The detection and study of tumor viruses with the electron microscope. Cancer Res 20:712, 1960

5. Green M: Oncogenic viruses. Ann Rev Biochem 39:735, 1970

6. Ruebner RJ, Todaro GJ: Oncogenesis of RNA viruses as determinants of cancer. Proc Nat Acad Sci 64:1087, 1969

7. Shope RE: Koch's postulates and a viral cause of human cancer. Cancer Res 20:1119, 1960

8. Hanafusa H: Avian RNA tumor viruses. In Becker FF (ed): Cancer: A Comprehensive Treatise, vol. 2. New York, Plenum Press, 1975, p 49

9. Baldwin RW, Price MR: Neoantigen expression in chemical carcinogenesis. In Becker FF (ed): Cancer: A Comprehensive Treatise, vol. 1. New York, Plenum Press, 1975, p 406

10. Gardner EJ, Richards RC: Multiple cutaneous and subcutaneous lesions occurring simultaneously with hereditary polyposis and osteomatosis. Am J Hum Genet 5:139, 1953

11. Wilson H: Carotid body tumors: familial and bilateral. Ann Surg 171:843, 1970

12. Jensen RD, Miller RW: Retinoblastoma: Epidemiologic characteristics. N Engl J Med 185:307, 1971

13. Falls HF, Neel JV: Genetics of retinoblastoma. Arch Ophth 46:367, 1951

14. Thompson H, Lyons RB: Retinoblastoma and multiple congenital anomalies associated with complex mosaicism with deletion of D chromosome and probably D/C translocation. Hum Chromosome Newsl No 15, 1965, p 21

15. Van Kempen C: A case of retinoblastoma, combined with severe mental retardation and a few other congenital anomalies, associated with complex aberrations of the karyotype. Manndschr Kindergeneeskd 34:92, 1966

16. Pruett RC, Atkins L: Chromosome studies in patients with retinoblastoma. Arch Ophth 82:177, 1969

17. Levene M: Congenital retinoblastoma and sarcoma botryoides of the vagina: report of a case. Cancer 13:532, 1960

18. Fraumeni JF Jr: Genetic factors. In Holland JF, Frei E III (eds): Cancer Medicine. Philadelphia, Lea and Febiger, 1973, p 7

19. Schimke RN, Hartmann WH, Prout TE, Riomorin DL: Syndrome of bilateral pheochromocytoma, medullary thyroid carcinoma, and multiple neuromas. N Engl J Med 279:1, 1968

20. Wander JV, Das Gupta TK: Neurofibromatosis. In Current Problems in Surgery, vol. 14. Chicago, Year Book Medical Publishers, 1977

21. Willis RA: Borderland of Embryology and Pathology, 2nd ed. London, Butterworth, 1962, p 341

22. Young DF, Eldridge R, Gardner WJ: Bilateral acoustic neuroma in a large kindred. JAMA 214:347, 1970

23. Lee DK, Abbott ML: Familial central nervous system neoplasia: Case report of a family with von Recklinghausen's neurofibromatosis. Arch Neurol 20:154, 1969

24. Epstein LL, Bixler D, Bennett JE: An incidence of familial cancer including three cases of osteogenic sarcoma. Cancer 25:889, 1970

25. McKusick VA: Genetic factors in intestinal polyposis. JAMA 182:271, 1962

26. Smith WG: The cancer-family syndrome and heritable solitary colonic polyps. Dis Colon Rectum 13:362, 1970

27. Li FP, Fraumeni JF Jr: Soft tissue sarcomas, breast cancer, and other neoplasms. A familial syndrome? Ann Intern Med 71:747, 1969

28. Fraumeni JF Jr, Vogel CL, Easton JM: Sarcomas and multiple polyposis in a kindred. A genetic variety of hereditary polyposis. Arch Intern Med 121:57, 1968

29. Li FP, Fraumeni JF Jr: Rhabdomyosarcoma in children: Epidemiologic study and identification of a familial cancer syndrome. J Nat Cancer Inst 43:1365, 1969

30. Miller RW: Deaths from childhood leukemia and solid tumors among twins and other sibs in the United States, 1960–1970. J Nat Cancer Inst 46:203, 1971

31. Turcot J, Despres JP, St Pierre F: Malignant tumors of the central nervous system associated with familial polyposis of the colon: Report of two cases. Dis Colon Rectum 2:465, 1959

32. Miller RW: Relation between cancer and congenital defects: an epidemiologic evaluation. J Nat Cancer Inst 40:1079, 1968

33. Miller RW, Fraumeni JF Jr, Manning MD: Association of Wilms' tumor with aniridia, hemihypertrophy, and other congenital malformations. N Engl J Med 270:922, 1964

34. Miller RW, Fraumeni JF Jr, Hill JA: Neuroblastoma: epidemiologic approach to its origin. Am J Dis Child 115:253, 1968

35. Fraumeni JF Jr, Miller RW, Hill JA: Primary carcinoma of the liver in childhood: an epidemiologic study. J Nat Cancer Inst 40:1087, 1968

36. Fraumeni JF Jr, Miller RW: Adrenocortical neoplasms with hemihypertrophy, brain tumors, and other disorders. J Pediat 70:129, 1967

37. Alexander P: The reactions of carcinogens with macromolecules. Adv Cancer Res 2:1, 1954

38. Alexander P, Horning ES: Observations on the Oppenheimer method of inducing tumors by subcutaneous implantation of plastic films. CIBA Foundation Symposium on Carcinogenesis, 1959, p 24

39. Bischoff F: Organic polymer biocompatibility and toxicology. Clin Chem 18:869, 1972

40. Bischoff F, Bryson G: Carcinogenesis through solid state surfaces. Progr Exp Tumor Res 5:85, 1964

41. Bryson G, Bischoff F: Polymer carcinogenesis. Symposium on Polymer Chemistry, American Chemical Society Western Regional Meeting, 1965

42. Burns WA, Kanhouwand S, Tillman L, Saini N, Herrmann JB: Fibrosarcoma occurring at the site of a plastic vascular graft. Cancer 29:66, 1972

43. Calnan JS: Assessment of biological properties of implants before their clinical use. Proc Roy Soc Med 63:1115, 1970

44. Carter RL, Roe FJC: Induction of sarcomas in rats by solid and fragmented polyethylene: experimental observations and clinical implications. Br J Cancer 23:401, 1969

45. Ott G: Fremdkorpersarkome. Exp Med Pathol Klin 32:1, 1970

46. Oppenheimer BS, Oppenheimer ET, Danishefsky I, Stout AP, Elrich FR: Further studies of polymers as carcinogenic agents in animals. Cancer Res 15:333, 1955

47. Oppenheimer BS, Oppenheimer ET, Stout AP, Willhite M, Danishefsky I: The latent period in carcinogenesis by plastics in rats and its relation to the precancerous stage. Cancer 11:204, 1958

48. Oppenheimer BS, Oppenheimer ET, Stout AP, Danishefsky I, Willhite M: Studies of the mechanism of carcinogenesis by plastic films. Acta Unio Int Contra Cancrum 15:659, 1959

49. Nothdurft H: Die experimentelle Erzeugung von Sarkomen bei Ratten und Mausen Durch Implantation von Rundscheiben aus Gold, Silber, Platin Oder Elfenbein. Naturwissenschaften 42:106, 1955

50. Nothdurft H: Uber die Sarkomauslosung durch Fremdkorperimplantationen bei Ratten in abhangigkeit von der Form der Implantate. Naturwissenschaften 42:106, 1955

51. Nothdurft H: Tumorezeugung durch Fremdkorperimplantation. Abhandl Deutsch Akad Wiss Derl Klasse Med 3:80, 1960

52. Nothdurft H: Unterschiedliche Ausbeuten an subcutanen Fremdkorpersarkomen der Ratte in Abhangigkeit von der Korperregion. Naturwissenschaften 49:18, 1962

53. Zollinger HU: Experimentelle Erzeugung maligner Nierenkapseltumoren bei der Ratte durch Druckreiz Plastic-Kapseln. Schweiz Z tschr allg 15:666, 1952

54. Milne J: Fifteen cases of pleural mesothelioma associated with occupational exposure to asbestos in Victoria. Med J Austral 2:669, 1969

55. Wagner JC, Berry G: Mesotheliomas in rats following inoculation with asbestos. Br J Cancer 23:567, 1969

56. Brand KG, Buoen LC: Polymer tumorigenesis: Multiple preneoplastic clones in priority order with clonal inhibition. Proc Soc Exp Biol Med 128:1154, 1968

57. Brand KG, Buoen LC, Brand I: Premalignant cells in tumorigenesis induced by plastic film. Nature 213(part 2):810, 1967

58. Brand KG, Buoen LC, Brand I: Carcinogenesis from polymer implants: New aspects from chromosomal and transplantation studies during premalignancy. J Nat Cancer Inst 39:663, 1967

59. Brand KG: Foreign body induced sarcomas. In Becker FF (ed): Cancer: A Comprehensive Treatise, vol. 1. New York, Plenum Press, 1975, p 486

60. Rubin LR, Bromberg BE, Walden RH: Long-term human reaction to synthetic plastics. Surg Gynecol Obstet 132:603, 1971

61. deCholnoky T: Augmentation mammaplasty: Survey of complications in 10,941 patients by 265 surgeons. Plast Reconstruct Surg 45:573, 1970

62. Dukes CE, Mitchley BCV: Polyvinyl sponge implants: experimental and clinical observations. Br J Plast Surg 15:225, 1962

63. Dutton J: Acrylic investment of intracranial aneurysms. Br Med J 2:597, 1959

64. Spence WT: Form-fitting plastic cranioplasty. J Neurosurg 11:219, 1954

65. Thompson RJ, Entin SD: Primary extraskeletal chondrosarcoma. Cancer 23:936, 1969

66. McDonald AD, Harper A, El Attar CA, McDonald JC: Epidemiology of primary malignant mesothelial tumors in Canada. Cancer 26:914, 1970

67. Roberts GH: Diffuse pleural mesothelioma: a clinical and pathological study. Br J Dis Chest 64:201, 1970

68. Staton MF, Wrench C: Mechanisms of mesothelioma induction with asbestos and fibrous glass. J Nat Cancer Inst 48:797, 1972

69. Oppenheimer ET, Willhite M, Stout AP, Danishefsky I, Fishman MM: A comparative study of the effects of embedding cellophane and polystyrene films in rats. Cancer Res 24:379, 1964

70. Johnson KH, Buoen LC, Brand I, Brand KG: Polymer tumorigenesis: clonal determination of histopathological characteristics during early preneoplasia; relationships to karyotypes, mouse strain, and sex. J Nat Cancer Inst 44:785, 1970

71. Johnson KH, Chobrial EKG, Buoen LC, Brand I, Brand KG: Intracisternal type A particles occurring in foreign-body-induced sarcomas. Cancer Res 35:1165, 1975

72. Johnson KH, Ghobrial HKG, Buoen LC, Brand I, Brand KG: Nonfibroblastic origin of foreign body sarcomas implicated by histologic and electron microscopic studies. Cancer Res 33:3139, 1973

73. Johnson FB: Studies on polymer implants in humans: plastics in surgical implants. In Special Technical Publication 386, American Society for Testing Materials, 1965, p 102

74. Martland HS: Occurrence of malignancy in radioactive persons. A general review of data gathered in the study of radium dial painters, with special reference to the occurrence of osteogenic sarcoma and the interrelationship of certain blood diseases. Am J Cancer 15:2435, 1931

75. Looney WB: Effects of radium in man. Science 127:630, 1958

76. Aub JC, Evans RD, Hempelmann LH, Martland HS: The late effects of internally deposited radioactive materials in man. Medicine 31:221, 1952

77. Marinelli LD: Radioactivity and the human skeleton. Am J Roentgenol 80:729, 1958

78. Evans RD: The effect of skeletally deposited alpha-ray emitters in man. Br J Radiol 39:881, 1966

79. National Academy of Sciences, National Research Council: The effects on populations of exposure to low levels of ionizing radiation. Report of the Advisory Committee on the Biological Effects of Ionizing Radiation. Washington DC, 1972

80. Bloch C: Post irradiation osteogenic sarcoma: Report of a case and review of the literature. Am J Roentgenol 87:1157, 1962

81. Finkel MP, Biskis BS: Experimental induction of osteosarcoma. In Hamburger F (ed): Progress in

Experimental Tumor Research. Basel, Karger, 1968, p 72

82. Upton AC: Physical carcinogenesis: radiation-history and sources. In Becker FF (ed): Cancer: A Comprehensive Treatise, vol. 1. New York: Plenum Press, 1975

83. Melief CJM, Schwartz RS: Immunocompetence and malignancy. In Becker FF (ed): Cancer: A Comprehensive Treatise, vol. 2. New York, Plenum Press, 1975

84. Schenk SA, Penn I: Cerebral neoplasms associated with renal transplantation. Arch Neurol 22:226, 1970

85. Schenk SA, Penn I: De-novo brain tumors in renal transplant recipients. Lancet 1:983, 1971

86. Penn I: The occurrence of cancer in immune deficiencies. Current Problems in Cancer. Vol. VI, No. 10, April, 1982

3

Classification

Tapas K. Das Gupta

The majority of malignant soft tissue tumors arise de novo. In the benign form these tumors seldom undergo malignant transformation, ie, only rarely do angiomas convert to malignant angioendotheliomas,[1] or do synovial sarcomas arise from benign preexisting tumors of the tendon sheath, or do lipomas become liposarcomas[1,2] (although some large lipomas may undergo xanthomatous or myxomatous degeneration, with liposarcoma developing many years later).[3,4] There are, however, certain disease entities that apparently are benign but on long-term followup show a high incidence of associated malignant tumors, a prime example being generalized neurofibromatosis.[5] Occasionally a tumor is histologically diagnosed as benign, but its behavior is characterized by local recurrence and distant dissemination. A reevaluation of the original histologic material usually shows that an incorrect diagnosis was made at the outset. Some tumors are histologically benign, but incomplete excision may result in local recurrence. Multiple recurrences may end up in malignant transformation.[2]

There are more than 50 different varieties of tumors and tumorlike conditions of the soft somatic tissues. Each is a separate entity and requires a specific plan of treatment. Therefore, even though the morphologic distinction of a given soft tissue tumor might at times be difficult and could be conjectural, every attempt should be made to establish an exact histologic diagnosis. The histologic classification becomes doubly difficult because most of these tumors are derived from primitive mesenchyme and have a tendency to undergo metaplasia under the stress of neoplasia. Before an attempt is made to develop a practical histogenetic classification of these tumors, it is appropriate to briefly trace the development of tissues from the primitive mesenchyme as well as elaborate on the term *metaplasia* in the context of somatc tissue tumors. Neoplasms arising from the nervous tissue are, strictly speaking, neither sarcomas nor sarcomatous conditions. However, most are clinically considered sarcomas or variants thereof, and thus are being included in this book.

The term mesenchyme embraces all the undifferentiated nonepithelial mesodermal tissue of the embryo or fetus. The derivatives of the mesoderm are (1) epithelium of the gonads; (2) mesothelium, the flat pavement epithelium or endothelium of the celomic cavities; and (3) mesenchyme (Greek: mesos = middle, enchyma = that which is poured in), the diffusely cellular precursors of the connective, vascular, skeletal, muscular, and hematopoietic tissues. The embryonic mesenchymal cells are fusiform or stellate, and their processes are in intimate contact with those of the adjacent cells, forming a network. Whether there is cell-to-cell continuity of protoplasm through these processes, so that the network is a syncytium, is unknown. The intercellular network is rich in mucoprotein. During the differentiation of mesenchyme into connective tissue, cartilage, and bone, distinctive substances are deposited in it—collagen and elastic fibers, chondroitin or osseomucin, and lime salts. The mesenchymal cells that line the blood vessels, lymph vessels, and celomic spaces are distinguished as endothelium, and celomic endothelium is called mesothelium. The distinction, although descriptively useful, is not absolute and is not of much help in interpreting the biologic behavior of tumors of the primitive mesenchyme. That the various kinds of tissues differentiated from mesenchyme are closely allied is shown not only by their common source in the embryo, but also by their regenerative growth in adult life, when they revert morphologically to the appearance of embryonic mesenchyme and may redifferentiate into other tissues. Thus, proliferating vascular and fibroblastic tissues may form cartilage, bone, smooth muscle, and hematopoietic cells—changes that are called metaplasia. The following paragraphs briefly summarize the developmental characteristics of the tissues derived from the primitive mesenchyme and the peripheral nervous tissue.

CONNECTIVE TISSUE

Fibrous, areolar, mucoid, and adipose tissues differentiate from the cellular mesenchyme. In the human embryo, most of the prospective fibrous tissues are still relatively cellular. The soft intercellular matrix is poor in collagen and rich in mucinous fluid. By the end of the second month of gestation, many of the main tendons, ligaments, fasciae, and other fibrous structures are plainly present as mesenchymal condensations, with appropriately orientated fibroblasts and increasing collagen. Fat cells first appear in the subcutaneous tissue during the fifth fetal month. Mesenchymal cells become plump and rounded. Multiple droplets of fat appear in their cytoplasm, and these enlarge and coalesce to form a single large droplet in each cell. However, Shaw[6] proposed that fat cells arise merely by fat storage in ordinary connective tissue cells, and some support for this concept can be found in adult tissue with metaplasia.

Chondrification in the mesenchyme begins in particular foci of perichondral centers; the cells here become separated by a mucinous intercellular matrix. The prechondral tissue quickly develops into embryonic cartilage with a hyaline basophilic matrix. In the human embryo, chondrification is well advanced by the seventh week (15 to 20 mm), each cartilage and bone being represented by its cartilaginous rudiment.[7]

Bursae and tendon sheaths develop as clefts in the mesenchyme and then undergo synovial differentiation.[8–10] They appear from the third month of gestation onward, although some do not develop until late fetal or postnatal life. The late development of some of these synovial structures indicates the importance of pressure and movement factors in their formation and prepares us for the metaplastic formation of false bursae over pressure points or under corns in adult life.[11]

VASCULAR OR ANGIOBLASTIC TISSUE

The earliest blood vessels are derived from angioblastic tissue, which differentiates from the mesenchyme in three regions: (1) the surface of the yolk sac; (2) the body of the stalk; and (3) the chorion.[12,13] In the yolk sac and base of the body stalk, small, more or less spherical groups of cells are found early in the third week of gestation. These are termed *blood islands*. It is generally believed that the peripheral cells of the islands become flattened and form the vascular endothelium, while the central cells convert into primitive red blood cells. Later, these small blood-containing spaces form a continuous network of small vessels.

All blood vessels, even the largest arteries and veins, begin as simple endothelial capillaries. The growth and differentiation of vessels can be observed in the living state in the developing limb buds or tails of tadpoles. A capillary plexus develops in a series of arcades from which new sprouts continuously grow into developing tissues. Certain vessels carrying an inflow of blood enlarge, acquire muscular coats by differentiation of smooth muscle fibers from surrounding mesenchymal cells, and become arteries. Other vessels with a return blood flow enlarge and become veins. By the end of the fourth week of gestation, as the rest of the body grows, the vascular system extends and undergoes increasing elaboration.

LYMPHATICS

The development of the lymphatics has always been a controversial topic. Sabin[14] and Lewis[15] believed them to be the outgrowths of a developing venous system. Other embryologists have theorized that the lymphatics develop in the local tissues by the confluence of mesenchymal spaces. In the human embryo of two to four months the lymphatics of the neck, mediastinum, and retroperitoneum are large, easily definable, thin-walled vessels.

MUSCULAR TISSUE

Smooth Muscle

Smooth muscle differentiates in situ from the mesenchyme surrounding the particular organ. This shows condensation and orientation of elongated cells in specific directions, circular or longitudinal with respect to the axis of the viscus or the vessel. As early as the sixth week, this process is evident in the walls of the intestine and many other viscera, but myogenesis from mesenchyme continues throughout the greater part of fetal life.[11]

Skeletal Muscle

Most of the classic writings on the embryology of the skeletal musculature assert, even today, that with the exception of certain muscles of the head and neck (which develop from branchial mesenchyme) and the limb muscles (which develop in situ from the mesenchyme of the limb buds), all somatic muscles are derived from myotomes. Each myotome divides into dorsal (epaxial) and ventral (hypaxial) regions, the former situated dorsolaterally to the developing vertebral column and the latter migrating ven-

trally in the body wall or somatopleure.[16] Willis,[17] however, questioned the validity of this concept. Based on histologic study of rhabdomyosarcoma, he suggested that some of the trunk musculature arises locally from the nonmyotonic mesenchyme.

In the differentiation of striated muscle, the primitive muscle cell, the rhabdomyoblast, may arise from either the somatic or nonsomatic primitive mesenchyme. Myoblasts multiply by mitosis, but further recruitment from the neighboring mesenchyme also occurs.[16] By the eighth week, however, the pale cytoplasm contains myofibrils, even with cross-striations. From the eighth week onward the rhabdomyoblasts continue to be differentiated and grow until after birth.

PERIPHERAL NERVOUS SYSTEM

The peripheral nerves and associated ganglia arise by migration of neuroblasts and the outgrowth of nerve fibers from two sources, the neural tube and the neural crest. The main contribution of the neural tube to the nervous system is the outgrowth of motor nerve fibers into the spinal and cranial nerves from neuroblasts in the basal laminae of the cord and the corresponding motor nuclei in the brain stem.

During the fourth week, the neural folds close to form the neural tube, with a longitudinal strip of special ectodermal tissue—the neural crest. The neural crest forms along the dorsal surface of the tube, between this surface and the overlying ectoderm. Its proliferating cells migrate ventrolaterally to form a large mass in each dorsolateral aspect of the neural tube from the mid-brain region downward, extending caudally as the neural tube itself elongates. From this mass arise the cranial and sensory nerve ganglia, the spinal posterior root ganglia being particularly prominent during the second month of gestation. Other cells migrate still further ventrally to form neuroblasts of the prevertebral and visceral autonomic ganglia, chromaffin cells of the adrenal medulla, organ of Zuckerkandl, renal and celiac ganglia, the neurilemmomal cells of Schwann, all the peripheral nerves, probably most of the melanoblasts of the skin and of the head and neck region, and possibly the branchial arch skeleton.

METAPLASIA

Metaplasia signifies transformation of an adult tissue of one kind into a differentiated tissue of another kind in response to abnormal circumstances. It is an acquired condition and must be distinguished from developmental heterotopia or heteroplasia.

Voluminous literature is available on the metaplastic formation of bone or cartilage in scars, hemorrhages, and inflammatory or degenerative lesions, but these topics will not be discussed here. Suffice it to point out that occasionally such metaplastic changes may create some clinical confusion concerning the diagnosis of a given soft tissue sarcoma. Notable among these are the ossification of scars, especially in the abdominal wall, which must be distinguished from desmoids; and the various types of myositis ossificans from extraskeletal osteosarcoma and chondrosarcoma.[18-25] The capacity of ordinary connective tissue to undergo transformation into adipose tissue has often been disputed. Lipoblasts have frequently been regarded as distinctive cell types.[26] However, some authors[27,28] accept the view that fat cells can form from connective tissue. Under the influence of tumorigenesis, metaplastic changes to adipose cells are sometimes seen. Liposarcomas often contain other kinds of connective tissue; lipo-

matous, fibromatous, cartilaginous, and myxomatous elements often coexist in the same tumor.[29]

Three distinct questions arise regarding muscular metaplasia: (1) Can new smooth muscle fibers be formed in adult tissue by transformation of nonmuscular cells? (2) Can cross-striated muscle fibers be so formed? (3) Can smooth muscle fibers be transformed into cross-striated fibers? The formation of smooth muscle from nonmuscular tissue in the adult occurs in some cases of endometriosis and in some mixed tumors of the endometrium. Willis[30] documented several instances of metaplastic smooth muscle fibers and striated muscle fibers in neoplastic endometrial stroma. Furthermore, rhabdomyosarcomas are occasionally encountered in adults in organs that normally contain no striated muscle, eg, breast[31,32] and lung.[33-35] In these cases it is much more likely that aberrant differentiation has taken place in tumor cells arising from some other mesenchymal tissue than it is that the tumor has arisen from long-dormant, developmentally heterotopic rhabdomyoblasts. However, regarding the question whether smooth muscle fibers can be transformed into striated fibers, Willis,[30] after extensively reviewing the subject, commented, "In spite of the suggestion, based on comparative histology, that two kinds of muscle may be akin

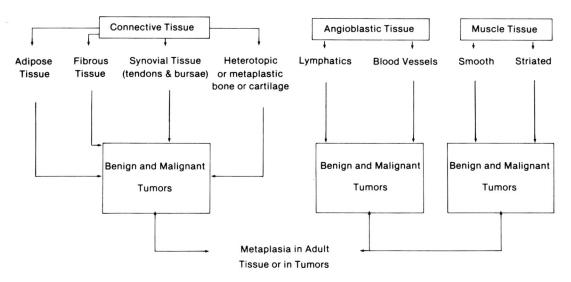

Figure 3.1. Primitive mesenchyme (ontogenesis of mesenchymal sarcoma).

TABLE 3.1. CLASSIFICATION OF SOFT TISSUE TUMORS

Tissue of Origin	Benign Tumors or Tumorlike Conditions	Malignant Tumors
Adipose tissue	Lipoma (solitary or multiple)	Liposarcoma
	Lipomatoses	
	Lipoblastoma	
	Hibernoma	
	Idiopathic lipopathies	
Fibrous tissue	Fibroma	Fibrosarcoma
	Fibromatoses	Malignant fibrous histiocytoma
	1. Juvenile variants	
	Congenital generalized fibromatosis	Malignant xanthogranuloma
	Fibromatous coli	Dermatofibrosarcoma protuberans
	Juvenile aponeurotic fibroma	
	Angiofibroma	
	Recurring digital tumors with	
	inclusion bodies	
	Progressive myositis	
	2. Adult variants	
	Keloid	
	Palmar and plantar fibromatoses	
	Penile fibromatosis	
	Idiopathic retroperitoneal fibrosis	
	Pseudosarcomatous fasciitis	
	Progressive myositis ossificans	
	Paradoxical fibrosarcoma of skin	
	Elastofibroma	
	Fibrous histiocytoma, with all its variants	
	Aggressive fibromatoses in all locations	
Muscle tissue		
A. Smooth muscle	Leiomyoma	Leiomyosarcoma
	Leiomyoblastoma	Hemangiopericytoma
	Glomus tumor	Rhabdomyosarcoma and all its variants
B. Skeletal muscle	Rhabdomyoma	

Peripheral nervous tissue

A. Tumors of schwannian origin	Schwannomas (neurilemomas) and/or neurofibromas, solitary type Similar tumors in association with von Recklinghausen's disease or other types of neurocutaneous syndromes	Malignant schwannoma (neurofibrosarcoma, solitary type) Malignant transformation in von Recklinghausen's disease or other types of neurocutaneous syndromes
B. Non-neoplastic traumatic masses	Traumatic neuromas	
C. Secondary neoplasms		Involvement of the peripheral nerves from other malignant tumors
D. Tumors of sympathochromaffin tissue	Ganglioneuroma (differentiated) Pheochromocytomas	Malignant ganglioneuromas (ganglioneuroblastomas) Neuroblastomas Malignant pheochromocytomas Neuroepitheliomas
E. Tumors of the cartoid body and allied structures	Cartoid body tumors Paragangliomas	Malignant cartoid body tumors Malignant paragangliomas

Synovial tissue

	Giant cell tumors of tendon sheath Xanthomas Ganglions	Malignant synoviomas Clear cell sarcoma of tendon sheath Epithelioid sarcoma

Angiomatous tissue

A. Vascular tissue	Hemangiomas Angiomatoses Benign hemangiopericytoma	Angiosarcoma Malignant hemangioendotheliomas Kaposi's sarcoma
B. Lymphatic tissue	Lymphangioma	Lymphangiosarcoma Extranodal lymphoma Extramedullary plasmacytoma

Heterotopic bone and cartilage

	Myositis ossificans Benign chondroma	Extraskeletal osteosarcoma Extraskeletal chondrosarcoma

Tissue of origin still unclear

	Granular cell myoblastoma Benign mesenchymoma	Malignant granular cell myoblastoma Alveolar soft-part sarcoma Malignant mesenchymoma Malignant fibrous mesothelioma

and therefore possibly interconvertible, the transformation of smooth to striated muscle remains unproven."

Metaplasia occurs only in proliferating cells. It is in many cases a form of regeneration accompanied by atypical differentiation. The multiplying cells of a regenerating tissue approach embryonic conditions, and metaplasia is evidence of resumed embryonic activity.

Figure 3.1 summarizes the ontogenesis of soft tissue sarcomas on the basis of embryologic data on the primitive mesenchyme. It is evident that all the adult components of the mesenchyme could be the primary site of a sarcoma. This common ancestry of all sarcomas obviously can create considerable difficulty in actual histogenetic classification. The problem becomes doubly difficult in those instances in which metaplasia is induced in the original adult tissue by neoplastic transformation. The tumor and tumorlike conditions of the peripheral nervous tissue, in contrast, have a different ancestry and can be distinguished from the mesenchymal tumors. In a number of instances, however, due to the contribution from the surrounding connective or muscle tissue, these tumors can mimic the histologic appearance of mesenchymal tumors, and the distinction is difficult to make by light microscopic examination alone.

With this background, we have classified the mesenchymal tumors and tumors arising from the peripheral nervous tissue (Table 3.1), based on Stout's[36,37] original classification, but with certain modifications in light of recent knowledge. Like most other classifications, this has its defects, especially since in some instances the cell of origin of some tumors still is in doubt. However, the clinician can use this as a ready reference for the management of these tumors and tumorlike conditions.

REFERENCES

1. Pack GT, Ariel IM: Tumors of the Soft Somatic Tissues. New York, Hoeber-Harper, 1958, p 44
2. Das Gupta TK, Brasfield RD: Soft tissue tumors: Classification and principles of management. CA 18:259, 1968
3. Schiller H: Lipomata in sarcomatous transformation. Surg Gynecol Obstet 27:218, 1918
4. Sternberg SS: Liposarcoma arising within subcutaneous lipoma. Cancer 5:975, 1952
5. Wander JV, Das Gupta TK: Neurofibromatosis. Current Problems in Surgery, vol 14. Chicago: Year Book Medical Publishers, 1977
6. Shaw HB: A contribution to the study of the morphology of adipose tissue. J Anat Physiol 36:1, 1902
7. Kernan JD Jr: The chondrocranium of a 20 mm human embryo. J Morphol 27:605, 1916
8. Black BM: The prenatal incidence, structure and development of some human synovial bursae. Anat Rec 60:333, 1934
9. Gray DJ, Gardner E: Prenatal development of the human knee and superior tibiofibular joints. Am J Anat 86:235, 1950
10. Gray DJ, Gardner E: Prenatal development of the human elbow joint. Am J Anat 88:429, 1951
11. Willis RA: The Borderland of Embryology and Pathology. London, Butterworth, 1958, p 54
12. Bloom W, Bartelmez GW: Hematopoiesis in young human embryos. Am J Anat 67:21, 1940
13. Hertig AT: Angiogenesis in the early human chorion and in the primary placenta of the macaque monkey. Contr Embryo 25:37, 1935
14. Sabin FR: On the origin of the lymphatic system from the veins and the development of the lymph hearts and thoracic duct of the pig. Am J Anat 1:367, 1902
15. Lewis FT: The development of the lymphatic system in rabbits. Am J Anat 5:95, 1906
16. Warwick R, Williams PL (eds): Gray's Anatomy, 35th ed. London, Longman, 1973, p 124
17. Willis RA: The Borderland of Embryology and Pathology. London, Butterworth, 1958, p 410
18. Nicholson GW: Heteromorphoses in the human body. Guy's Hosp Rep 71:75, 1922
19. Nicholson GW: Studies on tumour formation: Acquired tissue malformations. Guy's Hosp Rep 72:402, 1922
20. Keith A: Concerning the origin and nature of osteoblasts. Proc Roy Soc Med 21:1, 1927
21. von Seeman H: Über die Entstehungsbedingungen metaplastischer Knochenbildungen. Dtsch Z Chir 217:60, 1927
22. Huggins CB: The formation of bone under the influence of epithelium of the urinary tract. Arch Surg 22:377, 1931
23. Huggins CB: The phosphatase activity of transplants of the epithelium of the urinary bladder to the abdominal wall producing heterotopic ossification. Biochem J 25(pt 1):728, 1931
24. Lloyd-Williams IH: On a case of bony plaques developing in the skin. Br Med J 2:1055, 1929
25. Huggins CB, McCarroll HR, Blocksom BH Jr: Experiments on the theory of osteogenesis: the influence of local calcium deposits on ossification; the osteogenic stimulus of epithelium. Arch Surg 32:915, 1936
26. Cameron GR, Seneviratne RD: Growth and repair in adipose tissue. J Path Bact 59:665, 1947
27. Flemming W: Weitere Mittheilungen zur Physiologie der Fettzelle. Arch Mikv Anat 7:328, 1871
28. Clark ER, Clark EL: Microscopic studies of the new formation of fat in living adult rabbits. Am J Anat 67:255, 1940

29. Enzinger FM, Winslow DJ: Liposarcoma. A study of 103 cases. Virchows Arch Path Anat 335:367, 1962

30. Willis RA: Metaplasia. The Borderland of Embryology and Pathology. London, Butterworth, 1958, p 506

31. Sailer S: Sarcoma of the breast. Am J Cancer 31:183, 1937

32. Govan ADT: Two cases of mixed malignant tumour of the breast. J Path Bact 57:397, 1945

33. Cumming ARR, Shillitoe AJ: Ball-valve mitral obstruction by a sarcoma of a pulmonary vein. Br Heart J 19:287, 1957

34. McDonald S Jr, Heather JC: Neoplastic invasion of the pulmonary veins and left auricle. J Path Bact 48:533, 1939

35. Forbes GB: Rhabdomyosarcoma of bronchus. J Path Bact 70:427, 1955

36. Stout AP, Ariel IM: Panel on soft-part tumors. Proc Nat Cancer Conf, 1949, p 206

37. Stout AP: Tumors of the Soft Tissues. In Atlas of Tumor Pathology, Sect 2, Fasc 5. Washington DC, AFIP, 1953

4

Pathology of Soft Tissue Sarcoma

Tapas K. Das Gupta

Until recently, soft somatic tissue sarcomas, probably because of their rarity, did not arouse much enthusiasm for comprehensive study among pathologists and clinicians. Since the pioneering work of Ewing,[1] Stout,[2] Stout and Lattes,[3] and Pack and his associates,[4] however, attention has been increasingly focused on the nosology, natural history, and principles of management of these tumors. It has become apparent that they cannot and should not be lumped into the nonspecific category of "sarcomas," with the connotation that basically all have a similar biologic behavior. Rather, they should be histogenetically classified and their individual morphologic characteristics defined. Wherever such characterizations have been possible, the natural history of the tumor has been properly defined and the methods of management have become standardized. However, such classifications, although ideal, can be extremely difficult. Hare and Cerny[5] reported that 28 percent of their series of 200 cases could not be classified histogenetically. In Pack and Ariel's[6] series, 261 of 717 patients (36.4 percent) were found to have sarcomas of undetermined histogenesis.

With the routine use of special stains and histochemical studies at both light and ultrastructural levels, the morphologic classification of soft tissue tumors has now become easier.

The electron microscope alone provides solutions to some of the previously insoluble problems. Ultrastructural studies of normal mesenchymal cells of soft supporting tissues have revealed specific cytoplasmic characteristics and extracellular products indicative of specialized forms of cytodifferentiation that enable identification of cell types with reasonable certainty.[7-16] For the purposes of histogenetic study and classification, the ultrastructural cellular traits of normal mesenchymal cells appear to be retained in malignant neoplastic cells to a degree that has proved useful in diagnosis.[7,8,14,15,17-21]

Although electron microscopy has contributed significantly to the diagnosis of sarcomas, there are several overlapping features and variations that continue to hamper accurate histologic interpretation. For example, collagen production is not a certain indication that a given sarcoma is of simple fibrous tissue cell origin. The cells of neurogenic tumors, presumably derived from Schwann cells, also appear to be capable of formation of collagen fibrils. Similarly, endothelial cells in angiosarcomas do not resemble malignant mesenchymal cells; rather, their close intercellular junctions and desmosomes resemble those of other malignant epithelial cells. Thus a problem in cytologic identification between neoplastic endothelial and epithelial cells might arise even with electron microscopy. In highly anaplastic sarcomas it is frequently difficult to classify the origin of the malignant cell. Nevertheless, today ultrastructural confirmation of the light microscopic diagnosis of any given soft tissue sarcoma is almost mandatory.

In this chapter, an attempt is made to describe and discuss the structure, function, and pathologic aspects of the various forms of tumors and tumorlike conditions that arise in the soft somatic tissues. The classification of mesenchymal and neural tumors in Table 3.1, Chapter 3, forms the basis of the subsequent discussion.

TUMORS AND TUMORLIKE CONDITIONS OF ADIPOSE TISSUE

For a better understanding of tumor and tumorlike conditions of adipose tissue, it is appropriate to briefly describe the histogenesis and structure of both white and brown adipose tissue. Without such background information it is difficult to comprehend the complexities of these clinical entities.

Deposition of adipose tissue begins during the fifth month of intrauterine life. Keith[22] stated that certain granular cells of the connective tissue, especially of the subcutaneous layers, have the property of secreting fat, which appears first as diffuse droplets. These ultimately run together and produce the characteristic outline of the adipose cell. Fat reaches its greatest normal development just before and immediately after birth. At birth, a mass of tissue resembling the interscapular gland of hibernating mammals[23] is frequently found on each posterior triangle of the neck extending beneath the trapezius muscle. Adipose tissue is classified into two main types, *white* and *brown*, and the tumors and tumorlike conditions that arise in each type have distinctly different characteristics.

White Adipose Tissue

This term is applied to the white or yellowish-white fatty tissue that is widely distributed throughout the body. The mature adipose cell contains a single large droplet of neutral fat within a thin envelope of cytoplasm. The nucleus is compressed into a crescent shape within the thin rim of cytoplasm (Fig. 4.1). In well-nourished persons, the cells vary in size. In vivo, probably every adipose cell is in contact with a capillary. White adipose tissue appears to be one of the most highly vascularized tissues in the body.

Histogenesis. The origin of white adipose cells is still unclear. One view, which can be traced back to Flemming,[24] is that both the lobular and the more dispersed adipose tissues are formed by the accumulation of fat in unspecialized cells of connective tissue. This view has been widely

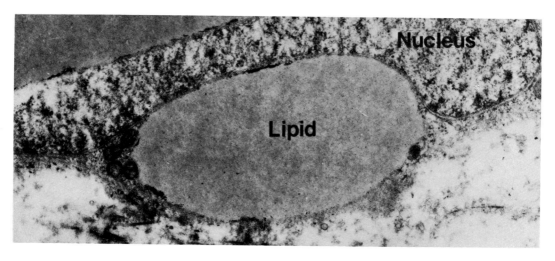

Figure 4.1. Electron micrograph of a mature human adipose cell. A single large droplet of lipid fat is compressing the nucleus into a crescent shape. (Original magnification ×31,360.)

supported, particularly by Clark and Clark,[25] who observed regular transformation of fat cells from fibroblasts in transparent chambers built into rabbit ears.

Toldt[26] and Wasserman[27] held that adipose tissues develop from a specialized anlage and proposed that each lobule of adipose tissue develops by enlargement and differentiation of a specific embryonic "primitive" organ composed of mesenchymal cells mingled with small blood vessels. Wasserman[27] suggested that, in the human embryo, lentiform areas of characteristic structure are separated from the surrounding connective tissue by a thin capsule. These lentiform areas consist of a network of capillaries and mesenchymal cells, and it is in these cells that fat appears. Both Dabelow[28] and Napolitano[29] provided supporting evidence for the thesis that, even at a very immature stage of development, white adipose cells have special structural features and can be distinguished from fibroblasts. Further support for this view stems from the appearance taken on by mature adipose cells in states of extreme nutritional depletion. Such cells

lose lipid and assume the form of embryonic adipose cells rather than fibroblasts.[30]

The number of adipose cells apparently increases in mature mammals. Sidman[30] found that in obese humans the amount of lipid per cell is elevated, but not sufficiently to account for an increase of 10 to 30 kg of body fat. The extra lipid, then, must be accommodated in new cells.[31,32]

A number of early reports in the tissue culture literature[33–35] described the accumulation of fat in cultured connective tissue cells. The relevance of these in vitro reports is uncertain, particularly since it is not yet known whether fatty fibroblasts are true adipose cells. However, transformation of adult fibroblasts into fatty fibroblasts cannot be ruled out. It appears that at least for the present the original concepts of Toldt[26] and Wasserman[27] are valid.

Structure. A living fat cell in white adipose tissue is a large, brilliant, spherical body. Every mature fat cell contains one large drop of fat that can be stained with such dyes as osmic acid

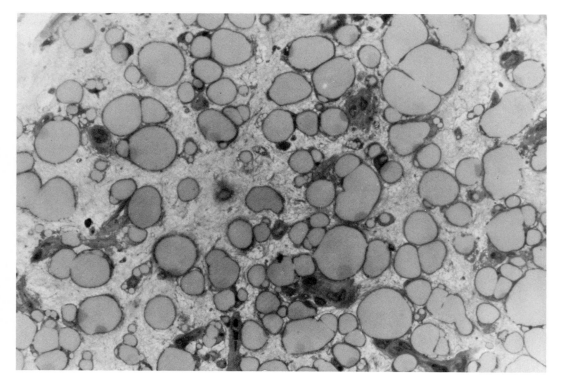

Figure 4.2. Mature adipose tissue, Araldite-embedded section. Osmiophilic lipid droplets are easily discernible. In some cells the peripherally placed nuclei are also visible. (Original magnification ×310.)

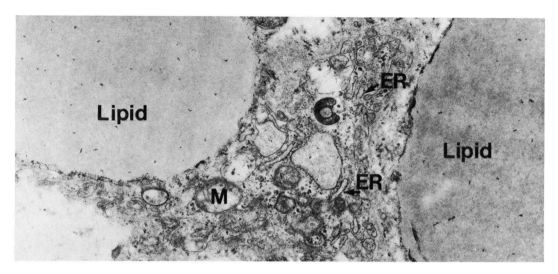

Figure 4.3. An adipose cell showing cytoplasmic details. ER represents endoplasmic reticulum and M is mitochondria. (Original magnification × 31,460.)

or Sudan black (Fig. 4.2). The cytoplasm is reduced to a thin membrane that surrounds the drop and is thickened in the part that contains the flattened nucleus with its central mass of chromatin. The composition of fat in a mature cell can range from simple lipid esters to compound lipids.

The amount of lipid present in a fat cell, its chemical composition, and the disproportionate volume in comparison to its cytoplasm make it difficult to process the tissue properly for ultrastructural study. Both Sheldon[36] and Napolitano[29] demonstrated that the fine structure of a fat cell is essentially the same as that of any other living cell (Fig. 4.3). The intracytoplasmic components are better discerned in fasting animals, owing to depletion of the cytoplasmic lipids.[36] Capillaries are in close proximity to the surface of white fat cells. In most instances they are separated by their respective basement membranes and small bundles of collagen. Neural elements, either myelinated or nonmyelinated, have infrequently been observed in the intercellular region of fat pads.[29]

Brown Adipose Tissue

Structure. This tissue is so named because of its color, which varies from rich reddish-brown to light tan. The color is contributed mainly by the high concentration of cytochrome pigments

in the mitochondria of the adipose cells. Some of the color represents hemoglobin, since the tissue is highly vascular. The species distribution, gross anatomy, and histologic structure have been well reviewed by Hammar,[37] Rasmussen,[23] and Johanason and Soderlund.[38] Brown adipose tissue is prominent in most hibernating and in many nonhibernating species of animals. Although masses of brown fat can be found in the neck, interscapular region, thorax, and axilla, in most species it is found along all the major blood vessels of the thoracic and abdominal cavities, extending to the proximal parts of the limbs. Brown-fat bodies are enclosed in a connective tissue capsule and are discretely localized.

The fat content of brown adipose cells can increase considerably. This fact raises the question of whether brown and white adipose tissues are separate in origin or represent two stages in the differentiation of one tissue. While there is room for dispute about the sources of white adipose cells, it is generally agreed that brown adipose cells arise from a specific anlage at particular body sites at certain times during fetal development. Brown adipose tissue is present only in certain sites in the body, and new areas do not develop in postnatal life.[30] With advancing age, however, the multivacuolar cells of brown adipose tissue are replaced by univacuolar cells, leading to the view that brown adipose tissue is no more than an immature form of white adipose tissue.[30] But when overfed animals are placed on a restricted diet, univacuolar brown adipose tissue cells revert to, and then keep, their multivacuolar form, whereas true white adipose tissue cells rapidly lose their fat altogether.

The human fetus clearly has brown adipose tissue, and the normal adult also has a small amount. In man, islands of cells of brown fat are best observed in the region of the neck, chest, and in the periadrenal fat tissue, which are the prominent sites in hibernating rodents.[26] Hibernomas usually occur in these sites. However, none of the studies thus far published has settled the question of whether the two kinds of adipose tissue are distinct from each other.

A normal brown adipose cell, in contradistinction to a white adipose cell, contains a number of small fat droplets. Ultrastructurally the cell cytoplasm is studded with myriads of mitochondria. The brown fat is richly innervated, and nonmyelinated fibers frequently are observed in the connective tissue septa separating the glandlike lobules. Axons may occur

in close apposition to brown fat cells. The resulting morphologic relationship is similar to that of the Schwann cell and its C fibers.[14] This observation by Napolitano is consistent with localizations of catecholamine in brown fat.[39,40] Dawkins and co-workers[39] postulated that cytoplasmic localizations of catecholamine, presumably noradrenalin, are clearly appropriate for the activation of lipase in the vicinity of fat droplets and lead to hydrolysis of triglyceride and subsequent oxidation of long-chain fatty acids. Romer[41] demonstrated the presence of corticosteroids and postulated that under certain conditions brown fat can take up the functions of the adrenal cortex.

Benign Neoplasms of White Adipose Tissue

Lipomas.

Macroscopic Findings. The gross appearance of lipomas found in the somatic tissues is essentially that of encapsulated fat. The fatty mass is usually yellow and semi-firm and is divided into smaller lobulations by fibrous strands that

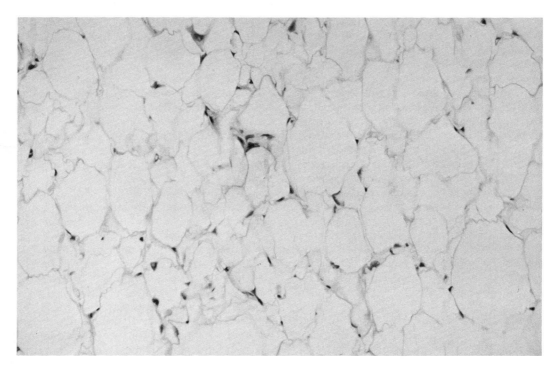

Figure 4.4. Solitary subcutaneous lipoma. Delicate fibrous septa and nutrient blood vessels can be easily seen. (H & E. Original magnification ×125.)

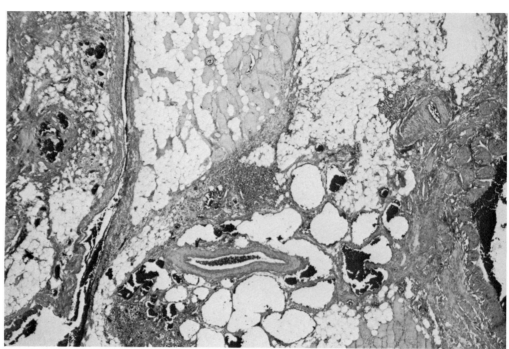

Figure 4.5. (A) Angiogram of an angiolipoma of the right calf of a 24-year-old man. Clinically this was thought to be a malignant tumor. **(B)** Angiolipoma showing multitude of capillaries within mature fatty tissue. The stroma shows the presence of fibroreticular material around the blood vessels. (H & E. Original magnification ×63.) A wide excision of the gross tumor, including gastrocnemius muscle, was performed. Although microscopic residual tumor was left behind during initial operation, patient has remained well 7 years.

B

A

traverse the tumor. The subcutaneous tumor is generally encapsulated by a thin fibrous layer; however, in the intermuscular variety the lipomatous tissue frequently extends or infiltrates along the muscle planes, a fact to be considered both from a diagnostic and a therapeutic standpoint—otherwise, an erroneous diagnosis of liposarcoma may be rendered.[42-44] When there is a comparatively small amount of fibrous tissue present, the tumor is semi-firm and it is difficult to cut sections. In contrast, in some tumors the fibrous tissue content is high and the tumor firm—these are called *fibrolipomas*. A typical lipoma is thinly encapsulated, presenting a greasy appearance and the yellow coloration of adipose tissue. Occasionally, hemorrhage and xanthomatous or myxoid degeneration may produce patchy discoloration and variegated appearance. Delicate fibrous septa intersect the lipoma and form an irregular supporting structure that carries nutrient blood vessels (Fig. 4.4). At times the vasculature of the lipoma is extensive, and the term *angiolipoma* is used (Fig. 4.5A and 4.5B). Angiolipomas are known to occur in all sites, including the viscera. Due

to their extensive vascularity, they sometimes tend to bleed and clinically may resemble sarcomas. Occasionally, bone formation (ossifying lipoma) and foci of chondrification also occur in lipomas (Fig. 4.6).

Microscopic Features. The tumor cells in common lipomas are usually large, spherical, and distended with fat; some are so laden with fat that the cytoplasm appears to be bound by a barely perceptible membrane surrounding a flattened nucleus (see Fig. 4.2). The cells may also be small, containing less fat, a proportionately greater amount of protoplasm, and a larger, ovoid, centrally placed nucleus. Lipomas have a fairly uniform cytologic appearance and are composed of a mixture of cells of different shapes and sizes, lying close together and sometimes arranged in small groups bound by fibroblasts and collagen. In angiolipomas, the fibrous tissue septa contain large numbers of blood vessels. These capillaries are lined by plump endothelial cells and are surrounded by immature and fusiform fat cells. Rasanen and co-workers[45] calculated the number of vascular channels and concluded that in angiolipomas the vascular

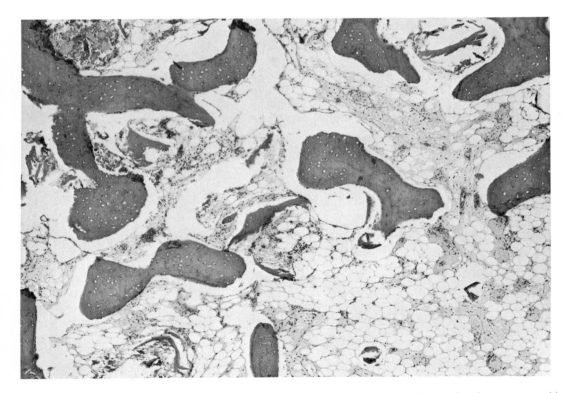

Figure 4.6. Osteolipoma: Islands of bone are formed within the stroma of a lipoma. This was found in a 65-year-old man with a long-standing history of a subcutaneous tumor in the forearm. (H & E. Original magnification ×63.)

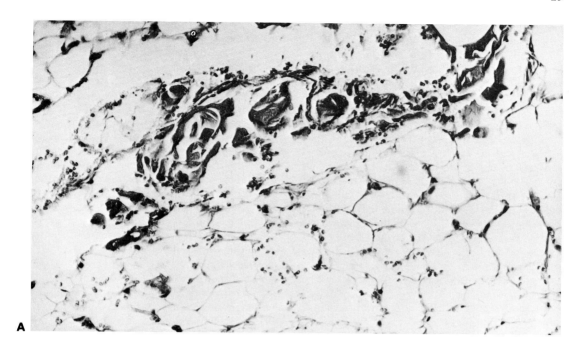

A

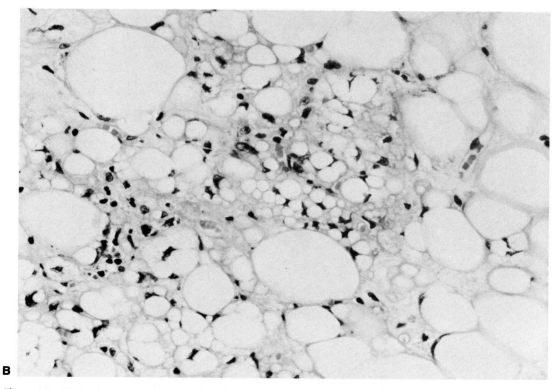

B

Figure 4.7. **(A)** A subcutaneous lipoma. This was a 5-cm mass in the gluteal region. The tumor was apparently totally excised. (H & E. Original magnification ×100.) Ten years later a 3-cm recurrent tumor was excised from under the scar of the previous operation. **(B)** This tumor was found to be a well-differentiated liposarcoma. (H & E. Original magnification ×250.)

component ranged from 15 to 40 percent of the fatty tissue.

Histochemistry of Lipomas. A subcutaneous lipoma is intensely stained by Sudan III and oil red 0. Red dyes are selectively absorbed by hydrophobic unsaturated triglycerides, cholesterol esters, and fatty acids. Common subcutaneous lipomas have an extremely low content of phospholipids.[46] Gellhorn and Marks[47] reported that the rate of acetate 1-^{14}C incorporation into mixed lipids of lipomas and normal subcutaneous adipose tissue from the same subject was faster in the tumor than in the normal tissue. These authors found that the distribution of radioactivity in lipid components of adipose tissue was about 1 percent of the total activity in free fatty acids, the remainder being in the triglycerides. They concluded that, in lipomas, a disturbance of lipid synthesis is a major factor in fat accumulation. Histochemical staining of enzymes in the common lipomas shows no apparent differences between normal white adipose tissue and lipomas.

Fine Structure of Lipomas. A fat cell from a lipoma seldom shows any variations in structure from a normal adult fat cell (see Figs. 4.1 and 4.3).

Malignant Change in Lipomas. Malignant change in a lipoma is extremely rare, and most liposarcomas arise as such ab initio. Wright,[48] in 1948, reported a case of liposarcoma arising in a lipoma, and accepted one other from Stout's[49] series. Since then, Sternberg[50] and Sampson et al.[51] have each reported a case of liposarcoma developing in a subcutaneous lipoma. In none of these cases did the tumor either recur or metastasize after excision. We have seen only one patient in whom a subcutaneous lipoma probably preceded the development of a liposarcoma (Fig. 4.7A and 4.7B).

Lipoblastomatosis. This is a benign tumor of fetal and embryonal adipose tissue, usually found in the extremities of infants and children. Although Jaffe[52] coined the term *lipoblastoma* in 1926 to describe tumors of immature fat cells, the existence of a benign lipoblastic tumor was

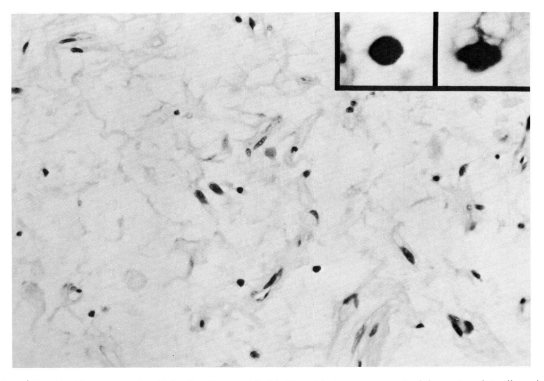

Figure 4.8. Lipoblastoma in the thigh of a 13-year-old girl. Note lobular arrangement of the mature fat cells and uniform cellular appearance within each lobule. The stroma is sparsely supplied with blood vessels. (H & E. Original magnification ×125.) Inset shows the different types of lipoblasts. (Original magnification ×600.)

not widely known until 1958, when Vellios and co-workers[53] described lipoblastomatosis as a benign lipoblastic tumor of the postnatal period. Shear[54] has since collected seven such cases. In 1975, Chung and Enzinger[55] reviewed 35 cases from the files of the Armed Forces Institute of Pathology and provided the basic morphologic criteria for these tumors.

The majority are lobulated and are found throughout the body, but most commonly in the extremities.[55] We have encountered only one such case, and that was in a 13-year-old girl with a tumor in the left thigh.

The microscopic features are characterized by a lobular arrangement of the tumor cells and a uniform cellular appearance within each tumor lobule (Fig. 4.8). Within each lobule the fat cells vary in the degree of differentiation. Mature fat cells are interspersed with various types of lipoblasts and spindled or stellate mesenchymal cells. Chung and Enzinger[55] found that histochemical studies of their material did not provide any diagnostic clues. These tumors probably represent a developmental anomaly.[56]

Malignant Neoplasms of White Adipose Tissue

Liposarcoma. Liposarcomas are relatively common mesenchymal neoplasms of the soft somatic tissues, described by Pack and Ariel[4] as constituting 14.6 percent of all sarcomas of the somatic tissues. Enzinger and Winslow[57] suggested that, among all mesenchymal tumors, liposarcomas are unsurpassed in their wide range of structure and behavior.

Virchow,[58] in 1857, first described a malignant tumor of the fatty tissue in a lower extremity. Following this description, a number of case reports appeared in the contemporary literature, emphasizing in particular the large size of these tumors.[4,59] Stout,[49] in 1944, analyzed 41 cases of liposarcoma and subsequently the subject was dealt with in detail by Pack and Pierson,[60] Enzinger and Winslow,[57] Reszel et al.,[61] Enterline et al.,[62] De Weed and Dockery,[59] and Das Gupta.[63]

Macroscopic Features. Primary liposarcoma is commonly situated deep in the intermuscular or periarticular planes, although subcutaneous locations are not uncommon. Smaller tumors appear to be encapsulated (pseudocapsule). The cut surface of these tumors, whether they are large or small, exhibits a variety of colors—white,

yellow, or red. In larger tumors, areas of necrosis, hemorrhage, and cyst formation are often seen (Fig. 4.9). Fibrous septa usually divide the tumors into distinct small lobules. The original primary tumor lies between, but does not invade, the muscle bellies. In contrast, recurrent liposarcomas do invade and infiltrate the surrounding tissue. In our early series,[63] 115 (48.7 percent) of 236 patients with liposarcoma had diffuse infiltrating tumors extending to the surrounding bones, muscles, and vessels. Rarely, liposarcomas are of multicentric origin; nine such cases have been treated by the Division of Surgical Oncology at the University of Illinois.

Microscopic Appearance. There is a diversity of opinion regarding classification of malignant adipose tissue tumors. Ewing[1] originally separated them into three cell types: adult, myxoid, and granular, relating the last group to brown fat. Stout[49] also classified them into three groups: (1) well-differentiated myxoid, in which the tumor is composed of adult fat cells, embryonal stellate cells, or spindle-shaped lipoblasts with cytoplasmic droplets that stain with Sudan III; (2) poorly differentiated lipoblasts, with various types of nuclei (this tumor carries a poor prognosis); and (3) the round cell type, in which the tumor cell is spherical, with a central nucleus and abundant foamy cytoplasm. Frequently, a fourth kind was seen that consisted of a mixed cell population. Enzinger and Winslow[57] modified Stout's classification and suggested the following four types: (1) myxoid, (2) round cell, (3) well-differentiated adult, and (4) pleomorphic.

The microscopic classifications of Ewing, Stout, and Enzinger and Winslow are all similar. Enzinger and Winslow suggested that their own classification was better for a prognostic guide. This classification is briefly described.

MYXOID TUMORS. According to Enzinger and Winslow,[57] this is the most common type of liposarcoma. These authors found a uniform myxoid pattern, with occasional transition to all other forms of liposarcoma. They aptly pointed out its close similarity to Wasserman's primitive fat organ. As in the primitive fat organ, the tumor is composed of three main elements: proliferating lipoblasts in various stages of differentiation, a plexiform capillary pattern, and a myxoid matrix. Because of this close similarity to primitive fat structure, the adult cells in certain myxoid liposarcomas are extremely difficult to distinguish from primitive mesenchyme and

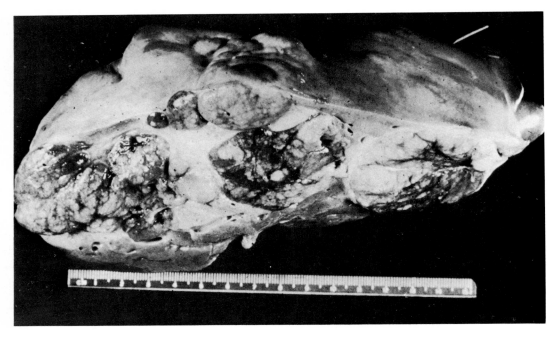

Figure 4.9. Cut section of a retroperitoneal liposarcoma. The cut surface shows the characteristic lobulated appearance of mature well-differentiated liposarcoma, with areas of hemorrhage.

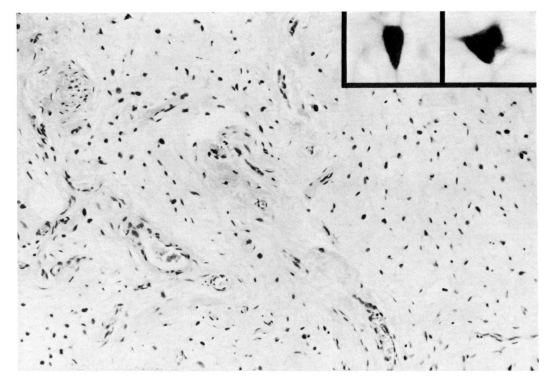

Figure 4.10. Myxoid liposarcoma. Vascular network, with the characteristic mucopolysaccharide-rich ground substance, is prominent. Close scrutiny shows anastomosing stellate and fusiform lipoblasts. (H & E. Original magnification ×125.) Inset depicts the morphology of these lipoblasts. (Original magnification ×600.)

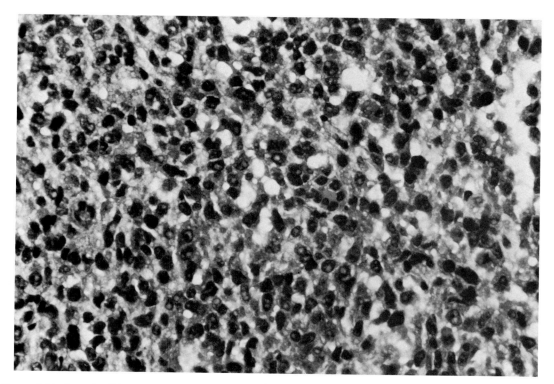

Figure 4.11. Round cell liposarcoma of the thigh in an 18-year-old girl. The uniform distribution of rounded cells and diminished intercellular material can be seen. Note fat-laden tumor cells and cells in mitosis. (H & E. Original magnification ×250.)

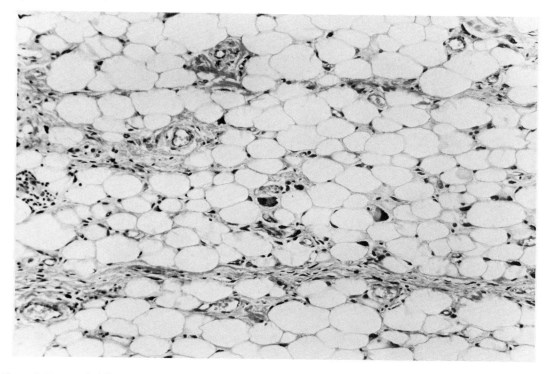

Figure 4.12. A well-differentiated liposarcoma of the right iliac fossa in an 80-year-old man. The tumor recurred twice before being treated by us for the third time. (H & E. Original magnification ×125.)

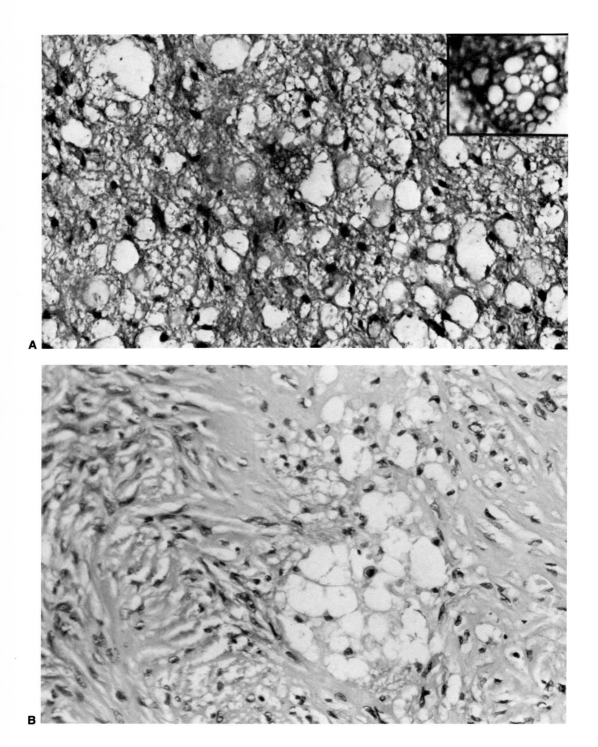

A

B

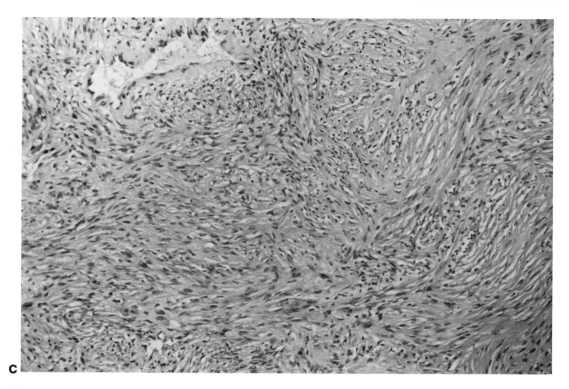

C

Figure 4.13. Pleomorphic liposarcoma from the thigh of a 55-year-old man. The disorderly growth pattern in the three areas of the same tumor is a characteristic feature of this type of tumor. **(A)** Area showing rich myxoid stroma with branching capillary network, a multilobulated lipoblast in the center. (H & E. Original magnification ×110.) Inset shows the characteristic features of malignant lipoblasts (Original magnification ×600.) **(B)** Tumor infiltrating the muscle. Lipoblasts and mitosis are visible. (H & E. Original magnification ×250.) **(C)** Area resembling fibrosarcoma. It is composed of uniform spindle cells containing pyknotic solitary nuclei and fibrillary cytoplasm. (H & E. Original magnification ×110.)

have sometimes been misinterpreted as mesenchymomas. The abundant capillary network is one of the characteristic features of this type of liposarcoma. The amount of myxoid matrix varies from tumor to tumor (Fig. 4.10). Anastomosing stellate and fusiform cells are arranged in an intricate loose network and are accompanied by a variable number of signet cells containing lipids.

ROUND CELL TUMOR. Enzinger and Winslow[57] considered that, although round cell tumors are closely related to the myxoid type, they deserve separate consideration because of their aggressive clinical course and frequency of metastases. In the great majority, the main characteristic is excessive proliferation of uniformly rounded cells (Fig. 4.11). Also, the intercellular myxoid material is diminished.

Ewing[1] considered round cell liposarcoma to be the malignant counterpart of a hibernoma.

This hypothesis does not seem logical in view of the locations reported and the frequent transition to other forms of the tumor.

WELL-DIFFERENTIATED LIPOSARCOMAS. The difficulty in distinguishing between a lipoma and the well-differentiated type of liposarcoma has been emphasized by numerous authors.[28,49,57,61,62] This tumor frequently is misdiagnosed as a benign deep-seated lipoma (Fig. 4.12). Fortunately, it is slow-growing and not likely to metastasize. Local recurrence is the rule for inadequately excised lesions, however. A distinction between the "lipomalike" form and the "sclerosing" form of well-differentiated liposarcomas has been proposed by Enzinger and Winslow,[57] but this description is more academic than practical.

PLEOMORPHIC TUMORS. The distinguishing features of pleomorphic tumors are the disorderly growth pattern, the extreme degree of cellular pleomorphism, and the giant cells (Fig. 4.13A to 4.13C). In some, the giant cells contain lipid droplets. In others, lipoblastic activity is limited, often confined to a few cells. The cellular pattern can range from rounded cells to large giant cells arranged in various configurations. These giant cells can be unicellular, with pyknotic nuclei or multinucleated, and both types can be found in the same field. Some tumors show polymorphic features, and areas resembling spindle cell fibrosarcomas can be seen (Fig. 4.13C). Therefore, it is apparent that a pleomorphic liposarcoma can mimic a number of other types of sarcoma, and it is essential to demonstrate the presence of lipoblasts to establish a prima facie diagnosis of liposarcoma.

The classification proposed by Enzinger and Winslow[57] is theoretically sound and can be used to estimate the biologic behavior of liposarcoma. Well-differentiated liposarcomas are commonly infiltrative and the incidence of local recurrence is higher than for distant metastasis. In contrast, poorly differentiated liposarcomas have a high potential for distant metastases. From a prac-

tical standpoint, however, it is clearly better to estimate the prognosis on the basis of tumor grade,[64] and today this method of prognostication is generally used. In tumors showing areas of varying microscopic features, prognostication must be based on the most undifferentiated area viewed.

Histochemistry. Histochemical studies of liposarcoma have been carried out by various workers,[49,57,65] and from their studies it is generally accepted that mucoid material is an integral part of liposarcoma. The mucoid substance is more abundant in the myxoid type than in the pleomorphic or poorly differentiated types and is essentially composed of acid mucopolysaccharides. In some cells, staining demonstrates periodic acid-Schiff-positive material, presumably glycogen. Fat stains show the presence of a large amount of neutral fat (Fig. 4.14). In poorly differentiated tumors, fat is not as well localized as in the differentiated types. A fine reticulin network is frequently present.

Electron Microscopy. Ultrastructurally, five cell types can be identified: multivacuolated tu-

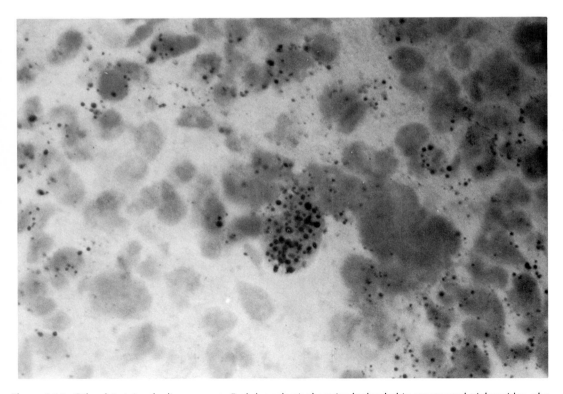

Figure 4.14. Oil red 0 stain of a liposarcoma. Red dye selectively stains hydrophobic unsaturated triglycerides, cholesterol esters, and fatty acids. (Oil immersion. Original magnification ×600.)

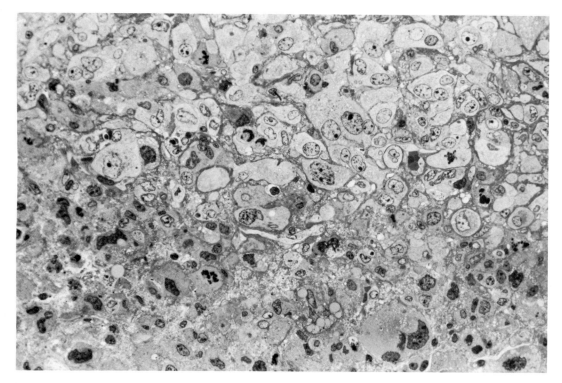

Figure 4.15. (A) One-micron Araldite-embedded section of a pleomorphic liposarcoma. Multivacuolated lipoblasts, stellate and round mesenchymal cells, and fibroblasts are easily discernible. Several cells show mitotic activity. (Toluidine blue, basic fuchsin. Original magnification ×375.)

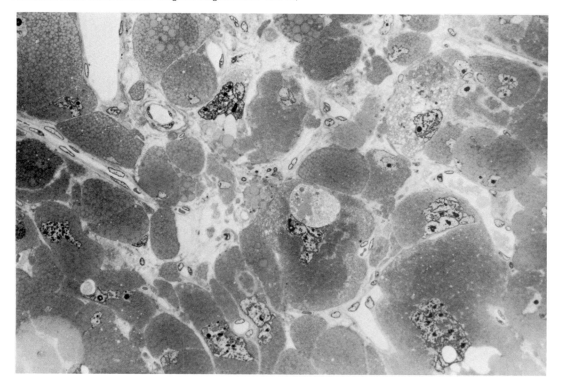

Figure 4.15. (B) One-micron section of a round cell liposarcoma. Note the variety of shapes and sizes of multivacuolated lipoblasts, some of which are in direct contact with the capillary lining. (Toluidine blue. Original magnification ×250.)

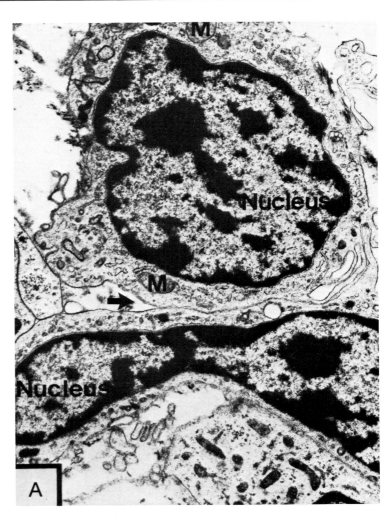

Figure 4.16. Electron micrographs of a round cell liposarcoma in the thigh of a 33-year-old male patient. **(A)** Two malignant adipocytes are in close proximity without desmosomal contact. Arrow shows the cell-to-cell contact. The upper cell has a round nucleus with scanty cytoplasm and no lipid inclusions. (Original magnification ×11,491.)

mor cell (liposarcoma cell), stellate mesenchymal cell, round mesenchymal cell, fibroblast, and normal fat cell (Figs. 4.15A, 4.15B, and 4.16A). The multivacuolated cells are large, with a peripheral nucleus and abundant cytoplasm containing lipid-laden inclusions, as well as other types of inclusions (Fig. 4.15A and 4.15B). Scarpelli and Greider[18] found some of these inclusions did not stain with Sudan black or oil red 0. Another characteristic feature of the cytoplasm is the abundance of microfilaments (Fig. 4.16B). In many of these tumor cells, multiple cytoplasmic inclusions and vacuoles that bear a certain resemblance to one another suggest that they might represent related stages of similar intracellular processes. Stellate and round mes-

enchymal cells have a similar appearance and are characterized by hyperchromatic nuclei and basophilic cytoplasm, one with cytoplasmic processes and the other without (Fig. 4.16C and 4.16D). The cytoplasm of these cells essentially differs from that of the multivacuolated cells by the absence of cytoplasmic inclusions (Fig. 4.16E). These three cell types probably are all malignant lipoblasts in different stages of evolution. The other two cell types, namely, fibroblasts and lipoblasts, have normal characteristics and can be easily identified.

Metastatic pattern of liposarcoma. Liposarcomas, like other soft tissue sarcomas, predominantly metastasize to the lung. Das Gupta[63] reported an overall incidence of 41 percent in a

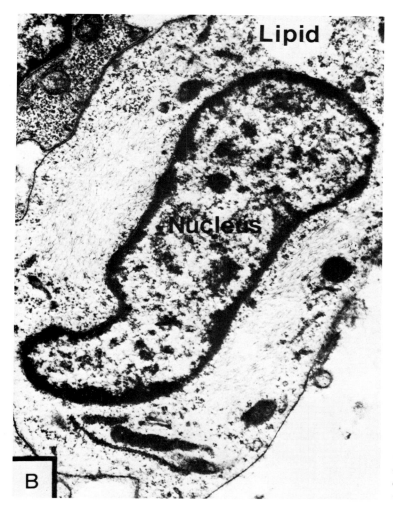

Lipid

Nucleus

B

Figure 4.16. (B) A tumor cell showing one lipid droplet, organelles, and filamentous matrix. (Original magnification ×14,833.)

series of 236 patients, of which 9.3 percent were found on routine postmortem examination. The liver is involved less frequently (only about 10 percent of cases). Metastases to various sites of the body are seen, including the brain, pleura, thyroid, pancreas, and spinal cord. Liposarcoma metastasizes to the gastrointestinal tract more frequently than any other type of sarcoma, usually to the colon (4 percent of all cases). Regional lymph node involvement is found in only 3 percent of the patients; however, this includes tumors located in close proximity to the regional nodes. In the agonal state or at postmortem, the incidence is much higher, ranging from 10 to 15 percent. Most of the nodal disease probably occurs by direct extension.

Brown Adipose Tissue Tumors

Benign. Hibernomas (lipomas of brown adipose tissue) are lipochrome-rich, tannish-brown, well-encapsulated solitary tumors.[65–67] They occur in adults,[68,69] and less commonly in adolescents[70] and children.[65,71] The tumors consist of masses of large, multiloculated, lipid-rich, closely aggregated round, oval, or polygonal cells containing sudanophilic granules and centrally placed nuclei (Fig. 4.17). The cells usually are arranged in a lobular fashion. These tumors are extensively supplied by capillary blood vessels. This pattern of blood supply is similar to that of the organs of hibernating lower mammals.

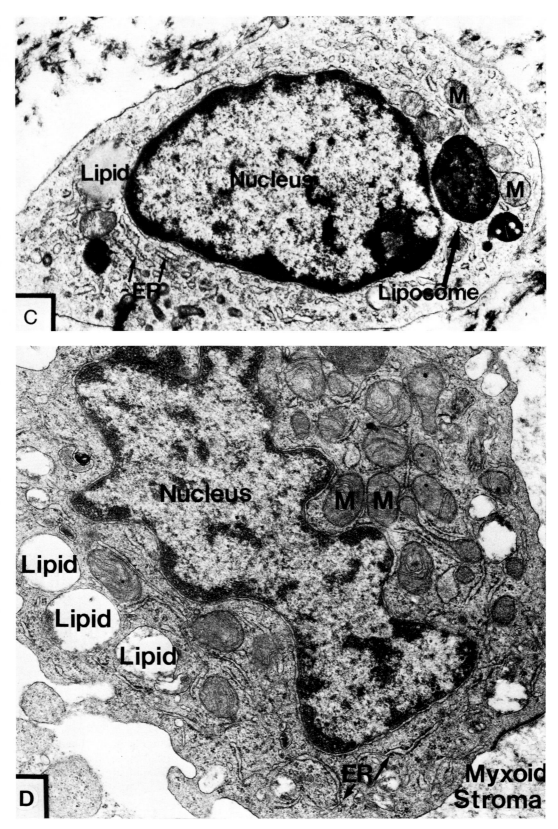

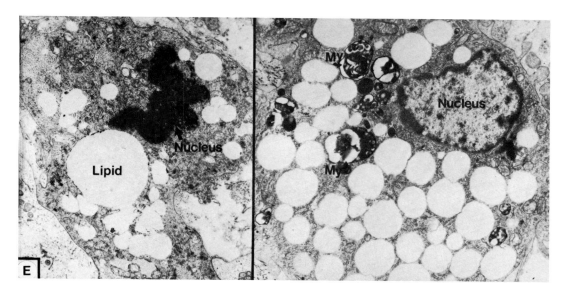

Figure 4.16. (E) Malignant lipoblast with large coalescing lipid droplets in the cytoplasm from a well-differentiated liposarcoma. Profiles of myelin figures (My) are frequently observed. (Original magnification ×14,214.)

Malignant. Primary malignant hibernoma or malignant transformation of a benign hibernoma has not yet been satisfactorily documented (Chapter 11). Symmers,[72] in 1944, described a case in a three-month-old boy who died of inanition. On postmortem examination extensive brownish-red nodules were noted throughout the abdominal cavity. Histologic examination suggested that they were brown fat. Pack and Ariel[4] speculated on the possibility of their being malignant hibernomas.

TUMORS OF THE FIBROUS CONNECTIVE TISSUE

Connective tissue originates from the embryonic primitive mesenchyme. Most prospective fibrous tissue is relatively well formed by the second month of intrauterine life. By the end of the second month, many of the main tendons, ligaments, fascia, and other fibrous structures are present as mesenchymal condensations and are identifiable. Fibrous connective tissue constitutes one of the major components of the extracellular compartment. For a better understanding of the diseases and neoplasms of fibrous connective tissue, adequate background information on the morphology and physiology of the extracellular compartment is necessary.

The realization of the presence of an extracellular compartment influencing the activity of cells has generated a body of information attempting to explain the morphology and function of this compartment. Today it is generally agreed that the extracellular compartment is truly an organ participating actively in many body functions as an autonomous unit. The major area germane to our consideration is that of the connective tissue elements of this compartment.

Figure 4.16. (C) An immature adipocyte with round nucleus. Scanty cytoplasm containing one large lipid droplet, mitochondria (M), and endoplasmic reticulum (ER). (Original magnification ×16,758.) **(D)** Lipoblast from a myxoid liposarcoma with multiple osmiophilic lipid droplets. These are usually composed of neutral lipids. The cytoplasmic processes in this cell are easily discernible. Note the myxoid stroma in the lower right corner of the micrograph. (Original magnification ×31,900.)

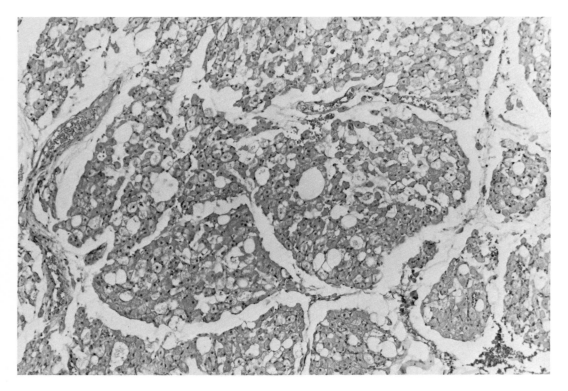

Figure 4.17. Hibernoma. Granular, round, or oval fat cells arranged in lobular fashion. (H & E. Original magnification ×65.) *(Courtesy of Dr. S. Sahgal, West Side VA Hospital, Chicago.)*

The components of adult connective tissue can be classified into several groups (Table 4.1). This table takes into consideration the origin of the respective component parts, whether derived locally or from the circulating plasma.[73] The connective tissue consists partly of structural units of local origin forming an enduring organization, and partly of materials in transit between the blood and cells of the region. Morphologic division of connective tissue into cells, fibers, and ground substance makes it simple to study the characteristics of each group (Fig. 4.18A to 4.18F).

Cells

The fibroblast is the characteristic cell in the connective tissue systems, but in specific tissues it appears in the guise of a chondroblast, an osteoblast, an odontoblast, or a synovioblast. These cells have in common the secretion of collagen, reticulin, elastin, various glycosaminoglycans, and glycoproteins.[73,74]

A mature fibroblast has an oval, eccentri-cally placed nucleus. The cytoplasm is characterized by dilated, rough-surfaced endoplasmic reticulum, a prominent perinuclear Golgi complex, multiple cytoplasmic granules, and polyribosomes (Fig. 4.18A). Fibroblasts grown in culture show all these characteristics, along with the dendritic processes.

Fibroblasts are considered to be the main source of fibrogenesis.[75-78] Extensive studies of the cytoplasmic granules within the fibroblast cytoplasm suggest that these granules are the site of metabolic activity leading to collagen formation.[78-81] Rough endoplasmic reticulum is also associated with fibrogenesis.[74,75] However, there is no clear-cut understanding of the role of each cytoplasmic component in fibrogenesis.

Fibrogenesis involves a number of sequential developmental steps. Mechanisms concerned in two of these have received particular attention in tissue culture investigations. One step concerns the determination of the size of the macromolecular particle of the fibrous protein collagen produced by the cell. The other

TABLE 4.1. ORGANIZATION AND COMPOSITION OF CONNECTIVE TISSUE

<u>Cells:</u>   Fibroblasts, chondroblasts, osteoblasts, synovioblasts, odontoblasts

<u>Fibers:</u>   Collagen fibers -- collagen
              Reticular fibers — reticulin
              Elastic fibers — elastin

<u>Ground substance:</u>

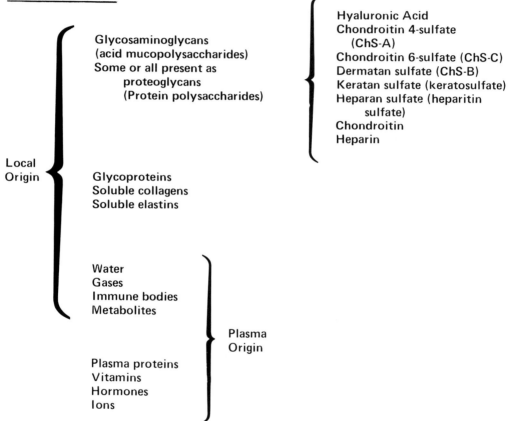

Local Origin
- Glycosaminoglycans (acid mucopolysaccharides) Some or all present as proteoglycans (Protein polysaccharides)
  - Hyaluronic Acid
  - Chondroitin 4-sulfate (ChS-A)
  - Chondroitin 6-sulfate (ChS-C)
  - Dermatan sulfate (ChS-B)
  - Keratan sulfate (keratosulfate)
  - Heparan sulfate (heparitin sulfate)
  - Chondroitin
  - Heparin
- Glycoproteins
  Soluble collagens
  Soluble elastins

Plasma Origin
- Water
  Gases
  Immune bodies
  Metabolites
- Plasma proteins
  Vitamins
  Hormones
  Ions

Courtesy of HR Catchpole: Connective tissue: Capillary permeability. In The Inflammatory Process, vol 2, 2nd ed. New York, Academic Press, 1973.

concerns localization of the site or sites where such particles become aggregated into a definitive fibril, and, as part of this, the mechanisms that are involved in the enlargement of individual collagen fibrils until their characteristic size for the particular tissue is attained.

The question of the relationship of the fibrous protein and collagen to cells has long been a controversial issue. In recent years, the development of organ culture techniques and the application of electron microscopy have provided considerable insight into the process of collagen formation.[82-86] Undoubtedly, collagen formation is an active process within the fibroblast cytoplasm (Fig. 4.18F).

Collagen is synthesized on polysomes attached to the endoplasmic reticulum, with the nascent chains vectorially oriented into the cisternae. Residues of collagen arise from enzymatic hydroxylation of specific prolyl and lysyl

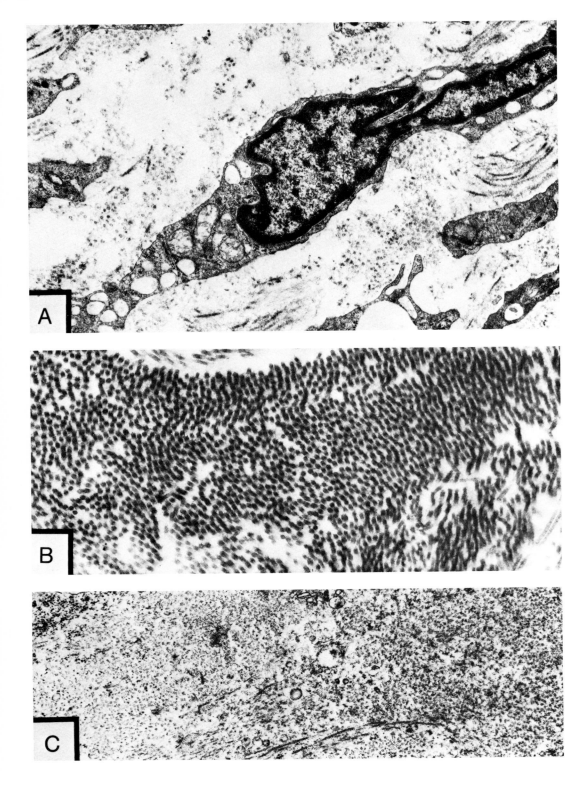

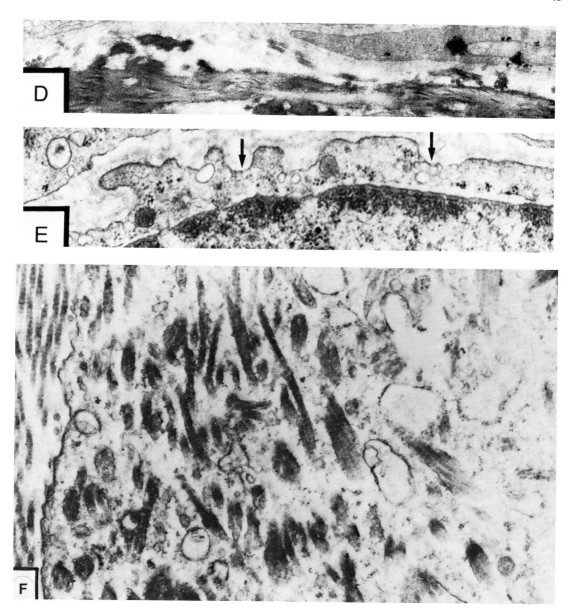

Figure 4.18. **(A)** A panoramic view of multiple normal human fibroblasts dispersed in a collagenous matrix. The nuclei are prominent and usually ovoid, but the shape depends on the plane of sectioning. The cytoplasm contains the usual organelles and is crowded with rough endoplasmic reticulum. (Original magnification ×6500.) **(B)** The mature collagen fibers are seen either in cross section or in different degrees of tangential or longitudinal sections. In the longitudinal section, the characteristic cross-striations can be identified. (Original magnification ×10,200.) **(C)** Reticulin fibers are usually similar to collagen fibers but are generally bunched together and are finer in texture. (Original magnification ×11,450.) **(D)** Elastic lamina of a medium-sized blood vessel. (Original magnification ×45,000.) **(E)** Profile of a basement membrane from an endothelial cell (Original magnification ×45,000.) **(F)** Cytoplasm of a fibroblast showing the presence of fibers in different stages of development (Original magnification ×54,625.)

residues in peptide linkage in the growing nascent chains. The transcellular movement and secretion of procollagen require energy, and the microtubular system is required for the translocations of the vacuolar elements. Once secreted from the cell, procollagen is enzymatically converted into collagen. The fibroblast secretes one or more enzymes (procollagen peptidase), which separate most of the nonhelical peptides from the ends of the precursor, generating tropocollagen, the triple helical molecule that retains only the abbreviated peptidases. Once generated, tropocollagen tends to come out of solution and aggregate in a specific manner to form collagen fibers.[84-88]

Fibers

Collagen. Collagen fibers are the principal structural components of connective tissue. They occur in the body as coarse bundles a few millimeters in diameter and can be seen under an electron microscope as fine fibrils with a diameter of 600 Å or less, showing a banded structure 640 Å in periodicity. The fundamental chemical unit of collagen that is shared with reticulin is a tropocollagen molecule consisting of three helically wound polypeptide chains.[88] Aggregations of tropocollagen molecules "in phase" lead first to various forms of soluble collagen and finally to relatively insoluble fibrillar collagen. The tropocollagen is a rodlike structure 3000 Å long and 15 Å wide; hydrogen bonding is responsible for both its internal stability and its capacity to react externally to form bundles, ie, cross-linking (Fig. 4.18B). Cross-linkings increase in number with age. Soluble forms of collagen are not seen with the electron microscope and can be classified as ground substance. Other compounds, such as saccharides, may participate in fiber formation. The amount of the carbohydrate-forming part of the intrinsic structure of collagen may be low (0.5–1.0 percent in tendon collagen) or quite high (10 percent or more in basement membrane collagen). Collagen has a high content of glycine (about 25 percent) and a low content of aromatic acid. Additionally, it contains two amino acids unique to this class of proteins: hydroxyproline and hydroxylysine.

Reticulin. Ultrastructurally these are similar to collagen fibers but are usually bunched and are finer in texture (Fig. 4.18C), with a characteristic distribution in close association with the basement membrane. Reticulin fibers show a strong affinity for silver stains, which has led to the idea that they are formed by the aggregation of tropocollagen molecules in a carbohydrate-rich material that creates these argyrophilic fibers.

Elastic. The major component of elastic fibers is the protein elastin, characterized by the presence of two amino acids specific to elastin: desmosine and isodesmosine.[89] These have fine structures that form bridges in a three-dimensional network. The resulting infinitely cross-linked structures are reminiscent of rubberlike polymers, whose behavior they mimic.[89] Elastin is the most important component of large blood vessel walls (Fig. 4.18D).

Ground Substance. The ground substance of connective tissue is all-inclusive of a larger, incompletely known variety of chemical substances constituting the matrix for the cells to rest on, and is contiguous with the basement membrane.[90] The ground substance is heterogenous (Table 4.1). It is convenient to divide the components into macromolecules and smaller molecular entities. The macromolecular group includes mucopolysaccharides or glycosaminoglycans, glycoproteins, basement membranes, soluble tropocollagens, and elastins not yet polymerized to fibrils, and, finally, serum proteins. In tissue, the acid mucopolysaccharides are complexed with proteins (proteoglycans) to different degrees, and, like fibrin, become relatively water-insoluble. The class of smaller molecular components includes metabolites, vitamins, hormones, gases (CO_2, O_2, N_2), ions, and water.

The ground substance is observed in light microscopic studies (preferably in cryostat vacuum-dried or freeze-dried sections combined with alcohol after fixation) as a homogeneous matrix staining metachromatically with toluidine blue, and pink to red with periodic acid-Schiff (PAS) stain. It is contiguous with the basement membrane of endothelial, epithelial, muscle, fat, and other cells. Because of fixation techniques, ultrastructural studies have been unsatisfactory, and in most instances only the collagen and reticulin fibers are visible.

A study of the distribution of intravenously injected ferrocyanide, which can be recognized because of subsequent formation of an electron-dense product, has yielded valuable information.[73] However, these studies, contrary to expectation, showed ferrocyanide present in discrete vacuoles of 1000 Å or less.[73] Therefore, it is not possible to consider ground substance as a colloidal homogeneous solution.

Basement Membrane. Basement membrane characteristically appears as a dense-staining line or sheet interposed between connective tissue and entoderm and highly differentiated mesodermal structures. It stains with PAS and is found contiguous with ground substance. Under the electron microscope, it appears as an electron-dense layer and is usually 300 to 500 Å wide, but may reach 3000 Å or more in a kidney glomerulus (Fig. 4.18E). Most of our knowledge of basement membrane composition is based on glomerular basement membrane. In the cell-free material obtained by differential centrifugation and sonication, fibrils are absent but analysis shows a collagenlike protein, together with associated carbohydrates containing about 7 to 10 percent neutral sugars. It is commonly thought that the basement membrane arises from the adjoining cells and has antigenic properties characteristic of the cells of probable origin. However, because of the chemical and antigenic complexity of the basement membrane at specific locations, a common origin for all types cannot as yet be proposed.[91]

Functions of Connective Tissue

The function of connective tissue ranges from the minimally extensible joining represented by the collagen-rich tendon, to the elastic recoil of an arterial wall in which elastin is the major connective component. Cartilage is a semi-rigid tissue marked by the presence of the strongly acidic, ion-binding but feebly hydrophilic chondroitin sulfate. The Wharton's jelly of the umbilical cord is composed of a network of collagen fibers embedded in a hydrophilic hyaluronic acid gel and is flexible and rubbery in texture. Skin connective tissue, containing roughly equivalent amounts of hyaluronic acid and chondroitin sulfate, shows considerable water-holding capacity. The limit, in an organized tissue, is reached in the vitreous body, being 99 percent or more water and dissolved substances, 0.1 percent collagen as an extremely fine network, and 0.15 percent hyaluronic acid. The structure is nevertheless self-supporting when physically intact. For the vitreous body, the sine qua non is transparency. The same holds true for the cornea, but here an external protective function is also required. It is composed of highly oriented collagen lamellae in a matrix of keratin and chondroitin sulfates. One senses the theme of adaptive evolution in which form and function may have made equal contributions. Other examples of connective tissue functional adaptation are bulk accommodation (uterus), relaxation (symphysis pubis), lubrication (joint interfaces), and the capacity to accumulate and release ions (cartilage, osteoid, and bone).

Changes in connective tissue occur with growth and differentiation. Apart from the manifold phenomena of embryonic induction, the remodeling of tissues as they increase in size implies lability of the extracellular elements.[74] The basement membrane of the skin appears to organize shortly after birth and to become progressively more prominent. Basement membranes tend to disappear after injury and are later regenerated. Striking connective tissue changes occur in the uterus during pregnancy. The process includes an increase in muscle mass, collagen content, and ground substance. Conversely, during involution, all these tissue elements are progressively and rapidly lost. Impairment of this involution process may be the reason for the induction of uterine "fibroids" (leiomyomas).

Hormones may produce an increase in organ size and vascularity and seem to include, as an integral part of this activity, effects on connective tissue morphology, water content, and ion distribution. Both male and female sex hormones have a large influence on the connective tissue. For example, in normal pregnancy there is an enormous accumulation of extrauterine fluid that must be regarded as physiologic edema. Recently, we showed the presence of steroid receptors in several types of human soft somatic tissue sarcomas.[92] The presence of estrogen, androgen, and glucocorticoid receptors in nongynecologic tumors of connective tissue origin, along with other tumors of diverse histogenesis, suggests that hormones probably play a much wider role in connective tissue physiology and in the induction and growth of tumors and tumorlike conditions than hitherto suspected.

The discovery of the connective tissue enzymes triggered much of the modern work on the nature of the ground substance. These enzymes are present in testis, many microorganisms, cercariae, snake venom, and leech digestive juices. By 1940, the substrates of the spreading factors had been recognized as being hyaluronic acid and chondroitin sulfates.[73] The role of these enzymes in the growth and spread of either primary neoplasms of the connective tissue or metastases from elsewhere has been studied. It appears that the spread of these transplantable tumors could in part be influenced by the depolymerizing enzymes (hyaluronidases). Currently, the role of the enzyme collagenase in tumors is being investigated. The exact role of the connective tissue enzymes in tumor growth and spread is unclear, but that they play an important role is beyond doubt.

In recent years, attention has been focused on the "growth factors." Both epidermal growth factor (EGF) and fibroblast growth factor (FGF) are being extensively evaluated.[93–95] The influence of these factors in normal organ development and aberrations thereof, as well as the influence on the biologic behavior of human fibrous tissue tumors, are areas of continued interest and research.

Tumors and tumorlike conditions of the connective tissues are not isolated instances of growth of a tumor in a given anatomic site; rather, they probably represent an alteration in one or more local or systemic factors. For example, aggressive fibromatosis occurs frequently among young women, and several types of fibromatoses are associated with various systemic conditions. Although no explanation for these correlations is yet available, it appears that all these tumors and tumorlike conditions should be reviewed from a new and more critical perspective.

The morphologic characteristics of tumors and tumorlike conditions of the connective tissue are described in the following section (Table 4.2). Before entering into a description of these individual types it is appropriate to comment on three points. The *first point* is recognition of the existence of a specific type of cell "histiocyte" in adult soft tissue tumors. Histiocytes are versatile in behavior and frequently can act either as true fibroblasts or as phagocytes. This versatility makes histologic classification of some of these tumors difficult. Therefore, it is becoming more and more customary to classify them, eg, dermatofibrosarcoma protuberans and some giant-cell tumors, as fibrous histiocytic tumors. The *second point* deals with the concept of "facultative fibroblasts." This term, first defined by Stout and Lattes,[3] reminds us that not all fibro-

TABLE 4.2. TUMORS OF THE CONNECTIVE TISSUE

Benign Tumors and Tumorlike Conditions	Histologically Benign but Clinically Malignant	Malignant Tumors
Fibroma	Dermatofibrosarcoma protuberans	Fibrosarcoma
Fibromatoses	Aggressive fibromatoses	Malignant fibrous histiocytoma
Juvenile type	Desmoids of the anterior abdominal wall	Malignant xanthogranuloma
Congenital, both localized and generalized		Malignant histiocytoma
Fibromatous coli	Extra-abdominal desmoids	Dermatofibrosarcoma
Juvenile aponeurotic fibroma		
Juvenile nasopharyngeal angiofibroma		
Recurring digital fibrous tumor with inclusions		
Progressive myositis fibroma		
Adult type		
Keloid		
Palmar and plantar fibromatosis		
Penile fibromatosis		
Idiopathic retroperitoneal fibromatosis		
Pseudosarcomatous fasciitis		
Progressive myositis ossificans		
Paradoxical fibrosarcomas of the skin		
Elastofibromas		
Fibrous histiocytomas with all their variants		

blastic cells in tumors or tumorlike conditions originate from preexisting fibroblasts. Under certain circumstances, mesothelial cells, Schwann cells, and lipoblasts can assume the characteristics of fibroblasts and take part in fibrogenesis. The *final point* is clinicopathologic. Although some tumors are histologically benign they should not be classified, without qualification, as benign tumors; clinically they are aggressive and can be fatal. Therefore, aggressive fibromatosis with all its variants must operationally be assumed to be of low-grade malignancy and must be treated accordingly (compare with Table 3.1, Chapter 3). The clinically useful terms "benign" and "malignant" do not describe the behavior of locally aggressive tumors satisfactorily.

Benign Tumors and Tumorlike Conditions

Benign tumors and tumorlike conditions fall into two categories: (1) the fibromas, which are pedunculated congenital malformations consisting of normal fibrous tissue; and (2) fibromatosis, a term that signifies proliferation of fibrous tissue and that, by definition, indicates a benign process. Frequently, it is self-limiting, but in some anatomic locations, by virtue of local extension, it can be complicating and, infrequently, fatal. The category of fibromatosis may include a large number of entities. For the sake of clarity these are divided into juvenile and adult variants, although they sometimes overlap.

Juvenile Variants.

Juvenile Congenital Fibromatosis. This is an extremely rare variant of juvenile fibromatosis. In this condition the infant is usually born with multiple localized areas of fibromas distributed all over the body; frequently, the infant does not survive long. In a still rarer localized form of the disease, the tumors, usually in the extremities, are known to spontaneously disappear in the course of a few weeks.

Fibromatous Coli. Another form of highly specialized fibromatosis, fibromatosis coli, is usually seen in the neck of newborns. Clinically, it is first recognized as a nodule in the sternomastoid muscle and the name "torticollis" is applied to these tumorlike conditions.

Juvenile Aponeurotic Fibroma. This is a highly specialized fibromatosis arising in the hands and feet of children.[96–98] It is prone to calcify and tends to infiltrate locally. Keasbey[97] first drew attention to this tumor; however, Lichtenstein and Goldman[98] have argued that these tumors are cartilaginoid in nature and that they are found in adults as well.

Juvenile Nasopharyngeal Angiofibroma. These are highly vascular tumors usually seen in the nasopharynx of young adults. Microscopically, they are a highly vascular type of fibrous tissue tumors (Fig. 4.19). The entire tumor is studded with new capillaries and occasional sinusoids. The absence of the elastic lamina is probably the cause of recurrent bleeding episodes, since these vessels do not contract.

Recurring Digital Fibrous Tumor with Inclusions. This rare form of juvenile fibromatosis is characterized by the occurrence of nodular tumors in the fingers and toes of young children. The single most important morphologic criterion is the presence of viruslike cytoplasmic inclusion bodies.

Progressive Myositis Fibrosa. In this type of fibromatosis, nodules develop in the muscles and subcutaneous tissue of infants. Probably these nodules at a later date give rise to myositis ossificans.

Adult Variants.

Keloid. A keloid is a type of hyperplasia of the fibrous tissue in a scar, usually associated with the swollen appearance of collagen fibers and degenerative changes (Fig. 4.20).

Palmar and Plantar Fibromatoses. These are clinical descriptions rather than specific pathologic findings (see Chapter 12 for description).

Penile Fibromatosis (Peyronie's Disease). This is a distinctive type of fibromatosis that hardens and deforms the penile shaft. No clear etiologic factor is known.

Idiopathic Retroperitoneal Fibrosis (Ormond's Disease). In this condition there is a definite proliferation of the retroperitoneal fibrous tissue accompanied by inflammatory cells and neovascularity.[99] Apparently the process starts in the pelvis and progresses cephalad. In many instances an erroneous diagnosis has been made and the underlying sarcoma or lymphoma has been missed.

Pseudosarcomatous Fasciitis. Konwaler, Keasbey, and Kaplan[100] first described this entity in 1955. This distinctive fibromatous tumor suddenly proliferates and infiltrates the sur-

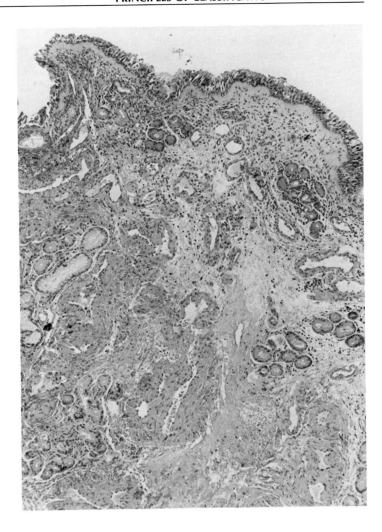

Figure 4.19. Juvenile nasopharyngeal angiofibroma. A rich network of thin blood vessels of varying sizes and contours are scattered in a stroma of collagen fibers. The vascular channels are usually lined by a single layer of endothelial cells. (H & E. Original magnification ×65.)

rounding tissue (Fig. 4.21). Its periphery is marked by many capillaries and by infiltrating inflammatory cells. The fact that it grows rapidly and that there is high mitotic activity often leads to a mistaken diagnosis of sarcoma.[101,102] A variant of this form in which the tumor infiltrates the periosteum has been described by Hutter and his associates.[103] A variant of pseudosarcomatous fasciitis is proliferative myositis, which is characterized by eosinophilic ganglion cells.

Progressive Myositis Ossificans. This unusual disease is characterized by localized bone formation within a muscle, and occasionally the entire muscle is replaced by the osteoid tissue. As mentioned earlier, probably the initial stage of this disease is progressive myositis.

Paradoxical Fibrosarcoma of Skin. In 1963, Bourne[104] described an entity that he termed paradoxical fibrosarcoma of the skin. However, Stout and Lattes[3] considered this entity a highly cellular fibromatosis or fibrous histiocytoma. The pathologic characteristics have since been reassessed.[105,106] Woyke et al.[106] also described ultrastructural studies of pseudosarcoma of the skin. All the data generated so far substantiate the opinion previously expressed by Stout and Lattes.[3] These tumors are predominantly found in the head and neck region.

Elastofibroma. In 1969, Jarvi et al.[107] described this benign entity, which is characterized by the presence of thick elasticlike fibers coating a reticulin matrix and conglomeration of elastic material (Fig. 4.22). This lesion usually

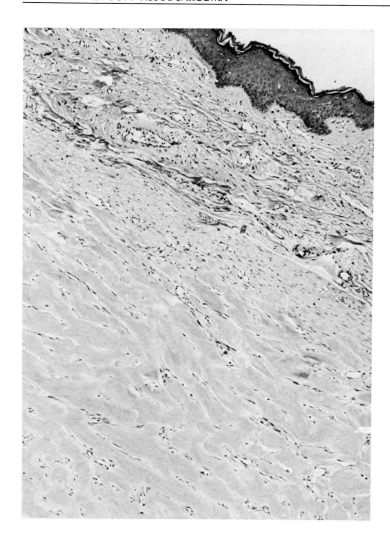

Figure 4.20. Keloid is characterized by the replacement of the dermis by scar tissue containing acellular dense collagenous tissue. (H & E. Original magnification ×40.)

arises in the scapular region and has never been known to recur. The elastic fibers can frequently be missed unless a special elastic tissue stain and reticulin stain are used. Although there is controversy as to the exact origin of this type of tumor,[107,108] it is probably a degenerative response to some form of trauma.

Myxoma. Myxomas occur in all parts of the body, including the heart. They vary from small subcutaneous tumors to large intermuscular types.[3,4] These tumors are composed of cells with elongated pyknotic nuclei and long, graceful cytoplasmic processes (Fig. 4.23). The ground substance stains with alcian blue or mucicarmine stains and the myxoid material can be digested by prior treatment with hyaluronidase.

Fibrous Histiocytic Tumors. Benign fibrous histiocytic tumors have recently been recognized as true clinicopathologic entities, and more and more such diagnoses are being rendered. Stout and Lattes[3] pointed out that a number of variants of this process are known to occur and, as such, several descriptive terms have appeared in the literature.

Fibrous Xanthoma. This tumor usually is covered by the epidermis and frequently extends to the subcutaneous tissue. It does not have a true capsule and local extension is seen on occasion. Histologically, fibroblasts, histiocytes, and reticulin fibers are found to grow in cordlike fashion without definitive architecture. Frequently, giant cells are found dispersed

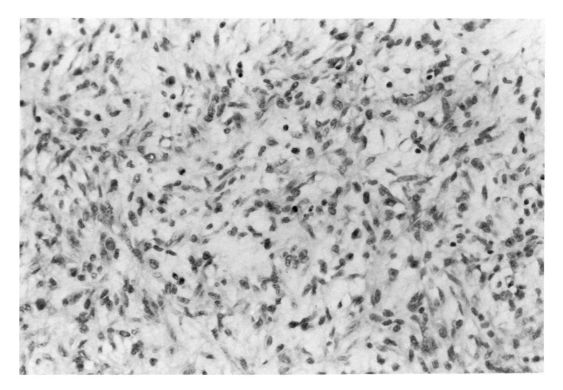

Figure 4.21. Pseudosarcomatous fasciitis. Note that the lesion consists of a number of capillaries, fibroblasts, histiocytes, and inflammatory cells scattered on a myxoid matrix. (H & E. Original magnification ×250.)

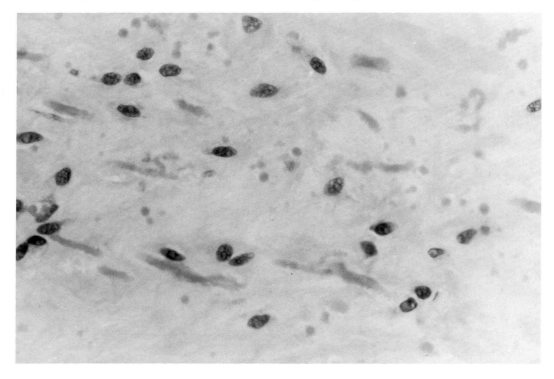

Figure 4.22. Elastofibroma dorsi. Microscopically these are characterized by the presence of broad areas of acellular connective tissue bands resembling abnormal elastic fibers. (H & E. Original magnification ×375.)

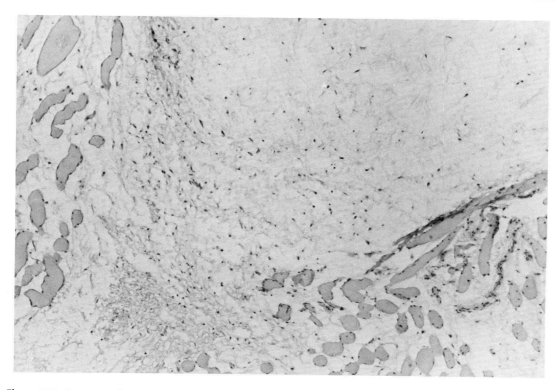

Figure 4.23. Intramuscular myxoma; note the fibrillar stellate cells with long fibrillar processes in a mucopolysaccharide-rich stroma. (H & E. Original magnification ×65.)

among these cordlike presentations (Fig. 4.24A and 4.24B).

Sclerosing Hemangioma. This common entity, because of its frequently brown coloration, requires differentiation from melanoma. Stout and Lattes[3] argued in favor of considering this tumor as of histiocytic origin (Fig. 4.25).

Giant Cell Tumor of the Soft Tissue (Tendon Sheath). This variant of fibrous histiocytoma is usually found in association with tendon sheaths of the hands and feet. The microscopic appearance varies according to location, the presence of fibroblasts, histiocytes, and giant cells (Fig. 4.26). Also, the length of time the tumor has been subjected to chronic trauma has an effect on its morphology. A variant of this tumor is villonodular synovitis described later in this chapter.

Nevoid Histiocytomas. These rare congenital lesions are multiple in nature and are usually found in the skin of the upper torso. There are several cases on record of spontaneous regres-sion.[3] No specific morphologic feature has ever been described.

Histologically Benign but Clinically Aggressive Tumors

In this category are two types of tumors: Dermatofibrosarcoma protuberans and aggressive fibromatoses (desmoids) of the anterior abdominal wall and extra-abdominal sites. The classification of these tumors is arbitrary and is resorted to with a view to proper management (Table 4.2).

Dermatofibrosarcoma Protuberans. The histogenesis of this relatively rare clinical entity has generated considerable confusion among pathologists. Taylor[109] considered it a sarcomatous tumor resembling keloid. Stout[110] considered it a fibrosarcoma of the skin. Taylor and Helwig[111] reviewed 115 cases and concluded this was a fibrous tissue tumor. O'Brien and Stout[112] later included dermatofibrosarcoma protuberans in

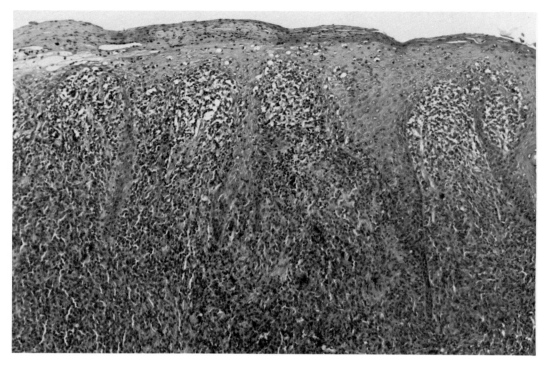

Figure 4.24. **(A)** Fibroblastic cells accompanied by reticulin fibers and histocytes are seen growing in cordlike fashion within the normal structure of the corium. The overlying corium is slightly thickened and is covered by intact epidermis. (H & E. Original magnification ×65.)

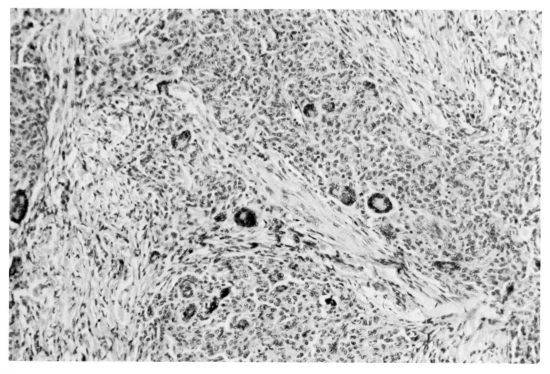

Figure 4.24. **(B)** An area showing the fibroblasts, histocytes, and giant cells. Some of the cells have a foamy cytoplasm. Characteristic examples of multinucleated epulis-type and Touton-type giant cells are obvious. (H & E. Original magnification ×125.)

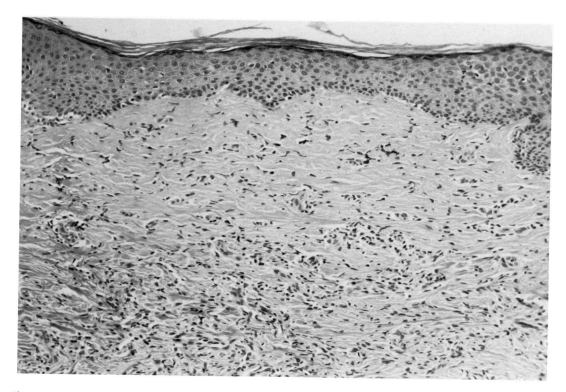

Figure 4.25. Sclerosing hemangioma (benign fibrous histocytoma). The tumor is composed of short spindle or oval cells clustering amid the capillaries. (H & E. Original magnification ×125.) *(Courtesy of Dr. S. Ronan, Departments of Pathology and Dermatology, University of Illinois Hospital.)*

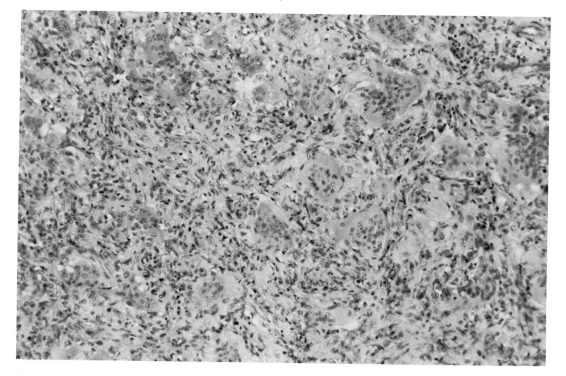

Figure 4.26. Benign giant cell tumor of soft tissues. Note the uniform round or oval histocytes and numerous multinucleated giant cells. (H & E. Original magnification ×125.)

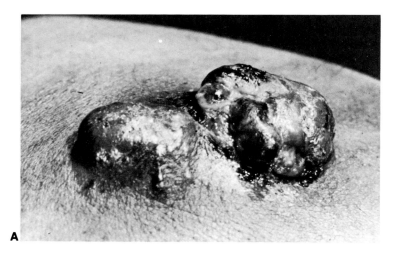

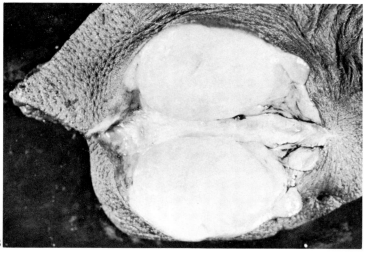

Figure 4.27. (A) A close-up of dermatofibrosarcoma protuberans showing the classical bossulated appearance. (B) Cut section of the smaller nodule. Note the glistening white colors and beginning of infiltration in the polar regions.

their group of storiform fibrous xanthomas. Today, it is generally agreed that these tumors are a variant of fibrous histiocytoma.[3] They occur in all parts of the body.

Macroscopic Pathology. Grossly, this tumor is firm and fibrous. Sometimes it is violaceous in color and on cut sections is often found to be infiltrating the surrounding skin and subcutaneous tissue (Fig. 4.27A and 4.27B).

Microscopic Pathology (Fig. 4.28). Dermatofibrosarcoma protuberans is a low-grade sarcoma of the dermis composed of spindle-shaped cells with the apparent ability to make collagen. There is often a relatively uninvolved zone immediately beneath the atrophic epidermis. Infiltration of subcutaneous tissue is the rule. The usual histologic pattern is one of interwoven fibrocellular fascicles comprised of somewhat uniform spindle-shaped cells and collagen. At points of intersection of the fascicles, there may be an acellular collagenous focus from which the fascicles appear to radiate. Stout[110] likened this appearance to a spiral nebula. It has been variously designated as storiform, stellate, whorled, cartwheel, twisted strip, or rosette-like. Myxoid areas may be prominent, particularly in recurrent lesions. At times, the intersecting fascicles may simulate a herringbone pattern. The stellate or cartwheel pattern has been given diagnostic emphasis by Penner[113] and by Taylor and Helwig,[111] who encountered it also in differentiated fibrosarcomas arising in the deeper subcutaneous tissue. Before a diagnosis of dermatofibrosarcoma protuberans is

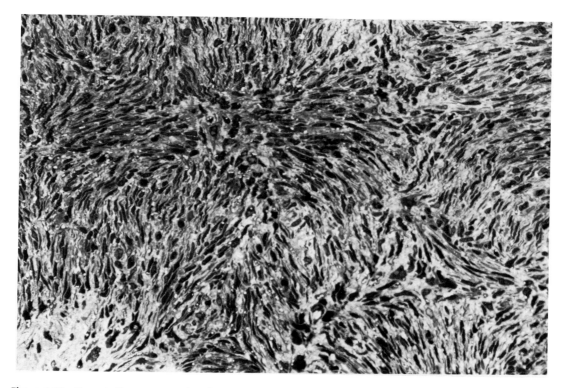

Figure 4.28. Dermatofibrosarcoma: The classic histologic pattern of interwoven fibrocellular fascicles radiating in a storiform or herringbone fashion is obvious in this Araldite-embedded 1-μm section. (Toluidine blue. Original magnification ×300.)

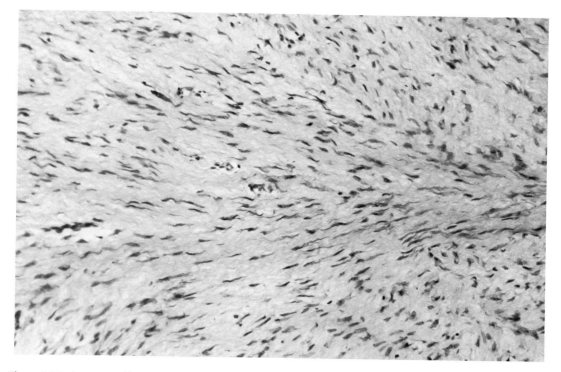

Figure 4.29. Aggressive fibromatosis of the abdominal wall (desmoid) is characterized by hypocellular bands of mature fibrous tissue. Similar histologic features are found in aggressive fibromatosis in all locations. (H & E. Original magnification ×125.)

made, it is perhaps better to consider the total clinicopathologic presentation than to rely solely on the histologic features.

In 1967, McPeak and co-workers[114] analyzed a series of 86 patients at Memorial Sloan-Kettering Cancer Center and concluded that the presence of a large number of mitotic figures (8 or more per 10-power field) is an indication of the metastatic potential of the tumor.

Aggressive Fibromatosis (Desmoids). Although the first microscopic description of desmoids was given in 1849 by Bennet,[115] the term desmoid tumors (Greek *desmos* = band or tendon) was first coined by Muller[116] in 1838. Des-

moidal tumors are found throughout the body, are of similar biologic behavior, have similar histopathologic characteristics, and are managed uniformly. However, traditionally two types are described, the first being abdominal wall desmoids and the second, the extra-abdominal wall variety.

Aggressive Fibromatosis of the Abdominal Wall. These tumors are circumscribed lesions located in the musculoaponeurotic structures of the anterior abdominal wall. Microscopically, the tumor consists of moderately hypocellular bands of mature fibrous tissue (Fig. 4.29) that infiltrate insidiously.

Desmoids of the anterior abdominal wall

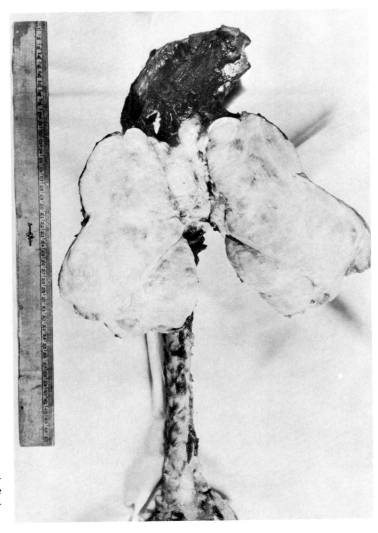

Figure 4.30. Aggressive fibromatosis of the extremity. The extensive infiltration of the tumor necessitated amputation.

are not known to metastasize either by the lymphatic or by the hematogenous route.

Extra-Abdominal Aggressive Fibromatosis. Macroscopically, extra-abdominal desmoid tumors are grossly circumscribed lesions located within musculoaponeurotic structures, assuming the characteristics of the anatomic region in which they arise. Their long axis is usually oriented in the direction of the fibers of the muscle bundles. The tumors are firm and rubbery and on cut section are grayish-white and trabeculated (Fig. 4.30). Aggressive fibromatosis, as the name implies, has a remarkable tendency to infiltrate the surrounding structures.

The microscopic appearance of aggressive fibromatosis is that of a fibroma in which bundles of striated muscles are often found in various stages of atrophy. The tumor consists of moderately hypocellular bands of mature fibrous tissue that infiltrate by extension between individual muscle fibers (Fig. 4.29). Abundant

collagenous fibers are arranged in large interwoven and sometimes fascicular bundles. Spindle-shaped fibroblasts with elongated normochromatic nuclei are dispersed between the collagen fibers.

The vascular supply of desmoids appears to be scanty. A capillary network, however, accompanies the proliferating fibrous tissue (Fig. 4.31A). In some lesions, a lymphocytic infiltrate may be found at the advancing periphery. In others, regenerating skeletal muscle fibers with centrally placed nuclei may give a false impression of tumor giant cells (Fig. 4.31B). It is not uncommon to find foci of myxomatous transformation, but metaplastic bone formation is less frequent (Fig. 4.31C). Histologic evidence of infiltration is commonly found (Fig. 4.32A to 4.32D). In certain instances aggressive fibromatoses might appear moderately cellular with hypertrophic fibroblasts containing hyperchromatic nuclei. However, mitoses are extremely

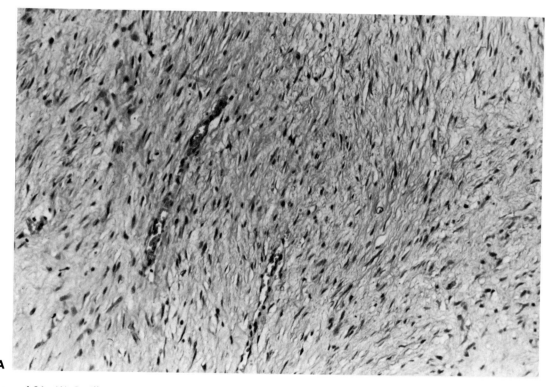

A

Figure 4.31. **(A)** Capillaries in proliferating fibrous tissue. (H & E. Original magnification ×100.) **(B)** Striated muscle fibers with myxomatous stroma. Note the degenerating muscle fibers with central nuclei and lymphocytic infiltration at the advancing edge. (H & E. Original magnification ×125.) **(C)** Aggressive fibromatosis showing metaplastic bone formation. (H & E. Original magnification ×250.)

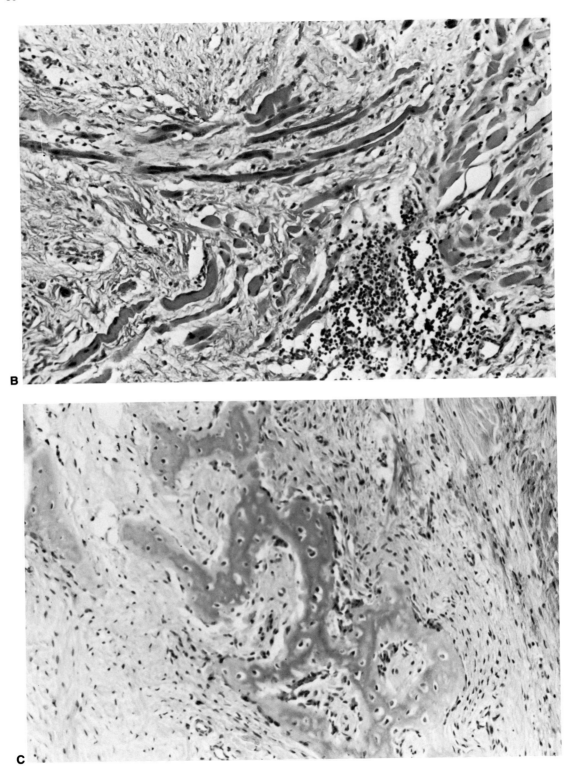

Figure 4.31. *Continued*

rare. The general architecture of a desmoid is distinctly different from that of a well-differentiated fibrosarcoma (Fig. 4.33).

Malignant Fibrous Tissue Tumors

Fibrosarcoma. At one time the diagnosis of fibrosarcoma was a catch-all diagnosis and many patients were thought to have fibrosarcoma when in fact the tumor was of a different histogenesis. Today, after all tumors composed of other types of cells capable of acting as facultative fibroblasts are excluded, the diagnosis of fibrosar-

coma is made less often. Sometimes, a microscopic diagnosis is indeed difficult, since the cellularity of a highly cellular fibromatosis frequently resembles that of a fibrosarcoma. Although fibrosarcomas may occur in all parts and organs of the body, they are most common in the extremities.

Macroscopic Findings. These tumors grow in an expansile fashion and usually present as a single gray, firm, round, or lobulated mass that is sharply delineated from the surrounding tissue. There is a pseudocapsule or a compression zone in which tumor invasion is frequently de-

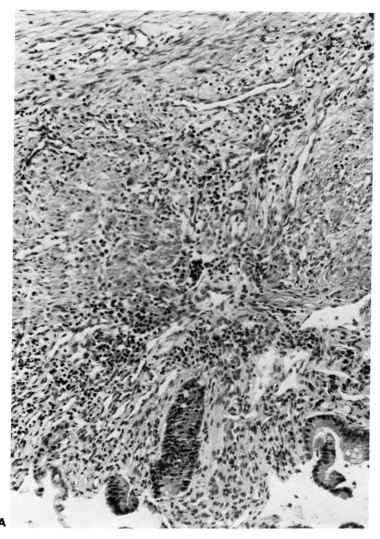

Figure 4.32. Infiltration of **(A)** wall of small intestine (original magnification ×100), **(B)** periosteum (original magnification ×100), **(C)** arterial wall (original magnification × 100), **(D)** pancreas (original magnification ×100).

A

62

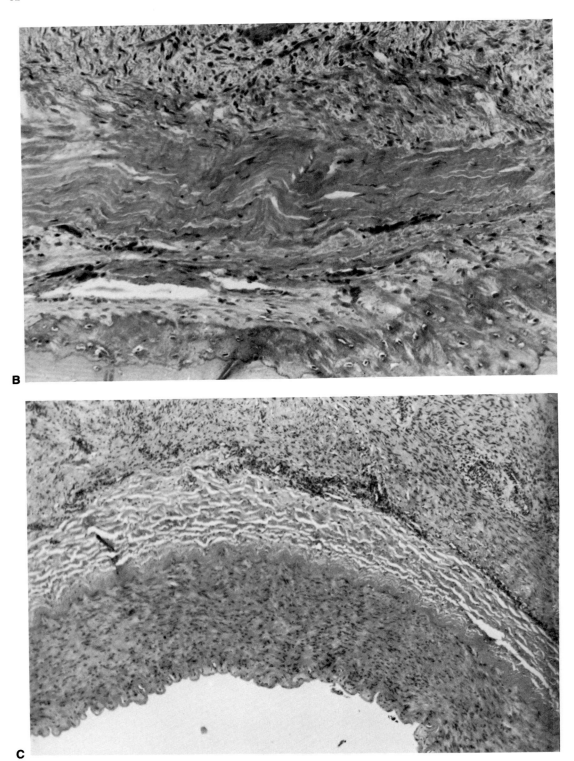

B

C

Figure 4.32. *Continued*

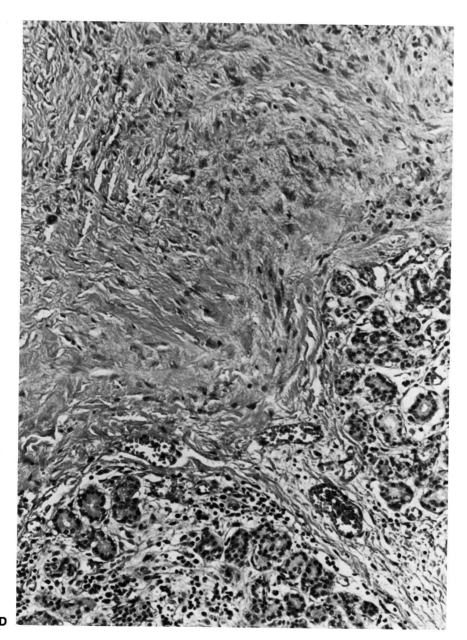

Figure 4.32. *Continued*

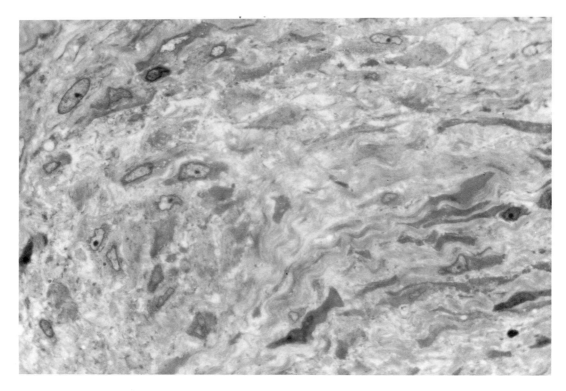

Figure 4.33. Cellular desmoid tumor with prominent nuclei, 1-μm Araldite section. (Toluidine blue and basic fuchsin stain. Original magnification × 600.)

monstrable (Fig. 4.34A and 4.34B). This tumor can attain enormous size; infrequently, it replaces a whole muscle compartment.

Microscopic Findings. The extracellular elements of fibrosarcomas are accompanied by varying amounts of collagen and reticulin. Such fibers and fibrils occur in strands and thick bands that can easily be seen in specially stained sections.

The microscopic features of fibrosarcoma have been conveniently classified into the differentiated and undifferentiated types. However, it is emphasized that such classification does not imply two distinct clinicopathologic entities, and frequently the histologic features of both types are found in two different areas of the same tumor.

Microscopically (Fig. 4.35A to 4.35C) these tumors are characterized by an interwoven texture of collagen and reticulin fibers, and dispersed between them are the fibrosarcoma cells. In the differentiated areas, intercellular collagen is abundant, and the nuclei of the fibrosarcoma cells are seldom in mitosis. The cytoplasm is scanty, acidophilic, and prolonged into long terminal processes or in spindling fashion. In contrast, the undifferentiated areas are richly cellular, with a few bands of collagen or reticulin displaying mitotic figures. The individual cells show large amounts of cytoplasm with oval nuclei. The presence of giant cells with single or multiple nuclei is not a rare occurrence.

Fibrosarcomas lend themselves to accurate histologic grading, which in turn influences treatment and prognosis.[64,117-119] The grading is based on the following criteria: (1) degree of tumor cellularity, (2) degree of cellular anaplasia, (3) production of ground substance, (4) prevalence of mitotic figures, and (5) the presence of giant cells. Grade 1 is the most differentiated and grades 3 and 4 are the least (see Chapter 5, Fig. 5.23). In areas of mixed differentiation, the tumor type should be classified according to the most poorly differentiated area. Based on this grading an accurate prognostication is possible; however, to obtain accurate

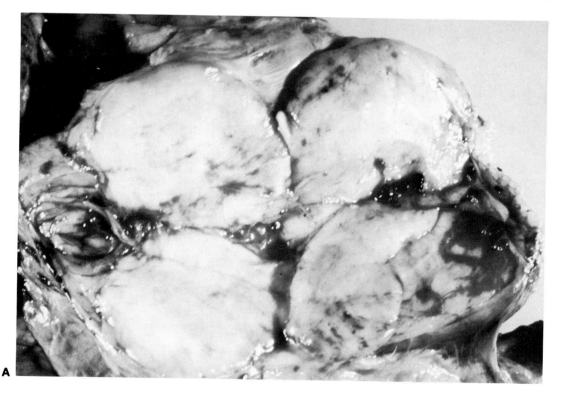

A

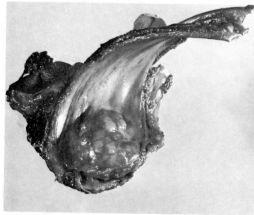

B

Figure 4.34. (A) A bilobed tumor of the posterior thigh has been bisected. Grayish-tan surface of the tumor is evident; an area of hemorrhage is also discernible. Note the apparent delineation from the surrounding soft tissue. (B) An unusual case of a fibrosarcoma of the chest wall viewed from the pleural surface. The extent of this tumor was not comprehensible from clinical examination of the tumor on the chest wall. Note the lobulated appearance of the tumor.

information, at least eight to ten tissue blocks must be sampled.[117]

Werf-Messing and van Unnik[120] proposed determination of the mitotic activity and/or the mitotic index, with the degree of fiber formation as a reliable basis for prognostication. They found that when the mitotic index was 11 or more, distant metastasis was invariably present. Although the technique of determining mitotic index as well as fiber formation is indeed excel-lent, in high-grade lesions (grade 4) mitoses might not occur uniformly, and this may lead to an erroneous interpretation. Therefore, scanning of a large number of sections and grading of the tumor by an experienced pathologist is probably a more practical way to correlate prognosis.

Ultrastructural study of the differentiated variety of fibrosarcoma shows the malignant myofibroblasts with mature collagen fibers (Fig. 4.36A). The malignant myofibroblastlike cells

66

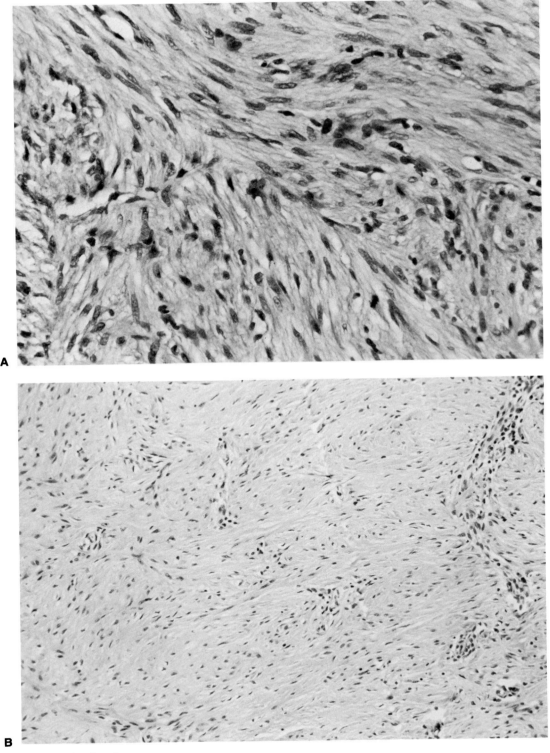

A

B

Figure 4.35. *Continued*

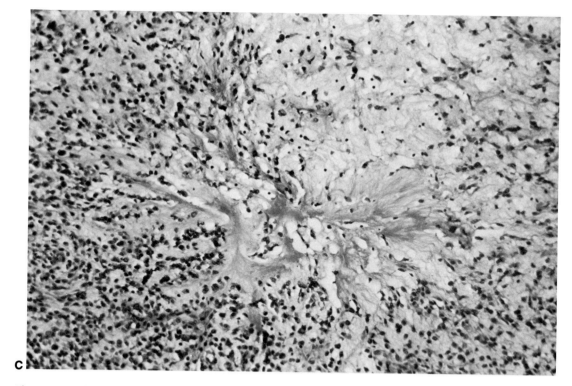

Figure 4.35. Fibrosarcoma: **(A)** Elongated fibrosarcoma cells are dispersed between a matrix interwoven with collagen and reticulin fibers; occasional mitosis can be seen. (H & E. Original magnification ×300.) **(B)** Well-differentiated fibrosarcoma, showing abundance of collagen with uniform distribution of fibrosarcoma cells. (H & E. Original magnification ×110.) **(C)** Undifferentiated areas of the tumor are richly cellular and the fibrosarcoma cells are seen with various shapes and configurations; a myxoid matrix in this micrograph is easily discernible. (H & E. Original magnification ×110.)

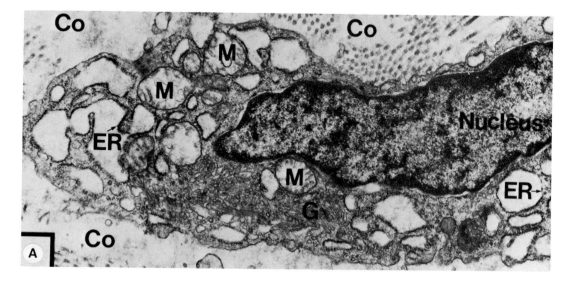

Figure 4.36. **(A)** Myofibroblast with mature collagenous stroma. The collagen fibers are seen both in tangential and longitudinal sections. Periodicity of collagen fibers appears to be normal. Cytoplasm shows abundance of rough endoplasm reticulum (ER) and mitochondria (M). Myofilament can be seen in the periphery of the cells. (Original magnification ×24,200.)

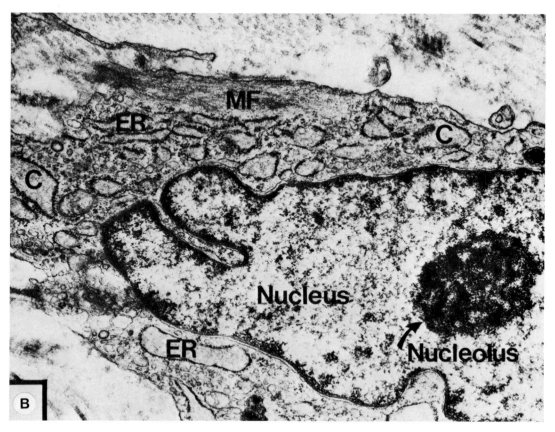

Figure 4.36. (B) High-power view of a myofibroblast. The nucleus has a prominent nucleolus. Cytoplasm is characterized by rough endoplasmic reticulum (ER) and swollen cisternae (C). In the peripheral part of the cytoplasm, characteristic bundles of myofilament (MF) are easily discernible. (Original magnification × 42,640.)

are basophilic and contain swollen cisternae filled with homogenous substances of moderate electron opacity. Myofilaments are seen in the peripheral part of the cell. The cytoplasm also contains a large number of rough endoplasmic reticula (Fig. 4.36B). In the pleomorphic variety, the spindle-shaped cells are seen to have a minimal degree of cell adhesion (Fig. 4.36C). A few collagen fibers are scattered in the intercellular spaces. The cytoplasmic characteristics of these malignant cells are similar to those of fibroblasts, with the exception of the intracytoplasmic myofilaments seen at the periphery of the cytoplasm. In tumors with extreme pleomorphism there are very few ultrastructural characteristics leading to a definitive diagnosis.

Metastases. Metastases from fibrosarcoma occur primarily via the bloodstream, and the most common viscus to be affected is the lung.

Distant metastasis is rare in patients with a well-differentiated or grade 1 fibrosarcoma, but the incidence becomes higher as the grade advances, particularly in grade 4. Regional node metastasis is rarely encountered. Metastasis can occasionally be found in viscera other than the lung, eg, the liver, stomach, pleura, and brain (Fig. 4.37).

Malignant Fibrous Histiocytoma (Malignant Fibrous Xanthoma or Fibroxanthosarcoma). In 1964, O'Brien and Stout[112] reviewed 1,516 cases, of which 979 were fibrous histiocytomas and so-called dermatofibrosarcoma protuberans, and 537 were giant cell tumors of the soft somatic tissues, including villonodular synovitis. They observed that although there had been a few case reports of malignant fibrous xanthoma, there was still some question as to whether a fibrous

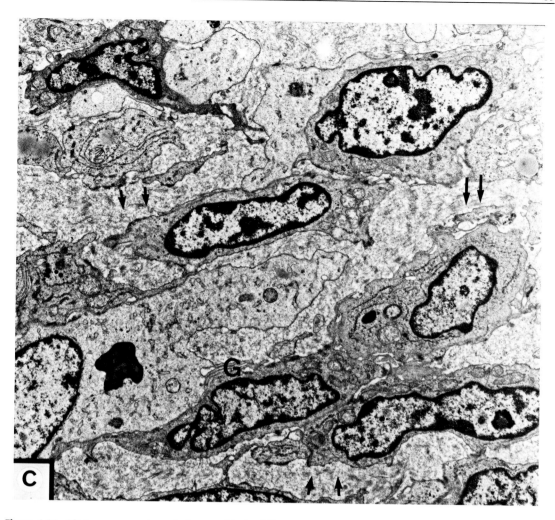

Figure 4.36. (C) Low-power view of pleomorphic (undifferentiated) fibrosarcoma. The spindle-shaped cells are numerous and are scattered all over the stroma, with minimal cell contact. Cytoplasm of most of the myofibroblasts shows peripheral myofilament bundles (arrows). (Original magnification ×42,000.)

xanthoma could indeed be termed malignant. O'Brien and Stout, however, were convinced that such a malignant tumor did exist and described 15 cases. Stout and Lattes,[3] in 1967, reclassified these tumors and called them malignant fibrous histiocytomas. Their classification and terminology are accepted by most authors.[96,101,112,121–126]

The histogenesis of malignant fibrous histiocytoma is still a matter of controversy. Some consider it to be of histiocytic origin.[96,125,127] Others suggest the origin is a primitive mesenchymal cell.[124] The tumor contains a broad spectrum of both fibroblastlike and histiocytelike cells.

Usually the tumor is composed of fibroblastlike spindle cells and round histiocytes arranged in a storiform pattern and interspersed with pleomorphic giant and inflammatory cells. Several variants from this norm have been recognized and named according to the predominant features. For example, when the stroma is myxoid, the tumor is termed *myxoid malignant fibrous histiocytoma.*[121] With osteoblastlike giant cells, it is called *malignant giant cell tumor of soft parts.*[128] With xanthoma cells and acute inflammatory cells, it is designated as *malignant xanthogranuloma, xanthosarcoma,* or *inflammatory fibrous histiocytoma.*[126,129,130]

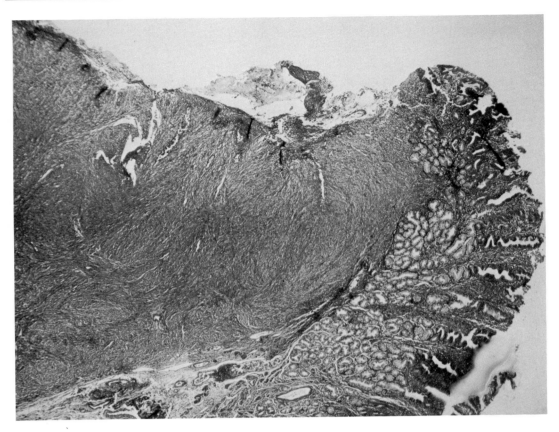

Figure 4.37. Fibrosarcoma metastatic to the stomach. Patient presented with upper gastrointestinal bleeding seven years after resection of a grade 3 tumor of the lower extremity. At the time of subtotal gastrectomy there was no obvious evidence of intra-abdominal extension. (Original magnification × 65.) *(Courtesy of B. Goldsmith, M.D.)*

Macroscopic Findings. Malignant fibrous histiocytomas grossly resemble any fibromatosis or fibrosarcoma. They arise in all parts of the human body, although the extremities constitute the most common site (Table 12.20, Chapter 12).

Microscopic Findings (Fig. 4.38A to 4.38E). The main histologic characteristics of malignant fibrous histiocytoma can be summarized as follows: (1) round histiocytes or histiocytelike cells, (2) spindle-shaped or fibroblastlike cells, (3) presence of fibrogenesis, (4) storiform pattern, (5) presence of both benign and tumor giant cells, (6) foamy cells, and (7) lymphocytes. Malignant fibrous histiocytoma has a variable morphologic pattern and frequently shows transitions from areas of highly ordered storiform pattern to progressively less differentiated areas. Weiss and Enzinger[123] described three patterns of microscopic presentation, namely, storiform, pleomorphic, and fascicular. They also found that in some instances a recurrent tumor varied from the original primary. These tumors frequently resemble malignant lymphoma, specifically reticulum cell sarcoma of soft parts[131] or malignant histiocytoma,[3] and, as Stout and Lattes[3] pointed out, sometimes can be distinguished only by the use of a reticulin stain.

Of the variants of malignant fibrous histiocytoma mentioned above, the myxoid and inflammatory variants require further elaboration. In 1977, Weiss and Enzinger[121] identified the myxoid variant. These tumors typically are encountered in the extremities, and the myxoid areas consist of widely spaced spindle and pleomorphic cells embedded in a matrix of mucopolysaccharides. These authors found that among all the subtypes of malignant fibrous his-

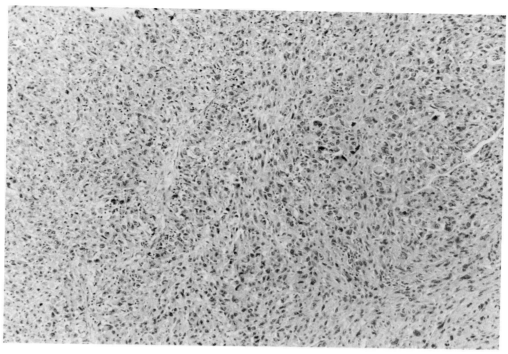

Figure 4.38. Malignant fibrous histiocytoma showing a wide range of histologic patterns. **(A)** Low-power view; both histiocytes and fibroblasts are identifiable. (H & E. Original magnification × 65.)

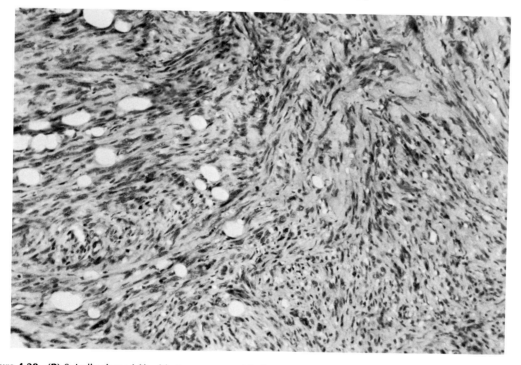

Figure 4.38. (B) Spindle-shaped fibroblasts are arranged in fascicular pattern. (H & E. Original magnification × 125.)

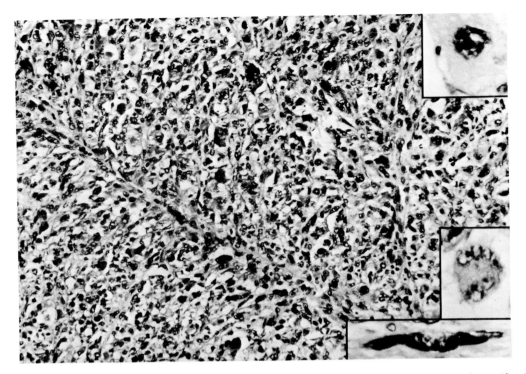

Figure 4.38. **(C)** Pleomorphic malignant fibrous histiocytoma showing cells in mitosis. (H & E. Original magnification ×250.) The insets show the variety of giant cells that can be encountered. (H & E. Original magnification ×400.)

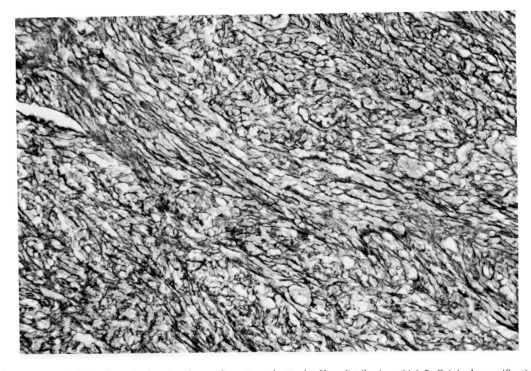

Figure 4.38. **(D)** Reticulin stain showing the configuration of reticular fiber distribution. (H & E. Original magnification ×125.)

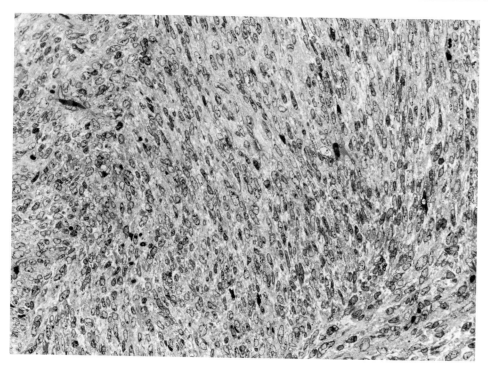

Figure 4.38. (E) One-micron-thick section showing the fibroblasts, histiocytes, giant cells, cells in mitosis, and scanty collageous stroma. (Toluidine blue. Original magnification ×250.)

tiocytomas, the myxoid variant carried a better prognosis for the patient from the standpoint of both local recurrence and metastases. The inflammatory variant[126] is characterized by diffuse neutrophilic infiltrates unassociated with tissue necrosis. The presence of this acute exudative reaction is a unique feature. Kyriakos and Kempson[126] also found interspersed foam cells, plasma cells, lymphocytes, and Reed-Sternberg-like cells. The clinical course of the inflammatory type is more aggressive than either the common type or the myxoid variant. The most significant microscopic factor influencing prognosis in the common type of malignant fibrous histiocytoma is the degree of cellularity. The more cellular the tumor, the less favorable the prognosis.

Electron Microscopy. Fu et al.[124] found that in each of their four cases, five cell types were clearly identifiable: the fibroblastlike cell, histiocyte cell, xanthomatous cell, multinucleated tumor giant cell, and an immature type resembling a reticulum cell (Fig. 4.39A to 4.39D). Naturally, the number of cells or their frequency is dependent on the portion of the tumor section

examined, xanthomatous and giant cells being the least common. The cells are attached to each other with several types of intercellular contacts. Typical *maculae adherentes* (desmosomes) may be found between fibroblastlike cells but very rarely between histiocytelike cells. The extracellular space consists mainly of a few well-formed collagen fibers, some immature collagen fibers, and a large number of fibers lacking in periodicity (Fig. 4.39A). The small blood vessels in the tumor have a continuous endothelium and are limited by a basal lamina. A relatively thick zone consisting of a pericyte process, collagen fibers, and microfibrils usually surrounds these vessels.

The fibroblasts have large, elongated nuclei with one or two nucleoli. The cytoplasm contains multiple cisternae of rough endoplasmic reticulum with well-developed Golgi zones, mitochondria, microfilaments (5 to 10 nm), and occasional lipid droplets. The histiocytes have oval nuclei, with a highly developed Golgi zone in the perinuclear area. The cytoplasm is characterized by the presence of an abundance of smooth endoplasmic reticulum, phagocytic vac-

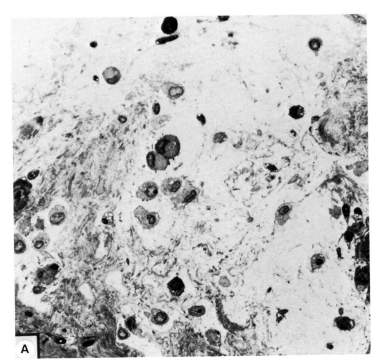

Figure 4.39. **(A)** One-micron section of malignant fibrous histiocytoma. Histiocytes are seen in clusters. Several multivacuolated cells and capillaries are scattered in a loose collagenous matrix. (Toluidine blue. Original magnification ×600.)

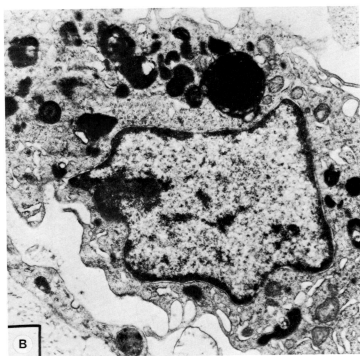

Figure 4.39. **(B)** One histiocyte from Figure 4.39A. These cells are characterized by an intensely vacuolated outer cytoplasmic fringe that corresponds to the many pseudopodlike processes. The cell body also contains a large variety of inclusion bodies originating from the enzymatic breakdown of phagocytized materials into secondary lysosomes and residual bodies. (Original magnification ×38,500.)

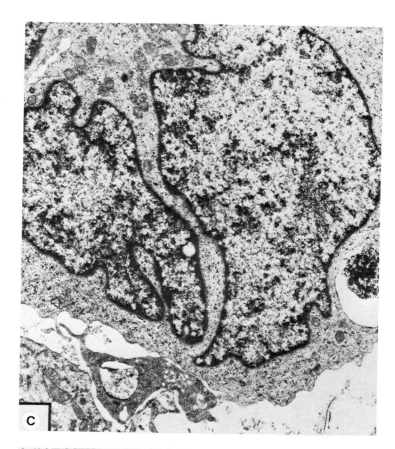

Figure 4.39. (C) A binucleated xanthomatous cell with a lipid inclusion. (Original magnification ×22,000.)

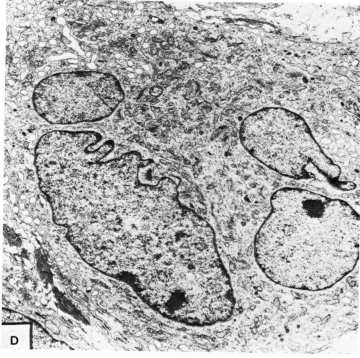

Figure 4.39. (D) Portion of a multinucleated giant cell. (Original magnification ×14,500.)

uoles, and multivesicular bodies. Frequently, membrane-bound bodies resembling lysosomes can be seen. In addition, the cell membranes are ruffled with numerous pseudopodia. The undifferentiated cells described by Fu et al.[124] are seen occasionally. These are small, ovoid cells with round nuclei and scanty cytoplasm, distinguishable from lymphocytes by their lysosomelike cytoplasmic structures. Xanthomatous cells are characterized by their empty, vacuolated cytoplasm or by lipid-filled bodies in the cytoplasm. Fu et al.[124] studied two of these tumors in tissue culture and subsequently processed the cells for light and electron microscopic study. They found that most of the tumor cells maintained similar morphologic characteristics.

Metastases. Soule and Enriquez[132] found metastases in 13 of their 33 patients with malignant fibrous histiocytoma (39 percent). Kempson and Kyriakos[125] reported only three instances in their 30 patients. O'Brien and Stout,[112] reported an incidence of 75 percent (10 of 15). Weiss and Enzinger[123] analyzed 200 cases, 196 of which were treated by wide local excision or amputation. Eighty two (42 percent) of the 196 patients had metastasis. The metastatic site was unknown in ten patients, but in the remaining 72 there was metastasis to the lung in 59 (82 percent) and to the lymph nodes in 23 (32 per-

cent). Liver, bone, brain, and other body sites were also involved (Table 4.3). The incidence of regional node metastases is difficult to assess in tumors of the extremities. O'Brien and Stout[112] found a 20 percent incidence; Weiss and Enzinger[123] suggested an overall figure of 12 percent. In our own series of 47 cases (Chapter 12), the incidence was 19 percent (8 cases).

Malignant fibrous histiocytoma is an aggressive tumor with a relatively high frequency of metastases, and therapeutic planning must take this factor into consideration. Weiss and Enzinger[123] emphasized the association of these tumors with various hematopoietic diseases, eg, leukemia, Hodgkin's disease, and non-Hodgkin's lymphoma. The relation of the hematopoietic disorders to the natural history of malignant fibrous histiocytoma remains to be elucidated.

Malignant Histiocytoma. Malignant histiocytomas have been classified as a separate histologic group of fibrous histiocytic tumors by Stout and Lattes,[3] Soule and Enriquez,[132] and other authors,[123,124,133] and they probably represent an undifferentiated form of fibrous histiocytoma. Kauffman and Stout[96] first described the existence of these tumors in children, and since then they have been reported in all age groups. They resemble reticulum cell sarcomas and can only

TABLE 4.3 INCIDENCE OF METASTASES IN MALIGNANT FIBROUS HISTIOCYTOMA IN FIVE SERIES*

Site of Metastases	O'Brien and Stout (15 patients, 1964)	Kempson and Kyriakos (30 patients, 1972)†	Soule and Enriquez (33 patients, 1972)†	Weiss and Enzinger (72 patients, 1978)	Das Gupta (42 patients, 1981)
Lymph nodes	3	1	13	23	8
Lung	7	3	Number not known	59	6
Liver	3	0	?	11	3
Bone	—	—	—	11	1
Brain	—	—	—	3	1
Other sites including nonregional nodes	9	2	2	37	4

*The numbers represent the number of patients with metastases. In patients with more than one site involvement each site has been counted separately.
†In the series reported by Kempson and Kyriakos and Soule and Enriquez the incidence of regional node metastases has not been clearly stated.

be differentiated from them by the use of reticulin stains, which show they have a paucity of reticulum fibers.

The metastatic pattern of these tumors is similar to that of anaplastic cancers and frequently they metastasize to the regional nodes and viscera.

Malignant Dermatofibrosarcoma Protuberans. In rare instances dermatofibrosarcoma protuberans metastasizes to the lungs and has been known to result in death. McPeak et al.[114] described five patients with hematogenous metastases in a series of 86 patients. We have encountered two such instances. It is difficult to pinpoint any specific microscopic criterion to serve as a basis for defining the metastatic potential of these tumors. McPeak and co-workers[114] considered a high mitotic index a good indication; however, a high mitotic rate alone should not be interpreted as a sign of malignancy. Usually, malignant dermatofibrosarcoma is encountered only in patients who develop multiple local recurrences following inadequate excision.

TUMORS ARISING IN MUSCLE TISSUE

The muscle tissue constitutes a major element of the body somite and phyllogenetically has been modified into smooth (involuntary), skeletal (voluntary), and cardiac muscle. A brief introductory summary of the embryology, histogenesis, histology, and tissue culture studies would help in understanding the pathologic findings of the tumors and tumorlike conditions of the muscles.

Smooth Muscle. Myogenesis appears in different organs and regions at different times, eg, *muscularis mucosae* develops much later than the main muscular coat in the gastrointestinal tract. In contrast, tracheal muscle is well developed by the eighth intrauterine week. The formation of smooth muscle in the uterus commences in the fourth or fifth month of intrauterine life and continues slowly during infancy and childhood, until just before puberty, when there occurs a great increase of muscle fibers, both in number and in size. Myogenesis in the uterus takes place by continued differentiation of fresh muscle fibers from an undifferentiated subepithelial zone of mesenchyme, the residue of which consti-

tutes the stroma of the adult endometrium, a tissue that retains myogenic power throughout life. Probably this is the reason for the development of endometrial sarcomas in women. Little is known of when effective contractility begins in the various muscular organs. However, the degree of differentiation of muscular coats of viscera and arteries suggests that they are capable of function from the second or third month of fetal life.

Histologic Appearance. Smooth muscle, otherwise known as nonstriated or involuntary muscle, differs considerably from the other two types of muscle. It is made up of mononucleate spindle-shaped cells varying in length up to 15 μm in the myometrium during pregnancy. In regions where a concentrated contraction in a particular direction occurs, these bundles lie parallel, eg, separated layers of the external musculature in the intestines. In muscular arteries, nonstriated muscles are present in thick sheets into which capillaries do not penetrate. Within a fasciculus, much of the surface of each cell is coated by a prominent basal lamina, and between and within the laminae, fine reticulin and collagen fibers form complex networks around each cell, which are separated, except at special points of contact, by a space of 40 to 80 nm.

Individual smooth muscle cells show a centrally placed elongated nucleus, with the cells weakly birefringent, indicating some degree of longitudinal orientation of the cell components. With the electron microscope, the cytoplasm of the cell is seen to consist of closely packed fine filaments lying parallel to the long axis of the cell (Fig. 4.40A). Although all the intracytoplasmic constituents are present predominantly in the conical part of the cytoplasm of these cells, most of the cytoplasm contains microfilaments (5 to 8 nm across) that resemble actin filaments of striated muscle. The plasma membrane of the muscle cell contains a number of pinocytotic vesicles, but a system of membranous channels similar to that of skeletal muscle appears to be lacking.

The sarcoplasm, collected in a zone surrounding the nucleus and in the septa between them, contains mitochondria, Golgi materials, and some glycogen. Fusiform densities occur at the sites of confluence of tracts or bundles of myofilaments and at the points where these insert upon the cell membrane. Myofilaments are for the most part organized into parallel bundles

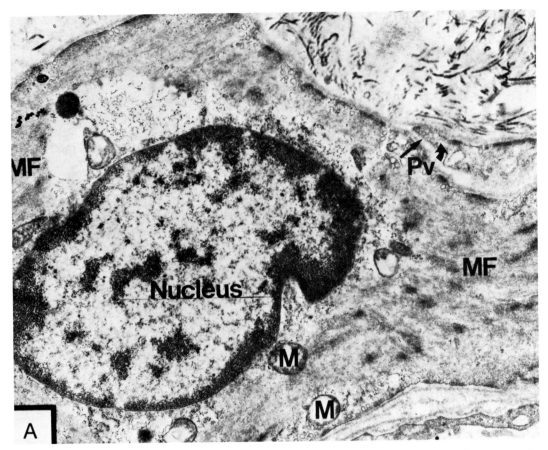

Figure 4.40. **(A)** Human normal smooth muscle cell (fallopian tube). The mitochondria and other cytoplasmic organelles occupy a perinuclear position. In the peripheral part of the cytoplasm are the myofilaments (MF), arranged along the longitudinal axis of the cell. These filaments appear to be inserted into the dense bodies. Pinocytotic vesicles (PV) are seen along the membrane. There are no transverse striations. (Original magnification ×31,892.)

oriented along the long axis of the cell. The fibrils are pulled or pushed out in different directions, crossing one another or fanning out at the periphery of the cell. It is suggested that contractility of smooth muscles is under the control of several internal and external factors.[134] Of interest is the data on hormonal influence[134] and the finding of an association of an acetylcholinelike substance in the activity of the smooth muscle grown in culture.

Striated or Skeletal or Voluntary Muscle. Although the classic concept that all voluntary muscles develop from paravertebral myotomes or branchial arches is still accepted by most embryologists and anatomists, the development of rhabdomyosarcomas in unlikely areas, such as the biliary tract,[135] leads one to question the validity of this age-old hypothesis. There appears to be sufficient pathologic[135] and experimental[136] evidence to modify the classic concept, insofar as to add, at least in part, that the somatic musculature is developed from the local nonmyotonic mesenchyme. This point should be borne in mind; otherwise, in some instances a diagnosis of rhabdomyosarcoma might be missed.

In the human embryo of six to seven weeks, the myotomes or other mesenchymal cells destined to become rhabdomyoblasts begin to undergo elongation and form condensed groups with their long axes parallel. They contain either one nucleus or (sometimes) two nuclei and show mitotic proliferation. In most situations the cytoplasm is devoid of fibrils. In the eight-week-old embryo, some of the rhabdomyoblasts are recognizable, showing the myofibrils with cross-striations. From the eighth week to the fifth month, and possibly still later, new rhabdomyoblasts continue to be differentiated from the mesenchyme. It is thought that from the fifth month onward, the nuclei take up their surface positions on the fibers, and the fibers acquire distinct sarcolemmal sheaths. Thus, during fetal life, voluntary muscle grows in four ways: (1) by differentiation of myoblasts from mesenchyme, (2) by mitotic proliferation of the myoblasts that have not yet become fibrillated, (3) by longitudinal division of young muscle fibers, and (4) by progressive enlargement of fibers, the last becoming relatively more and more im-

portant as the fetus grows. In postnatal life, under normal conditions the growth of muscle is mainly due to the enlargement of the fibers.

Willis[135] reported that although muscle primordia receives the nerves by the eighth week, the first appearance of motor end plates in muscle is much later (at 20 weeks in the tongue and at 26 to 28 weeks in the limbs). Innervation, though not essential for the development of vertebrate skeletal muscle, is essential for its maintenance. Adult muscles deprived of their nerve supply suffer atrophy and eventually disappear.

Histologic Appearance. Under the light microscope, skeletal muscles appear as closely packed cylinders in longitudinal sections, but with either circular, elliptical, or polygonal profiles in cross-section. The flattened nuclei of

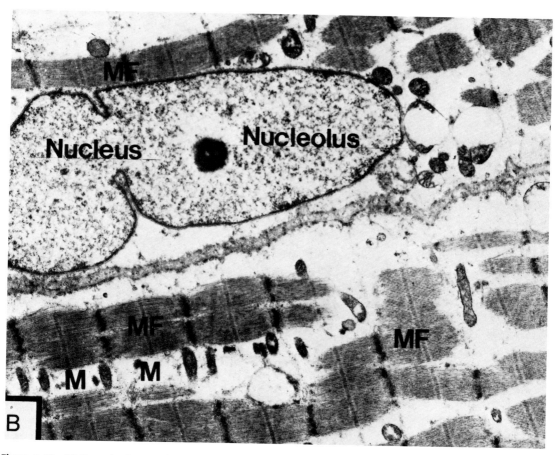

Figure 4.40. (B) Part of a human skeletal muscle cell (sartorius). All the characteristics of a voluntary muscle cell nucleus, with longitudinal arrangement of mitochondria along the contractile elements (MF), are easily discernible. (Original magnification ×14,732.)

muscle fibers lie peripherally in the zone immediately beneath the cell membrane or sarcolemma; their cytoplasm or sarcoplasm is divided into longitudinal bands or myofibrils each about 1 mm in diameter. In transverse sections these myofibrils frequently appear aggregated in small groups. In longitudinal sections the myofibrils are seen to be traversed by striations apparently continuous right across the fiber. Myofibrils vary in their staining characteristics and optical properties, and on the basis of these characteristics several bandlike structures can be identified. The significance and behavior of these bands have been described by Huxley and Hanson.[137]

On electron microscopic examination (Fig. 4.40B), each myofibril in longitudinal section is seen to be composed of longitudinally disposed myofilaments. In the resting muscle these are divided transversely by the Z bands into serially repeating regions termed sarcomeres, each about 2.5 μm long. Two types of myofilaments, one thin (5 nm) and the other thick (12 nm), have been identified. These are supposedly actin and myosin, respectively.

The morphology of the rhabdomyoblast has been investigated in skeletal muscles grown in tissue culture, and most of the observations made by electron microscopic examination of fixed tissue specimens have been confirmed. However, the major accomplishment of tissue culture has been a clearer understanding of the histogenesis of rhabdomyoblasts.[138,139] Konigsberg[138] found that skeletal muscle cells in culture pass through a series of morphologic changes resulting in fibrogenesis. Probably a similar mechanism is the underlying reason an anaplastic rhabdomyosarcoma sometimes resembles fibrosarcoma.

Cardiac Muscle. The development and morphogenesis of cardiac musculature has been investigated extensively and valuable data obtained. However, since tumors of the heart muscle are rare, a detailed discussion is beyond the scope of this treatise.

The foregoing summary of the embryology, histogenesis, histology, and tissue culture studies of smooth and skeletal muscle fibers forms the background for the succeeding description of tumors of myogenic origin.

Tumors of the Smooth Muscles

Leiomyomas. Leiomyomatous tumors constitute the most common form of primary mesenchymal tumors of the gastrointestinal tract[140-144]

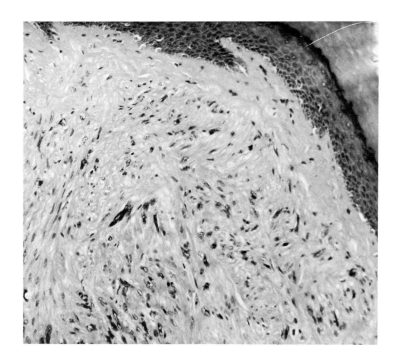

Figure 4.41. Cutaneous leiomyoma composed of long, slender, smooth muscle cells arranged in fascicles. Note the long atypical nuclei. (H & E. Original magnification × 125.)

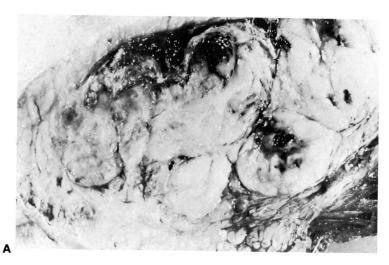

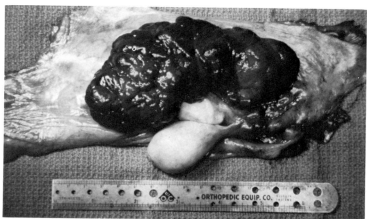

Figure 4.43. (A) Cut section of a leiomyosarcoma of an extremity. Note peripheral hemorrhagic areas. **(B)** Polypoid type of leiomyosarcoma of the esophagus. In this instance, both benign leiomyoma and leiomyosarcoma were found in the same location. *(Courtesy of Drs. H. Wiedemar and D. deCamara, Cook County Hospital, Chicago.)*

Macroscopically these tumors are seldom larger than 2 to 3 cm, are usually brown, and have a rubbery consistency.

Microscopically they consist of large, round or oval cells and abundant pale cytoplasm. In a phosphotungstic acid-hematoxylin (PTAH)-stained section, the cross-striations are readily seen (Fig. 4.47A and 4.47B). Under the electron microscope, the scant stroma contains numerous epithelial-lined capillaries supported by delicate bundles of collagen. Muscle cells comprise almost the entire cell population. The cytoplasm of the cardiac variant is filled with glycogen and a well-developed system of smooth vesicles and agranular endoplasmic reticulum (glycogen tumors). Myofilaments of varying width are found in the periphery of the cytoplasm. Biologically

these are benign tumors and have no relation to rhabdomyosarcomas.

Rhabdomyosarcoma. Rhabdomyosarcomas arise in relation to the skeletal muscle in adults and juveniles. However, the tumor is occasionally seen in anatomic locations not known to have an abundance of rhabdomyoblasts; for example, in organs such as the bladder,[181] urethra,[182] prostate,[148] spermatic cord,[182] vagina,[183,184] uterus,[3,4,148] round ligament,[148] breast,[148] bronchus,[185] palate,[186–188] tonsil,[186–188] tongue,[186–188] nasopharynx,[186–188] orbit,[3,4,148,189,190] eustachian tube,[190] middle ear,[191] and common bile duct.[192,193]

It is customary to classify rhabdomyosarcomas into three different groups: (1) *embryonal,* which usually affect children, occasionally ad-

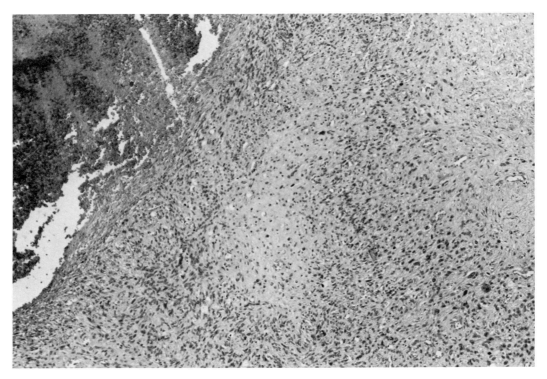

Figure 4.44. Leiomyosarcoma. **(A)** Low-power view provides the general appearance of the elongated cells growing in fascicular manner; area of hemorrhage and necrosis in the left corner. (H & E. Original magnification ×65.)

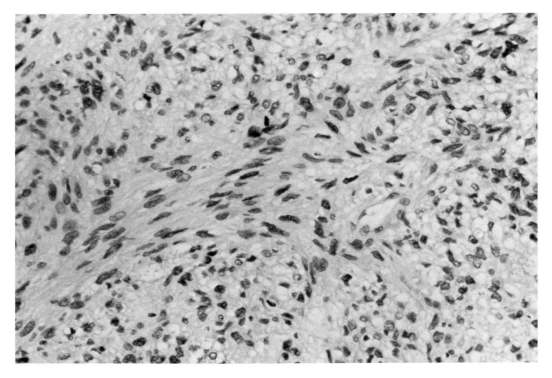

Figure 4.44. **(B)** Higher-power view of long, blunt, elongated nuclei with pallisading, a characteristic appearance of leiomyosarcoma. One cell is in mitosis. (Original magnification ×125.)

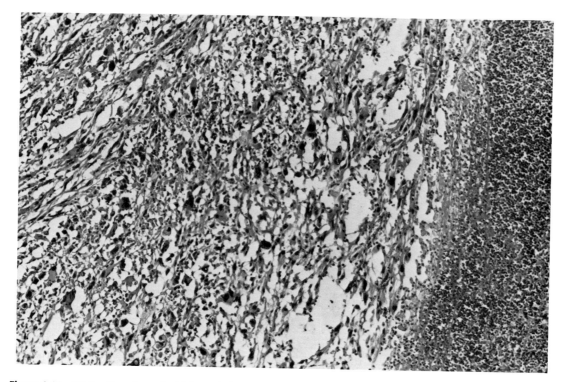

Figure 4.44. **(C)** Another view of a high-grade leiomyosarcoma, of the right arm. Areas of hemorrhage and multiple cells in mitosis, with scanty stroma and tumor giant cells, are seen. (Original magnification ×65.)

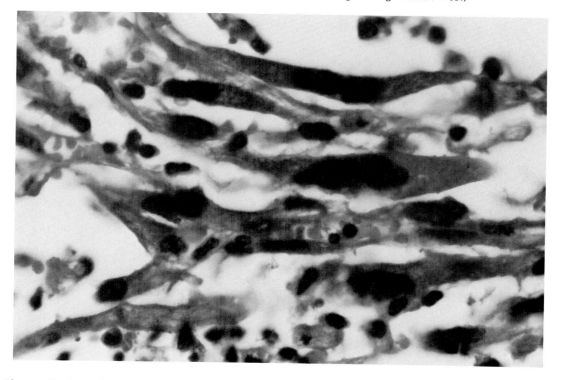

Figure 4.44. **(D)** Higher-power of 4.44C. Smooth muscle cells with longitudinally oriented myofibrils are discernible. (Original magnification ×600.) This patient died within two years of definitive therapy.

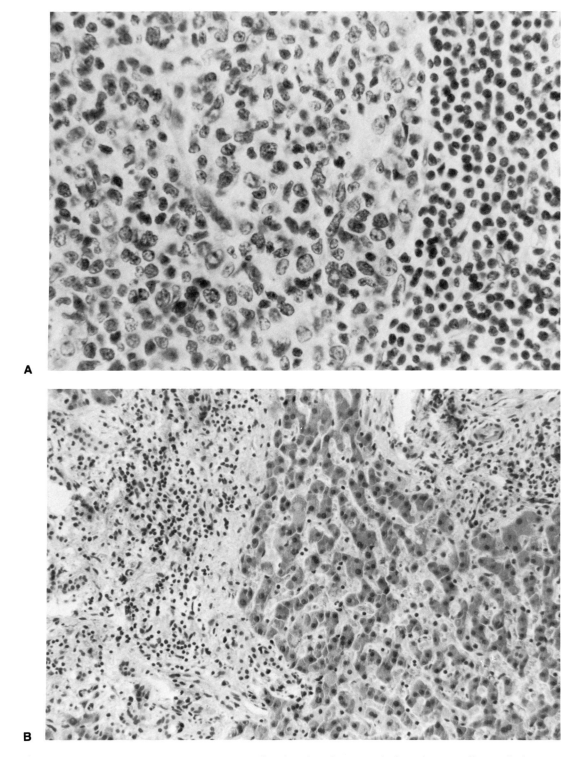

Figure 4.45. **(A)** Leiomyosarcoma metastatic to axillary lymph node. Patient had an elective axillary node dissection for a leiomyosarcoma of the arm. (H & E. Original magnification ×250.) **(B)** Metastatic leiomyosarcoma to liver. (H & E. Original magnification ×250.)

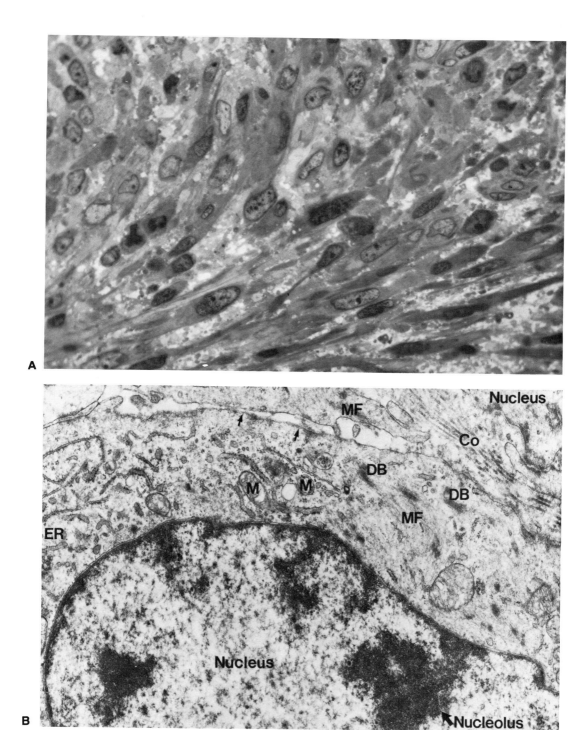

Figure 4.46. (A) Araldite-embedded 1-μm-thick section of a leiomyosarcoma in the arm of a 55-year-old man. The longitudinal arrangement of the smooth muscle cells is obvious. (Toluidine blue and basic fuschin. Original magnification ×600.) (B) Malignant smooth muscle cell from a patient with a retroperitoneal leiomyosarcoma. In this micrograph, the major part of one malignant smooth muscle cell, with myofibrils located peripherally within the cytoplasm, is seen. The myofibrils (MF) appear to be inserted into the dense bodies (DB) and the cell membrane (arrows). Cytoplasm contains mitochondria (M) and endoplasmic reticulum (ER). In the top of the micrograph, cytoplasm of another muscle cell is identifiable. No desmosomal contacts between these two cells are present. (Original magnification ×35,240.)

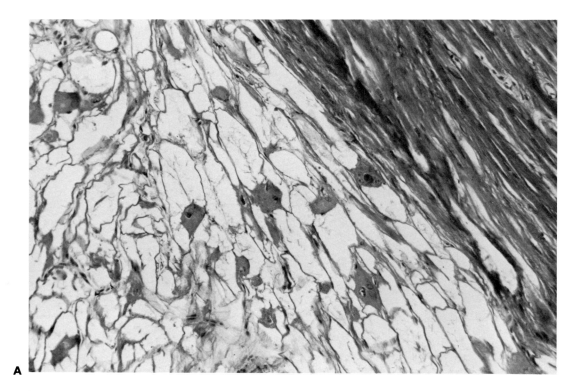

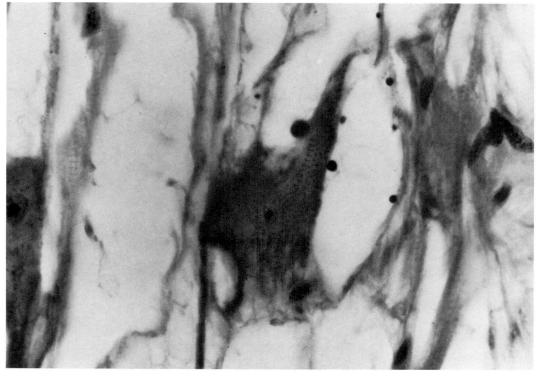

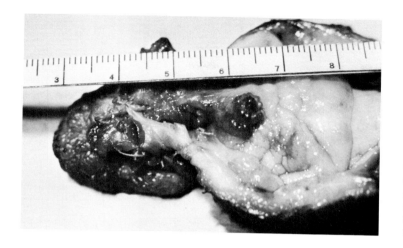

Figure 4.48. Specimen of urinary bladder and vagina of 4-month-old girl. The primary tumor originated in the urinary bladder and protruded through the urethra to the vagina. The presentation was mistakenly considered a vaginal botryoid sarcoma and inadequately excised. Following recurrence within two months, patient was referred to us (see Table 13.13, Chapter 13 for further clinical details).

olescents, and rarely adults; (2) *pleomorphic*, which are composed of pleomorphic elements, are usually found in adults, and arise in relation to skeletal muscle (only rarely do these occur in children); (3) *alveolar*, in which the tumors show a distinct alveolar pattern and are found in all age groups.

Embryonal Rhabdomyosarcoma (Sarcoma Botryoides). This tumor occurs predominantly in children and is most common in the region of the head and neck. When it arises near the mucosal surfaces it tends to become lobulated and resembles a bunch of grapes; hence, the descriptive term *botryoid* sarcoma.

MACROSCOPIC FINDINGS. Embryonal rhabdomyosarcoma has no characteristic gross feature by which it can be diagnosed, except in locations such as the vagina, anus, nose, palate, or external ear, where the presenting edge truly resembles a cluster of grapes (Fig. 4.48). In all other locations it resembles any other circumscribed tumor and seldom attains a size of more than 5 cm.

MICROSCOPIC FINDINGS (FIG. 4.49A TO 4.49D). The embryonal rhabdomyoblast may be small and rounded, with acidophilic cytoplasm, or it may be larger and elongated, with cross-striations and acidophilic cytoplasm. Usually a high rate of mitoses is observed in each high-power field. The botryoid tumors generally have a layer of small, rounded rhabdomyoblasts, two to four cells thick, with high mitotic activity.

ELECTRON MICROSCOPY (FIG. 4.50A AND 4.50B). Nuclei with prominent nucleoli demonstrate light-staining chromatin with narrow peripheral compact margination. Immature rhabdomyoblasts manifest a complex cytoplasmic structure with an abundance of organelles and membranes. The overall morphologic appearance resembles that of an immature rhabdomyoblast grown in tissue culture.[194] The mitochondria are usually large, with a clear matrix and a parallel array of cristae. Endoplasmic reticulum varies in quantity and in organization from numerous small cisternae of smooth endoplasmic reticulum to large clefts lined with rough endoplasmic reticulum. The quantity and type of cytoplasmic fibers are directly proportional to the stage of maturation of the rhabdomyoblast under study (Fig. 4.50C). In the mature rhabdomyoblast, fully formed intracytoplasmic fibers are apparent. Most authors[194–198] have not been able to find the I and Z bands in the myoblasts.

PATTERNS OF METASTASES. Embryonal rhabdomyosarcoma can metastasize to the regional nodes.[186,188,199,200] The great majority, of course, metastasize via the bloodstream, the lungs being

Figure 4.47. **(A)** Rhabdomyoma of the heart. Note arrangement of round cells supported by their stromal trabecula. (H & E. Original magnification ×125.) **(B)** High-power view with phosphotungstic acid-hematoxylin stain. The cross striation within the muscle fibers is easily seen. (Original magnification ×375.) *(Courtesy of Dr. S. Teas, Medical Examiner's Office, Chicago.)*

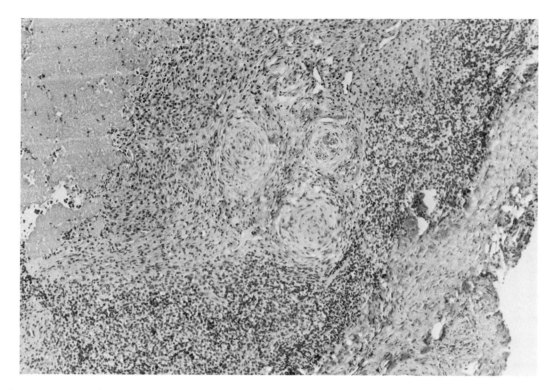

Figure 4.49. (A) Embryonal rhabdomyosarcoma. The rhabdomyoblasts are circular in shape. The left-hand corner of the micrograph shows hemorrhage and necrosis; and on the right, infiltration of the surrounding muscle bundles can be seen. (H & E. Original magnification ×65.)

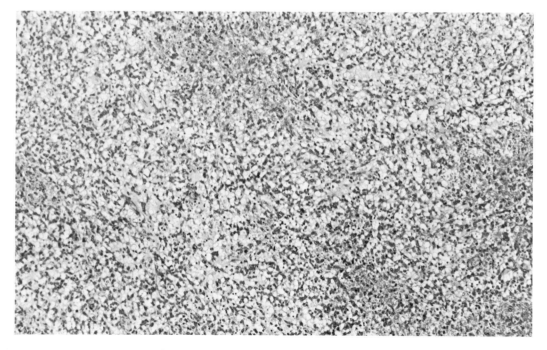

Figure 4.49. (B) Embryonal rhabdomyosarcoma showing a multitude of round cells and areas of myxomatous degeneration. (H & E. Original magnification ×65.)

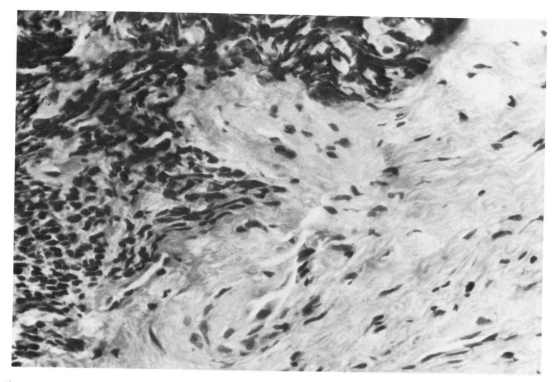

Figure 4.49. **(C)** Infiltration of surrounding muscle in an extremity rhabdomyosarcoma. (H & E. Original magnification ×125.)

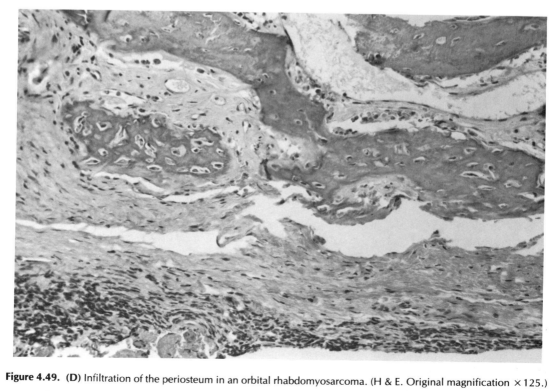

Figure 4.49. **(D)** Infiltration of the periosteum in an orbital rhabdomyosarcoma. (H & E. Original magnification ×125.)

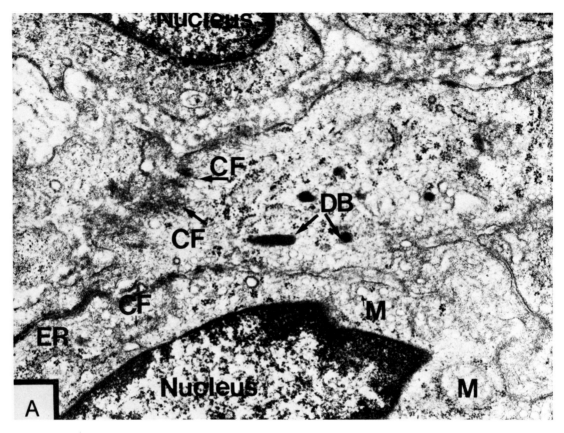

Figure 4.50. (A) Immature malignant rhabdomyoblast, showing various cytoplasmic contents, smooth membrane system, occasional rough endoplasmic reticulum (ER), large mitochondria (M), attempts at cytoplasmic filament formation (CF), and a few dense inclusion bodies (DB). (Original magnification × 34,420.)

the most common site.[201] Hepatic metastases as the initial evidence of systemic involvement has been occasionally observed. In the agonal stage, however, all organ systems can be involved.

Pleomorphic Rhabdomyosarcoma (Adult Type). Pleomorphic rhabdomyosarcoma is most commonly found in adults and most often in the extremities.

MACROSCOPIC FINDINGS. The tumor is usually deep-seated within the musculature (Fig. 4.51). It can attain large size and frequently infiltrates the surrounding tissue. The cut sections of the tumor are usually reddish-appearing, and often the central part shows hemorrhage or necrosis or both.

MICROSCOPIC FINDINGS (FIG. 4.52A AND 4.52B). The tumor varies so much in pattern and cellularity that, unless convincing evidence of rhabdomyoblasts is shown, the diagnosis is open to question. The rhabdomyoblasts may be rounded or strap-shaped, with more than two nuclei arranged in tandem; they may be racquet-shaped with one nucleus; or they may take the shape of a giant cell. These rhabdomyoblast giant cells are usually well preserved and rarely have pyknotic nuclei. They may have large and irregularly shaped vacuoles, peripherally arranged, producing "spider-web" cells. The cell cytoplasm tends to be acidophilic and, in differentiated cells, cross-striations or myofibrils are seen. The diagnosis of highly pleomorphic rhabdomyosarcoma is often difficult under the light microscope, and electron microscopy should be used in doubtful cases.

ELECTRON MICROSCOPY. The electron microscopic findings of these tumors are similar to those of the embryonal variety just described. The presence of mature rhabdomyoblasts with all the cellular characteristics, and of rhabdomyosarcoma giant cells, aids in establishing an

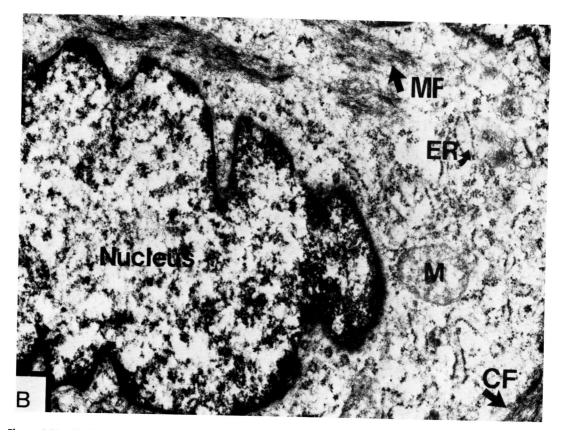

Figure 4.50. (B) More mature malignant rhabdomyoblast; formed myofibrillar structures (MF) are evident. (Original magnification ×23,520.)

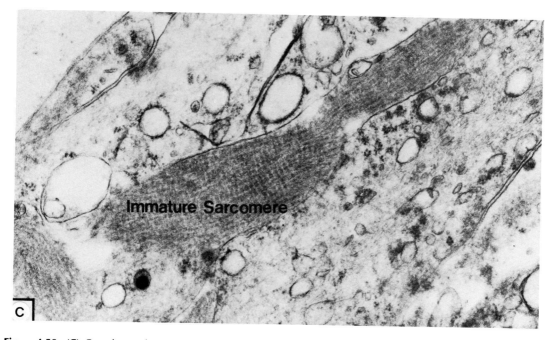

Figure 4.50. (C) Cytoplasm of a neoplastic rhabdomyoblast showing an attempt at sarcomere formation. (Original magnification ×46,351.)

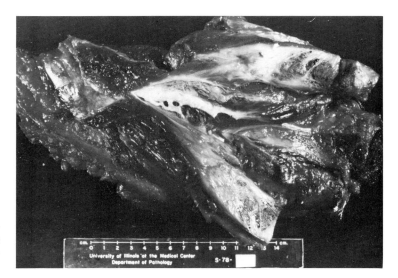

Figure 4.51. Cut section of a pleomorphic rhabdomyosarcoma of the lower extremity, with areas of hemorrhage and necrosis.

accurate diagnosis. In poorly differentiated tumors a careful search for Z-bands in tumor cells is a valuable step in diagnosis.

METASTATIC PATTERN. Pleomorphic rhabdomyosarcoma, like the embryonal variety, metastasizes to the regional nodes and the lungs. The incidence of regional node metastases, however, is less frequent than in the embryonal variety. In the late stages of the disease it can metastasize to the pleura, lungs, bones, subcutaneous tissue, kidney, adrenals, pancreas, ovaries, and even the brain.

Alveolar Rhabdomyosarcoma. Alveolar rhabdomyosarcoma usually occurs in children and adolescents but can be encountered in all age groups. It is found more frequently in the extremities, although it can occur in any part of the body. As in the other two types, the tumor infiltrates the surrounding tissues.

MACROSCOPIC FINDINGS. This tumor can attain any size. The transected tissue is firm, grayish-white, and usually shows central necrosis or cystic degeneration.

MICROSCOPIC FINDINGS. The cells are round or oval, of moderate size, and apparently unattached to each other. They are contained within spaces lined by the fibrous tissue septa. Frequently, the cells cling to these septa and mimic a pseudoglandular or an alveolar pattern, hence the name (Fig. 4.53A to 4.53C). Occasionally the cells proliferate and the alveolar pattern is destroyed. The architecture resembles a neuroblastoma or a malignant lymphoma. As men-

tioned before, the presence of the rhabdomyoblast, with all its characteristics, determines the diagnosis.[202]

The incidence of regional node involvement is almost as high as in the embryonal type (Fig. 4.54). Enzinger and Shiraki[203] found 36 of 110 patients (33 percent) to have regional node metastases. In five of their patients the diagnosis of the primary tumor was made after biopsy of the palpable regional nodes. In our group of 12 patients, four (33 percent) had regional node metastases.

TUMORS DERIVED FROM NERVOUS TISSUE

Most nerve fibers are present in muscles and skin by the second month of intrauterine life, but effective functional innervation takes much longer to develop. Appreciation of the structure and function of mammalian nervous tissue began with the pioneering investigations of Ramon y Cajal,[204] Schwann,[205] del Rio Hortega,[206] His,[207] Sherrington,[208] and Le Gross Clarke[209] in the earlier part of this century, culminating in the description of synapses and synaptosomes by Eccles[210] in the 1950s. Since then there has been an explosion of knowledge in this area. A description of these elegantly designed studies, the results obtained, and the conclusions drawn, although a fascinating and romantic study in themselves of the evolution of knowledge in

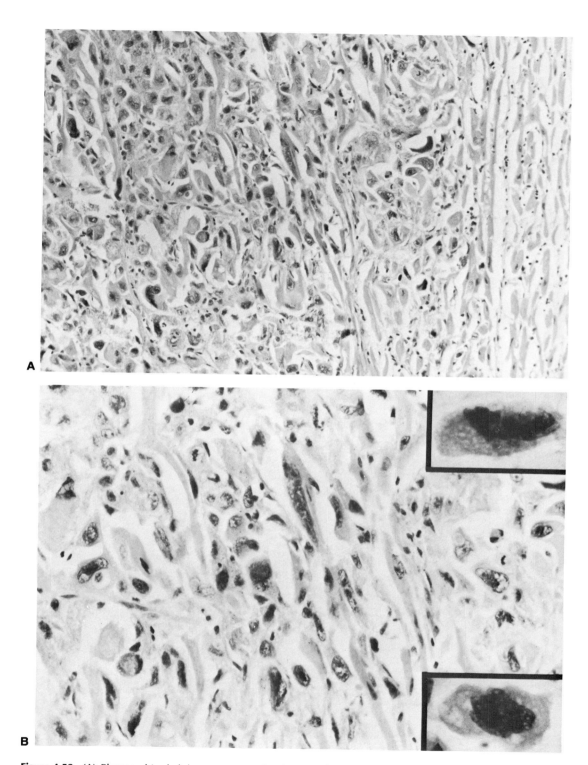

Figure 4.52. (A) Pleomorphic rhabdomyosarcoma showing a wide variety of sizes and shapes of the cells. (H & E. Original magnification ×125.) (B) Higher-power view showing the spindle-shaped cells and tumor cells. (H & E. Original magnification ×250.) Inset shows cross striations in malignant rhabdomyoblast. (Original magnification ×600.)

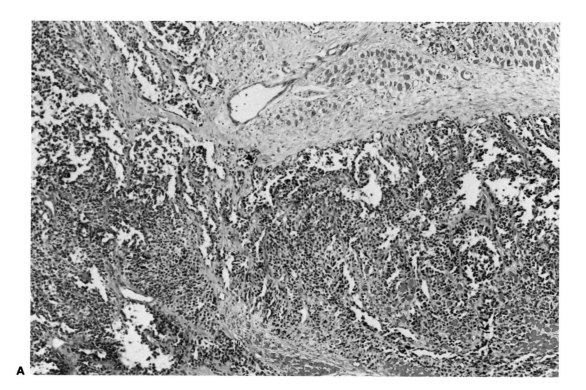

A

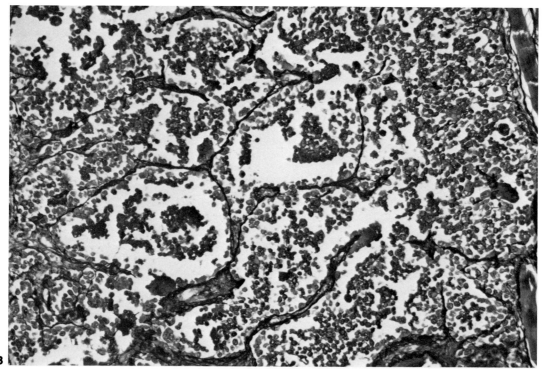

B

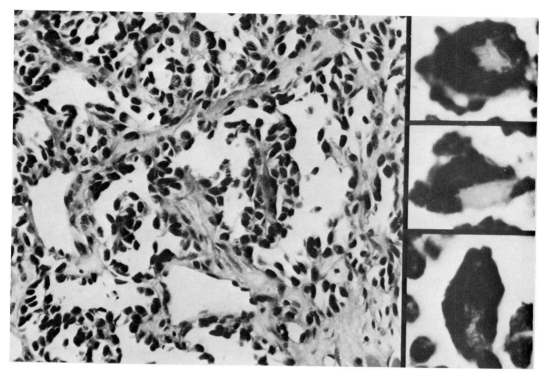

Figure 4.53. **(A)** Alveolar arrangement of an extremity alveolar rhabdomyosarcoma. Infiltration of surrounding structures is apparent. (Original magnification ×65.) **(B)** Reticulin stain outlining the alveolar pattern; unattached rhabdomyoblasts are lying loose within the center of the alveolus. (Original magnification ×125.) **(C)** Under high power, the cellular morphology of the rhabdomyoblasts is apparent. (H & E. Original magnification ×250.) Inset shows the tumor giant cells. (Original magnification ×600.)

human biology, is not germane to a section on the pathology of neoplasms of the peripheral nerves. However, it is desirable to have a brief summary of the structure and function of normal peripheral nervous tissue as a point of reference for a better appreciation of the pathologic anatomy of the tumors of the nervous system.

The peripheral nervous system comprises the cerebrospinal and autonomic system of nerves and their associated ganglia-containing nerve cell bodies, together with the cellular and connective tissue elements that ensheath them.

The structure of the sensory ganglia of the dorsal spinal nerve roots and the corresponding ones on the trunk of the trigeminal, facial, glossopharyngeal, and vagus nerves are similar to those of neurons and do not require elaborate description. The autonomic ganglia, in contrast, have a different structure, since their cell bodies are multipolar with dendritic processes that re-

ceive synapses from incoming preganglionic visceral motor fibers. Autonomic ganglia are found in the paravertebral sympathetic chains, near the roots of the great visceral arteries in the abdomen, and near, or embedded within, the walls of various viscera. Autonomic ganglion cells may also be highly modified, as in the case of *chromaffin cells* of the adrenal medulla in which the axon is absent.

The nerve trunks and their principal branches are composed of roughly parallel bundles of nerve fibers comprising the efferent and afferent axons, ensheathing Schwann cells, which in some cases produce myelin. These bundles of nerve fibers are surrounded by connective tissue sheaths at different levels of organization. The fibers are grouped together within a trunk in a number of fascicles, each of which may contain from a relatively few to many hundreds of nerve fibers (Fig. 4.55A and 4.55B).

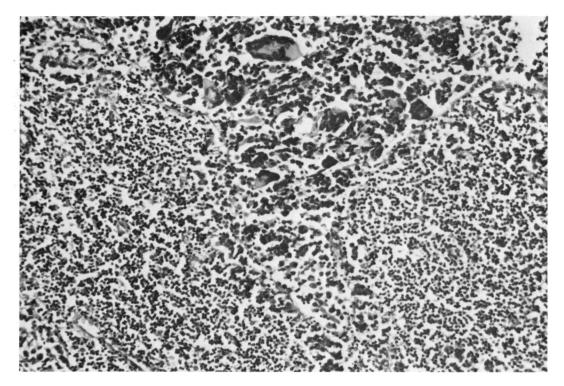

Figure 4.54. Axillary lymph node metastases from a primary alveolar rhabdomyosarcoma of the lower end of the arm. (H & E. Original magnification × 125.) Patient is a 28-year-old man, five years postoperative, treated with excision of primary tumor and a simultaneous axillary node dissection. He also received adjuvant chemotherapy (see Chapter 8 for details).

A dense, irregular connective tissue sheath, the epineurium, surrounds the whole trunk, and a similar but less fibrous perineurium encloses each fasciculus. Between these two spaces lies the loose delicate connective tissue network, the endoneurium. These connective tissue planes serve as convenient access for the vasculature of the peripheral nerves that run parallel to the nerve fibers in the endoneurial spaces.

The epineurium is a collagenous adventitial coat with little regular organization; the perineurium, in contrast, has a regular structure of highly flattened laminae of fibroblasts alternating with fine collagenous sheets running in various directions within the sheath (Fig. 4.55A). On the basis of total fiber diameter (ie, axon, as well as its myelin sheath) and the rate of impulse conduction, the fibers in mixed peripheral nerves have been classified into three major types: A, B, and C. The A fibers, the largest, consist of various myelinated somatic afferent and efferent fibers; class B are composed of the myelinated preganglionic fibers of the autonomic nervous system; and class C, nonmyelinated sensory fibers.

Schwann cells are the chief nonexcitable cells of the peripheral nervous system, enfolding and enwrapping axons over most of their surfaces (Fig. 4.55B). Morphologically, Schwann cells vary with the type of fiber, but generally the nucleus tends to be heterochromatic and ellipsoidal, and the cytoplasm is rich in mitochondria, microtubules, and microfilaments, in addition to prominent lysosomes and well-developed rough endoplasmic reticulum. The basement membrane is found on the external surface, except where it lies adjacent to a nerve cell process. It is a continuous sheath over the abutting Schwann cells at the node of Ranvier, a gap where the axolemma is exposed. The Schwann cells have been found not only to provide mechanical support to the nerve cells but also to take part in a myriad of physicochemical activities.

All the larger axons are incorporated in a

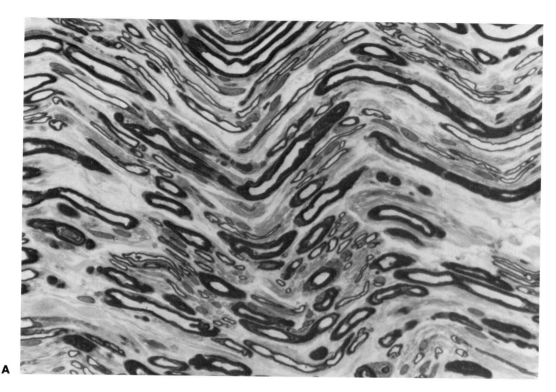

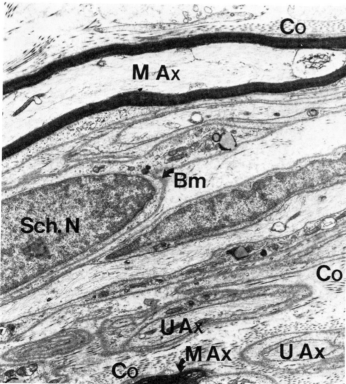

Figure 4.55. **(A)** One-micron-thick section of a normal human sciatic nerve. Myelinated fibers are easily discernible. (Osmium tetroxide stain. Original magnification ×80.) **(B)** Low-power electron micrograph of the same nerve showing the myelinated axons (MAx) and unmyelinated axons (UAx) in different profiles, Schwann cells (Sch.N), with basement membrane (Bm), and the interstitial collagen fibers (Co). (Original magnification ×6,026.)

myelin sheath and are termed myelinated fibers (Fig. 4.55A and 4.55B). The fatty composition of the myelin is responsible for the glistening whiteness of the peripheral nerves and white matter centrally. Axons smaller than 0.5 to 1.0 μm generally lack these sheaths and are therefore termed nonmyelinated fibers. In routine light microscopic sections the lipids are removed and the myelin sheath appears as a vacuolated zone between the axon and the cytoplasm and the nucleus of the Schwann cell. Special stains are required to neutralize myelin; there is no difficulty in distinguishing these structures by electron microscopy.

Schwann cells, autonomic ganglia, chromaffin cells, and other nerve structures can be grown in tissue culture. Schwann cells are known to have myelinating properties even in vitro,[211] and chromaffin cells produce catecholamines.[212] When these cells are fixed and studied under the electron microscope, the ultrastructural characteristics of the cultured cell appear the same as in the fixed tissue specimens.

This brief background on the embryologic and structural aspects allows us to classify the tumors and tumorlike conditions of the peripheral nervous tissue (see Table 3.1, Chapter 3). A purist might possibly take exception to some finer points in this classification, but from a clinicopathologic standpoint such a classification is essential, or else the principles of management of these conditions can never be properly defined.

Benign Tumors of Schwann Cell Origin

Solitary Benign Schwannomas, Neurilemomas, Perineuronal Fibroblastomas, Acoustic Neuromas. These solitary, benign, slow-growing encapsulated tumors are composed of Schwann cells in a collagenous matrix. They can originate in cranial (acoustic neuroma), peripheral, or autonomic nerves. Schwannomas can occur either in association with von Recklinghausen's disease or, occasionally, in patients who exhibit no evidence of genetic predeterminations.

Benign solitary tumors arising in the peripheral nerves develop in practically every anatomic region. There is still some controversy over the cellular origin of schwannomas and neurofibromas, creating considerable confusion as to the classification and terminology of peripheral nerve tumors. Although connective tissue fibers, especially collagen, are conspicuous in neurofibromas, and although fibroblasts can be demonstrated in cutaneous neurofibromas, these tumors are derived from Schwann cells. Waggener,[213] in an ultrastructural study of benign neurilemomas and neurofibromas, demonstrated that these tumors are derivatives of Schwann cells. Thus, Stout's[214] original suggestion to consider all localized benign peripheral nerve tumors as neurilemomas seems to be practical.

Macroscopic Findings. These tumors can vary in size from a few millimeters to more than 20 cm. The small tumors are usually white, fusiform, firm, circumscribed, and encapsulated (Fig. 4.56A), whereas the larger ones are irregularly lobulated, and grayish- or yellowish-white. Cut sections of larger tumors show occasional cystic areas and some of these cysts contain hemorrhagic fluid. When the nerve of origin is recognized, the tumor usually projects from one side and is adherent to the nerve (Fig. 4.56B). Frequently, the nerve of origin is not found.

Microscopic Findings. According to the morphology of the tumor cells and their spatial arrangements, two types of tissues have been described. In type A tissue of Antoni, the texture is compact and composed of interwoven bundles of long bipolar spindle cells, which in cross-section are seen to be narrow cylinders with tapering ends. The cells have oval or rod-shaped nuclei containing variable amounts of chromatin and inconspicuous nucleoli. In places, the cells form a typical palisading arrangement, with their nuclei in a well-organized pattern. Such foci are termed verocay bodies (Fig. 4.56C). Type B tissue is distinguished by its loose texture and the polymorphism of the tumor cells. Both are highly specific structures of neurilemomas (Fig. 4.56D). Type B distribution is commonly, but not invariably, present in all schwannomas. With hematoxylin-eosin or Alcian blue stains, the matrix stains poorly, or not at all. Vessels in schwannomas are usually prominent, with thick, hyalinized walls. Some of the vessels, particularly large sinusoidal channels, may contain recent or organized thrombi. Lipid-filled foam cells and hemosiderin-laden macrophages, lymphocytes, and mast cells may be found in large numbers, usually around blood vessels.

The electron microscopic appearance of benign schwannomas is characterized by the presence of multiple Schwann cells, with both myelinated and unmyelinated axons interspersed

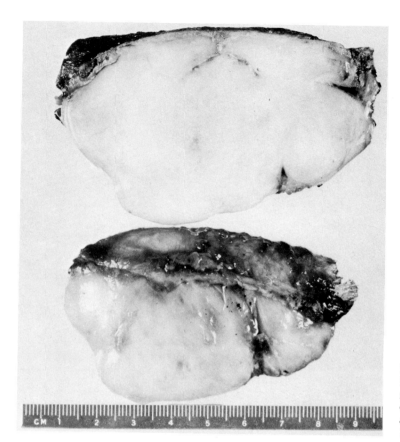

Figure 4.56. (A) Cut section of a benign schwannoma showing the glistening white surface. A capsule can be easily seen. *(Figs. 4.56A,C, and D Courtesy of Cancer 24:355, 1969.)*

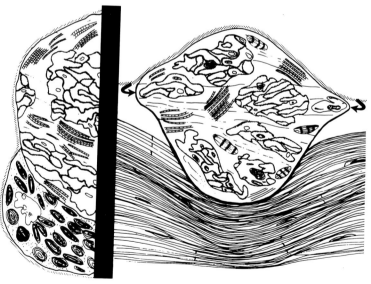

Figure 4.56. (B) Diagrammatic rendition of a benign schwannoma compressing the adjacent nerve fiber as it increases in size. The tumor is encapsulated and the main cellular components are neoplastic Schwann cells. The arrows show the plane through which these tumors can be enucleated with relative ease. *(Modified from Weller and Cervos-Navarro, 1977.)*

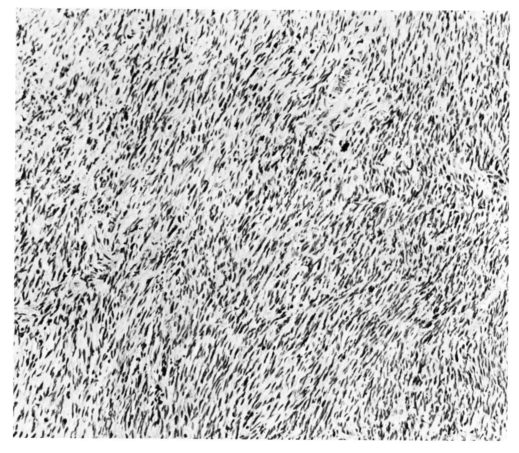

Figure 4.56. (C) Benign schwannoma showing type A tissue of Antoni. Note compact arrangement of interwoven bipolar spindle cells. (H & E. Original magnification × 100.)

between the interstitial collagen matrix (Fig. 4.56E). Along with Schwann cells a number of fibroblasts, macrophages, lymphocytes, and mast cells are also found within these tumors.

In recent years attention has been focused on the presence of mast cells in normal peripheral nerves and in peripheral nerve tumors (Fig. 4.57A and 4.57B). Gamble and Goldby[215] found mast cells in the peripheral nerves of a variety of mammals, including man. Ultrastructural study has demonstrated a large number of mast cells in peripheral nerve tumors.[216,217] The function of mast cells in these tumors is not clearly understood but several possibilities have been suggested. Csaba and associates[218] proposed that mast cells inhibit tumor growth by neutralizing tumor polysaccharides. Simpson,[219] in contrast, postulated that epithelial hyperplasia is the

probable cause of local increase in mast cells. The increase in mast cell population may also be related to the increase in endoneurial collagen following nerve degeneration.[220-223] The true significance of these cells, however, remains unexplained.

Several variants of schwannoma are encountered in any survey of a large series. One variant, the cellular schwannoma, requires more clarification, since this type might be misinterpreted as a malignant tumor. Cellular schwannomas are characterized by hypercellularity and nuclear atypism (Fig. 4.58); however, structural characteristics of Antoni types A and B are preserved. Mitoses are occasionally seen, but the prognosis for cellular schwannomas is the same as for all other benign solitary schwannomas.

The totipotential characteristics of the

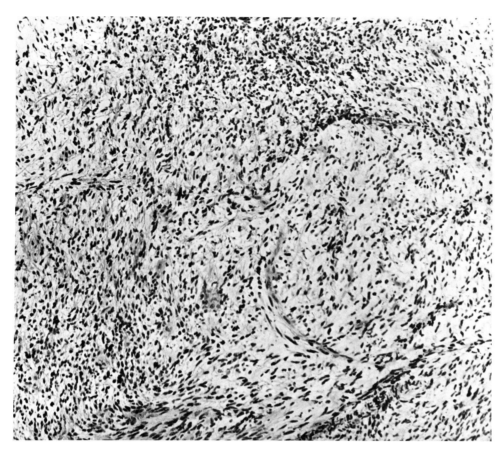

Figure 4.56. (D) Type B is characterized by loose texture and polymorphism of tumor cells. (H & E. Original magnification ×100.)

Schwann cell have recently been reemphasized.[224–229] It is well known that peripheral nerve tumors can undergo metaplastic changes. The most common benign secondary elements seen in these tumors are cartilage and osteoid, whereas secondary malignant changes include foci of rhabdomyosarcoma, chondrosarcoma, osteogenic sarcoma, and liposarcoma. Woodruff[225] described five nerve sheath tumors containing glands lined with columnar epithelium and mucicarminophilic material. The development of such foci within the substance of nerve sheath tumors is best explained by the multipotential ability of the Schwann cell.

Most investigators believe that encapsulated schwannomas are benign and do not undergo malignant transformation. Only a few documented case reports are found in the literature.[230] We agree with Russell and Rubenstein[231] that documentation of malignant transformation of an apparently benign schwannoma is extremely difficult.

Solitary Neurofibromas. Neurofibromas are still considered by most pathologists to be a distinct entity and are defined as benign, slow-growing, encapsulated tumors originating in the Schwann cells of a peripheral nerve. Harkin and Reed[232] argued that these tumors differ from solitary schwannomas both microscopically and clinically. However, the clinical behavior of a benign solitary neurofibroma and benign solitary schwannoma is indistinguishable.[230]

A typical neurofibroma of the skin is circumscribed, compresses the adjacent dermis, and is separated from the epidermis by a band

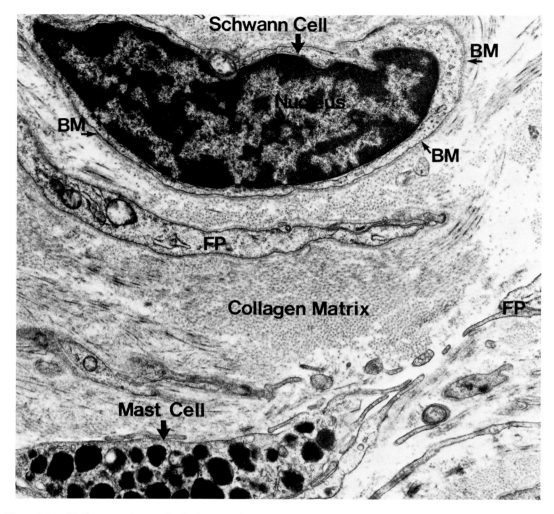

Figure 4.56. **(E)** Electron micrograph of a benign schwannoma. Note Schwann cell with its basement membrane (BM), the interstitial collagen matrix, cytoplasmic process of a fibroblast (FP), and a mast cell with its characteristic granules. (Original magnification ×21,300.)

of dermis. These characteristics are not found in neurofibromas located in the deeper tissues and they are macroscopically indistinguishable from solitary schwannomas. The prominent intercellular component of a neurofibroma is composed of numerous collagen fibrils and a nonorganized matrix. The proportion of interstitial collagen in a subcutaneous neurofibroma is higher than in a corresponding solitary schwannoma and microscopic distinction between the two can usually be made. Schwann cells are still the principal cells, and the tumor develops because of their proliferation.

Schwannomas and Neurofibromas Associated with von Recklinghausen's Disease. It is appropriate at this point to describe some of the salient pathologic features of von Recklinghausen's neurofibromatosis. Von Recklinghausen's disease is a hereditary disorder characterized by abnormal cutaneous pigmentations and multiple skin tumors. Frequently, patients with this disease have associated neural and epithelial tumors and several syndromes of the neuroendocrine axis. The subject has been extensively dealt with in our previous publications.[233,234]

Neurofibromatosis is generally considered

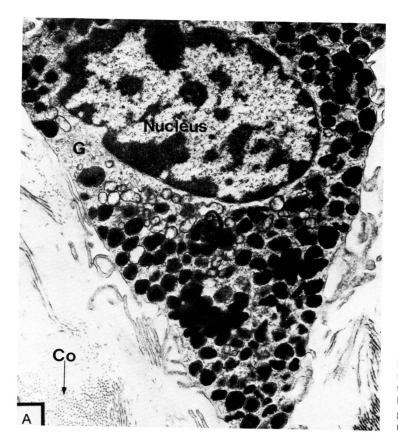

Figure 4.57. (A) Mast cell in a benign schwannoma (neurofibroma) from a patient with von Recklinghausen's disease. Cytoplasmic granules are mostly intact. (Original magnification ×14,732.)

to be a primary disorder of neural crest derivation, with secondary support from the mesenchymal elements. However, a controversy remains as to whether the neural and mesenchymal components of this disease are interrelated or arise independently.

Both pigmentary disturbances and neural tumors will be described in this section.

Café-au-Lait Spots. The pigmentation associated with neurofibromatosis is macular in nature and histologically consists of an abnormal deposition of melanin in the basal layers. The characteristic color of this pigmentation has led to the descriptive term of café-au-lait spots, which are essentially equal to large malpighian freckles with melanosis of the basal layers.

The pigmentation in neurofibromatosis is comparable to the pigmented spots in Albright's syndrome.[235] The salient cytologic feature of the pigmentary disturbance in neurofibromatosis is the presence of giant pigment granules in either malpighian cells or melanocytes; such granules are demonstrated in both café-au-lait spots and in normal skin.[218,236] Neither the chemical nature nor the fine structure of these pigmented granules is clear. They may vary in size, either filling the whole cell or ranging down to units just at the limit of resolution of the light microscope (0.5 μm). Frequently, they occur in melanocytes and can be seen in preparations not treated with DOPA. The DOPA reaction, however, enhances their color. In the hyperpigmented lesions of neurofibromatosis, more melanin granules are present in the basal layer than in the surrounding nonpigmented skin. The presence of these giant granules is an important criterion for differentiating between café-au-lait spots occurring in neurofibromatosis, in Albright's syndrome, or in normal subjects.

The question that always perplexes the clinician and the pathologist is the significance of these café-au-lait spots. Although histologically these are hyperpigmented areas and characterize von Recklinghausen's disease, unlike active

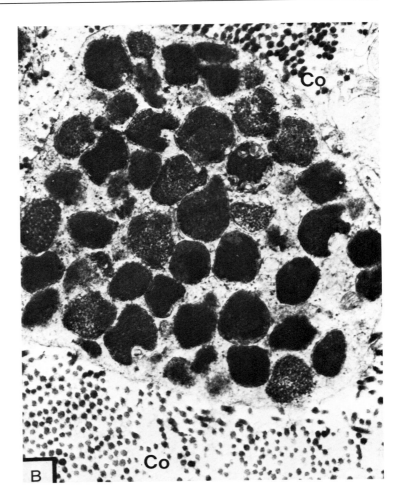

Figure 4.57. (B) Mast cell cytoplasm from a malignant schwannoma. Note granules in various stages of degranulation. (Original magnification ×46,699.)

junctional nevi, they do not undergo change during the patient's lifetime.

Giant pigmented nevi and bathing-trunk nevi are associated with leptomeningeal melanocytosis in about 20 percent of the cases, and with melanoma in approximately 10 percent.[237] Although the majority of cases of bathing-trunk nevi are not associated with von Recklinghausen's disease, giant pigmented nevi do sometimes occur in this disease. Reed and associates[237] recognized the clinical and sometimes microscopic similarity to neurofibroma but considered giant pigmented nevi and neurofibromatosis to be separate and distinct entities. Their opinion is not universally shared.[233,238–241] Histologically, the giant pigmented nevi often include several varieties, such as compound nevi, blue nevi, and spindle cell nevi. Brasfield and Das Gupta[233] found histologic characteristics

ranging from neurofibroma to plexiform neuroma in the tissues underlying the giant bathing-trunk nevi. Additionally, multiple hamartomatous areas of collagen, fat, and neural tissue are also present.[234] About one-fourth of the lesions are classified as neuroid or schwannian. They respond positively to the histochemical test for cholinesterase and contain abundant mast cells.[237]

Conway[238] had two patients with neurofibromatosis in his 40 patients with extensive nevi. Crowe and associates[239] found three patients with extensive nevi of the bathing-trunk type in a series of 233 patients. In Brasfield and Das Gupta's study,[233] 26 patients were unequivocally known to have been born with the stigmata of von Recklinghausen's disease. Of these 26, four had giant bathing-trunk nevi at birth, and melanoma developed in one. In the University of

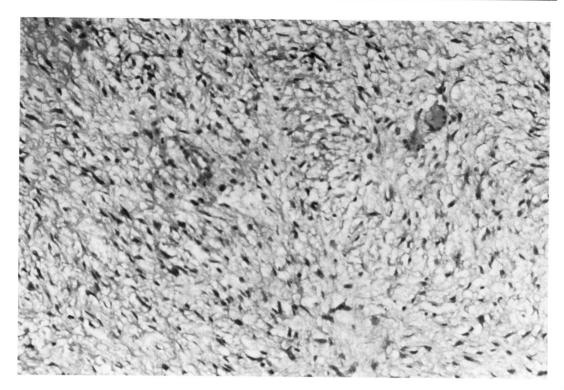

Figure 4.58. Cellular schwannoma in a woman of 55 years. This was initially thought to represent a malignant schwannoma. Careful scrutiny of all areas demonstrated the presence of Antoni A and B types of presentation. (H & E. Original magnification ×100.) Patient has remained well, without local recurrence, since a minor excision eight years ago.

Illinois series, one patient had a congenital bathing-trunk nevus which developed into melanoma at the age of 11 years (Chapter 14).

Benign Nerve Sheath Tumors Associated with von Recklinghausen's Disease. Benign cutaneous and subcutaneous neurofibromas are the hallmarks of von Recklinghausen's disease. Because of a common cell of origin, some authors[232] have classified all benign nerve sheath tumors under a single name. However, the clinical characteristics of plexiform neuroma are so distinct that these tumors should be classified separately.

From comparative neuropathology studies, it is apparent that neurofibromas in conjunction with neurofibromatosis are found in numerous species of animals.[234] In cattle, neurofibromas occur chiefly in the peripheral nerves, with acoustic neuromas and bone dysplasias observed only rarely. Neurofibromas that undergo sarcomatous transformation are found in horses. Extraocular tumors are usually inconspicuous in goldfish; however, malignant transformation occurs in 10 to 15 percent.

The unifying cell that is common to all benign nerve sheath tumors is the Schwann cell. The neurofibromas of von Recklinghausen's disease are schwannian in origin. To avoid conceptual difficulties, Feigin and Popoff[242] defined a peripheral Schwann cell as one capable of producing peripheral myelin, whatever other properties it might have and without regard to its origin. These authors postulated that some cells might also be related to nonmyelinated axons. The sheath cells are sometimes described as forming two classes of cells: the *Schwann cells* and the *endoneurial fibroblasts,* though this distinction is not readily evident with light microscopy. Under the electron microscope, approximately 90 percent of the cells of a normal human peripheral nerve appear to be uniform

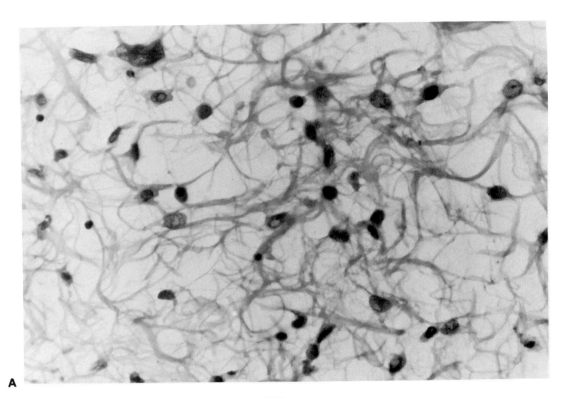

A

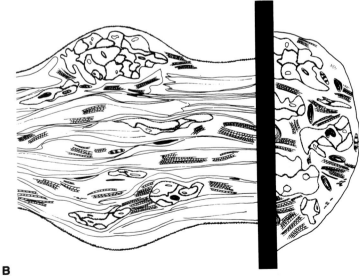

B

Figure 4.59. **(A)** Neurofibroma from a patient with von Recklinghausen's disease. Note the fusiform bipolar or multipolar tumor cells with long, slender processes. Some of these processes are branched as well. (H & E. Original magnification ×375.) **(B)** Diagrammatic rendition of the growth of a neurofibroma within a peripheral nerve. The haphazard growth pattern within the nerve makes it virtually impossible to enucleate this tumor, unlike its solitary counterpart (Fig. 4.56B). (*Modified from Weller and Cervos-Navarro 1977.*)

and intimately related to myelin and axons and have a basement membrane (see Figs. 4.55 and 4.56); therefore, they can be considered as Schwann cells.[221,222] A similar basement membrane is present around the perineural cell.[243] Myelin is demonstrated ultrastructurally to consist of a spiral of Schwann cell membranes. The Schwann cell is also capable of producing reticulin and collagen, as well as mimicking the activity of a macrophage.

Although a certain amount of confusion still exists in the interpretation of the histogenesis of tumors of neurogenic origin, the prevailing opinion is that these tumors are neoplastic transformations of neuroectodermal Schwann cells, ie, schwannomas, neurofibromas, or plexiform neurofibromas.[231,244] Ultrastructurally, the presence of a basement membrane around the tumor cells establishes their Schwann cell character and excludes fibroblastic origin. Mast cells are usually more numerous in neurofibromas and schwannomas associated with von Recklinghausen's disease.

The neurofibromas in von Recklinghausen's disease are characterized by an irregular overgrowth of Schwann cells associated with an exuberance of reticulin and collagen and by penetration by nerve fibers. However, a distinction between neurofibroma and schwannoma associated with von Recklinghausen's disease is not clear-cut, since the morphologic features of both lesions frequently blend into each other (Fig. 4.59A and 4.59B). The presence of melanin pigment on the overlying epidermis is a common feature of neurofibroma. Sometimes a neurofibroma contains groups of cells full of melanin, and some such lesions are related to cellular blue nevi.[240] Histochemical study of neurofibromas and schwannomas has shown the presence of cholinesterase.

Plexiform Neurofibroma. A plexiform neurofibroma is considered diagnostic of neurofibromatosis.[232] It may affect a large nerve trunk or small terminal branches (Fig. 4.60A and 4.60B). Its borders are usually poorly defined. The tumorous nerve may be surrounded by normal tissue or by lymphangiomatous-hemangiomatous tissue, with redundancy and hyperpigmentation of the overlying skin (Fig. 4.60C). The resulting elephantoid appearance may also be associated with either hyperplasia or hypoplasia of underlying bones. In a plexiform neurofibroma, the elements of a normal nerve are present but arranged in a grotesquely distorted and bizarre fashion. If a large nerve is affected, it will show poorly defined swellings that are soft and elastic in texture, whereas the cut surface is usually opalescent, whitish, and devoid of the whorled texture of the schwannoma. Histologically, the swellings consist of a myxoid material that contains small round cells with a stellate cytoplasm separating cords of Schwann cells containing the neurons (Fig. 4.60D and 4.60E).

The tendency of the neurofibromas of von Recklinghausen's disease to become malignant is generally accepted, but the incidence of such transformation is not well documented. Hosoi[245] calculated that about 13 percent undergo some form of malignant change. Malignant transformation was found in 29 percent of our pa-

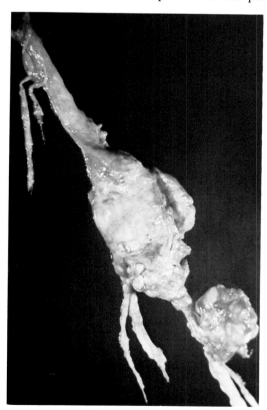

Figure 4.60. **(A)** Dissected sciatic nerve from a 28-year-old woman with malignant schwannoma arising in the lower part of the nerve, prior to division. The larger mass was malignant. Note smaller pedunculated plexiform neuroma and the beaded appearance of the lower branches. She was treated by a major amputation (dissection of sciatic nerve performed by J. Wander, M.D.).

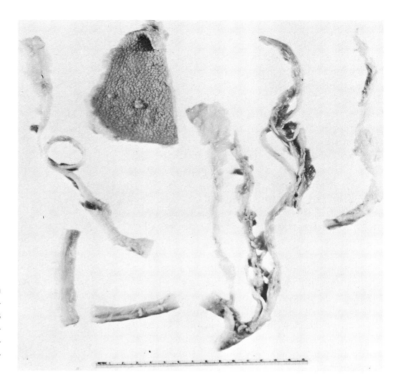

Figure 4.60. **(B)** A composite of an elephantoid skin with a small neurofibroma and dissected cutaneous nerves showing the beading characteristic of plexiform neurofibroma of von Recklinghausen's disease.

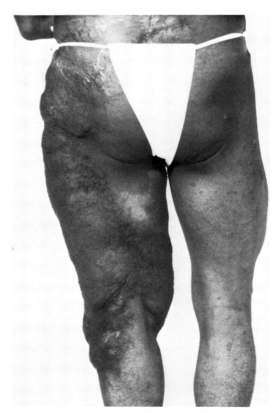

Figure 4.60. **(C)** Hyperpigmentation and redundancy of skin overlying a plexiform neurofibroma of long duration.

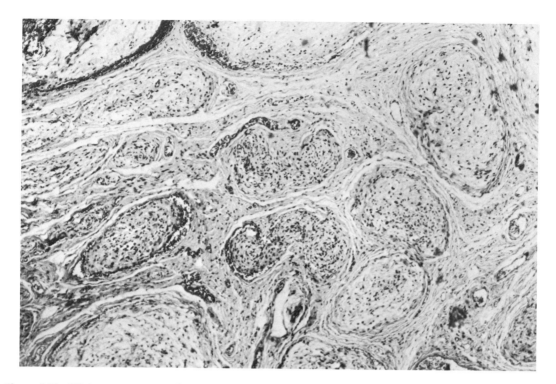

Figure 4.60. **(D)** Low-power view of a plexiform neurofibroma showing the proliferating Schwann cells arranged in bundles separated by fibrous tissue. (H & E. Original magnification ×80.)

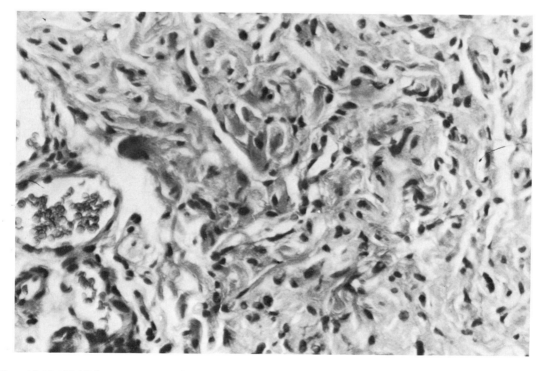

Figure 4.60. **(E)** Higher-power view of sciatic nerve showing preserved myelinated fibers and plump spindle cells embedded in a fibrillary myxomatous background. (H & E. Original magnification ×250.) *(Fig. 4.60A and 4.60D courtesy of Current Problems of Surgery, vol. 14, no. 2, 1977.)*

tients.[233,234] Malignancy is suggested by a rapid increase in size and shape of the tumor. Russell and Rubenstein[231] pointed out that components of both morphologic types blended into a single tumor may individually show histologic evidence of malignancy. Although in some patients the malignant form seems to arise de novo, usually a malignant transformation is preceded by a few recurrences of a seemingly benign neurofibroma or a plexiform neurofibroma. More than one malignant lesion may occur in a patient with von Recklinghausen's disease.[233]

Involvement of the central nervous system is basic to von Recklinghausen's disease and often has been termed the central form of the disease. A variety of neoplasms, including gliomas (glioblastomas, ependymomas, and oligodendrogliomas), meningiomas, and schwannomas can occur in the brain, spinal cord, and meninges.[233,234] Pack and Ariel[4] estimated that the incidence of central nervous system involvement might be 5 percent. The two most commonly encountered intracranial anomalies are the gliomas of the optic nerve and the acoustic neuromas of the auditory nerve. A nerve growth-promoting factor has been isolated in patients with both the central and peripheral forms of the disease.[246,247] It appears that this biologic marker probably can be used in evaluating the nature and degree of progression of von Recklinghausen's disease.

Malignant Tumors of Schwann Cell Origin

Malignant Schwannoma. A malignant schwannoma is of nerve sheath origin. It infiltrates locally and also metastasizes. As with its benign counterpart, a large number of synonyms are found in the literature, eg, malignant neurinoma, malignant neurilemoma, and neurogenic sarcoma, to name a few. However, there is sufficient justification to consider these tumors to arise from Schwann cells, and they are either malignant schwannomas or malignant neurilemomas.[231,244,248] A malignant schwannoma can be found either sporadically or in association with von Recklinghausen's neurofibromatosis.

Harkin and Reed[232] classified malignant peripheral nerve sheath tumors into the following four groups: (1) malignant schwannoma, (2) malignant epithelioid schwannoma, (3) nerve sheath fibrosarcoma, and (4) malignant melanocytic schwannoma. According to these au-

thors, group 1 tumors were associated with plexiform neuroma. Groups 2 and 3 were found to be highly malignant. In view of their rarity, little is known about group 4. The histologic features of groups 1 and 3 frequently overlap, and assignment of a given tumor to one or the other category was sometimes arbitrary. Such classifications are of little clinical value. It appears, therefore, that once the histogenetic type of a given tumor has been properly arrived at as being of schwannian origin, a grading according to the degree of anaplasia would be of more clinical significance than such histologic subclassifications.

Solitary Malignant Schwannoma. Malignant solitary schwannomas arising in the peripheral nerves develop in practically every anatomic region. To avoid confusion concerning the histogenesis of primary malignant tumors of the peripheral nerves, D'Agostino and co-workers[249,250] included only tumors that could be shown to arise from major peripheral nerves. This selection was rigorous and excluded a number of patients who might possibly have had malignant schwannomas. Not all schwannomas arise in large, named, peripheral nerves. A number occur in smaller branches, and the relationship is often overlooked. However, true malignant peripheral nerve neoplasms are rare.[214]

MACROSCOPIC FINDINGS (FIG. 4.61A TO 4.61C). The tumors arising from large peripheral nerves are usually fusiform and appear to be surrounded by a capsule. Although the nerve appears to enter and traverse the neoplasm, it is impossible to trace it in the tumor. The emergence is obvious in a large peripheral nerve, but in the mediastinum or in smaller nerves this feature is not discernible. The cut surface may have a faint-to-marked whorled pattern such as that of a uterine leiomyoma. Areas of cystic degeneration or hemorrhage appear in large tumors. Gross extension of the tumors for significant distances within a nerve is frequently observed. The author has encountered patients in whom the primary tumor arose in the sciatic nerve in the pelvis and extended through the sciatic notch to the posterior thigh to form a palpable mass (Fig. 4.61A). D'Agostino et al.[250] described one patient in whom the tumor extended all through the median nerve.

MICROSCOPIC FINDINGS (FIG. 4.62A TO 4.62D). These tumors are composed of plump spindle cells. Mitoses are frequently found, and the nuclei are hyperchromatic and vary in size.

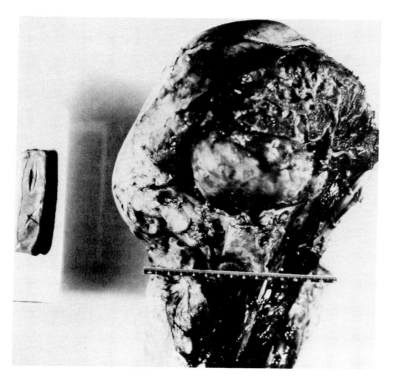

Figure 4.61. (A) Malignant schwannoma of the buttock. This tumor was first palpated and visible in the buttock, but actually a part of it was intrapelvic, extending through the sciatic notch and requiring a hemipelvectomy.

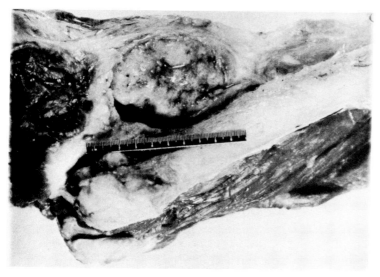

Figure 4.61. (B) Cut surface of a malignant schwannoma infiltrating the muscle planes. *(Courtesy of Annals of Surgery 175:86, 1972)*

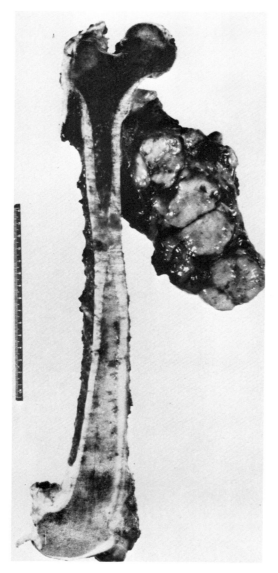

Figure 4.61. (C) Malignant schwannoma adherent to the femur. The tumor had infiltrated the linea aspera. A hip joint disarticulation was performed. Patient is still disease-free four years later.

The pattern of interlacing bundles of tightly packed cells is commonly seen. There is usually a marked uniformity of cell type, producing a monotonous microscopic pattern. Infiltration of the epineurium occurs almost invariably. Infiltration of the perineurium and extension along the fascicles is common enough that the clini-

cian must take this fact into consideration before planning definitive primary therapy.

Electron microscopic examination of malignant solitary schwannomas, like the benign type, shows a large array of Schwann cells, fibroblasts, giant cells, macrophages, and mast cells (see Figs. 4.57A and 4.57B and 4.62D), but a general disorganization is evident. The Schwann cell cytoplasm is frequently in various stages of myelin production. The tumor giant cells and multiple nuclei are common features. Macrophages are seen with a variety of ingested material, probably disintegrated myelin. The collagen matrix is scanty compared with that in the benign variety.

Malignant Schwannoma Associated With von Recklinghausen's Disease. The general morphologic and histologic characteristics of these tumors are similar to those of solitary malignant schwannoma. The malignant neoplasm that develops along the course of a peripheral nerve is often well demarcated and fusiform (see Fig. 4.60A). Some are lobulated, and those that extend through an intervertebral foramen assume an hourglass shape. The tumor usually infiltrates the surrounding tissues and the epineurium.

Microscopically, malignant schwannomas associated with von Recklinghausen's disease on close scrutiny can be distinguished from their solitary counterparts. They consist predominantly of fusiform elements lightly packed in interlacing bundles, closely resembling fibrosarcomas (Fig. 4.63A). Coarse reticulin fibrils may extend in parallel rows among the spindle cells, but adjacent cells may be entwined by delicate fibrils, as in fibrosarcoma. Collagen fibers are usually scanty and mitoses are common. Frequently, there are foci of pleomorphism, and giant cells of the mononucleate or multinucleate type may be distributed sparingly or plentifully throughout the tumors. In highly anaplastic tumors, bipolar spindle cells and stellate cells are sometimes observed. Electron microscopic examination of these tumors shows that they are more pleomorphic than are solitary malignant schwannomas, with still less interstitial collagen and fewer Schwann cells in varying degrees of maturation. There is an increased incidence of mast cells, macrophages, and lymphocytes (Fig. 4.57A and 4.57B and Fig. 4.63B).

Nerve sheath fibrosarcomas are also frequently associated with von Recklinghausen's

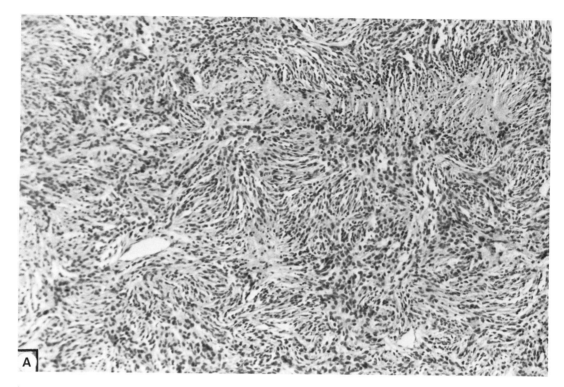

Figure 4.62. (A) Malignant schwannoma. The tumor cells are uniform and spindle-shaped, with less collagenous matrix. Multiple blood vessels are also seen. There appears to be a monotony of pattern. Although the tumor is malignant, an Antoni type A presentation still can be seen. (H & E. Original magnification ×63.)

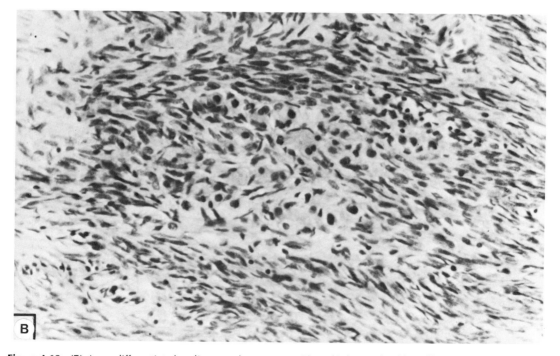

Figure 4.62. (B) An undifferentiated malignant schwannoma with multiple ganglionlike cells and a general disorganization. (H & E. Original magnification ×110.)

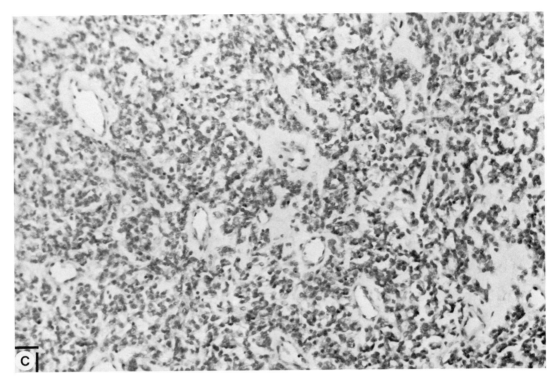

Figure 4.62. **(C)** Malignant schwannoma. The cells appear to be epithelioid in nature and are arranged haphazardly. Prominent blood vessels with thick walls are obvious. No area shows the characteristic Antoni A or B configuration. (H & E. Original magnification ×125.) The tumor was excised from the ulnar nerve of a 54-year-old man.

disease. The tumor cells are thought to be fi-broblasts. The matrix may be mucinous and, on purely morphologic grounds, a diagnosis of fi-bromyxosarcoma can be forwarded. Fre-quently, such tumors are indistinguishable from common types of fibrosarcoma, even under an electron microscope.

Tumors of Tissues Secondarily Involving Peripheral Nerves

Metastases or direct invasion of the perineural spaces is seen in advanced cases of malignancy. In some patients, the direct extension to the adjoining nerve is the only evidence that the presenting tumor is malignant. The mechanism of paralysis in a peripheral nerve was experi-mentally investigated by Kashef and Das Gupta.[251] These authors found that the primary pathologic change in the sciatic nerves of rats in the presence of Walker 256 carcinosarcoma was segmental demyelination, which appears in most clinical settings to be the initial cause

of nerve deficit. However, in long-standing tu-mors, Wallerian degeneration is often found in the peripheral nerves distal to the tumors (Fig. 4.64A to 4.64C). In the carcinomatous neuro-myopathy sometimes seen in patients with ter-minal pulmonary cancer, a patchy loss of mye-linated fibers has been observed. Croft and co-workers[252] have alluded to an immune theory to explain this phenomenon of carcinomatous neuromyopathy in man. It is apparent that fur-ther investigation is in order to explain some of these riddles.

Traumatic Neuroma. Traumatic neuroma, or amputation neuroma, is defined as a prolifer-ative non-neoplastic mass found at the site of trauma to a peripheral nerve. It is caused by entrapment of a cluster of Schwann cells, axons, and fibroblasts in a collagenous matrix.

Macroscopic Findings. The fully developed lesion is characterized by a fusiform enlarge-ment that bridges the defect in a severed nerve

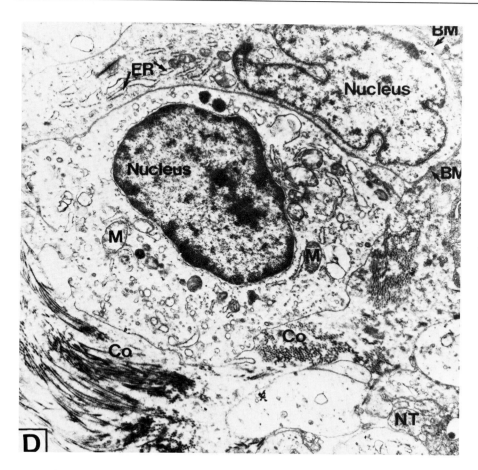

Figure 4.62. (D) Electron micrograph from a patient with solitary malignant schwannoma. Profiles of two Schwann cells with basement membrane (BM) are easily recognizable. The cells are in a scanty collagenous matrix (Co). A nerve terminal (NT) can be easily recognized. (Original magnification ×16,109.)

or by a bulbous expansion of the end of an amputated nerve. The nerve fibers disappear in a white, dense, fibrous scar.

Microscopic Findings. In the active phase of growth, the proximal and distal nerve stumps are surrounded by a mucinous matrix that is continuous with the endoneurium and perineurium. In well-formed lesions, Schwann cell cords containing axons thicken, undergo partitioning, and are transformed into compact bundles of nerve fascicles (Fig. 4.65). Perineurium condenses around each fascicle and the adjacent tissue is converted to dense fibrous tissue. In the late stage, the whole architecture consists of tangled axons in a dense collagenous matrix, and frequently only Schwann tubes are seen, with no recognizable axons.

The Sympathochromaffin System

In the peripheral nervous system, tumors of nerve cell origin occur predominantly in the region of the sympathetic trunk. Sympathogonia are stem cells not only of the sympathoblasts and sympathetic ganglion cells, but also of the chromaffin cells found in the chromaffin tissue dispersed throughout the human body. Thus, two types of tumors occur that correspond to the dichotomy in the development of sympathogonia: (1) sympathetic tumors arising from neuronal cell lines, and (2) pheochromocytomas arising from chromaffin cells. Biochemical studies show that sympathetic tumors are able to synthesize and secrete catecholamines, a well-known characteristic of pheochromocytomas. The amount of catecholamines stored in indi-

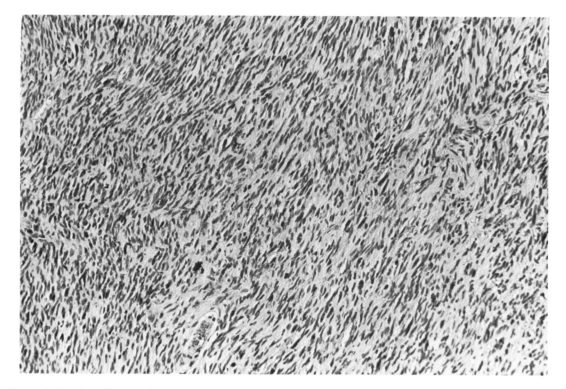

Figure 4.63. (A) Malignant schwannoma in von Recklinghausen's disease. The individual cells as well as the overall architecture resemble a fibrosarcoma. (H & E. Original magnification ×250.)

vidual tumors is, however, variable.[253] It appears that, in spite of the diversity of clinicopathologic features of the strict sympathetic tumors and the classical pheochromocytomas, both share a common ancestry and can be classified as tumors of the sympathochromaffin system. A brief description of the chromaffin system precedes the description of these tumors.

The expression *chromaffin system* is an arbitrary but convenient term to bring together various groups of cells which, like those in the adrenal medulla, contain cytoplasmic granules with an affinity for certain salts of chromic acid.[212] Such cells are described as chromaffin elements, or pheochromocytes. There is evidence that these cells are derived, in company with sympathetic neurons, from a common source in the neural crest, and that the ultimate cell groups so derived preserve considerable topographical relationship with various components of the sympathetic moiety of the autonomic nervous system. Chromaffin cells in the adrenal medulla secrete adrenalin and noradrenalin and are innervated

by preganglionic sympathetic fibers, but how far these features are true of chromaffin cells in other situations is not clear. In addition to the medulla of the adrenal gland, the chromaffin tissue includes (1) groups of cells known as paraganglias, (2) para-aortic bodies, and (3) small masses of chromaffin cells scattered irregularly and variably among the ganglia of the paravertebral sympathetic chains, splanchnic nerves, and the great (prevertebral) autonomic plexuses. Coupland[212] described the distribution of the chromaffin tissue in the newborn infant (Fig. 4.66).

The chromaffin cells of the adrenal medulla synthesize and secrete noradrenalin and adrenalin into venous sinusoids, the release being under preganglionic sympathetic control.[212] In several species of mammals these substances have been identified in two distinct cell types, the noradrenalin-storing cells, which are usually situated more peripherally, and those that store adrenalin, which are centrally located.[254] Chromaffin cells are columnar and arranged in

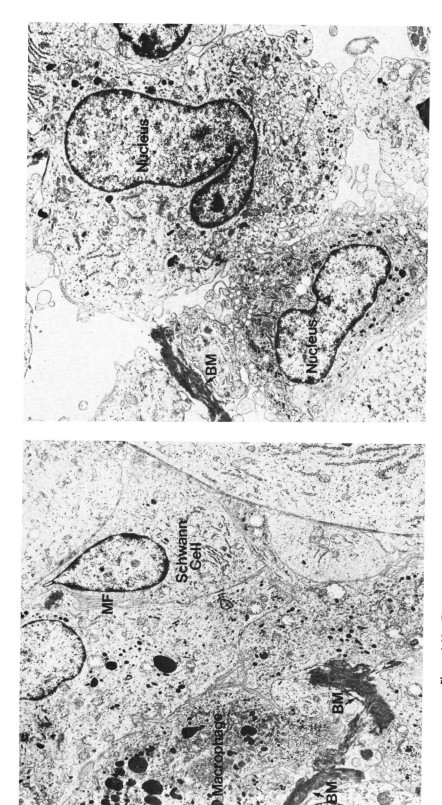

Figure 4.63. (B) A panoramic view of a malignant schwannoma associated with von Recklinghausen's disease. Left, one macrophage with various cytoplasmic inclusions and fragmented basal membranes (BM) is prominent. However, in the upper right, a Schwann cell is in the process of infolding its membranes (MF), the initial step in the process of myelination. (Original magnification ×8,185.) Right, various cells in a relatively scanty stroma are present. The cell with a kidney-shaped nucleus is identifiable as a neoplastic Schwann cell. (Original magnification ×6,122.)

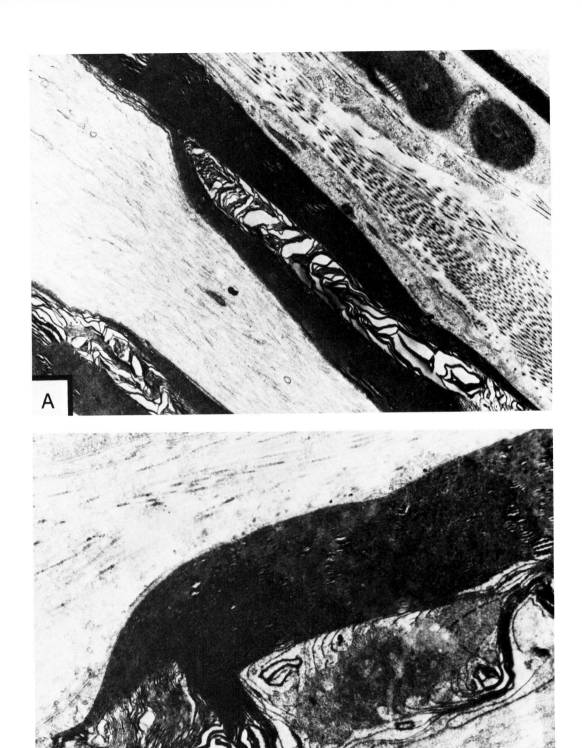

Figure 4.64. *Continued*

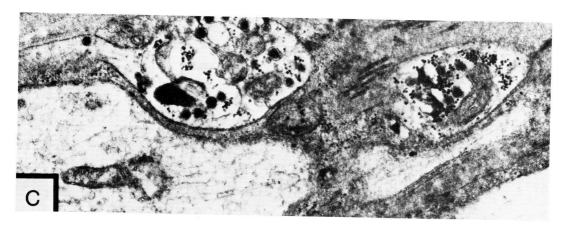

Figure 4.64. Sciatic nerve from a patient with a recurrent liposarcoma of the left iliac fossa infiltrating the lateral wall of the pelvis. Patient was treated by a hemipelvectomy and is doing well eight years later. During her first visit to the University of Illinois Hospital, a sciatic nerve deficit was noted. These electron micrographs were taken from the distal sciatic nerve about 5 cm beyond the gross tumor. **(A)** Initiation of segmental changes in the Schmidt-Lanterman incisures at the node of Ranvier. (Original magnification ×19,735.) **(B)** The process of segmental demyelination is apparent. (Original magnification ×34,720.) **(C)** Early phase of Wallerian degeneration can also be seen. (Original magnification ×34,720.)

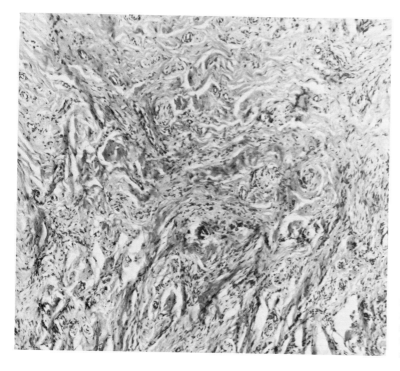

Figure 4.65. Micrograph of a traumatic neuroma. Thick axons are seen surrounded by dense fibrous tissue. (H & E. Original magnification ×63.)

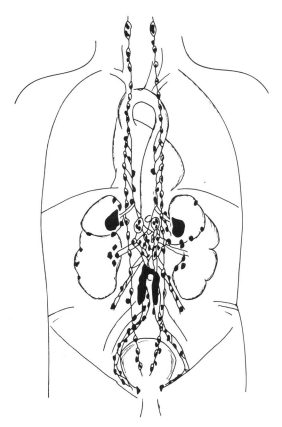

Figure 4.66. Diagram of the distribution of chromaffin tissue in the newborn infant. *(Modified from RE Coupland, 1965.)*

rows one cell thick along the margins of venous sinusoids. The cytoplasm of the chromaffin cell is basophilic and ultrastructurally shows a well-developed granular endoplasmic reticulum, mitochondria, and Golgi complex. Numerous secretory vesicles are also present. In noradrenalin-storing cells, these are typically rounded or ellipsoidal bodies which, after treatment with aldehyde and osmium, are highly electron-dense. In adrenalin-storing cells, after similar treatment the vesicles have a paler appearance, often with a clear zone between the granular contents and the binding membrane.[254] In the human adrenal cells both types of vesicles have been found, presuming that both may be secreted from the same cell.[255] The chromaffin cells of the adrenal medulla develop and migrate from the neural crests (sympathochromaffin tissue). The chromaffin reaction in the cell is positive in the fifth

month of fetal life, but adrenalin is present as early as the third month.[212]

Paraganglia. The paraganglia are spherical masses of chromaffin cells about 2 mm in diameter, each lying inside or embedded in the capsule of a ganglion of the sympathetic trunk. In the adult they are generally represented by microscopic remnants only.

The Para-Aortic Bodies (Organs of Zuckerkandl). The para-aortic bodies progressively develop during fetal life and attain their maximum size in the first three years of postnatal life, by which time the largest take the form of 1-cm elongated bodies lying on each side of the abdominal aorta in the region of origin of the inferior mesenteric artery. They are usually united across the aorta in the form of an H. The constituent cells undergo dispersal and atrophy and by age 14 are usually disintegrated.[212] They consist of masses of polygonal chromaffin cells secreting noradrenalin. Other small collections of chromaffin cells are found in fetuses, but these usually regress with age and in adults only microscopic evidence remains. The function of these chromaffin nests remains unclear.

Carotid Bodies. The two carotid bodies are reddish-brown ellipsoidal structures situated on each side of the neck in close relation to the carotid sinus. Each is about 5 to 7 mm in length and 2.5 to 4 mm in width and varies slightly in position, either posterior to the bifurcation of the common carotid artery or wedged between the commencements of the internal and external carotid arteries. They are attached to, and sometimes partially embedded in, the adventitial layer of these arteries.

The carotid body first appears as a condensation of the mesenchyme around the third pharyngeal arch artery. Its initial nerve supply is mainly from the glossopharyngeal nerve to the third arch. Other similar small bodies are found near the arteries of the fourth and sixth pharyngeal arches; thus, they are close to the arch of the aorta, the ductus arteriosus, and the right subclavian arteries, and are supplied by the superior cervical ganglion and the vagus nerve.

A strong fibrous capsule invests the carotid body, and septa from this capsule pass into the organ and divide it into lobules. Each lobule consists of masses of large polyhedral epithelioid cells (glomus cells or chief cells) and supporting cells, among which are interspersed networks of sinusoidal blood vessels.[256] Each glomus cell contains a large, pale-staining nucleus and a pale, finely granular cytoplasm. The main nerve supply of the carotid body is the carotid branches of the glossopharyngeal nerve, the branches from the superior cervical ganglion, and the vagus nerve. The organ itself is richly innervated by myelinated and nonmyelinated axons. The unmyelinated nerve endings can form groups. One group terminates in close contact with sinusoid synaptic end bulbs containing 50-nm cholinergic-type clear vesicles associated with the surfaces of glomus cells.[256] Stimulation of the glomus cells alters the chemoreceptor activity in the carotid body.

Electron microscopy of a normal carotid body shows that the glomus cell cytoplasm is characterized by the presence of abundant membrane-limited, osmiophilic granules with generally rounded profiles. These granules range from 100 to 150 nm in outer diameter. Some are separated by a clear zone.

Tympanic Body (Glomus Jugulare). This is a small ovoid body about 0.5 mm long and 0.25 mm wide that is located in the adventitia of the upper part of the superior bulb of the internal jugular vein. Its structure is similar to that of the carotid body. It may consist of two or more masses related to the tympanic branch of the glossopharyngeal nerve or the auricular branch of the vagus, as these nerves lie in their canals in the petrous part of the temporal bone.

Coccygeal Body (Glomus Coccygeum). This body is about 2.5 mm long. It is located anterior or immediately inferior to the apex of the coccyx at the termination of the median sacral vessels that supply afferent and efferent branches to the organ, and is closely related to the ganglion impar of the sympathetic trunk.

Tumors of the Sympathochromaffin System

The tumors of the sympathochromaffin system can be classified as either benign or malignant (see Table 3.1, Chapter 3). The benign tumors are (1) ganglioneuromas, (2) pheochromocytomas, (3) carotid body tumors, and (4) nonchromaffin paragangliomas. The malignant tumors are (1) malignant ganglioneuromas, (2) neuroblastomas, (3) malignant pheochromocytomas,

(4) malignant carotid body tumors, and (5) malignant nonchromaffin paragangliomas.

Benign Tumors.

Ganglioneuroma. This is a comparatively rare benign tumor in which ganglion cells, neurofibrils, and neurilemma cells occur in varying proportions. These tumors are well known for their ability to mature and become quiescent. In order of decreasing frequency, these tumors are found in the posterior mediastinum, lumbar region, adrenal medulla, and neck.[257–260] Infrequently, they have been found in other locations.[261] Since there is little evidence that mature ganglion cells multiply, it is presumed that during formation a ganglioneuroma is composed of immature neuroblasts. Thus, in a rapidly growing tumor, even if the biopsy specimen suggests a mature ganglioneuroma, a diagnosis of benign tumor should seldom be made.

MACROSCOPIC FINDINGS. A ganglioneuroma is a firm, well-demarcated, usually encapsulated tumor, occasionally of large dimensions. The cut surface is grayish-white and often resembles leiomyosarcoma. Although some of these tumors, notably the mediastinal, attain a large size and extend into the surrounding tissue, infiltrative activity has not been reported.

MICROSCOPIC FINDINGS. Mature ganglion cells are the characteristic feature of these tumors. Ganglion cells may occur singly or in clusters and are scattered haphazardly throughout the tumor tissue (Fig. 4.67). Occasionally a ganglioneuroma structurally resembles a normal ganglion. There is an abundant dense stroma, which may contain stainable neurofibrils as well as collagen fibers, but the stromal pattern may vary considerably and arrangements reminiscent of neurofibromas may be seen. In some instances there is evidence of calcification of individual cells or groups of ganglion cells.

ELECTRON MICROSCOPY. The tumor cells have large nuclei with prominent nucleoli measuring up to 2 μm in diameter. There is abundant cytoplasm, which contains a complex arrangement of various organelles and inclusions. Mitochondria are present in large numbers and are sometimes irregularly shaped. Some are enormous, with short cristae. Both rough and smooth endoplasmic reticulum, with a well-developed Golgi complex, are frequently seen.[253]

Numerous granules of different shapes and sizes are present in the cytoplasm. The small membrane-bound granules are uniform in size

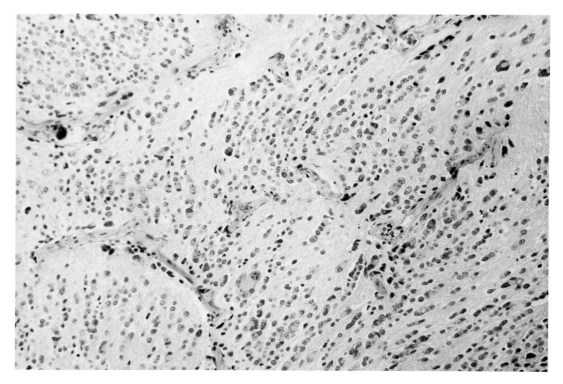

Figure 4.67. Ganglioneuroma showing the characteristic fibrillary tissue and ganglion cells. (H & E. Original magnification ×125.) *(Micrograph courtesy of Dr. L. McDonald, Department of Ophthalmology, University of Illinois, Chicago.)*

and shape, are about 100 nm in diameter, and resemble catecholamine granules. They are distributed throughout the perinuclear region and are frequently associated with the Golgi complex. The larger osmiophilic granules are ovoid, with diameters ranging from 250 to several hundred nanometers. Both types of granules are intermingled and frequently coalesce to form larger masses. Multivesicular bodies up to 300 nm are also seen in the cytoplasm of tumor cells.

Much of the space between tumor cells is filled with bundles of cell processes of varying length, some of which are surrounded by Schwann cells. Although multiple myelinated and unmyelinated axons are seen, typical synapses have not yet been described.[262] Interspersed between these cell processes, collagen fibers and other cells such as fibrocytes or fibroblasts are occasionally observed.

Pheochromocytoma. Pheochromocytomas arise in the adrenal glands in approximately 90 percent of patients, but they can arise wherever sympathochromaffin tissue is found (Fig. 4.66).

MACROSCOPIC FINDINGS. Some pheochromocytomas are small spherical or ovoid masses, usually 1 to 2 cm in diameter but sometimes larger. Size and function, however, are not directly related, since small tumors may be pharmacologically as active as large ones. The larger pheochromocytomas are well demarcated, smooth, and lobulated. The cut surface is brownish-gray, and areas of local hemorrhage are common. In smaller lesions, unless a well-formed capsule separates the tumor, it is difficult to distinguish an area of local hyperplasia of the adrenal medulla from a tumor.

MICROSCOPIC FINDINGS. The microscopic features of pheochromocytomas correspond well to those of normal adrenal medulla. Frequently medullary hyperplasia so resembles a pheochromocytoma that distinction between them becomes impossible. Most tumors consist of delicate, richly vascular connective tissue that supports large or small solid alveoli, whorls, cords, or sheets of tumor cells (Fig. 4.68). The cells of a pheochromocytoma are intimately re-

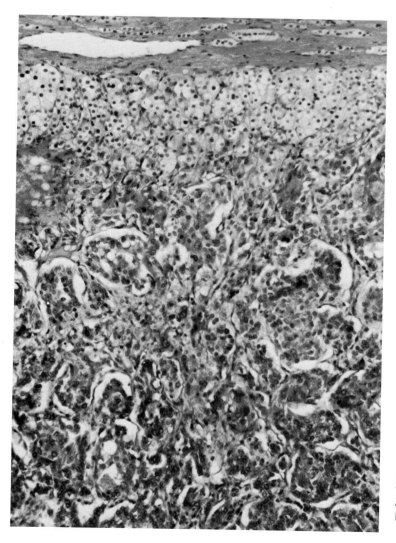

Figure 4.68. Pheochromocytoma. This was a functioning tumor. Nests of tumor cells are easily identifiable. (H & E. Original magnification ×125.)

lated to thin-wall blood vessels and sinusoids, often lined by tumor cells. The tumor cells are usually larger than normal medullary cells (20 to 30 μm), conspicuously granular, and sometimes vacuolated or foamy. The nucleus is eccentrically placed, hyperchromatic, and often large. This nuclear pleomorphism is a distinguishing feature. These cells stain dark with bichromate salts or chromic acid.

ELECTRON MICROSCOPY. The tumor cells resemble adrenal medullary cells. In most areas the plasma membranes are in close apposition and the cells are clustered into sheets and nests; however, in some areas the cells are separated by a rich, collagenous, interstitial tissue. The cytoplasm of the tumor cells contains numerous mitochondria and both smooth and granular endoplasmic reticulum. The characteristic feature, however, is the presence of osmiophilic dense-cored vesicles, which are the site of localization of catecholamines and have been extensively studied.[253]

Carotid Body Tumors. Tumors of the carotid body are rare. The majority are solitary, usually oval, superficially lobulated, and seldom exceed a few centimeters in diameter. They are resilient and occasionally hard and fibrous, but ordinarily they vary from rubbery to soft; they often are firmly adherent to the carotid bifurcation.

MICROSCOPIC FINDINGS. Essentially the tumor consists of a complex framework of blood vessels between which there is a richly cellular, predominantly epithelioid parenchyma. The tumor cells are aggregated in small solid nests, columns, and strands in close relation to the delicate sinusoids and numerous capillary channels (Fig. 4.69). Frequently the organoid pattern is repeated and the alveolar pattern is sharply outlined in sections stained for reticulin. The individual tumor cells retain the cytologic features common to normal pheochromocytes.

ELECTRON MICROSCOPY. Electron microscopy of carotid body tumors shows that the tumor consists of polygonal cells. The nuclei are generally spherical or oval and occupy either a central or peripheral position. The cytoplasm is rich with mitochondria and both smooth and rough-surfaced endoplasmic reticulum. The cytoplasmic granules usually are of two sizes. The smaller membrane-bound granules are about 0.1 μm and spherical and consist of a central electron-dense core that is separated by a clear zone from the enveloping membrane. The larger variety morphologically is similar to the smaller one, except for the size (0.4 to 0.5 μm). The

interstitium of carotid body tumors consists of the usual collagen material, and occasionally some nerve fibers.

Nonchromaffin Paraganglioma. These slow-growing tumors are histologically similar to carotid body tumors and are usually found either in the glomus jugulare or in the retroperitoneal space. Because of their position behind the tympanic membrane or in the external auditory meatus, glomus jugulare tumors are frequently covered by squamous epithelium. Histologically, these tumors are indistinguishable from carotid body tumors.

Malignant Tumors.

Malignant Ganglioneuroma (Ganglioneuroblastoma). Malignant ganglioneuroma probably represents an intermediate degree of differentiation in the gamut of tumors designated as neuroblastoma, malignant ganglioneuroma, or ganglioneuroblastoma. Some authors have used these terms interchangeably. Operationally, tumors resembling neuroblastoma, with moder-

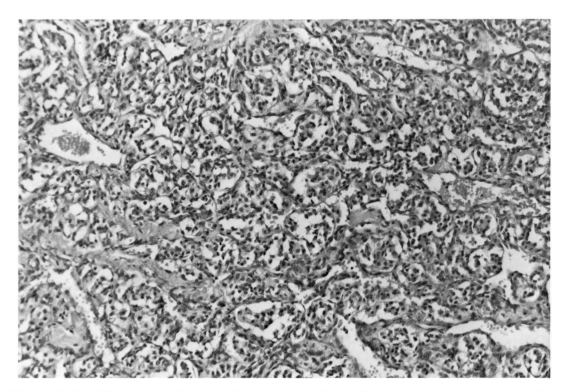

Figure 4.69. Carotid body tumor. The tumor cells are arranged in alveolar fashion around vascular channels lined by endothelial cells. (H & E. Original magnification ×125.) *(Courtesy of Dr. S. Sahgal, Department of Pathology, West Side Veterans Administration Hospital, Chicago.)*

ate differentiation of the cellular elements located outside the retroperitoneum, may be designated as malignant ganglioneuromas. One of the common sites is the neck.[263-265] Malignant ganglioneuroma arising in the vagus nerve has also been described.[266]

The tumors are usually ovoid and of fleshy consistency. They are indistinguishable from neuroblastoma on light microscopic examination. The tumor cells, which are small and rounded, show varying degrees of pleomorphism. However, ganglion cells are seen interspersed within a rough collagen matrix. Electron microscopy reveals that these tumor cells resemble the cells in pheochromocytoma, with large nuclei and prominent nucleoli. The cytoplasm contains secretory granules containing catecholamines. The interstitium is usually cluttered with unmyelinated axons of varying size and is either partially or completely surrounded by Schwann cell cytoplasm.

Neuroblastoma (Ganglioneuroblastoma). Neuroblastoma, although rare, is one of the most common forms of childhood malignancies. This tumor has been observed in fetuses, newborns, and in infants only a few weeks old.[56,267-269] Infrequently, it occurs in adolescents or adults.[270] It has also been observed in association with some congenital anomalies[267,271] and with von Recklinghausen's disease.[148,272,273]

MACROSCOPIC FINDINGS. Neuroblastomas grow as large, rounded or lobulated, demarcated, soft, vascular, reddish-gray to yellow masses of solid but easily fragmented tissues. Occasionally they are bilateral and, when they arise near the spine, have a dumbbell appearance. Frequently, there is local infiltration. Necrosis, hemorrhage, and cyst formation within the substance are common.

MICROSCOPIC FINDINGS. Neuroblastomas are composed of small, round, or slightly elongated cells with oval hyperchromatic nuclei (Fig. 4.70 A and 4.70B). Cellular pleomorphism is a characteristic feature of neuroblastoma. Frequently, areas of totally undifferentiated cells (sympathogonia) and mature ganglion cells are observed in the same tumor. In areas of undifferentiated tumor cells, distinction between a neuroblastoma and an anaplastic lymphosarcoma can be difficult. A distinguishing feature of neuroblastoma, however, is that the lymphocytelike cells are characteristically arranged in a rosette formation. In more differentiated tumors (ganglioblastomas, sympathicoblastomas), the cells

have more cytoplasm, and the short processes of the unipolar or bipolar tumor cells can be demonstrated by silver impregnation techniques.

ELECTRON MICROSCOPY. There is a remarkable similarity in the fine structure of neuroblastoma and malignant ganglioneuroma.[253,274] Three major ultrastructural types (A, B, and C) can be distinguished in neuroblastoma. In undifferentiated tumors, type A predominates, whereas in most of the common varieties all three types are encountered in the same tumors.

In type A, the tumor cells are loosely attached to one another and the cell surfaces are relatively smooth, with fine undulating surfaces devoid of interdigitations; a few desmosomes, however, are apparent. The nuclei are round, elliptical, or polygonal, have a rim of cytoplasm around the nucleus, and contain a few organelles.

In type B areas, the tumor cells are separated by numerous islands of cytoplasm that are actually tangential sections of cytoplasmic processes. Occasionally, several cells are arranged in a rosettelike fashion. The nuclei in type B cells are smaller, with a larger cytoplasmic rim containing well-developed endoplasmic reticulum and organelles. In contrast to type A, there is a myriad of cytoplasmic processes and invagination.

The cells of type C areas have polymorphic nuclei with prominent nucleoli. There is more cytoplasm associated with these cells than with types A and B. The cytoplasm is characterized by the presence of dense-cored vesicles ranging from 100 to 400 nm in diameter. Numerous unmyelinated axons are also seen in type C areas.

The tumor cells and the cytoplasmic processes in neuroblastoma lack a basement membrane, even where their cell surfaces border a perivascular space. Amorphous homogenous material containing scanty collagen fibers and large numbers of microfibrils fill the intercellular spaces; microfibrillary bundles with characteristic periodic striation are also seen.[253]

Neuroblastoma has the highest rate of spontaneous regression of any solid tumor in man.[253,275] It is characterized by a spectrum of varying degrees of maturation of the tumor cells. At one end of the spectrum is a highly undifferentiated small cell (type A) and at the other end are ganglioneuromas composed solely of mature cell types. Therefore, the histopathol-

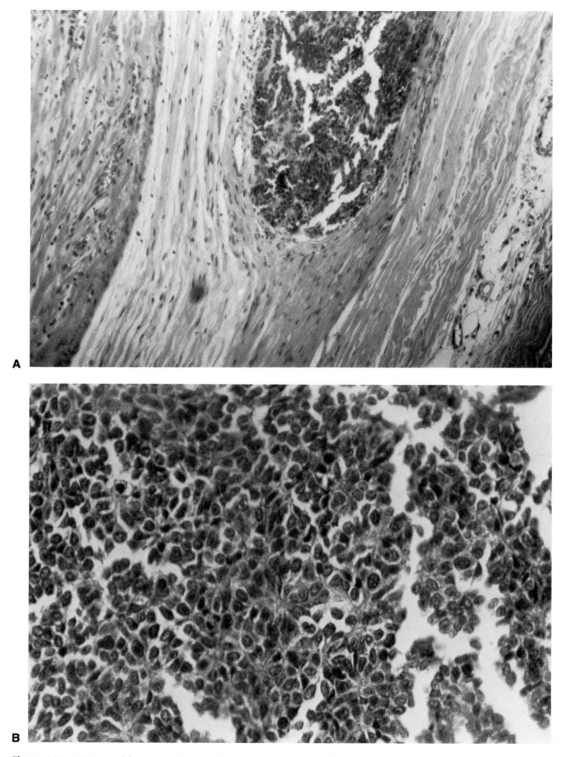

Figure 4.70. **(A)** Neuroblastoma arising in the peroneal nerve of a 25-year-old man. Note the localized area of the tumor along the course of the nerve. (H & E. Original magnification ×65.) **(B)** Same tumor under higher power showing the classical rosette formation. (H & E. Original magnification ×300.)

ogist is left with the responsibility of correlating morphologic features with the biologic behavior of these tumors. In 1968, Beckwith and Martin[276] proposed such a correlation. Their work has since been corroborated by McKinen[277] and by Hughes and co-workers.[278] In contrast, Lauder and Aherne[279] suggested that the prognosis was not related to maturation, but to the degree of lymphocytic infiltration within the tumor.

Histologic grading has been done on the basis of the proportional presence of differentiated versus undifferentiated cells. Beckwith and Martin[276] proposed a quantitative classification, whereas McKinen[277] and Hughes and co-workers[278] proposed a simple histologic grading. It seems that by either of these methods similar conclusions can be reached. The histologic grading proposed by Hughes and co-workers, being more practical, is described in this section.

The tumors can be classified as follows: *Grade 1* tumors show a mixed pattern of undifferentiated cells and mature ganglion cells. *Grade 2* tumors show a mixed pattern of undifferentiated cells and some cells show evidence of partial differentiation toward ganglion cells, as indicated by any of the following: (1) vesicular nuclei, (2) the presence of nucleoli, (3) increased cytoplasmic nuclear ratio, (4) formation of the cytoplasmic process. *Grade 3* tumors are totally undifferentiated.

Most authors[148,276–278] have found that with grade 1, the survival rate is excellent and with grade 3, poor. Hughes et al.[278] reported only three-year crude survival and found that of 13 patients with grade 1, 9 (69 percent) survived; of 22 with grade 2, only 9.1 percent survived; and out of 48 with grade 3, only 6.2 percent survived. In Beckwith and Martin's[276] series, the patients were classified in finer detail and quantitatively. The 5-year survival rate was as follows: with grade 1, 5 out of 5 patients; with grade 2, 3 out of 4; with grade 3, 4 of 13 (30 percent); and finally, with grade 4, only 1 of 28 (25 percent).

The majority of these tumors in children younger than 2 years of age are either grade 1 or 2. In older children the tumors are more undifferentiated and carry an unfavorable prognosis.[279]

Malignant Pheochromocytoma. This tumor is so rare that there is some controversy as to its very existence. In general, if a pheochromocytoma proves fatal, it is attributable to the action of pressor amines. Although in some tumors the microscopic characteristics of hyperchromatic nuclei, giant cells, immature cells, and many mitoses are occasionally seen, there is no evidence that these features are indicative of a clinically malignant neoplasm. The presence of distant metastases, the tissues of which are chromaffin-positive in locations where chromaffin tissue ordinarily does not occur, is the only proof of a malignant pheochromocytoma.[148]

Malignant Carotid Body Tumors. Malignant carotid body tumors are rare.[280] The microscopic criteria generally used to distinguish between a benign and malignant tumor are not reliable. Occasionally, local infiltration might be considered as a sign of low-grade malignancy. If strict criteria for both microscopic and clinical behavior of a malignancy are applied, the majority of reported malignant carotid body tumors will be found to be benign.

Malignant Nonchromaffin Paraganglioma. The histogenesis of these tumors is still unclear. Some authors believe that histologically they resemble alveolar soft tissue sarcoma and should be so classified (see section later in chapter).

TUMORS AND TUMORLIKE CONDITIONS OF SYNOVIAL TISSUE

Synovial membrane is a derivative of the embryonic mesenchyme lining the nonarticular parts of the synovial joints, the synovial bursae, and the synovial tendon sheaths.[135,281]

In the human embryo at five weeks the skeletal blastema of each limb is a continuous unsegmented core of condensed mesenchyme. In this core the prechondral and, later, cartilaginous centers of individual bones differentiate and extend. As they approach each other, parts of the undifferentiated blastema are left between them. These are the interchondral discs, the rudiments of the future joints. From these discs develop all the joint tissues, including the synovial membrane. Where the synovial and cartilaginous tissues are continuous, distinction between the two, and also between them and the neighboring tissues, is indefinite. The close histogenetic kinship of fibrous, osseous, cartilaginous, and synovial tissue is nowhere better displayed than in these junctional tissues of joints. Here the normal histologic features might show many metaplastic changes of mesenchymal tissues.

In postnatal life, the synovial tissue is a pink, smooth, moist, shiny membrane lining the nonarticular parts of the synovial joints, bursae, and tendon sheaths. Although the free surfaces are formed by cells, they are not aligned in a continuous layer. Rather, they are intermittently arranged and embedded in surrounding collagenous tissue. This provides the nidus for synovial cells away from the actual joint cavity.[135,281] The inner surface of the synovial membrane is occasionally lined with synovial villi; elsewhere, the membrane is thrown into numerous folds projecting into the joint cavity. An accumulation of adipose tissue is characteristic of synovial membrane.

Structurally, synovial membrane varies considerably in different regions, but essentially it consists of a cellular intima resting upon a vascular connective tissue, subintima (subsynovial tissue). The subintima is loose and areolar but often contains organized laminae of collagen and elastin fibers running parallel to the membrane surface, between which are scattered fibroblasts, macrophages, lipoblasts, and mast cells, frequently contributing to confusion in the diagnosis of these tumors. The subintimal adipose cells that accumulate as fat pads are arranged in compact lobules surrounded by fibroelastic interlobular septa. In contrast, where the synovial membrane lines intrinsic ligaments or intercapsular tendons, the subintima is difficult to distinguish as a separate zone, since it is formed of fibrous tissue that merges with that of the adjacent capsule or tendon.

A *synovioblast* is the stem cell for all types of synovial cells. Ultrastructurally, two cells types, A and B, have been recognized,[282] but cells with intermediate characteristics are common, and perhaps the differences described merely reflect stages of functional activity rather than distinct cell lineages (Fig. 4.71).

Type A synovial cells predominate and are characterized by surface filopodia, plasma membrane invaginations, and associated micropinocytotic vesicles. Their cytoplasm contains numerous mitochondria, varieties of lysosomes, a system of cytoplasmic filaments, a particularly prominent Golgi apparatus, and associated smooth-walled vesicles, but profiles of endoplasmic reticulum are scanty. Neighboring cells are separated by distinct gaps, but where they approach closely their surfaces may be complex and interdigitated. Synovial type A cells are the sites of hyaluronate synthesis.[281] In type

B synovial cells, most of the above characteristics are poorly developed; however, they contain a wealth of rough endoplasmic reticulum, varying from small, round, or oval profiles to a large, flattened, intercommunicating cisternae, together with scattered free cytoplasmic ribosomes. Both cell types contain glycogen deposits, but lipid inclusions are rare, as are perinuclear centrioles.

The tumors and tumorlike conditions are distinctive growths that reproduce many of the histologic and cytologic features of normal synovial tissue. These features include the coexistence of pleomorphic synovial cells and fibroblastic tissue, indications of the persistence of developmental clefts and crypts, the formation of spaces and papillary processes lined by synovial cells, and the presence of mucopolysaccharides and extracellular mucin. However, a number of authors[122,283-286] believe that the term implies only that neoplastic mesenchymal cells have reached a characteristic pattern of differentiation resembling the morphology of synovial membrane.

Although most benign growths of the synovial tissue are structurally characteristic and simple in form, the existence of a truly benign neoplasm of the synovial tissue has been questioned. Jaffe[287] preferred to regard these growths as hyperplastic inflammatory responses rather than true neoplasms. It is well known that arthritic overgrowths of the synovial tissue around a knee joint are often difficult to distinguish from true neoplasms. Frequently these lesions have a villous configuration and contain giant cells, lipid-laden phagocytes, and hemosiderin. For these lesions, the term *pigmented villonodular synovitis* was introduced.[287] But whether true neoplasms arise in these florid hyperplastic villous reactions of synovial tissue, or how many of the so-called benign synoviomas are only tumorlike conditions, is still a matter of controversy. Although this histologic question is intriguing, the clinical significance of such a discussion is important only insofar as determining whether these lesions require any treatment, whether after excision there is a tendency for recurrence, and finally, whether there is any evidence that some or any of these tumors, at any stage of their evolution, become malignant.

Frequently these tumefactions are seen as a single solid tumor in and around a joint and tendon sheath, and excision becomes necessary to rule out the possibility of a malignant tumor.

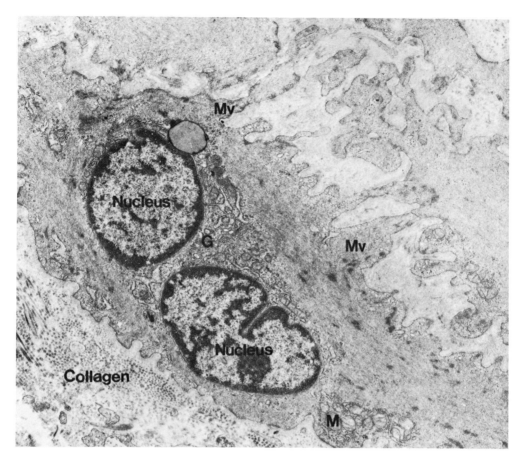

Figure 4.71. Electron micrograph of a human synovial membrane showing the predominant cell types. Type A cytoplasm contains occasional inclusion bodies, mitochondria (M). The cytoplasm is uniquely devoid of rough-surfaced endoplasmic reticulum. Type B cell cytoplasm is characterized by relative abundance of rough-surfaced endoplasmic reticulum. In this micrograph, subsynovial tissue is not seen. (Mv = microvilli, G = Golgi zone. Original magnification ×22,800.)

The anatomic relationship of the growth to the surrounding tendon sheaths and joints determines the completeness of its removal, thereby influencing the likelihood of recurrence. Tumors that recur almost invariably have a high degree of cellularity, and there are infrequent reports of malignancy developing in the recurrence of previously histologically benign lesions.[148] However, malignant transformation of a villonodular synovitis is highly unlikely.

From this morass of cytologic detail it is probably appropriate to seek a clinically acceptable classification of tumor and tumorlike conditions relating to synovial tissue. A simplified classification is given below:

A. Benign tumorlike conditions
  1. Synovioma
  2. Villonodular synovitis
  3. Giant cell tumors
  4. Ganglion
B. Malignant Tumors
  1. Synovial sarcoma (malignant synovioma)
  2. Clear cell sarcoma of tendon sheaths
  3. Giant cell tumor of soft tissue
  4. Epithelioid sarcoma

Benign Tumorlike Conditions

Synovioma (Fig. 4.72). Infrequently a localized swelling around the knee joint is encountered.

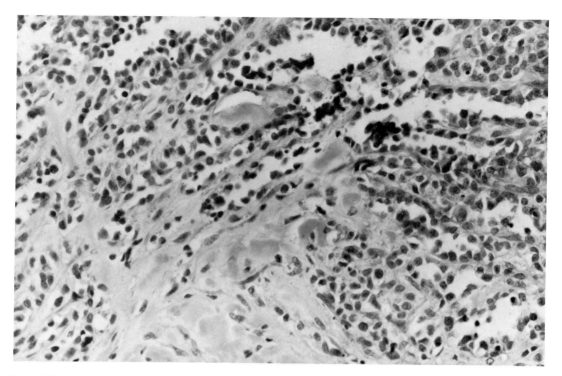

Figure 4.72. Benign synovioma. Photomicrograph of a well-delineated tumor of the joint showing slitlike spaces lined by cuboidal cells with bland nuclei. (H & E. Original magnification × 250.)

Morphologically these tumors consist of fibrous stroma in which mature synovial cells are interspersed. The clefts are reminiscent of the synovial spaces in the joint capsule and the overall histologic appearance is somewhat similar to that of synovial sarcoma. There is some controversy as to whether this entity should be separately classified or is indeed a form of villonodular synovitis.

In a strict sense, the following three tumorlike conditions cannot be classified as synovial tumors, since villonodular synovitis and giant cell tumors are variants of a fibrous histiocytoma (discussed earlier in chapter), and a ganglion is not even a true tumor. However, these three lesions are all benign, they arise in close association with tendons and joints, and they clinically resemble a synovial tumor. For these reasons, all three entities are operationally grouped in the category of benign synovial tumors.

Villonodular Synovitis. This is a relatively common entity frequently seen in conjunction with the flexor tendons of the fingers, the wrist, the toes, and the ankles, but seldom around a large, weight-bearing joint. These lesions can be single or multiple and frequently take the shape of the tendon with which they are associated or to which they are attached. Depending on the local extension, the incidence of recurrence can be high. Although the general histologic appearance is similar to that of localized benign synoviomas, these lesions exhibit a preponderance of inflammatory cells (Fig. 4.73A and 4.73B). Hemosiderosis is almost a constant accompaniment. The presence of iron lends the characteristic color to these tumors.

Giant Cell Tumor. This fibrous growth is variable in appearance, depending upon the number of fibroblasts and multinucleated giant cells of the foreign body type (see Fig. 4.26).

Ganglion. This is a cystic swelling of the tendon sheaths of the joint capsules, especially of the tendons of the hands and the feet. Mainly it is of myxoid tissue. Sometimes the high con-

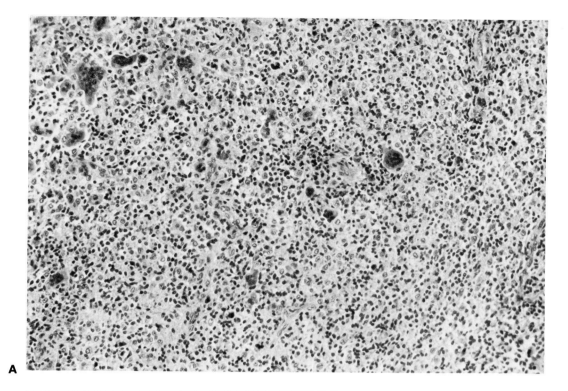

A

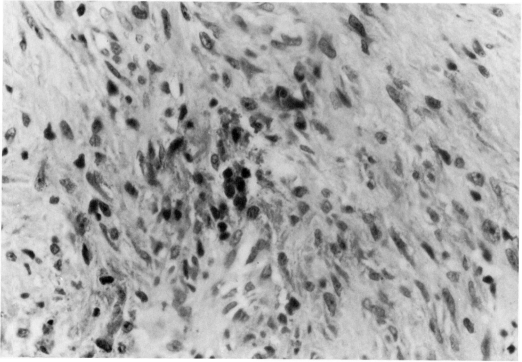

B

Figure 4.73. **(A)** Villonodular synovitis. Note the blending of histiocyte foam cells, stromal round cells, and inflammatory cells. A few giant cells are scattered throughout the field. (H & E. Original magnification ×125.) **(B)** Higher power, showing the fibrous stroma with loose scattering of histiocytes and hemosiderin granules. (H & E. Original magnification ×375.)

tent of mucopolysaccharides leads to the development of multilocular cysts obliterating the peripheral cells.

Malignant Tumors

Synovial Sarcoma (Malignant Synovioma). These relatively rare tumors usually arise from the soft tissues of the extremities of young adults.[283–285,288] Frequently they are found around joints, tendons, and bursae, but some are relatively remote from a specific joint, eg, those in the neck,[289–291] chest, or abdominal wall,[283,292] or even the larynx.[293] Common sites for synovial sarcoma include the wrist, the ankle, the hands and feet, the shoulder region, and the hip and knee.[148,283–285,288,294] Seldom do these tumors arise from the lining of a joint cavity, and if the synovial membrane is involved, it is usually due to direct extension.[148,194]

Macroscopic Appearance (Fig. 4.74A and 4.74B). The appearance of these tumors depends on the site of origin, the duration, and the rate of growth. In general, they are limited by a pseudocapsule of compressed and attenuated adjacent tissue. They develop as a firm, lobulated, gray or light brown mass of varying size that grows chiefly by expansion, and they can be predominantly vascular. In bulky tumors, areas of necrosis or cystic spaces containing a jellylike amorphous material are common.

Light Microscopy Features (Fig. 4.75A to 4.75C). The pattern is striking because usually the tumors are extremely pleomorphic. A distinctive feature of synovial sarcoma is the differentiation into pseudoglandular cystlike cavities and clefts devoid of basement membrane. Frequently, the cells lining these spaces secrete a periodic acid-Schiff (PAS)-positive and mucicarminophilic material. This material is hyaluronic acid and probably represents attempts by the synovioblasts to form synovial structures.[3] Pseudoglandular spaces are more common in well-differentiated tumors than in the undifferentiated types resembling fibrosarcoma, and a prolonged search of different areas of the tumor is often required before these pathognomonic histologic features can be identified. The cells filling the spaces between these clefts are spindle-shaped, show mitoses, are accompanied by reticulin fibers, and resemble fibroblasts.

Electron Microscopy (Fig. 4.76A to 4.76D). Examination of ultrathin sections usually reveals a distinct biphasic cell population, the columnar

epitheliumlike cells forming the pseudoglandular structures and the stromal cells resembling fibroblasts. In a low-power view, the epithelial stroma junction is differentiated by a discrete basement membrane of varying thickness. Roth and associates[290] calculated that the thickness varies from 1500 to 5500 Å. In undifferentiated tumors, the basement membrane is frequently disrupted, with resultant contiguity of stromal and epithelial type cells.[295]

The epithelial type cells are usually of different cytoplasmic density and, according to the degree of osmiophilia, can be classified into light and dark cells (types A and B); frequently an intermediate variety is encountered.

The light cells (type A) contain an oval nuclei with evenly dispersed chromatin. The cytoplasm of these cells has an abundance of smooth-surfaced endoplasmic reticulum. Fine granular material within the dilated spaces of rough endoplasmic reticulum is commonly observed. Microfilaments, which are a frequent accompaniment to the epithelial type cells, are usually found in abundance in the light cells.

The dark cells (type B) contain irregularly shaped nuclei with coarse chromatin clumping. The general cytoplasmic morphology of these cells is similar to that of their counterpart, but there is less osmiophilia. However, few differences are noted on close scrutiny. In the cytoplasm of the dark cells, there is less concentration of endoplasmic reticulum, resulting in a lesser concentration of fine granular material within the dilated spaces. There is also a general diminution of microfilaments and microtubules in these cells. Desmosomes and interdigitating cytoplasmic processes are frequently seen.

Synovial cell sarcomas involve regional nodes, albeit less frequently than has been reported.[296] The incidence of nodal involvement is shown in Table 15.2, Chapter 15. However, these data reflect the incidence during the entire natural history of the disease. Therefore, as a general guideline it can be assumed that the incidence of regional metastases is higher in locally advanced cases and in highly pleomorphic tumors.

Clear Cell Sarcoma of Tendons and Aponeuroses. This entity was first described by Enzinger[297] in 1965. Its uniform, distinctive clinical and morphologic pattern distinguishes it from other groups of tenosynovial tumors.[122]

Clear cell sarcomas are slow-growing and

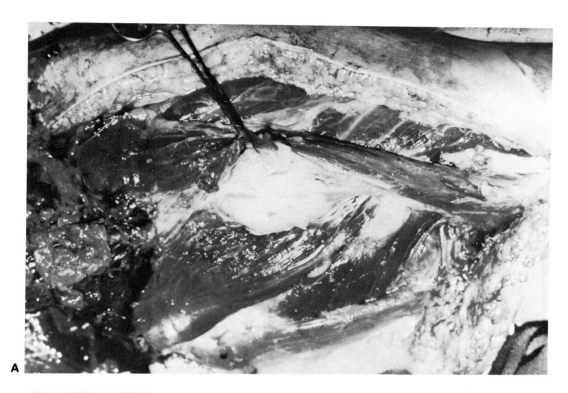

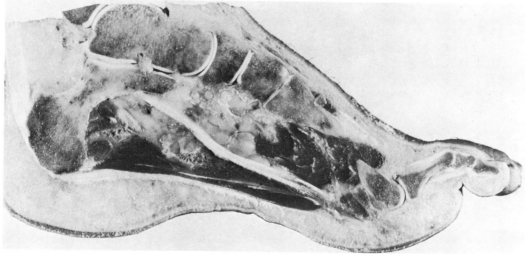

Figure 4.74. **(A)** Recurrent synovial sarcoma of the medial thigh in a 31-year-old woman. The lesion was locally excised six months previously. A hip joint disarticulation with groin dissection and adjuvant chemotherapy was the treatment. Note tumor infiltrating the adductor group of muscles. Proximally the tumor extended up to the base of the femoral triangle. Patient has lived free of disease for seven years. **(B)** Sagittal view of the bisected specimen of synovial sarcoma of the left foot. The tumor has extended to several compartments. *(Fig. 4.74B courtesy of Drs. R.M. Barone and S. Saltzstein of San Diego, Ca.)*

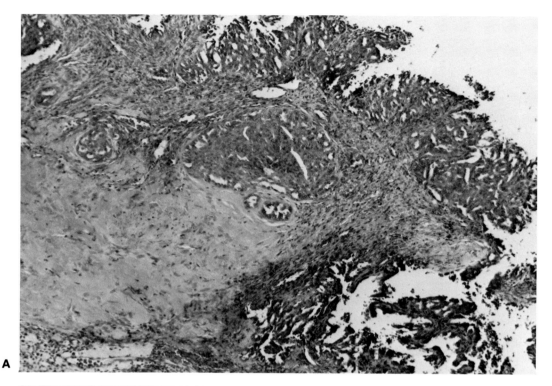

A

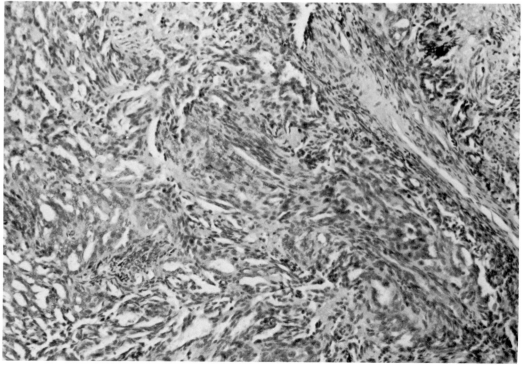

B

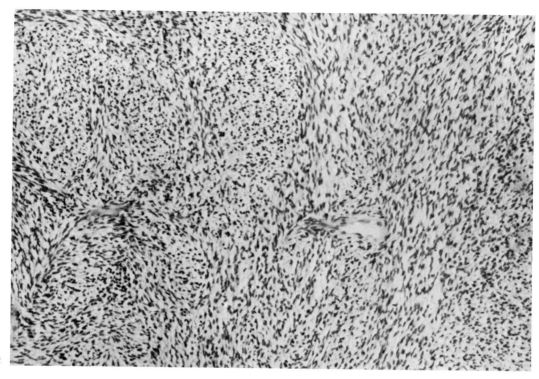

C

Figure 4.75. Synovial cell sarcoma. **(A)** The papillary nature of tumor is apparent. (Original magnification ×65.) **(B)** Two types of cells can be seen: cuboidal cells forming or trying to form glands, which are engulfed by spindle-shaped cells. (H & E. Original magnification ×250.) **(C)** After five years the tumor recurred and only the spindle cells were noted (original magnification ×125), making it monophasic.

are commonly seen in association with tendons and aponeuroses around the knee and ankle joints.[122,297–303] According to Enzinger,[297] they have a predilection for young women. Because these tumors are intimately adherent to the surrounding tendons and aponeuroses, simple local excision usually leaves behind a residue of the tumor, with resultant local recurrence and metastases.

The overall microstructure of these tumors resembles that of synovial sarcoma (Fig. 4.77). However, the lack of a classic biphasic pattern and the overall rarity of the pseudoglandular clefts favor a diagnosis of clear cell sarcoma of the tendon sheaths. The monotony of the microscopic appearance with the disappearance of PAS-positive material following diastase treatment separates these tumors from the classic types of synovial sarcoma.

A variant of clear cell sarcoma of the tendon sheath and aponeurosis is infrequently encoun-

tered. In this variant, intracytoplasmic pigment has been noted.[298–303] Hoffman and Carter[300] found the intracytoplasmic pigment in their patients to be melanin. Similar findings of melanin production by tumor cells have been reported by others.[299,302,303] We have also encountered one such patient. The presence of melanin certainly confuses the issue of histogenesis. An origin from neural crest cells associated with a peripheral nerve is worthy of consideration[298] but, for the present, cannot be substantiated. The biologic behavior of this variant is similar to that of synovial cell sarcoma.

Electron microscopic examination of some of these tumors shows that they closely resemble synovial sarcomas.[298,302] Kubo[301] found two types of epithelial-like cells with basement membrane and stromal cells resembling fibroblasts. Although the cell of origin should be further investigated, it is suggested that from a clinical standpoint these tumors be considered,

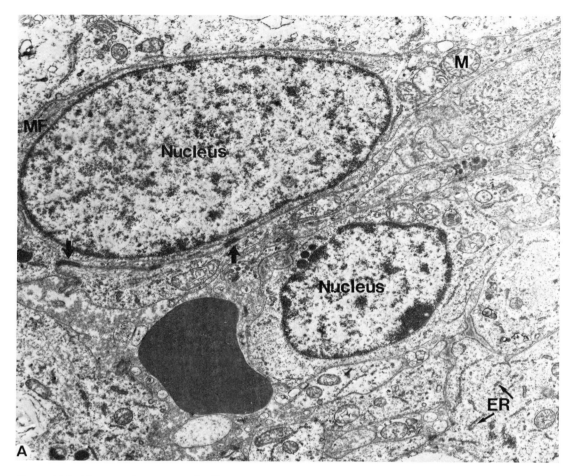

Figure 4.76. (A) Monophasic synovial cell sarcoma. In this micrograph, profiles of two type A cells are seen. The cytoplasm is characterized by an abundance of microfilaments (MF) and smooth membrane system. Also note the quality of fine granules in the rough endoplasmic reticulum (ER). A number of inclusion bodies resembling lysosomes are apparent. The two cells are connected by means of multiple desmosomes shown by arrows. Profiles of cytoplasmic processes are apparent. (Original magnification ×31,900.)

for the time being, as a variant of synovial sarcoma and their cell of origin be operationally assumed to be synovial.

Malignant Giant Cell Tumor of Soft Tissues (Fig. 4.78A and 4.78B). Malignant giant cell tumor of the soft tissue resembles a giant cell tumor of the bone and tendon sheath. In 1972, Guccion and Enzinger[304] analyzed 32 cases and delineated the clinical pathologic features and biologic behavior of these tumors. The patient age is usually between 41 and 80 years. These tumors occur predominantly in males; pain and

the presence of a mass are the two most common complaints. The most important laboratory finding is roentgenographic evidence of a soft tissue mass eroding the cortex of the adjacent bone. These tumors are classified into superficial and deep. The superficial tumors are usually less than 5 cm, while the deep ones can grow up to 30 cm. They may be bossulated or oval, with a pseudocapsule. The tumor is tan, with areas of hemorrhage and necrosis. Foci of bone are occasionally noted at the edge.

Histologically this tumor is characterized by pleomorphic multinucleated giant cells, mononuclear histiocytes, and bizarre to pleo-

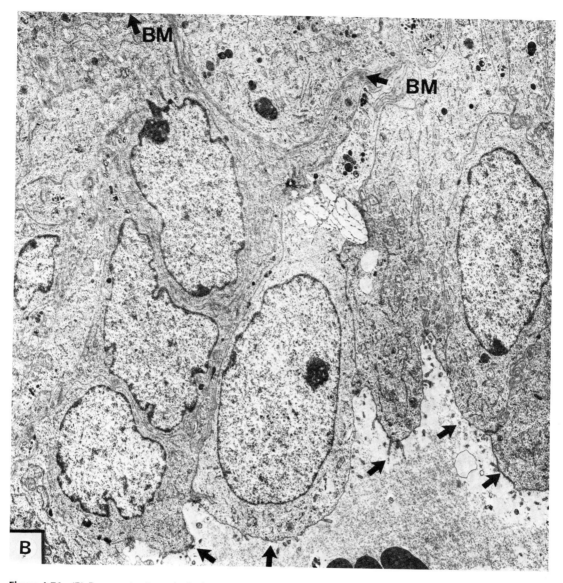

Figure 4.76. (B) Panoramic view of a biphasic synovial cell sarcoma. Both type A and type B cells are apparent. The basal lamina is discrete and can be seen in the upper part (BM) of the micrograph. The lower part of the micrograph shows that several epithelioid cells containing microvilli (arrows) are bordering the cleftlike lumen. The lumen is filled with amorphous material. (Original magnification ×22,000.)

morphic fibroblasts, either arranged around large vascular spaces or clumped in a nodular fashion. The multinucleated giant cells are thought to be neoplastic rather than reactive because of their presence in distant metastasis and blood vessels. They may have formed by fusion or amitotic division, or by phagocytosis of their mononuclear precursor; they contain hemosiderin and osteoid bodies. The osteoid bodies stain best by phosphotungstic acid-hemotoxylin. Chondroblastic and osteoblastic differentiation with formation of cartilage and bone is occasionally observed (Fig. 4.78B).

The formation of bone makes it difficult to

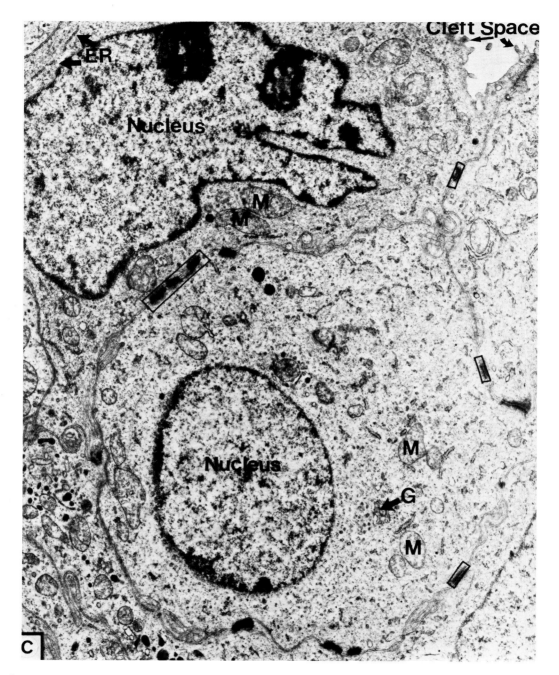

Figure 4.76. **(C)** Higher power. Note the multiple desmosomal contacts (marked by boxes) that type A cells have with surrounding cell processes and one type B cell above. Prominent Golgi zone (G) in the type A cells is easily seen. Upper right-hand corner shows microvilli (arrows) lining a cleft space. (Original magnification ×30,800.)

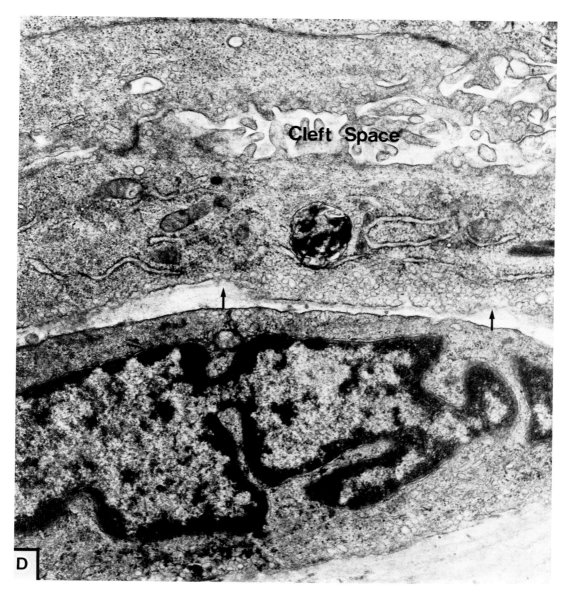

Figure 4.76. **(D)** Higher-power view showing the protruding microvilli in the cleftlike space of a biphasic synovial cell sarcoma. (Original magnification ×46,460.)

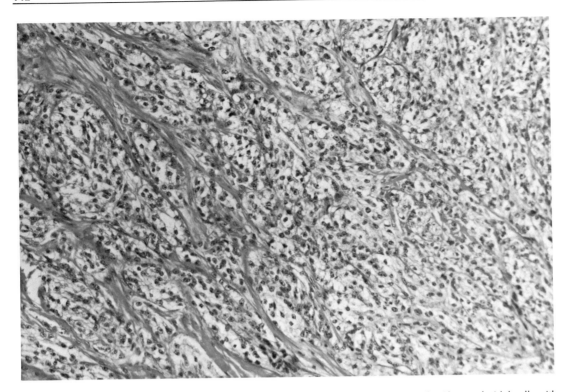

Figure 4.77. Clear cell sarcoma of tendon sheath. The tumors are composed of clusters of uniform cuboidal cells with clear or finely granular cytoplasm and well-delineated cell border. (H & E. Original magnification ×125.)

differentiate these tumors from the osteocytic variety of osteogenic sarcoma with numerous giant cells. For the present, these tumors should be considered a variant of synovial cell sarcoma.

Epithelioid Sarcoma. This is an unusual tumor often confused histologically with several other neoplasms, including malignant melanoma, granulomatous lesions, and, occasionally, metastatic adenocarcinoma.[97,305–308] In 1970, Enzinger[307] analyzed 62 cases and named this entity epithelioid sarcoma. This descriptive term is now generally accepted.

Epithelioid sarcoma is commonly seen as a subfascial or subcutaneous lesion, usually originating in the extremities. Infrequently, it occurs in the trunk and scalp, and two cases have been reported arising in the penile shaft.[309]

Macroscopic Appearance. The appearance of these tumors varies according to their location. When they occur in the vicinity of a tendon near a joint, multiple nodular tumors along the course of the tendon sheath are observed. When lo-

cated deep in the subcutaneous tissue, there is no characteristic feature other than a relatively diffuse tumor.

Light Microscopy (Fig. 4.79A to 4.79C). The microscopic appearance of these lesions has been well described by Enzinger,[307] Santiago et al.,[310] Gabbiani et al.,[311] and Pratt et al.[305] In general, the histologic appearance of epithelioid sarcomas can be divided into the following five types: (1) granulomatous, (2) pseudocarcinomatous pattern, (3) melanomalike appearance, (4) angiosarcomatous, and (5) undifferentiated sarcomatous pattern. Either all or most of these features can be seen in different areas of a given tumor. Santiago and associates[310] suggested that the angiosarcomatous pattern probably represents a fixation artifact. Cytologically the tumor cells are large, round, or polygonal, with abundant eosinophilic cytoplasm and round or oval nuclei with prominent nucleoli. Poorly differentiated spindle cells with collagenous ground substance are interspersed throughout the tumor.

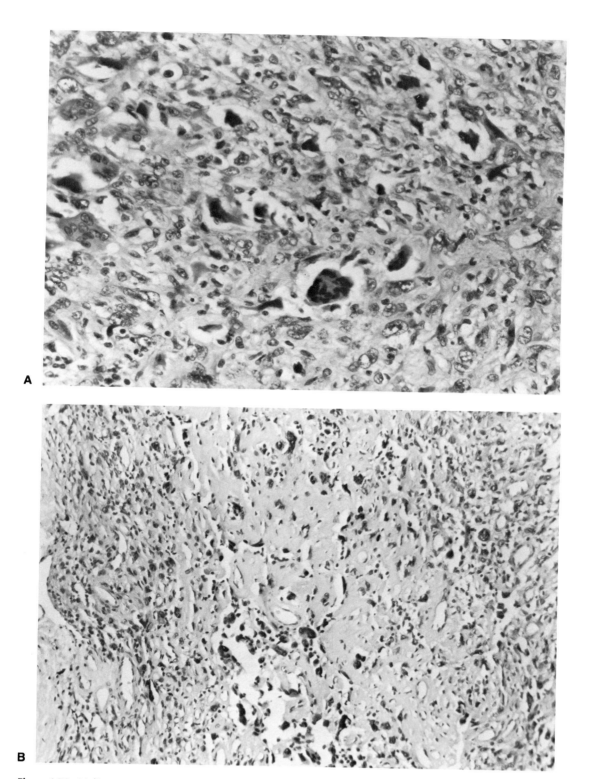

Figure 4.78. Malignant giant cell tumor. **(A)** The tumor consists of multinucleated giant cells, pleomorphic mononuclear histocytes, and fibroblasts. (H & E. Original magnification ×250.) **(B)** Low power, showing osteoblastic differentiation. (H & E. Original magnification ×125.) *(Courtesy of Dr. P. Szanto, Department of Pathology, Cook County Hospital, Chicago.)*

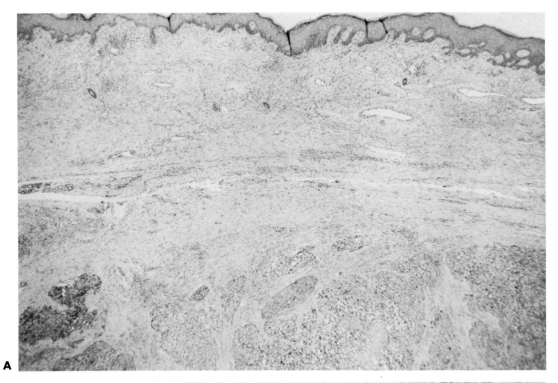

A

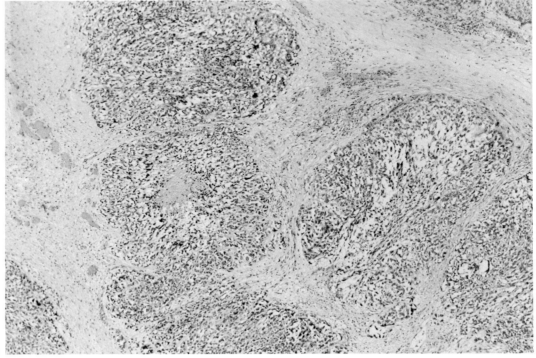

B

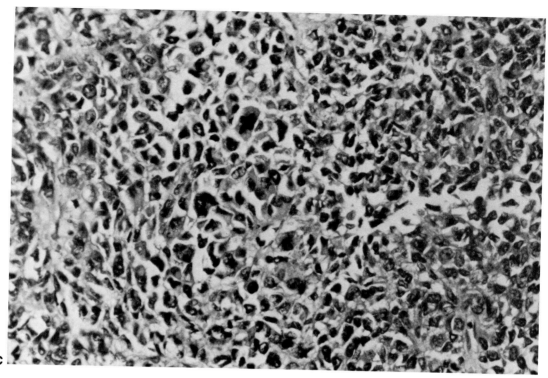

Figure 4.79. Epithelioid sarcoma. **(A)** The tumor is usually located close to the skin. (H & E. Original magnification ×25.) **(B)** The microscopic architecture is clear in relatively higher power. The tumor is composed of clusters of clear oval cells with central necrosis. The necrosis is obvious in the cluster at left. (H & E. Original magnification ×40.) **(C)** Higher power, same area, showing pleomorphic nuclei and abnormal mitosis. (H & E. Original magnification ×250.)

Electron Microscopy. Ultrastructural studies of these tumors have been published by Enzinger,[307] Gabbiani et al.,[311] Frable et al.,[312] and by Bloustein and associates.[313] These tumors consist of epithelial like cells similar to those found in normal synovial membrane,[282] synovial sarcoma,[290,295] and clear cell sarcomas of the tendon sheaths and aponeurosis.[302] On the basis of these studies and the clinical features (see Table 15.7, Chapter 15), epithelioid sarcoma can be considered as another variant of synovial sarcoma.

TUMORS AND TUMORLIKE CONDITIONS OF THE VASOFORMATIVE TISSUES

Primitive angioblastic tissue differentiates from the mesenchyme in the chorionic end of the body stalk and in the mesoderm lining the chorion. The cells of the mesoderm give rise to solid strands of angioblasts, each of which coalesces and eventually becomes blood vessels. The earliest blood vessels, therefore, develop at several separate sites. From the walls of these vessels buds grow outward, become canalized, and anastomose with neighboring vessels, forming a rich vascular network. By the end of the fourth week, the human embryo has a well-developed vascular system with a beating heart.[135] Willis[135] found that in the healing of granulation tissue, embryonic methods of new vessel formation come into operation. A similar phenomenon probably can explain the histogenesis of some of the benign and malignant vascular angiomas.

There are two divergent views as to the initial stages of development of the lymphatic system.[135] In the early part of this century it was thought that lymphatic spaces commence as clefts in the mesenchyme and that their living cells take on the characteristics of the endothelium. These spaces coalesce and form a network from which the lymph sacs, eg, cisternae chyle, develop. In 1969, Kampmeier[314] concluded that the balance of argument is in favor of their developing independently of the venous system. In the human embryo of two to four months the lymphatics of the neck, mediastinum, and retroperitoneum are relatively large, easily identifiable, thin-walled vessels. In hamartomas of the lymphatic system these spaces are unusually enlarged and become clinically important.

Tumors and Tumorlike Conditions of the Vascular System

Vascular tissue can be the site of several types of benign and malignant neoplasms. They can be classified as follows:

A. Benign
  1. Hemangioma
  2. Angiomatoses
  3. Benign hemangiopericytoma (smooth muscle origin)
  4. Glomus tumor (glomangioma)

B. Malignant
  1. Angiosarcoma (malignant hemangioendothelioma)
  2. Malignant hemangiopericytoma (smooth muscle origin)
  3. Kaposi's hemangiosarcoma

Benign Tumors.

Hemangioma. The exact nature of hemangiomas has been a matter of concern over the years. They appear to be hamartomatous disorders. The term *hamartoma* signifies a tumorlike, but primarily non-neoplastic, malformation or inborn error of tissue development characterized by an abnormal mixture of tissues indigenous to the part, with an excess of one or more of the component structures constituting the tissue. Although the excessive tissue in hamartomas is essentially malformational and not neoplastic, it sometimes gives rise to a true neoplasm.[135] That hemangiomas are not true tumors is shown by the following observations: (1) Most are congenital or appear soon after birth, eg, birthmarks. Visceral angiomas, however, are usually discovered later in life, although a number of these tumors, along with systemic angiomatosis, are diagnosed in children (see Fig. 16.8, Chapter 16). (2) No sharp line of demarcation can be drawn between "angiomas" and

acknowledged vascular malformations, eg, cirsoid aneurysms. (3) The common angiomas do not grow disproportionately and indefinitely as true neoplasms do. Most grow along with the tissues of the part and do not involve a greater territory than the original part affected. Indeed, some, such as strawberry nevi, spontaneously regress after an initial burst of growth.[315] Accidental complications, such as traumatic hemorrhage, inflammation, thrombosis, or cystic changes, might cause an angioma to suddenly change in size and suggest malignant transformation of a preexisting benign tumor. Hemangiomas are discussed below as benign tumors.

The histopathologic findings of these lesions are difficult to describe without a review of the normal histologic appearance of the blood vessels.[316–318] The capillaries are composed of a lining of endothelial cells, a supporting sheath of reticulin and fibroblasts, and pericytes scattered over the outer surface of the sheath (Fig. 4.80). The capillaries consist of a tube lined by a single layer of polygonal endothelial cells which show variations in their fine structure and intercellular junctions. Surrounding the endothelial tube is usually a typical glycoprotein basal lamina, which at isolated points over the capillary splits to enclose flattened or branching perivascular cells (pericytes). The exact nature of pericytes is not understood. The basal lamina usually merges into an adventitial layer of fine reticular tissue, with occasional fibroblasts or mast cells, that borders the perivascular spaces. Variations in all these features form the basis of a variety of classifications, but broadly, a capillary may be considered as either continuous or fenestrated.[319]

Angiomas have been classified according to their composition (Fig. 4.81A and 4.81B). A hemangioma comprised of capillaries alone is termed a *capillary hemangioma.* In this variety the capillaries are arranged haphazardly, and if they are widely dilated the resulting tumor is called a *cavernous hemangioma.* Sometimes capillary angiomas in infants and children show proliferation of the endothelial layer. Stout and Lattes[3] coined the term *benign hemangioendothelioma* for these lesions. However, this distinction is not of great significance except for interpreting the most unusual form of malignant hemangioendothelioma.

Angiomatosis. Infrequently, angiomas are found to arise in a multitude of tissues. They are observed as a large dilation of vascular spaces

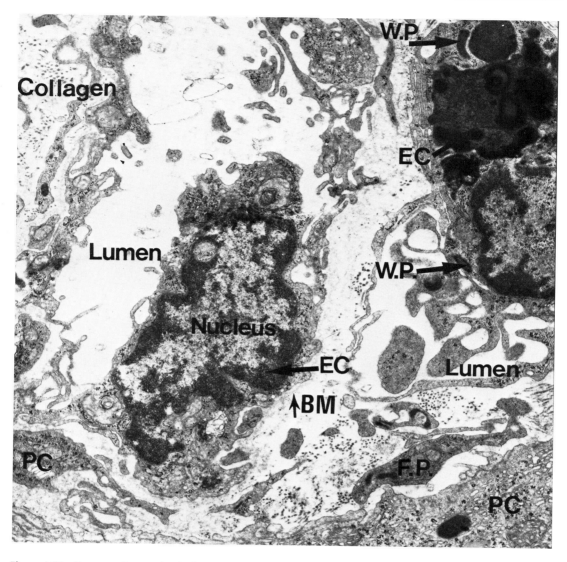

Figure 4.80. Electron micrograph of a human capillary from the skin showing the continuous endothelial lining, the endothelial cell (EC), pericyte (PC), and the basal lamina (BM). The endothelial cell contains Weibel-Palade bodies (WP). Several cytoplasmic processes of fibroblasts (FP) are also seen. (Original magnification ×15,000.)

both in the somatic tissues and in the viscera. This widespread distribution suggests a common developmental error. A description of these entities will be found in the section dealing with the clinical features of angiomas (Chapter 16).

Benign Hemangiopericytoma. Pericytes, referred to above, can proliferate as rounded or elongated cells just outside the reticulin sheath of the capillary and develop into a hemangiopericytoma. This tumor has been observed in

many parts of the body and in a number of viscera, including the brain.

Glomus Tumor (Glomangioma). This tumor, commonly seen as a painful nodule in the subungual regions, was first accurately described by Masson.[320] Glomus tumors seldom are larger than a few centimeters and are sporadically found elsewhere in the body.[321–323] Of the viscera, the stomach,[179,324–326] heart,[148] and uterus[327] are the three organs in which glomus tumors have been described. Intraosseous variants are occasionally seen in the terminal phalanges.[328]

The lesion is usually circumscribed and often limited by a well-defined fibrous capsule. The majority of glomus tumors are characterized by a collection of thick-walled vessels, between which are interspersed innumerable unmyelinated axons. Different degrees of glomus cell proliferation and varying ratios of cellular-to-vascular elements are exhibited by these tumors (Fig. 4.82A and 4.82B). The morphologic characteristics of these cells are similar to those of pericytes. Based on in vitro studies, Murray and Stout[329] concluded that these cells probably are pericytes. However, in recent years the actual histogenesis of glomus tumors[178,330–335] has been reassessed. Ultrastructural studies by Venka-

tachalam and Greally,[21] Murad and co-workers,[178] Toker,[335] and Tarnowski and Hashimoto[336] all tend to show that, morphologically, glomus cells resemble smooth muscle cells. All these authors concluded that with the recent ultrastructural evidence in hand these tumors should not be classified as hemangiopericytomas, but rather as smooth muscle tumors of the blood vessels.

Malignant Vascular Tumors. Confusion has been created with the use of several different terms to describe what is probably the same clinical entity. The term malignant hemangioendothelioma, coined by Mallory,[337] signifies a malignant vascular tumor in which the endothelial cells are dominant. Perhaps the designation of

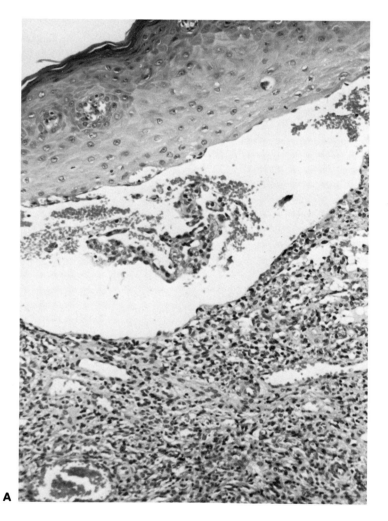

Figure 4.81. **(A)** Capillary hemangioma of the skin. All the capillaries are well developed and are full of red blood cells. Note the compression of dermal structures. (H & E. Original magnification ×125.) **(B)** Cavernous hemangioma; large blood spaces are lined by single layer of endothelium. (H & E. Original magnification ×125.)

A

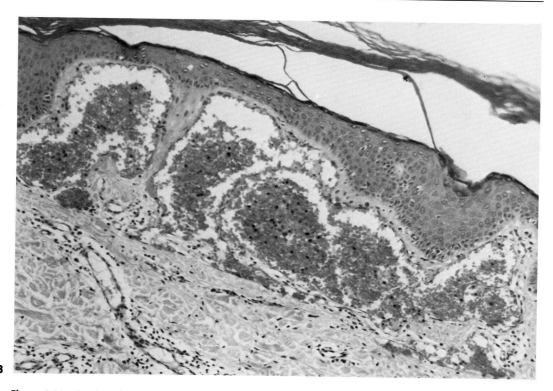

B

Figure 4.81. *Continued*

angiosarcoma would be more appropriate for all malignant tumors of the endothelium, recognizing that a histologic variant is hemangioendothelioma. However, the biologic behavior is the same, and hence the management is the same.

Angiosarcoma (Malignant Hemangioendothelioma). These tumors are found more frequently in the viscera[338-341] and bones[342,343] and less often in the soft tissues.[228,344,345] Of the soft tissue types, angiosarcoma of the breast[346] is probably the most common.

MACROSCOPIC FINDINGS. These tumors are extremely vascular. Frequently, however, either due to thrombosis or to the unusual proliferation of the endothelial lining, the cut surface consists of large, cystlike cavities.

MICROSCOPIC FINDINGS (FIG. 4.83A AND 4.83B). The microscopic variations found in this tumor are striking. These tumors in general are composed of anastomosing capillary channels lined by an aggregation of atypical endothelium. Sometimes the lining consists of one layer of polygonal or round cells, but frequently it

consists of heaped-up masses several layers thick. The proclivity for anastomoses of these vascular channels is sometimes such that the area acquires a papillary pattern. Extension into the surrounding tissues by the budding of capillary-like elements is also commonplace at the margins of angiosarcoma in which the central areas are more highly cellular and have a solid structure. In the so-called splenic hemangioendotheliomas, multinucleated giant cells are frequently seen. This occasionally complicates the microscopic diagnosis because of their similarity to choriocarcinoma. Sometimes hormonal determinations become necessary for a correct diagnosis.

ELECTRON MICROSCOPY (FIG. 4.83C AND 4.83D). Ultrastructural examination of the tumor shows the following characteristics: (1) *Vasculature.* There is an overgrowth of endothelial cells, manifested by an overall increase in vasculature without conspicuous changes in the endothelial lining. The numerical increase in endothelial cells is evident when these cells almost clog the lumen by bridging across it. (2)

Tumor cells. The cells lying between vascular channels throughout much of this tumor show considerable variability in morphology. The cells are scattered randomly and intercellular attachments are seldom seen. Cytoplasmic microfilaments are frequently observed, although inclusions of any type are rare. (3) *Interstitial matrix.* The interstitial matrix is composed of fine fibrillar or flocculent material.

Malignant Hemangiopericytoma. Malignant hemangiopericytoma is a rare form of tumor that grows slowly, remains well encapsulated for a long time, and occurs in all parts of the body,[342,347-358] including the mediastinum[350] and brain.[333]

MACROSCOPIC FINDINGS. This tumor has no specific macroscopic characteristics. Occasionally in larger tumors, cut surfaces show areas of necrosis, cyst formation, and hemorrhage (Fig. 4.84A and 4.84B).

MICROSCOPIC FINDINGS. A rich vasculature consisting of endothelial channels surrounded by round, ovoid, or fusiform, sometimes pale-staining cells (Fig. 4.84C and 4.84D) is the prominent feature of hemangiopericytoma. Although the histologic appearance is subject to considerable variation, all hemangiopericytomas have three main characteristics: (1) numerous vessels lined by apparently normal endothelium separated from the tumor cells by a layer of collagenous tissue; (2) proliferating parenchymal cells disposed as whorls or mantles around the connective tissue cuffs; and (3) a distinctive reticulin pattern.[148]

At the ultrastructural level the cells show extreme variations in shape and size from one

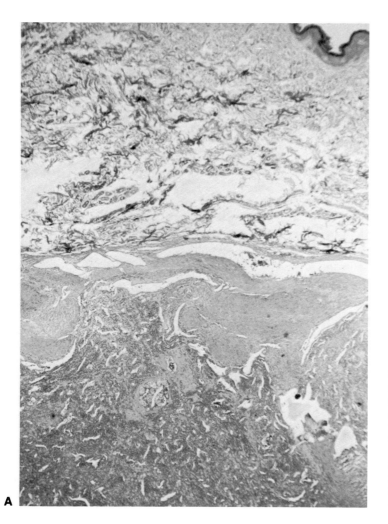

Figure 4.82. (A) Small foci of a subcutaneous glomus tumor. The glomus cells are arranged in cords along the blood spaces. (H & E. Original magnification × 25.) **(B)** Glomus cells arranged in layers lying in a hyaline matrix. (H & E. Original magnification × 125.) *(Courtesy of Dr. S. Ronan, Departments of Pathology and Dermatology, University of Illinois Hospital.)*

A

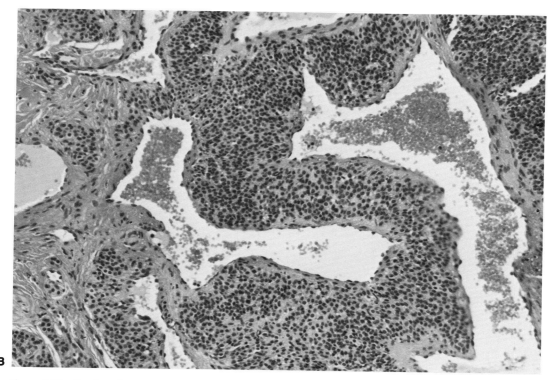

B

Figure 4.82. *Continued*

area to another. In one part the predominating cells are elongated, with irregular, large, and elongated nuclei. Other areas show ovoid cells with marked irregularity of the nuclear membrane. The intercellular spaces are filled with light osmiophilic material resembling basement membrane. The tumor cells have no basement membrane of their own and are separated from the endothelial cells by the basement membrane of the endothelial cells. The cytoplasm contains rough-surfaced endoplasmic reticulum with a moderate number of fine cristae. A few electron-dense granules may be present in the cytoplasm of tumor pericytes. In a few places, collagen fibers are seen in close proximity to tumor cells (Fig. 4.85A to 4.85C).

The histogenesis of malignant hemangiopericytoma, as with its benign counterpart (discussed earlier in chapter), is clouded with controversy.[21,178,330-336] Present data suggest that probably these tumors should be classified as malignant smooth muscle tumors.

It is frequently difficult to correlate histologic grading with prognosis, since many of these innocuous-looking tumors are found to have metastasized,[348,349] sometimes to the regional nodes but more commonly by vascular spread.

Kaposi's Disease (Kaposi's Sarcoma). Kaposi's disease was first described in 1872.[353] Since then, much interesting information has accrued regarding this entity.[354-357] Typically, in Kaposi's disease, multiple, purple, usually vascular, nodules first develop within the dermis of the distal part of the lower extremities. However, variations of the disease are immense. Involvement of the surrounding soft tissues, regional nodes, bones, and viscera is seen as well.

The histologic appearance of Kaposi's lesions varies considerably with the stage of the disease. In general, the lesion is composed of capillaries showing free anastomoses, and the space between the vessels is filled with red blood cells and lined with spindle-shaped cells and reticulin fibers (Fig. 4.86A to 4.86C). The microscopic appearance appears to be related to the duration of the tumor and has no particular prognostic significance.

Electron microscopic examination of Kaposi's sarcoma shows that the tumor is composed mainly of two cell types, hypertropic en-

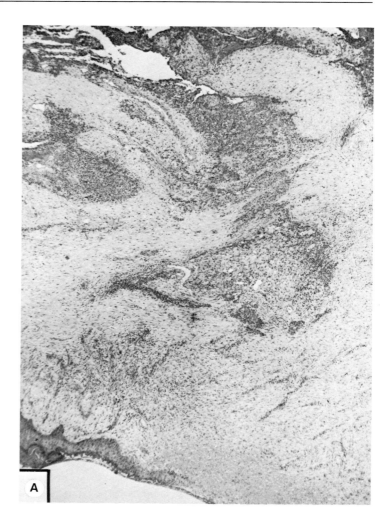

Figure 4.83. (A) Angiosarcoma of the soft tissues. Part of the skin can be seen in the lower left-hand corner. (H & E. Original magnification ×25.) (B) Close-up of the area seen in the upper left-hand corner of Figure 4.83A. Plump cuboidal tumor cells are seen projecting into the lumen in a papillary fashion. (H & E. Original magnification ×250.) (C) Micrograph of an angiosarcoma of the extremities. The neoplastic endothelial cells (Ec) are protruding into the lumen, almost obliterating it. Proliferating endothelial cells are haphazardly scattered throughout, with the usual cytoplasmic components. (Original magnification ×17,140.) (D) Higher-power view of a malignant endothelial cell protruding into the lumen. Note the cytoplasmic microfilaments (MF). Also note the intact basal lamina (BM) in this micrograph. (Original magnification ×20,540.)

dothelial cells and phagocytic fibroblasts. The endothelial cells show small numbers of lysosomes with sparsely distributed ferritin. The remaining characteristics of endothelial cells are well preserved. The fibroblasts, in contrast, resemble macrophages with numerous cytoplasmic phagosomes and ferritin-containing organelles. The interstitial area, as in other types of malignant vascular tumors, is clear with scanty collagen.

Histochemical studies show moderate localization of alkaline phosphatase, acid phosphatase, nonspecific esterases, and intense reaction to aminopeptidase activity. No phosphorylase activity is seen.[358]

Although electron microscopic studies show

that most of the malignant cells resemble endothelial cells, the cell of origin of Kaposi's sarcoma is still debated.[359,360] Dayan and Lewis,[361] using silver impregnation techniques, proposed that Kaposi's sarcoma originates from the reticuloendothelial tissue and might be related to Burkitt's lymphoma. The good response to alkylating agents in Kaposi's sarcoma[362] has continued to provide some justification for this hypothesis.

Tumors or Tumorlike Conditions of the Lymphatic System

These tumors or tumorlike conditions can be classified as follows:

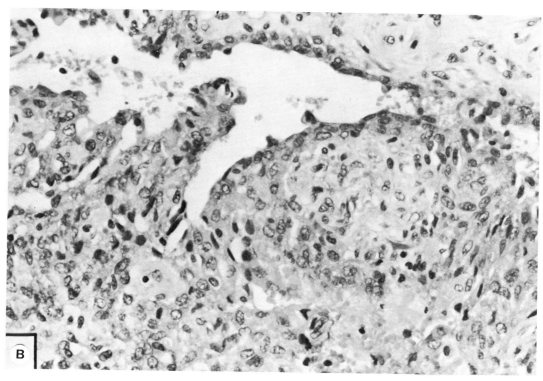

Figure 4.83. *Continued*

A. Benign
  1. Lymphangioma
  2. Cystic hygroma
  3. Omental and retroperitoneal cysts
B. Malignant
  1. Lymphangiosarcoma
  2. Lymphangiomyomatosis
  3. Extranodal lymphoma
  4. Extramedullary plasmacytoma

Benign.

Lymphangioma. A lymphangioma, like its vascular counterpart, the angioma, is not a true neoplasm but a hamartomatous malformation. However, for the sake of clarity, it will be discussed here. Proliferation of lymphatic vessels is less common than in the blood vessels. Generally, lymphangiomas are present at birth as diffuse proliferations that ultimately give the associated structures a grotesque appearance, eg, gigantism of an extremity. In another form, cystic dilations of enormous size are found, especially in the neck, giving rise to the term cystic hygroma. Infrequently, this type of cyst is found in the omentum and mesentery. Microscopically, the lesion is seen to consist of a honeycomb formed of large and small thin-walled cysts separated by bands of fibrous tissue (Fig. 4.87).

Malignant.

Lymphangiosarcoma. In 1948, Stewart and Treves[363] first recognized the syndrome of postmastectomy lymphangiosarcoma, ie, the development of lymphangiosarcoma associated with chronic postmastectomy lymphedema. Since then a number of cases have been reported.[364-367] Similar sarcomatous lesions also occur in patients with idiopathic edema of an extremity.[368,369]

Lymphangiosarcoma is recognized by its characteristic blue-red or purplish well-defined macular or papular cutaneous lesions in an edematous extremity.

The microscopic appearance of the tumor usually consists of a disorderly growth of vascular channels and fibroblastic proliferations;

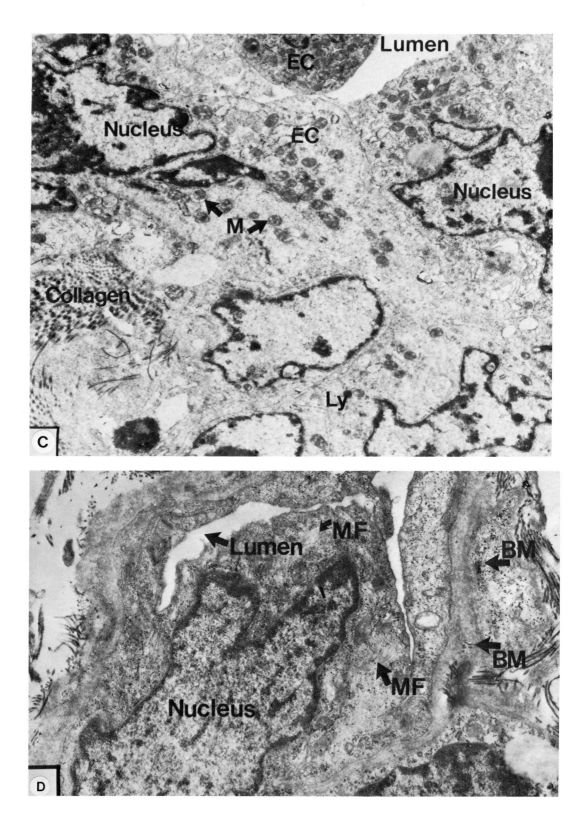

Figure 4.83. *Continued*

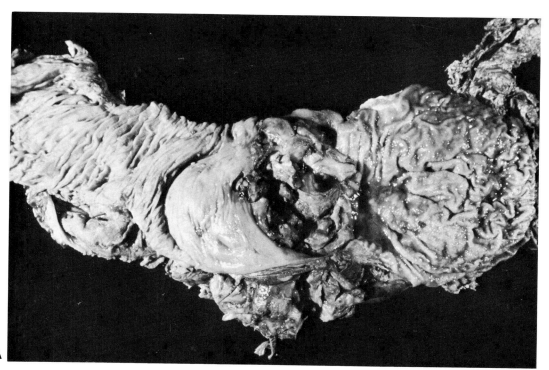

A

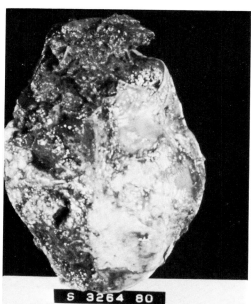

S 3264 80

B

Figure 4.84. This recurrent hemangiopericytoma of the anterior abdominal wall was removed from a 26-year-old man. He required excision of the anterior wall, part of the right lobe of the liver, the head of the pancreas, duodenum, and 60 percent of the stomach and transverse colon. **(A)** Specimen of resected anterior abdominal wall with tumor invading first part of the duodenum. This was the cause of preoperative upper gastrointestinal bleeding. After a disease-free interval of four years, he had intra-abdominal recurrence. **(B)** Tumor is invading the spleen. **(C)** Hemangiopericytoma, showing a multitude of vascular channels. The crowding of the neoplastic cells is outside the walls of the vascular spaces. (H & E. Original magnification ×125.) **(D)** Higher-power view, showing the predominantly oval and spindle-shaped pericytes. Apparently, normal endothelium is separated from the malignant cells by an amorphous collagenous matrix. (H & E. Original magnification ×375.)

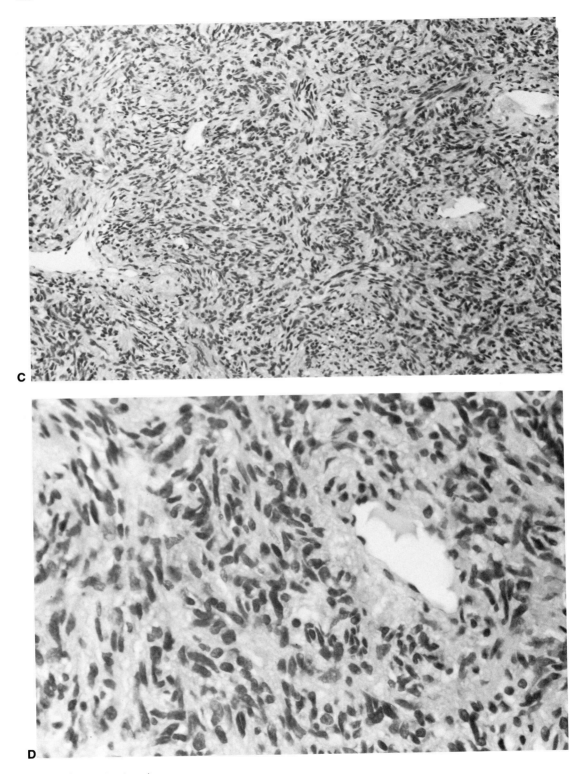

C

D

Figure 4.84. *Continued*

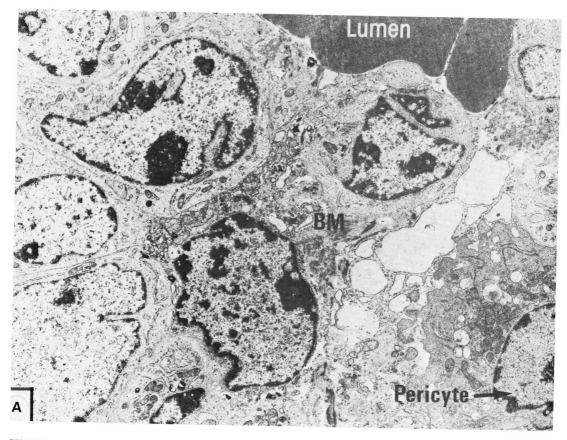

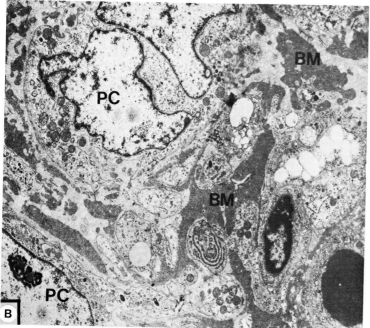

Figure 4.85. (A) Low-power view of a hemangiopericytoma. A capillary filled with two attenuated RBCs is surrounded by neoplastic pericytes. Note the thin discontinuous basal lamina surrounding the neoplastic pericytes. Cytologic details of pericytes are obvious. (Original magnification ×10,470.) **(B)** Another low-power view from a patient with recurrent pelvic hemangiopericytoma. Note the haphazard distribution of basal lamina. (Original magnification ×7,013.) **(C)** A neoplastic pericyte in higher power. Note the relation of the pericyte with the endothelial cell. This is from a 20-year-old woman with an atypical hemangiopericytoma of the groin.

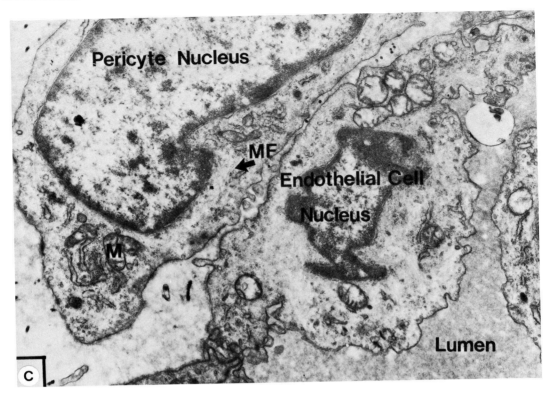

Figure 4.85. *Continued*

these fibroblastlike cells infiltrate the surrounding tissues (Fig. 4.88A and 4.88B). It is often difficult to arrive at an exact histologic diagnosis from the microscopic picture alone. However, armed with the clinical information that the lesion arises in an edematous extremity, the diagnosis becomes simple.

Lymphangiomyomatosis. This is a rare condition[370,371] characterized by proliferation of the smooth muscle fibers that participate in the formation of lymphatic channels throughout the body. The clinical presentation, however, is usually manifested by chylothorax, dyspnea, and pneumothorax.[372] The extrapulmonary symptoms include chylous ascites and edema of the extremities (Chapter 17).

Extranodal Lymphomas. Although the vast majority of malignant lymphomas arise primarily in the hematopoietic system, occasionally malignant lymphoma of the soft somatic tissue is encountered (Fig. 4.89). The diagnosis is made on histologic examination of the biopsy specimen. Reticulum cell sarcomas are distinguished from histiocytomas by demonstration

of reticulin fibers. However, an accurate diagnosis is often difficult.

Extramedullary Plasmacytoma. This is a rare entity, but the pathologic diagnosis is relatively easy, since the tumor is chiefly composed of plasma cells in various stages of development (Fig. 4.90A and 4.90B).

TUMOR AND TUMORLIKE CONDITIONS ARISING IN HETEROTOPIC BONE AND CARTILAGE

The histogenesis of either extraskeletal osteogenic sarcoma or chondrosarcoma is still unclear. Probably most of this is related to osseous or cartilaginous metaplasia of soft tissues. Metaplastic ossification is known to occur in voluntary muscles[135] and in other locations.[135] Huggins[373] stressed the concept of metaplasia of connective tissue into bone as a result of unknown influences. In 1940, Binkley and Stewart[374] made an extensive study of the morphogenesis of extraskeletal osteogenic sarcoma and pseudo-osteosarcoma. They proposed that the most important underlying causes of the development of the tumors were localized vascular stasis and concomitant tissue anoxia. Brookes,[375] in 1966, produced experimental osteogenesis by elevation of carbon dioxide tension and red cell count. It appears, therefore, that histologic[373] and experimental[375] evidence is available to support the concept of metaplasia of connective tissue cells into bone. Willis[135] found that new bone or cartilage formation has been described in all tissues of the body.

The bony metaplasia in voluntary muscles, or myositis ossificans, is not, strictly speaking, a tumor; however, because of an occasional clinical presentation of what resembles a tumor, this entity is briefly described. Metaplastic ossification occurs in skeletal muscles in two forms: localized myositis ossificans and a progressive generalized form of unknown cause.

The localized form is usually the result of chronic trauma. The most celebrated form of this entity is so-called "rider's bone," which is seldom seen nowadays. Microscopically the histologic picture of new bone extending into in-

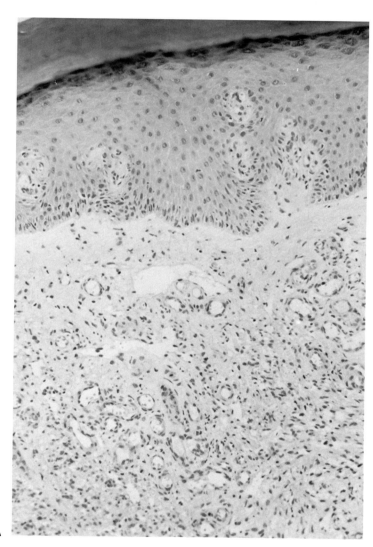

A

Figure 4.86. **(A)** Cutaneous nodule of Kaposi's sarcoma. In the dermis, multiple capillaries with intervening spindle-shaped cells can be seen. (H & E. Original magnification ×125.) *(Courtesy of Dr. S. Ronan, Departments of Pathology and Dermatology, University of Illinois.)* **(B)** The dermis showing the capillaries with malignant spindle-shaped cells. These are filled with RBCs. (H & E. Original magnification ×375.) **(C)** Kaposi's sarcoma involving the small intestine. (H & E. Original magnification ×65.)

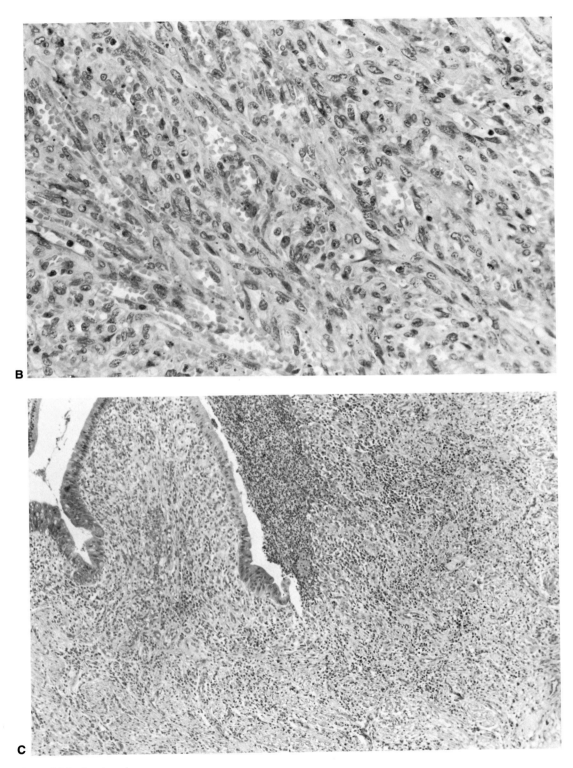

Figure 4.86. *Continued*

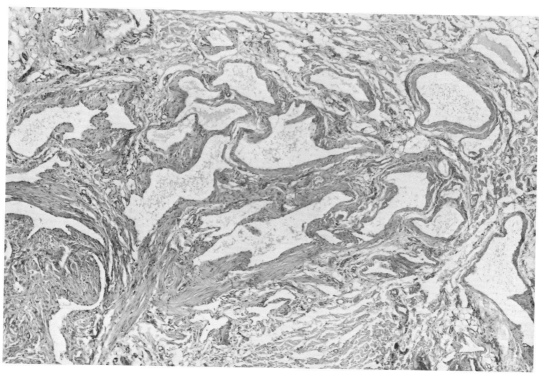

Figure 4.87. Lymphangioma showing the honeycomb appearance of thin-walled cystic spaces filled with amorphous material. (H & E. Original magnification × 40.)

flamed fibrosing muscle is diagnostic. Care must be taken not to confuse this benign self-limiting entity with osteosarcoma.

A rare progressive form of this disease is described in Chapter 18.

Extraskeletal Osteogenic Sarcoma. Extraosseous osteogenic sarcoma is indeed rare. Since the original description by Boneti[376] in the year 1700, only a handful of documented cases have been reported.[98,374,377–380]

Macroscopic Findings (Fig. 4.91). These tumors are usually surrounded by a tough connective tissue capsule that is intimately adherent to surrounding structures, making dissection extremely difficult. The overlying skin is occasionally ulcerated. The size of the tumor varies. The color of the cut surfaces of the tumors ranges from red to grayish-white to yellowish-white; often several combinations can be seen in different areas of the same tumor. Areas of hemorrhage and necrosis are common. The central

part is usually cystic, whereas the periphery is firm. Rarely, specks of calcification or bone formation can be seen. The remarkable ability of this tumor to infiltrate the surrounding muscles, tendons, and adipose tissue should be borne in mind during gross examination of the tumor. In rare instances, the lesion is in contact with the periosteum of the underlying long bone.

Microscopic Findings (Fig. 4.92A to 4.92C). A striking histologic feature is the nodular arrangement of the tumor. The nodules are quite cellular and contain both spindle and giant cells, frequently arranged in cords similar to those in fibrosarcoma. The nuclei in the spindle cells vary in shape, size, and staining quality, and frequently are hyperchromatic. Although the degree of cellular pleomorphism and the number of giant cells vary from field to field, there is uniform cellular morphology throughout the tumor. Tumor giant cells with multiple nuclei are most commonly seen in the fibrous part of the tumor. In some instances, 25 or more nuclei are

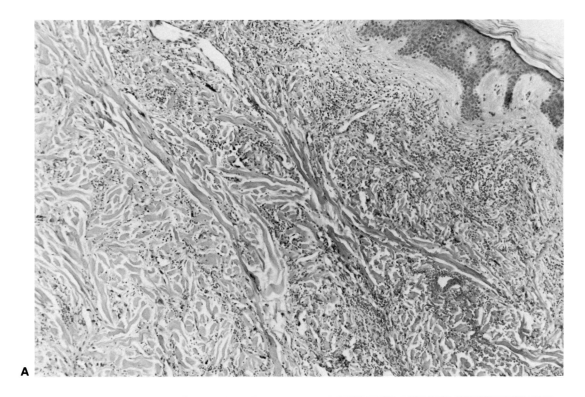

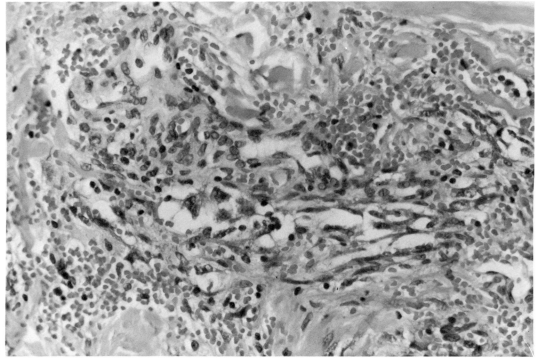

Figure 4.88. (A) Postmastectomy lymphangiosarcoma. A focus of disorderly growth of vascular channels lined by atypical spindle-shaped cells is seen invading the skin. (H & E. Original magnification ×65.) **(B)** Lymphatic channels of various sizes are lined by pleomorphic endothelial cells. (H & E. Original magnification ×250.)

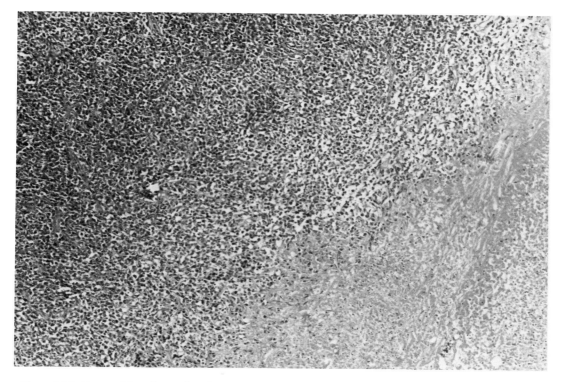

Figure 4.89. Extranodal malignant lymphoma of the subcutaneous tissue. (H & E. Original magnification ×65.)

present in a single giant cell. Mitoses are occasionally observed.

Bone formation can be seen in all parts of the tumor, and often a transformation zone from fibrous stroma can be demonstrated. Calcification of osteoid and fibrous tissue can also be observed at various sites in the lesion. Vascularity is not a marked feature, and frequently blood vessels are not seen in several sections. Malignant cells may invade and penetrate the capsule, extending into the surrounding tissue. However, invasion of blood vessels by tumor cells does not commonly occur.

Extraskeletal Chondrosarcoma (Fig. 4.93A to 4.93C). Malignant cartilaginous tumors not connected with bone are exceedingly rare. Stout and Verner[381] described seven cases. These tumors resemble chondrosarcomas of the bone, except that they frequently exhibit conspicuous areas of stellate and round cells set in a poorly differentiated myxomatous matrix, with relatively few foci of hyaline cartilage.[381–384] Enzinger and Shiraki[382] reviewed a series of 34 patients

and, on the basis of their light microscopic findings, described the tumors as multinodular, consisting of small, uniform, rounded or elongated cells with a narrow eosinophilic cytoplasm. The cells are arranged in cords, strands, nests, or clusters. The myxoid ground substance stains deep red with mucicarmine, blue with alcian blue, and deep purple with aldehyde-fuchsin. These staining reactions are not altered by pretreatment with hyaluronidase.[382]

These tumors sometimes resemble myxoid liposarcomas and careful histologic criteria must be used for a correct diagnosis.[382]

Extraskeletal Ewing's Sarcoma (Fig. 4.94A and 4.94B). In 1975, Angervall and Enzinger[385] described the clinicopathologic features of an uncommon extraskeletal neoplasm resembling Ewing's sarcoma of the bone. These tumors occur mainly in young adults[385,386] and are aggressive. Microscopically they consist of solidly packed small, round or ovoid, uniform cells arranged in sheets of lobules separated by strands of fibrous connective tissue. The nucleus of the

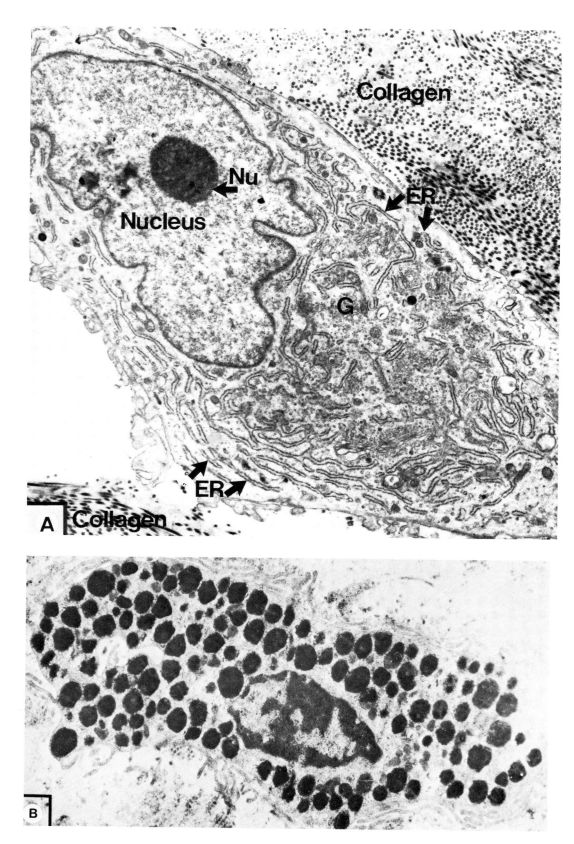

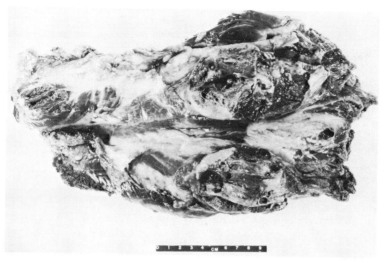

Figure 4.91. Cut section of extra-skeletal osteosarcoma. The primary tumor was excised from the posterior thigh. Note the infiltrating quality of this tumor. Multiple muscle bundles have been infiltrated on the right. An area of hemorrhage is clearly visible on the upper right corner.

tumor cells contains a finely divided chromatin, a distinct nuclear membrane, and frequently a minute nucleolus. The scanty, ill-defined cytoplasm contains varying amounts of glycogen. Sometimes the histologic picture is dominated by a "peritheliomatous" pattern, or by large areas of necrosis or hemorrhage. The lungs and the skeleton are the two most common sites of metastases.[385]

TUMORS AND TUMORLIKE CONDITIONS OF UNDETERMINED HISTOGENESIS

Although more and more variants of soft tissue tumors are being classified, there are still several for which the histogenesis has not been defined. In benign tumors or tumorlike conditions, the necessity for such classification is not acute, but in the malignant variety, further investigation is essential. For the present, all these tumors are classified into benign and malignant types as follows:

A. Benign
   1. Granular cell myoblastoma
   2. Benign mesenchymoma
B. Malignant
   1. Alveolar soft part sarcoma (malignant granular cell tumor)

2. Malignant mesenchymoma
3. Malignant granular cell myoblastoma
4. Malignant fibrous mesothelioma

Benign

Granular Cell Tumor (Myoblastoma). In 1926, Abrikossoff[387] first described a group of tumors arising in the muscles of the tongue, lip, and leg. In view of the presence of granular cells and the close proximity of these tumors to the tongue musculature and other striated muscles, he assumed these tumors to be of myoblastic origin. With the description of more and more of these tumors, the proposed myoblastic histogenesis has now come under serious doubt.[148,388–392] Because of their sometimes intimate relationship with, and their occasional presence within, nerve bundles, the granular elements of the myoblastoma cells have been considered to be of neural derivation from Schwann cells or fibroblasts of peripheral nerve sheaths. Pearse,[390] on the basis of histochemical studies, suggested that these tumors are granular cell perineural fibroblastomas, within the cells of which a lipid-containing complex has accumulated. A Schwann cell origin has been suggested by several other authors,[17,389] and this concept probably has some degree of validity. It does not lessen the possibility that these granular cells have histiocytic capacities, since

Figure 4.90. (A) A plasma cell from a solitary subcutaneous extramedullary plasmacytoma of the scapular region in a 56-year-old woman. Profiles of endoplasmic reticulum (ER), and Golgi zones (G) are apparent. (Original magnification ×15,080.) Following excision of this 8 × 6 × 7 cm soft tissue mass, her protein electrophoresis became normal. **(B)** Mast cell from the same patient. (Original magnification ×13,690.)

Schwann cells are facultative fibroblasts and can have phagocytic properties. Although schwannian origin is an attractive and probably a tenable hypothesis, it would probably be imprudent at present to classify granular cell myoblastomas as peripheral nerve tumors.

Granular cell myoblastomas appear as solitary small nodules with well-defined but not sharply demarcated boundaries. The microstructure of these lesions is characterized by irregularly arranged strands, solid clumps, and nests of large, granular, round or polyhedral, faintly acidophilic cells with vesicular or densely chromatic nuclei (Fig. 4.95). The cluster of cells is surrounded by variable amounts of collagenous tissue or reticulin fibers interspersed with nerve fibers. Frequently, the granular cells are in close apposition to nerve bundles. The histochemistry of these cells may vary considerably from that of muscle cells.

The granular cells of myoblastoma resemble the congenital epulis of the newborn. Stout and Lattes[3] considered these as variants of granular cell myoblastoma.

Benign Mesenchymoma. Benign mesenchymomas are circumscribed rare tumors usually encountered in the region of the kidney and perirenal tissue,[3] although they can occur elsewhere in the body.[3] These tumors are composed of a mixture of mesenchymal tissues in addition to fibrous tissue. They are recognizable by the haphazard distribution of adipose tissue, smooth muscle cells, and blood vessels (Fig. 4.96). They have a a tendency to locally infiltrate, thereby giving a false impression of malignancy.

Malignant

Alveolar Soft Part Sarcoma (Malignant Granular Cell Tumor). One of the groups of sarcomas of undetermined histogenesis is the alveolar soft tissue sarcoma, first described by Christopherson, Foote, and Stewart in 1952.[393] Characteristically, these slow-growing but definitely malignant tumors are usually found in young adults, more often in women. In 1951, Smetana and Scott[394] described a group of 14

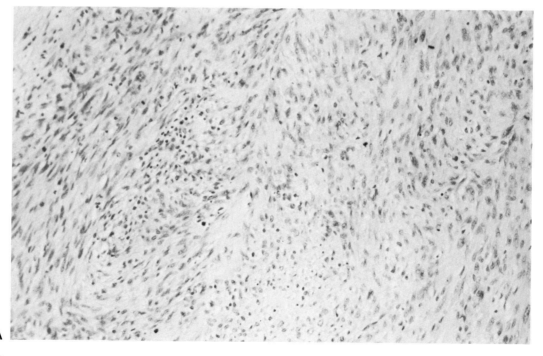

A

Figure 4.92. (A) Extraskeletal osteosarcoma. The tumor is highly cellular with scanty stroma, but arrangement resembles that of a fibrosarcoma. (H & E. Original magnification ×125.) **(B)** The nuclei of spindle cells are hyperchromatic, with giant cells and immature osteoid formation. (H & E. Original magnification ×125.) **(C)** High-power view, showing the profile of a malignant osteoblast. (H & E. Original magnification ×375.)

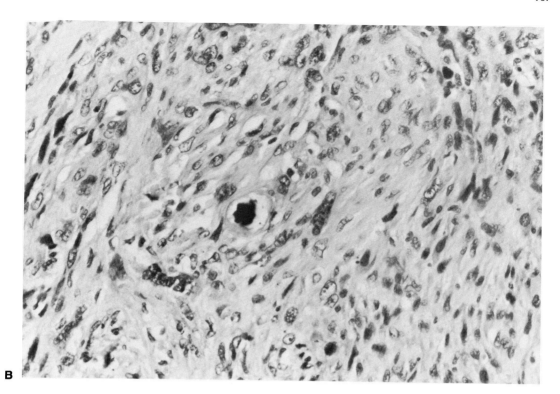

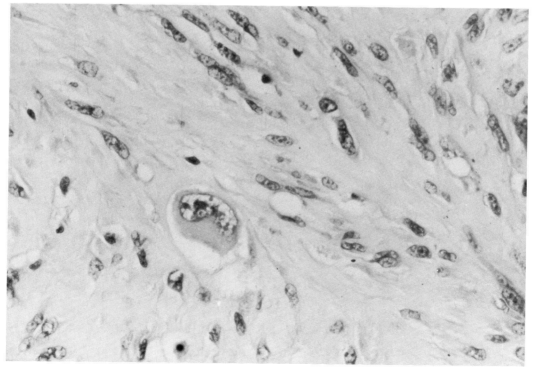

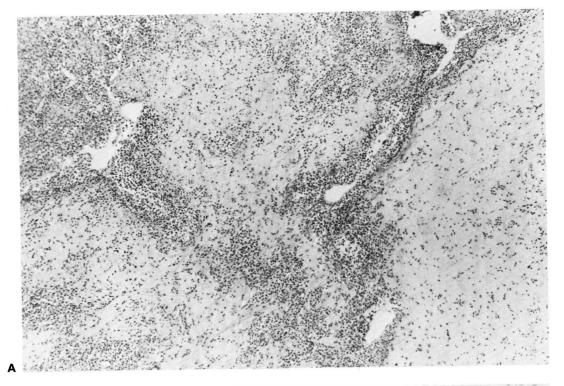

A

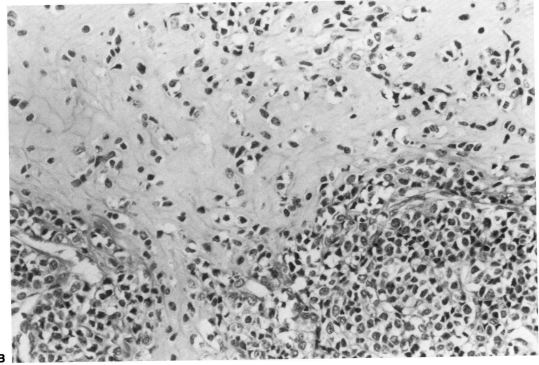

B

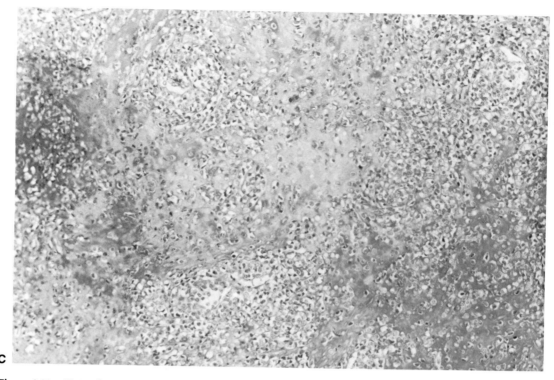

C

Figure 4.93. (**A**) Uniform distribution of homogenous undifferentiated mesenchymal cells and chondrocytes. (H & E. Original magnification ×65.) (**B**) The majority of malignant mesenchymal cells are either oval or spindle-shaped, intimately interspersed with pleomorphic clumped chondrocytes. (H & E. Original magnification ×250.) (**C**) Alcian blue stain showing the myxoid ground substance. (Original magnification ×125.)

similar cases with a distinct organoid pattern resembling that of a carotid body neoplasm (discussed earlier in this chapter). They considered these tumors to be homologous to branchial chemodectomas and called them malignant nonchromaffin paragangliomas. Since then, lesions of identical appearance with organoid structure have been reported by other authors.[3,395,396] Although there is disagreement concerning the histogenesis, and consequently the taxonomy and terminology, there is no doubt that these tumors have a distinctive histologic appearance and constitute a rare group of malignant tumors.

The organoid endocrinelike pattern is a striking and uniform microscopic feature of alveolar soft part sarcoma. The tumor cells are arranged in rounded or cordlike discrete groups bound by collagen fibers (Fig. 4.97A and 4.97B). The individual cells are round and contain distinctive granules in the cytoplasm. These gran-ules are always diastase-resistant and PAS-positive.

Shipkey and associates,[397] by electron microscopic examination, observed unique cytoplasmic crystals in cellular components. These crystals in osmium-tetroxide-fixed tissues show a lattice pattern. More recently, the detailed electron microscopic findings have been described.[398,399]

Ultrastructurally, the nuclei exhibit moderate amounts of chromatin and usually contain a solitary nucleolus. The mitochondria tend to be arranged in clusters, frequently separated from one another by strands of coarse endoplasmic reticulum. The Golgi structures are well developed. All tumor cells contain a varying number of intracytoplasmic crystalline inclusions exhibiting a variety of geometric configurations. These are, for the most part, bound by a solitary limiting membrane. Their internal structure is comprised of parallel laminary fil-

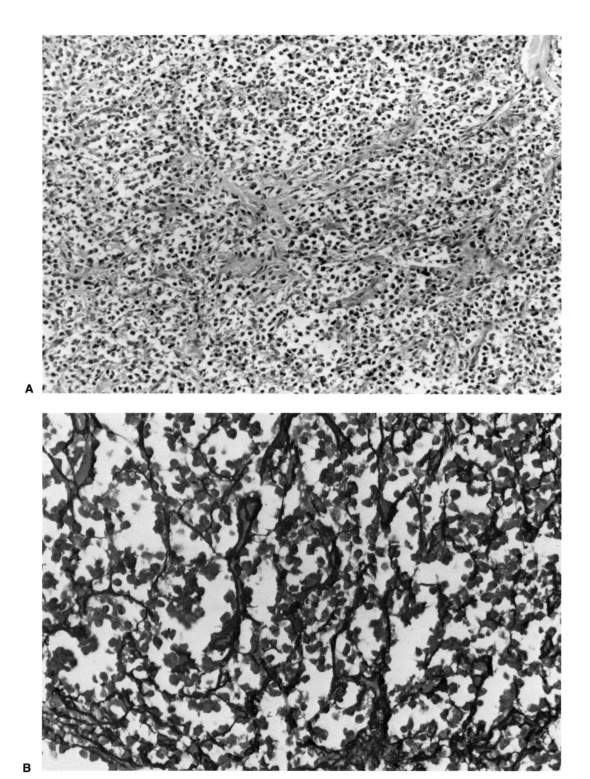

Figure 4.94. **(A)** Monomorphic, predominantly round cells are arranged in sheets in a rich vascular stroma. (H & E. Original magnification × 125.) **(B)** Reticulin stain showing the spatial arrangement of the tumor cells. (Original magnification × 125.)

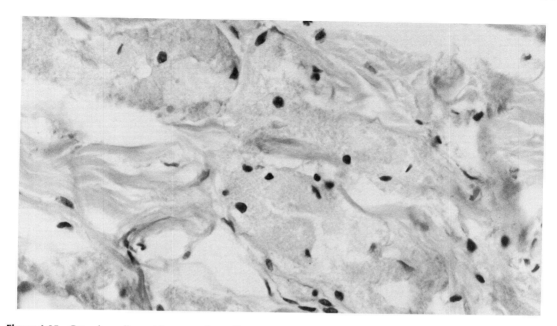

Figure 4.95. Granular cell myoblastoma. The cells are uniform, well defined, and granular, with pyknotic nuclei. (H & E. Original magnification ×250.)

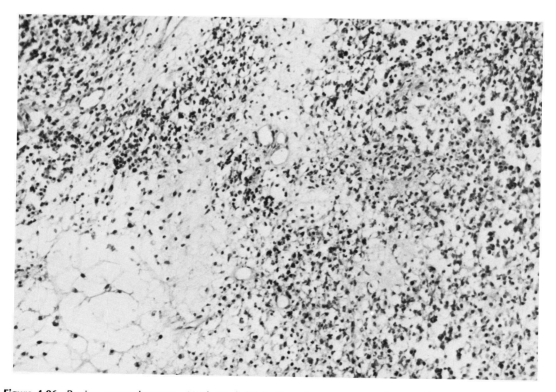

Figure 4.96. Benign mesenchymoma. Haphazard distribution of various types of mesenchymal cells can be easily recognized. (H & E. Original magnification ×125.)

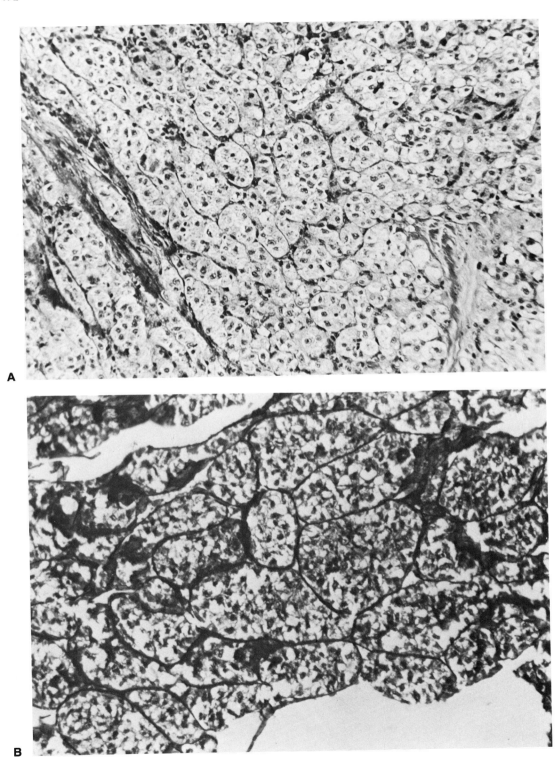

Figure 4.97. *Continued*

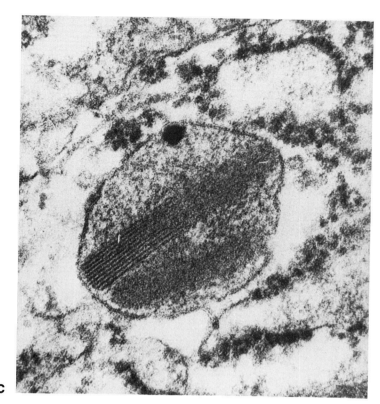

C

Figure 4.97. **(A)** Alveolar soft part sarcoma. The discrete rounded arrangement (organoid) is obvious. (H & E. Original magnification ×125.) **(B)** Reticulin stain clearly showing the organoid pattern. (Original magnification ×125.) **(C)** The classical intracytoplasmic, crystalline, membrane-bound inclusion. Note the parallel laminary filament. (Original magnification ×45,600.)

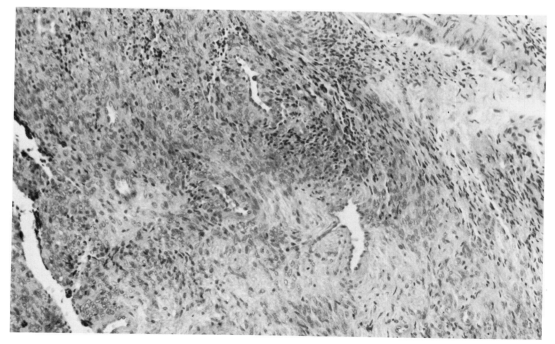

Figure 4.98. A malignant mesenchymoma showing the characteristics of a number of cell types. (H & E. Original magnification ×125.)

aments measuring 36–90 Å in thickness and are arranged with a periodicity of 58–100 Å. In some, a cross-grid arrangement or square filamentous arrays are evident (Fig. 4.97C).

Fisher and Reidbord[398] compared the ultrastructural features of alveolar soft part sarcoma with those of granular cell myoblastoma, melanoma, carotid body tumors, and alveolar rhabdomyosarcoma. They found sufficient cytomorphologic evidence at the ultrastructural level to consider these tumors a unique type of rhabdomyosarcoma. Obviously, until this histogenetic controversy is resolved, these tumors will remain histologically unclassifiable. Welsh and co-authors,[399] in 1972, argued that, while alveolar soft part sarcoma and nonchromaffin paraganglioma share a close homology and thus a related histogenesis, they are different entities. They further argued that malignant granular cell myoblastoma exhibited so many structural differences that it was completely unrelated. Unni and Soule[400] have confirmed the observation of Welsh and his associates.

Malignant Mesenchymoma (Fig. 4.98). This is a descriptive term applied to those soft tissue sarcomas in which there are two or more unrelated malignant elements. In the past, the term was frequently used for tumors with extreme pleomorphism. Today, this diagnosis is seldom rendered.

Malignant Granular Cell Myoblastoma. The malignant variety of granular cell myoblastoma is indeed rare.[390,391] Cadotte,[401] in 1974, found only 22 case reports with valid data. We have encountered one such patient. The clinical history is summarized in Table 19.2, Chapter 19. Metastases via both the lymphatics and the bloodstream have been observed.

Malignant Fibrous Mesothelioma. Several acceptable cases have been recorded, primarily in the pleura[3,148,402] and the peritoneum.[148,403] In recent years the association of asbestos exposure and pleural mesotheliomas has generated considerable interest in these tumors, but because of their rarity and their anatomic location they are seldom treated as malignant fibrous tissue tumors.

The tumors arising in relation to serous surfaces show either a predominantly spindle cell or epithelial cell appearance. The two cell types can be found together (as in synovial cell sarcoma) or can be distributed in separate areas of a given tumor. Thus, some areas resemble spindle cell fibrosarcoma and some show other mesenchymal characteristics. The cytoplasm of the epithelial cells is basophilic and mitosis is seldom encountered.

REFERENCES

1. Ewing J: Neoplastic Diseases, 4th ed. Philadelphia, Saunders, 1940
2. Stout AP: Atlas of Tumor Pathology. Tumors of the soft tissues. Firminger HI (ed). Series 2, Fasc 5. Washington D.C., AFIP, 1967
3. Stout AP, Lattes R: Atlas of Tumor Pathology. Tumors of the soft tissues. Firminger HI (ed). Series 2, Fasc 2. Washington D.C., AFIP, 1967
4. Pack GT, Ariel IA: Tumors of the Soft Somatic Tissue. A Clinical Treatise. New York, Hoeber-Harper, 1958
5. Hare HF, Cerny MJ Jr: Soft tissue sarcoma. A review of 200 cases. Cancer 16:1332, 1963
6. Pack GT, Ariel IA: Tumors of the Soft Somatic Tissues. Chap 24: Sarcomas of undetermined histogenesis. New York, Hoeber-Harper, 1958, p 673
7. Lazarus SS, Med S, Trombetta LD: Ultrastructural identification of a benign perineurial cell tumor. Cancer 41:1823, 1978
8. Feiner H, Kaye GI: Ultrastructural evidence of myofibroblasts in circumscribed fibromatosis. Arch Path 100:265, 1976
9. Cameron DA: The fine structure of bone and calcified cartilage. A critical review of the contribution of electron microscopy to the understanding of osteogenesis. Clin Orthop 26:199, 1963
10. Peach R, Williams G, Chapman JA: A light and electron microscopic study of regenerating tendon. Am J Path 38:495, 1961
11. Porter KR, Pappas GD: Collagen formation by fibroblasts in the chick embryo dermis. J Biochem Cytol 5:153, 1959
12. Huxley HE: The structure of striated muscle. In Nachmansohn D (ed): Molecular Biology. New York, Academic Press, 1960
13. Palade GE: Blood capillaries in the heart and other organs. Circulation 24:368, 1961
14. Napolitano LM: Observations on the fine structure of adipose cells. Ann NY Acad Sci 137:34, 1965
15. Zimmerman LE, Font RL, Ts'o MOM, Fine BS: Application of electron microscopy to histopathologic diagnosis. Trans Am Acad Ophth Otolaryngol 76:101, 1972
16. Stembridge VA, Luibel FJ, Ashworth CT: Soft tissue sarcomas: Electron microscopic approach to histogenetic classification. South Med J 57:772, 1964
17. Fisher ER, Wechsler H: Granular cell myoblastoma—a misnomer: Electron microscopic and histochemical evidence concerning its Schwann cell derivation and nature (granular cell schwannoma). Cancer 13:936, 1962

18. Scarpelli DG, Greider MH: A correlative cytochemical and electron microscopic study of a liposarcoma. Cancer 15:776, 1962
19. Nystrom SHM: Electron microscopical structure of the wall of small blood vessels in human multiforme glioblastoma. Nature 184:65, 1959
20. DeRobertis E, Setelo JR: Electron microscope study of cultured nervous tissue. Exp Cell Res 3 (Suppl 2):433, 1952
21. Venkatachalam MA, Greally JG: Fine structure of glomus tumor: Similarity of glomus cells to smooth muscle. Cancer 23:1176, 1969
22. Keith A: Human Embryology and Morphology, 6th ed. London, Edward Arnold and Company, 1948
23. Rasmussen AT: The so-called hibernating gland. J Morphol 38:147, 1923
24. Flemming W: Weitere Mittheilungen zur Physiologie der Fettzelle. Arch Mikr Anat 7:328, 1871
25. Clark ER, Clark EL: Microscopic studies of the new formation of fat in living adult rabbits. Am J Anat 67:255, 1940
26. Toldt C: Lehubuch der Gewebelehre mit voraugsweiser Berucksichtingung des menschlichen Korpers, 3rd ed. Stuttgart, F Enke, 1888, p 724
27. Wasserman E: The concept of the "fat organ." In Rodahl K and Issekutz B (eds): Fat as a Tissue, Symposium Monograph. New York, McGraw-Hill, 1962, p 22
28. Dabelow A: Anat Anz, Erg Heft Band 104, Verh Anat Ge, 54 Vers, Frieburg I Br 83–96, 1957
29. Napolitano L: The differentiation of white adipose cells. An electron microscope study. Cell Biol 18:663, 1963
30. Sidman RL: Adipose tissue. In Willmer EN (ed): Cells and Tissues in Culture, Methods, Biology and Physiology, vol 2. New York and London, Academic Press, 1965
31. Thomas LW: The chemical composition of adipose tissue of man and mice. Quart J Exper Physiol 47:179, 1962
32. Hellman B, Hellerstrom C: Cell renewal in the white and brown fat tissue of the rat. Acta Path Microbiol Scandinav 51:347, 1961
33. Latta JS, Bucholz DJ: The effects of insulin on the growth of fibroblasts in vitro. Arch Exper Zellforsch 23:146, 1939
34. Burkhardt L: Beobachtungen an explantiertem Fettgeweb. Arch exper Zellforsch 16:187, 1934
35. Trowell OA: The culture of mature organs in a synthetic medium. Exper Cell Res 16:118, 1959
36. Sheldon H: The fine structure of the fat cell. In Rodahl K and Issekutz B (eds): Fat as a Tissue, Symposium Monograph. New York, McGraw-Hill, 1962
37. Hammar JA: Zur Kenntniss de Fettgewebes. Arch Mikr Anat 45:512, 1902
38. Johanason L, Soderlund S: Intrathoracic lipoma. Acta Chir Scandinav 126:558, 1963
39. Dawkins MJR, Duckett S, Pearse AGE: Localization of catecholamines in brown fat. Nature 209:1144, 1966
40. Wirsen C, Hamberger B: Catecholamines in brown fat. Nature 214:625, 1967
41. Romer TE: Corticosteroids in brown fat by a histochemical method. J Histochem 12:646, 1964
42. Dionne GP, Seemayer TA: Infiltrating lipomas and angiolipomas revisited. Cancer 33:732 1974
43. Enzinger FM, Harvey DA: Spindle cell lipoma. Cancer 36:1852, 1975
44. Kindblom L-G, Angervall L, Stener B, Wickbom I: Intermuscular and intramuscular lipomas and hibernomas. Cancer 33:754, 1974
45. Rasanen O, Nohteri H, Dammert K: Angiolipoma and lipoma. Acta Chir Scandinav 133:461, 1967
46. Weller RO, Baylis OB, Abdulla YH, Adams CWM: The electron histochemical demonstration of phosphoglyceride. J Histochem Cytochem 13:690, 1965
47. Gellhorn A, Marks PA: The composition and biosynthesis of lipids in human adipose tissues. J Clin Invest 40:925, 1961
48. Wright CJE: Liposarcoma arising in a single lipoma. J Path Bacteriol 60:483, 1948
49. Stout AP: Liposarcoma—malignant tumor of lipoblasts. Ann Surg 119:86, 1944
50. Sternberg SS: Liposarcoma arising within a subcutaneous lipoma. Cancer 5:975, 1952
51. Sampson CC, Saunders EH, Gree WE, Larey JR: Liposarcoma developing in a lipoma. Arch Path 69:506, 1968
52. Jaffe RH: Recurrent lipomatous tumor of the groin. Arch Path 1:381, 1926
53. Vellios F, Baez JM, Shumacker HB: Lipoblastomatosis: A tumor of fetal fat different from hibernoma. Report of a case, with observations of the embryogenesis of human adipose tissue. Am J Path 54:1149, 1958
54. Shear M: Lipoblastomatosis of the cheek. Br J Oral Surg 5:173, 1967
55. Chung EB, Enzinger FM: Benign lipoblastomatosis: An analysis of 35 cases. Cancer 32:482, 1975
56. Willis RA: The Pathology of the Tumours of Children. Pathological Monographs II. Edinburgh, Oliver and Boyd, 1962, p 100
57. Enzinger FM, Winslow DJ: Liposarcoma. A study of 103 cases. Virchows Arch Path Anat 335:367, 1962
58. Virchow R: Edin Fall von bosartigen, Zum Theil in der Form des Neurouns auftretende Fettgeschwulsten. Virchows Arch Path Anat 11:281, 1857
59. De Weed JH, Dockery MD: Lipomatous retroperitoneal tumors. Am J Surg 84:397, 1952
60. Pack GT, Pierson JC: Liposarcoma. A study of 105 cases. Surgery 36:687, 1954
61. Reszel PA, Soule EH, Coventry MB: Liposarcoma of the extremities and limb girdles. J Bone Joint Surg 48-A:229, 1966
62. Enterline HT, Culberson JD, Rochlin DB, Brady LW: Liposarcoma: A clinical and pathological study of 53 cases. Cancer 13:932, 1960
63. Das Gupta TK: Tumors and Tumorlike Conditions of the Adipose Tissue. Current Problems in Surgery. Chicago, Year Book Medical Publishers, March 1970
64. Manual for Staging of Cancer. Chicago, American Joint Committee for Cancer Staging and End Result Reporting, 1978

65. Kauffman SL, Stout AP: Lipoblastic tumors of children. Cancer 12:912, 1959
66. Sutherland JC, Callahan WP Jr, Campbell GL: Hibernoma: A tumor of brown fat. Cancer 5:364, 1952
67. Leiphart CJ, Nudelman EJ: Hibernoma masquerading as a pheochromocytoma. Radiology 95:659, 1970
68. Jennings RC, Behr G: Hibernoma (granular cell lipoma). J Clin Path 8:310, 1955
69. Mesara BW, Batsakis JG: Hibernoma of the neck. Arch Otolaryngol 85:95, 1967
70. Brines OA, Johnson MH: Hibernoma: a special fatty tumor. Am J Path 25:467, 1949
71. Inglis K: The so-called interscapular gland and tumours arising therein. J Anat Physiol 61:452, 1927
72. Symmers D: Spindle and giant cell sarcoma arising from unidentified precordial bodies. Arch Path 37:180, 1944
73. Catchpole HR: Connective tissue: Capillary permeability. In Zweifach BW, Grant L, McCluskey RT (eds): The Inflammatory Process, vol 2, 2nd ed. New York, Academic Press, 1973
74. Movat HZ, Fernando NVP: The fine structure of connective tissue. 1. The fibroblast. Exp Mol Path 1:509, 1962.
75. Kulonen E, Pikkarainen (eds): Biology of Fibroblast. New York, Academic Press, 1973
76. Daniel MR, Glauert AM, Dingle JT, Lucy JA: The action of vitamin A (retinol) on the fine structure of rat dermal fibroblasts in culture. Strangeways Research Laboratory Reports, 1965, p 13
77. Davis R, James DW: Electron microscopic appearance of close relationships between adult guinea-pig fibroblasts in tissue culture. Nature 194:695, 1962
78. Fitton Jackson S: Connective tissue cells. In Urachet J, Mirsky AE (eds): The Cell, vol 6. New York, Academic Press, 1964
79. Ramachandran GN (ed): Treatise on Collagen, vol 1, Chemistry of Collagen. New York, Academic Press, 1967
80. Gross J: Collagen biology, structure, degradation and disease. Harvey Lect 68:351, 1974
81. Gallop PM, Paz MA: Post-translational protein modifications, with special attention to collagen and elastin. Physiol Rev 55:418, 1975
82. Cameron DA: The fine structure of osteoblasts in the metaphysis of the tibia of the young rat. J Biophys Biochem Cytol 9:883, 1961
83. Bornstein P, Piez KA: Collagen: Structural studies based on the cleavage of methionyl bonds. Science 143:1353, 1965
84. Bornstein P: The biosynthesis of collagen. Ann Rev Biochem 143:567, 1974
85. Goldberg B, Sherr CJ: Secretion and extracellular processing of procollagen by cultured human fibroblasts. Proc Nat Acad Sci 70:361, 1973
86. Gross J: The behavior of collagen units as model in morphogenesis. J Biophys Biochem Cytol 2 (suppl):261, 1956
87. Doyle BB, Hukins DWL, Hulmes DJS, Miller A, Woodhead-Galloway J: Collagen polymorphism: Its origins in the amino acid sequence. J Mol Biol 91:79, 1975

88. Veis A, Brownell AG: Collagen biosynthesis. Crit Rev Biochem 2:417, 1975
89. Ross R, Bornstein P: Elastic fibers in the body. Sci Am 224:44, 1971
90. Balazs EA (ed): Chemistry and Molecular Biology of the Intercellular Matrix, vol 2: Glycosaminoglycans and Proteoglycans; vol 3: Structional Organization and Function of the Matrix. New York, Academic Press, 1970
91. Kefalides NA: In Balzas EA (ed): Chemistry and Molecular Biology of the Intercellular Matrix, vol 1. New York, Academic Press, 1970, p 553
92. Chaudhuri PK, Walker MJ, Beattie CW, Das Gupta TK: Presence of steroid receptors in human soft-tissue sarcomas of diverse histological origin. Cancer Res 40:861, 1980
93. Dodson JW, Hay ED: Secretion of collagen by corneal epithelium. II. Effect of the underlying substratum on secretion and polymerization of epithelial cell products. J Exp Zool 189:51, 1974
94. Gospodarowicz D, Greenburg G, Birdwell CR: Determination of cellular shape by the extracellular matrix and its correlation with control of cellular growth. Cancer Res 38:4155, 1978
95. Cohen M, Tayler JM: Epidermal growth factor chemical and biological characterization. Recent Prog Hormone Res 30:533, 1974
96. Kauffman SL, Stout AP: Histiocytic tumors (fibrous xanthoma and histiocytoma) in children. Cancer 14:469, 1961
97. Keasbey LE: Juvenile aponeurotic fibroma (calcifying fibroma). A distinctive tumor arising in the palms and soles of young children. Cancer 6:338, 1953
98. Lichtenstein L, Goldman RL: Cartilage tumors in soft tissues, particularly in the hand and foot. Cancer 17:1203, 1964
99. Mitchison MJ: The pathology of idiopathic retroperitoneal fibrosis. J Clin Path 23:681, 1970
100. Konwaler BE, Keasbey L, Kaplan L: Subcutaneous pseudosarcomatous fibromatosis (fasciitis). Am J Clin Path 25:241, 1955
101. Chung EB, Enzinger FM: Proliferative fasciitis. Cancer 36:1450, 1975
102. Culbertson JD, Enterline HT: Pseudosarcomatous fasciitis: A clinicopathological entity. Report of three cases. Ann Surg 151:235, 1960
103. Hutter RVP, Stewart FW, Foote FW: Fasciitis: A report of 70 cases with follow-up proving benignity of the lesion. Cancer 15:992, 1962
104. Bourne RG: Paradoxical fibrosarcoma of the skin (pseudosarcoma): A review of 13 cases. Med J Aust 50(1):504, 1963
105. Finlay-Jones LR, Nicol P, Ten Seldam REJ: Pseudosarcoma of the skin. Pathology 3:215, 1971
106. Woyke S, Domagala W, Olszewski W, Korabiec M: Pseudosarcoma of the skin. An electron microscopic study and comparison with the fine structure of the spindle-cell variant of squamous carcinoma. Cancer 33:970, 1974
107. Jarvi OH, Saxen AE, Hopsu-Havu VK, Wartiovaara JJ, Vaissalo VT: Elastofibroma—a degenerative pseudotumor. Cancer 23:42, 1969
108. Barr RJ: Elastofibroma. Am J Clin Path 45:679, 1966

109. Taylor RW: Sarcomatous tumors resembling in some respects keloid. J Cutaneous Genitourinary Dis 8:384, 1890

110. Stout AP: Fibrosarcoma; the malignant tumors of fibroblasts. Cancer 1:30, 1948

111. Taylor HH, Helwig EB: Dermatofibrosarcoma protuberans. Cancer 15:717, 1962

112. O'Brien JE, Stout AP: Malignant fibrous xanthomas. Cancer 17:1445, 1964

113. Penner DW: Metastasizing dermatofibrosarcoma protuberans. Cancer 4:1083, 1951

114. McPeak CJ, Cruz T, Nicastri AD: Dermatofibrosarcoma protuberans: An analysis of 86 cases—five with metastasis. Ann Surg 166:805, 1967

115. Bennet JH: On cancerous and cancroid growths. Edinburgh, Southerland and Knox, 1849, p 176

116. Muller J: Uber den feinern Bau und die Formen der Krankhaften Greschwiilste. Berlin, Reimer, 1838, p 80

117. Pritchard DJ, Soule EH, Taylor WF, Ivins JC: Fibrosarcoma. A clinicopathological and statistical study of 199 tumors of the soft tissue and trunk. Cancer 33:888, 1974

118. Soule EH, Geitz M, Henderson ED: Embryonal rhabdomyosarcoma of the limbs and limb girdles. Cancer 23:1336, 1969

119. Suit HD, Russell WD, Martin RG: Sarcoma of soft tissue: clinical and histopathological parameters and response to treatment. Cancer 35:1978, 1975

120. Werf-Messing BV, Van Unnik JAM: Fibrosarcoma of the soft parts. Cancer 18:1113, 1965

121. Weiss SW, Enzinger FM: Myxoid variant of malignant fibrous histiocytoma. Cancer 39:1672, 1977

122. Hajdu SI, Shiu MH, Fortner JG: Tenosynovial sarcoma: a clinicopathological study of 136 cases. Cancer 39:1201, 1977

123. Weiss SW, Enzinger FM: Malignant fibrous histiocytoma. An analysis of 200 cases. Cancer 41:2250, 1978

124. Fu YS, Gabbiani G, Kaye GI, Lattes R: Malignant soft tissue tumors of probable histiocyte origin (malignant fibrous histiocytomas): General considerations and electron microscopic and tissue culture studies. Cancer 35:176, 1975

125. Kempson RL, Kyriakos M: Fibroxanthosarcoma of the soft tissues. A type of malignant fibrous histiocytoma. Cancer 29:961, 1972

126. Kyriakos M, Kempson RL: Inflammatory fibrous histiocytoma: An aggressive and lethal lesion. Cancer 37:1584, 1976

127. Ozzello L, Stout AP, Murray MR: Cultural characteristics of malignant histiocytomas and fibrous xanthomas. Cancer 16:331, 1963

128. Guccion JG, Enzinger FM: Malignant giant cell tumor of soft parts. An analysis of 32 cases. Cancer 29:1518, 1972

129. Kahn LB: Retroperitoneal xanthogranuloma and xanthosarcoma (malignant fibrous xanthoma). Cancer 31:411, 1973

130. Rosas-Uribe A, Ring AM, Rappaport H: Metastasizing retroperitoneal fibroxanthoma (malignant fibroxanthoma). Cancer 26:827, 1970

131. Shrikhande SS, Sirsat MV: Reticulum cell sarcoma and malignant histiocytoma of soft tissue. Ind J Cancer 9:265, 1972

132. Soule EH, Enriquez P: Atypical fibrous histiocytoma, malignant fibrous histiocytoma, malignant histiocytoma and epithelioid sarcoma. A comparative study of 65 tumors. Cancer 30:128, 1972

133. Langsam LB, Fine G, Ponka JD: Malignant histiocytomas. Arch Surg 113:473, 1978

134. Murray MR: Muscle. In Willmer EN (ed): Cells and Tissues in Culture, Methods, Biology and Physiology, vol. 2, Chap. 8. New York, Academic Press, 1965, p 311

135. Willis RA: The Borderland of Embryology and Pathology. London, Butterworth, 1958, p 411

136. Murray MR: Skeletal muscle tissue in culture. In Bourne GH (ed): Structure and Function of Muscle. New York, Academic Press, 1960, p 111

137. Huxley HE, Hanson J: Changes in the cross-striation of muscle during contraction and stretch and their structural interpretation. Nature 173:973, 1954

138. Konigsberg I: Clonal analysis of myogenesis. Science 140:1273, 1963

139. Reporter MC, Konigsberg IR, Strehler BL: Kinetics of accumulation of creatine phosphokinase activity in developing embryonic skeletal muscle in vivo and in monolayer culture. Exp Cell Res 30:410, 1963

140. Berg J, McNeer G: Leiomyosarcoma of the stomach: A clinical and pathological study. Cancer 13:25, 1960

141. Lavin P, Hajdu SI, Foote FW: Gastric and extragastric leiomyoblastomas. Cancer 29:305, 1972

142. Quan SHQ, Berg JW: Leiomyoma and leiomyosarcoma of the rectum. Dis Colon Rect 5:415, 1962

143. Yannopoulos K, Stout AP: Smooth muscle tumors in children. Cancer 15:958, 1962

144. Gray SW, Skandalakis JE, Shepard D: Smooth muscle tumors of the esophagus: collective review. Internat Abstr Surg 133:205, 1961

145. Barnes HM, Richardson PJ: Benign metastasizing fibroleiomyoma. J Obstet Gynecol, Brit Common 80:569, 1973

146. Darby AJ, Papadki L, Beilby JOW: An unusual leiomyosarcoma of the uterus containing osteoblast-like giant cells. Cancer 36:495, 1975

147. Rothbard MF, Markham EH: Leiomyosarcoma of the cervix: Report of a case. Am J Obstet Gynecol 120:853, 1974

148. Ashley DJB: Evans' Histological Appearance of Tumors, vol 1, 3rd ed. Edinburgh, Churchill Livingstone, 1978, p 30

149. Stout AP: Solitary cutaneous and subcutaneous leiomyoma. Am J Cancer 29:435, 1937

150. Stout AP, Hill WT: Leiomyosarcoma of the superficial soft tissues. Cancer 11:844, 1958

151. Golden T, Stout AP: Smooth muscle tumors of the gastrointestinal tract and retroperitoneal tissue. Surg Gynecol Obstet 73:784, 1941

152. Melicow PJ: Primary tumors of the retroperitoneum: A clinicopathologic analysis of 162 cases. Review of the literature and tables of classification. J Internat College Surgeons 19:401, 1953

153. Smith BH, Dehner LP: Sarcoma of the prostate gland. Am J Clin Path 58:43, 1962

154. Light HG, Peskin GW, Ravdin IS: Primary tumors of the venous system. Cancer 13:818, 1960
155. Thijs LG, Kroon TAJ, Vanheeuwen TM: Leiomyosarcoma of the pulmonary trunk associated with pericardial effusion. Thorax 29:490, 1974
156. Silbar JD, Silbar SJ: Leiomyosarcoma of the bladder: three case reports and review of the literature. J Urol 73:103, 1955
157. Yannopoulos K, Stout AP: Primary solid tumors of the mesentery. Cancer 16:914, 1963
158. Werner JR, Klingensmith W, Denko JV: Leiomyosarcoma of the ureters: Case report and review of literature. J Urol 82:68, 1959
159. Jenkin DG, Subbuswany SG: Leiomyosarcoma of the spermatic cord. Br J Surg 59:408, 1972
160. Craig JM: Leiomyoma of female breast. Arch Path 44:314, 1947
161. Miles AEW, Waterhouse JP: A leiomyosarcoma of the oral cavity with metastasis to lymph glands. J Path Bact 83:551, 1962
162. Hendrick JW: Leiomyoma of thyroid gland: Report of a case. Surgery 42:597, 1957
163. Evans DMD, Sanerkin NG: Primary leiomyosarcoma of bone. J Path Bact 90:348, 1965
164. Stout AP: Bizarre smooth muscle tumors of the stomach. Cancer 15:400, 1962
165. Martin JF, Bazin F, Feroldi J, Cabanne F: Tumours myoides intramurales de l'estomac: Consideration microscipiques a propos de 6 cas. Ann Anat Path (Paris) 5:484, 1960
166. Kurman RJ, Norris HJ: Mesenchymal tumors of the uterus. VI. Epitheloid smooth muscle tumors including leiomyoblastoma and clear cell leiomyoma. Cancer 37:1853, 1976
167. Rywlin AM, Reecher L, Benson J: Clear cell leiomyoma of the uterus. Cancer 17:100, 1964
168. Gerszten E, Kay S: Light and electron microscopic study of a leiomyoblastoma of the duodenum. Am J Dig Dis 14:350, 1969
169. Salazar H, Totten RS: Leiomyoblastoma of the stomach. An ultrastructural study. Cancer 25:176, 1970
170. Corong JL: Gastric leiomyoblastoma: A clinical and ultrastructural study. Cancer 34:711, 1974
171. Johnson S, Rundell M, Platt W: Leiomyosarcoma of the scrotum: A case report with electron microscopy. Cancer 41:1830, 1978
172. Panabokke RG, Attygalle LS: Leiomyosarcoma of the skin. Br J Dermatol 79:305, 1967
173. Pritchett PS, Fu YS, Kay S: Unusual ultrastructural features of a leiomyosarcoma of the lung. Am J Clin Path 63:901, 1975
174. Akwari OE, Dozois RR, Weiland LH, Bears OH: Leiomyosarcoma of small and large bowel. Cancer 42:1384, 1979
175. Aaro LA, Symmonds RE, Dockerty MB: Sarcoma of the uterus: A clinical-pathological study of 177 cases. Am J Obst Gynecol 94:101, 1966
176. Tarnowski WM, Hashimoto K: Multiple glomus tumors: An ultrastructural study. J Invest Dermat 52:474, 1969
177. Hahn MJ, Dawson R, Esterly JA, Joseph DJ: Hemangiopericytoma: An ultrastructural study. Cancer 31:255, 1973
178. Murad TM, von Haam E, Murphy MSN: Ultrastructure of a hemangiopericytoma and a glomus tumor. Cancer 22:1239, 1968
179. Appelman HD, Helwig EB: Glomus tumors of the stomach. Cancer 24:230, 1969
180. Moran JJ, Enterline HT: Benign rhabdomyoma of the pharynx. A case report and review of the literature and comparison with cardiac rhabdomyoma. Am J Clin Path 42:174, 1964
181. Mostofi RK, Morse WH: Polypoid rhabdomyosarcoma (sarcoma botryoides) of bladder in children. J Urol 67:681, 1952
182. Tanimura H, Furuta M: Rhabdomyosarcoma of the spermatic cord. Cancer 22:1215, 1968
183. Salm R: Botryoid sarcoma of the vagina. Br J Cancer 15:220, 1961
184. Hilgers RD, Malkasian GD, Soule EH: Embryonal rhabdomyosarcoma (botryoid type) of the vagina: A clinicopathologic review. Am J Obstet Gynecol 107:484, 1970
185. Forbes GG: Rhabdomyosarcoma of bronchus. J Path Bacteriol 70:427, 1955
186. Masson JK, Soule EH: Embryonal rhabdomyosarcoma of the head and neck. Report on eighty-eight cases. Am J Surg 110:585, 1965
187. Dito WR, Batsakis JG: Intraoral pharyngeal and nasopharyngeal rhabdomyosarcoma. Otolaryngology 77:123, 1963
188. Donaldson SS, Castro JR, Wilbur JR, Jesse RH: Rhabdomyosarcoma of head and neck in children. Combination treatment by surgery, irradiation and chemotherapy. Cancer 31:26, 1973
189. Jones IS, Reese AB, Draut J: Orbital rhabdomyosarcoma: An analysis of 62 cases. Am J Ophthalmol 61:721, 1966
190. Horn RC, Enterline HT: Rhabdomyosarcoma: A clinicopathological study and classification of 39 cases. Cancer 11:181, 1958
191. Deutsch M, Leen R, Mercado R: Rhabdomyosarcoma of the middle cranial fossa. Cancer 31:1193, 1973
192. Farinacci RJ, Fairchild JP, Sulak MH, Gilpatrick CW: Sarcoma botryoides (form of embryonal rhabdomyosarcoma) of common bile duct: Report of two cases. Cancer 9:408, 1956
193. Horn RC, Yakovac WC, Kaye R, Koop CE: Rhabdomyosarcoma (sarcoma botryoides) of the common bile duct. Report of a case. Cancer 8:468, 1955
194. Corbeil LB: Differentiation of rhabdomyosarcoma and neonatal muscle cells in vitro. Cancer 20:572, 1967
195. Morales AR, Fine G, Horn RC Jr: Rhabdomyosarcoma: An ultrastructural appraisal. Path Ann 7:81, 1972
196. Toker C: Embryonal rhabdomyosarcoma: An ultrastructural study. Cancer 21:11964, 1968
197. Horvat BL, Caines M, Fisher ER: The ultrastructure of rhabdomyosarcoma. J Clin Path 53:555, 1970
198. McAllister RM, Nelson Rees WA, Johnson EY, Rongey RW, Gardner MB: Disseminated rhabdomyosarcomas formed in kittens by cultured human rhabdomyosarcoma cells. J Nat Cancer Inst 47:603, 1971
199. Pack GT, Eberhart WF: Rhabdomyosarcoma of skeletal muscle. Report of 100 cases. Surgery 32:1023, 1952
200. Stout AP: Rhabdomyosarcoma of skeletal muscle. Ann Surg 123:447, 1946

201. Hajdu SI, Koss LG: Cytologic diagnosis of metastatic myosarcomas. Acta Cytol 13:545, 1969
202. Chung A, Ringus J: Ultrastructural observations on the histogenesis of alveolar rhabdomyosarcoma. Cancer 41:1355, 1978
203. Enzinger FM, Shiraki M: Alveolar rhabdomyosarcoma: An analysis of 110 cases. Cancer 24:18, 1969
204. Ramon y Cajal S: Histologie du Systeme Nerveux de L'Hoome et des vertebres 2 vols (1909–1911). London, Oxford University Press, 1928
205. Schwann TH von: Microscopical Researches into the Structure and Growth of Animals and Plants. Translated by Henry Smith. London, Sydenham Society, 1847
206. del Rio Hortega P: Le nevroglie et le troisieme element des centres nerveuc. Bull Soc Sci Med Biol Montpellier Vol 5, 1924
207. His W: Zur Geschichte des Menslichen Ruckenmarks und der Nerven wurzlen. Abh Gesch Math 13:477, 1887
208. Sherrington CS: The Integrative Action of the Nervous System. New Haven, Yale University Press, 1947
209. Le Gross Clark WE: The Anatomical Patterns on the Essential Basis of Sensory Discrimination. Oxford, Clarendon Press, 1947
210. Eccles JC: The Physiology of Synapses. Berlin, Springer-Verlag, 1964
211. Murray ME: Nervous tissue in vitro. Chap 9, In Willmar EN (ed): Cells and Tissues in Culture, Methods, Biology and Physiology, vol. 2. New York, Academic Press, 1965, p 373
212. Coupland RE: The Natural History of the Chromaffin Cell. London, Longmans, 1965
213. Waggener ID: Ultrastructure of benign peripheral nerve sheath tumors. Cancer 19:699, 1966
214. Stout AP: Tumors of the peripheral nervous system. In: Atlas of Tumor Pathology, vol. 2, part 6. Washington DC, AFIP, 1949
215. Gamble HJ, Goldby S: Mast cells in peripheral nerve trunk. Nature 189:766, 1961
216. Pineda A: Mast cells: Their presence and ultrastructural characteristics in peripheral nerve tumors. Arch Neurol 13:372, 1965
217. Isaacson P: Mast cells in benign nerve sheath tumors. J Path 119:193, 1976
218. Csaba G, Acs T, Horvath C, Mold K: Genesis and function of mast cells: Mast cells and plasmacyte reaction to induced homologous and heterologous tumors. Br J Cancer 15:327, 1961
219. Simpson WL: Distribution of mast cells as a function of age and exposure to carcinogenic agents. Ann NY Acad Sci 103:4, 1963
220. Gambel HF, Eames RA: An electron microscopic study of the connective tissues of human peripheral nerves. J Anat 98:665, 1964
221. Nathaniel EJH, Pease DC: Degenerative changes in rat dorsal roots during Wallerian degeneration. J Ultrastruct Res 9:511, 1963
222. Nathaniel EJH, Pease DC: Collagen and basement membrane formation by Schwann cells during nerve regeneration. J Ultrastruct Res 9:550, 1963
223. Ramon y Cajal S: Degeneration and Regeneration of the Nervous System, 2nd ed. New York, Hafner, 1959
224. Woodruff JM, Chernick NL, Smith M, Millet WB, Foote FW: Peripheral nerve tumors with rhabdomyosarcomatous differentiation (malignant "triton" tumors). Cancer 32:426, 1973
225. Woodruff JM: Peripheral nerve tumors showing glandular differentiation (glandular schwannoma). Cancer 37:2399, 1976
226. Bricklin AS, Ruston HW: Angiosarcoma of venous origin arising in radial nerve. Cancer 39:1556, 1977
227. Usui M, Ishii S, Yamawaki S, et al: Malignant granular cell tumor of the radial nerve: An autopsy observation with electron microscopic and tissue culture studies. Cancer 39:1547, 1977
228. Kuo TT: Observation of nervous tissue in a Wilm's tumor: Its histogenetic significance. Cancer 39:1105, 1977
229. Krumerman MS, Stingle W: Synchronous malignant glandular schwannomas in congenital neurofibromatosis. Cancer 41:2444, 1978
230. Das Gupta TK, Brasfield RD, Strong EW, Hajdu RI: Benign solitary schwannomas (neurilemomas). Cancer 24:355, 1969
231. Russell DS, Rubenstein LJ: Pathology of Tumors of the Nervous System, 3rd ed. Baltimore, Williams and Wilkins, 1971, p 311
232. Harkin JC, Reed RJ: Tumors of the peripheral nervous system. In: Atlas of Tumor Pathology, Series 2, Fasc 3. Washington, DC, AFIP, 1969
233. Brasfield RD, Das Gupta TK: Von Recklinghausen's Disease: A clinical pathologic study. Ann Surg 175:86, 1972
234. Wander JV, Das Gupta TK: Neurofibromatosis. Current Problems in Surgery, vol 14, no. 2. Chicago, Year Book Medical Publishers, 1977
235. Albright F et al: Syndrome characterized by osteitis fibrosa disseminata, areas of pigmentation and endocrine dysfunction with precocious puberty in females. N Engl J Med 217:727, 1937
236. Jimbow K, Szabo G, Fitzpatrick TB: Ultrastructure of giant pigment granules (macromelanosomes) in the cutaneous pigmented macules of neurofibromatosis. J Invest Dermat 61:300, 1973
237. Reed WB, Becker SW Sr, Becker SW Jr, Nicke WR: Giant pigmented nevi, melanoma and leptomeningeal melanocytosis: A clinical and histopathological study. Arch Dermat 91:100–119, 1965
238. Conway H: Bathing trunk nevus. Surgery 6:585, 1939
239. Crowe FW, Schull WJ, Neel JV: A Clinical, Pathological, and Genetic Study of Multiple Neurofibromatosis. Springfield (Ill), Thomas, 1956
240. Pack GT, Davis J: Nevus giganticus pigmentosus with malignant transformation. Surgery 49:347, 1961
241. Rook A, Wilkinson DS, Ebling FJG: Textbook of Dermatology. Oxford, Blackwell, 1972, p 164
242. Feigin I, Popoff N: Regeneration of myelin in multiple sclerosis. The role of mesenchymal cells in such regeneration and in myelin formation in the peripheral nervous system. Neurology 16:364, 1966

243. Feigin I: The nerve sheath tumor, solitary and in von Recklinghausen's disease: A unitary mesenchymal concept. Acta Neuropath (Berlin) 17:188, 1971

244. Rubinstein LJ: Tumors of the Central Nervous System, Fasc. 6, Washington DC, AFIP, 1972

245. Hosoi K: Multiple neurofibromatosis (von Recklinghausen's disease) with special reference to malignant transformation. Arch Surg 22:258, 1931

246. Schenkein I, Bueker ED, Helson L, Axelrod F, Davis J: Increased nerve-growth stimulating activity in disseminated neurofibromatosis. N Engl J Med 290:613, 1974

247. Siggers DC, Boyer SH, Eldrige R: Letter—Nerve-growth factor in disseminated neurofibromatosis. N Engl J Med 292(21):1134, 1975

248. Das Gupta TK, Brasfield RD: Solitary malignant schwannomas. Ann Surg 171:419, 1970

249. D'Agostino AN, Soule EH, Miller RH: Primary malignant neoplasms of nerves (malignant neurilemomas in patients without manifestations of multiple neurofibromatosis (von Recklinghausen's disease). Cancer 16:1003, 1963

250. D'Agostino AN, Soule EH, Miller RH: Sarcomas of the peripheral nerves and somatic soft tissues associated with multiple neurofibromatosis (von Recklinghausen's disease). Cancer 16:1015, 1963

251. Kashef R, Das Gupta TK: Segmental demyelination of peripheral nerves in the presence of malignant tumours. Br J Cancer 21:411, 1967

252. Croft PB, Henson RA, Urich H, Wilkinson PC: Sensory neuropathy with bronchial carcinoma: A study of four cases showing serological abnormalities. Brain 88:501, 1965

253. Weller RO, Cervos-Navarro J: Pathology of Peripheral Nerves. London, Butterworth, 1977, p 188

254. Coupland RE, Pyper AS, Hopwood DA: Method for differentiating between noradrenaline- and adrenaline-storing cells in the light and electron microscope. Nature 201:1240, 1964

255. Brown WJ, Barjas L, Latte H: The ultrastructure of human medulla with comparative studies of white rats. Anat Rec 169:173, 1970

256. Biscoe TJ: Carotid body: Structure and function. Physiol Rev 51:437, 1971

257. Olson JL, Salyer WR: Mediastinal paragangliomas (aortic body tumor): A report of four cases and a review of the literature. Cancer 41:2405, 1978

258. Kay S, Montague JW, Dodd RW: Non-chromaffin paraganglioma (chemodectoma) of thyroid region. Cancer 36:582, 1975

259. Olsen JR, Abell MR: Non-functional, non-chromaffin paragangliomas of the retroperitoneum. Cancer 23:1358, 1969

260. Stout AP: Ganglioneuromata of the sympathetic nervous system. Surg Gynecol Obstet 84:101, 1947

261. Dahl WV, Waugh JM, Dahlin DE: Gastrointestinal ganglioneuromas: Brief review with report of duodenal ganglioneuroma. Am J Path 33:953, 1957

262. Yokoyama M, Okad K, Takayasa H, Yamada R: Ultrastructural and biochemical study of benign ganglioneuroma. Virchows Arch Path Anat 361:195, 1973

263. deLorimer AA, Bragg KV, Linden G: Neuroblastoma in childhood. Am J Dis Child 188:441, 1969

264. Young LW, Rubin P, Hanson RE: The extra-adrenal neuroblastoma: High radiocurability and diagnostic accuracy. Am J Roentgenol Rad Ther Nucl Med 108:75, 1970

265. Dawson DA: Nerve cell tumors of the neck and their secretory activity. J Laryngol Otol 84:203, 1970

266. Pack GT, Ariel IM, Miller TRA: Malignant ganglioneuroma of the ganglion nodosum of the vagus nerve. Arch Surg 67:545, 1953

267. Koyoumdjian AO, McDonald JJ: Association of congenital renal neuroblastoma with multiple anomalies including unusual oropharyngeal cavity (imperfect buccopharyngeal membrane). Cancer 4:784, 1951

268. Horn RC, Koop CE, Kisen Wetter WB: Neuroblastoma in childhood. J Lab Invest 5:016, 1956

269. Birrier WF: Neuroblastoma as a cause of antenatal death. Am J Obst Gynecol 82:1388, 1961

270. Marsden HG, Steward JK: Tumors in children. Recent Results in Cancer Research, #13. Berlin, Springer-Verlag, 1968

271. Sy WM, Edmandson JH: The developmental defects associated with neuroblastoma—etiologic implications. Cancer 22:234, 1968

272. Knudson AG, Amromin GD: Neuroblastoma and ganglioneuroma in a child with multiple neurofibromatosis. Cancer 19:1022, 1966

273. Bolande RP, Towler WF: A possible relationship of neuroblastoma to von Recklinghausen's disease. Cancer 26:162, 1970

274. Greenberg R, Rosenthal I, Fall GS: Electron microscopy of human tumors secreting catecholamines: Correlation with biochemical data. J Neuropath Exp Neurol 179:475, 1969

275. Everson TC, Cole WH: Spontaneous Regression of Cancer. Philadelphia, Saunders, 1966

276. Beckwith JB, Martin RB: Observations on the histopathology of neuroblastomas. J Pediat Surg 3:106, 1968

277. Mckinen J: Microscopic patterns as a guide to prognosis of neuroblastoma in childhood. Cancer 29:1637, 1972

278. Hughes M, Marsden HB, Palmer MK: Histologic patterns of neuroblastoma related to prognosis and clinical staging. Cancer 34:1706, 1974

279. Lauder I, Aherne W: The significance of lymphocytic infiltration in neuroblastoma. Br J Cancer 26:321, 1972

280. Brown JW, Burton RC, Dahlin DC: Chemodectoma with skeletal metastases. Report of two cases. Mayo Clinic Proc 42:551, 1967

281. Ghadially FN, Roy S: Ultrastructure of Synovial Joints in Health and Disease. London, Butterworth, 1969

282. Barland P, Novikoff AB, Hamerman D: Electron microscopy of the human synovial membrane. J Cell Biol 14:207, 1962

283. Cadman NL, Soule EH, Kelly PJ: Synovial sarcoma. An analysis of 134 tumors. Cancer 18:613, 1965

284. Mackenzie DH: Synovial sarcoma: A review of 58 cases. Cancer 19:169, 1966

285. Ariel IM, Pack GT: Synovial sarcoma: Review of 25 cases. N Engl J Med 268:1272, 1963

286. Ichinose H, Powell L, Hoerner HE, Derbes VJ, Byers JF: The potential histogenetic relationship of the peripheral nerve to synovioma. Cancer Res 39:4270, 1979

287. Jaffe HL: Tumors and Tumorous Conditions of the Bones and Joints. London, H. Kimpton, 1958, p 584

288. Van Andel JG: Synovial sarcoma: A review and analysis of treated cases. Radiol Clin Biol 41:145, 1972

289. Krugman ME, Rosin HD, Toker C: Synovial sarcoma of the head and neck. Arch Otolaryngol 98:53, 1973

290. Roth JA, Enzinger FM, Tannenbaum M: Synovial sarcoma of the neck: A followup study of 24 cases. Cancer 35:1243, 1975

291. Attie JN, Steckler RM, Platt N: Cervical synovial sarcoma. Cancer 25:785, 1970

292. Hale JE, Calder ILM: Synovial sarcoma of the abdominal wall. Br J Cancer 24:471, 1970

293. Miller LH, Sanatella-Latimer L, Milly T: Synovial sarcoma of the larynx. Tr Am Acad Ophth Otolaryngol 80:488, 1975

294. Haagensen CD, Stout AP: Synovial sarcoma. Ann Surg 120:826, 1944

295. Gabbiani G, Kaye GI, Lattes R, Jajoni G: Synovial sarcoma: Electron microscopic study of a typical case. Cancer 28:1031, 1971

296. Weingrad DN, Rosenberg SA: Early lymphatic spread of osteogenic and soft tissue sarcomas. Surgery 84:231, 1978

297. Enzinger FM: Clear cell sarcoma of tendons and aponeuroses—an analysis of 21 cases. Cancer 18:1163, 1965

298. Budreaux D, Waisman J: Clear cell sarcoma with melanogenesis. Cancer 41:1387, 1978

299. Bearman RM, Noe J, Kempson RL: Clear cell sarcoma with melanin pigment. Cancer 36:977, 1975

300. Hoffman GJ, Carter D: Clear cell sarcoma of tendons and aponeuroses with melanin. Arch Path 95:22, 1973

301. Kubo T: Clear cell sarcoma of patellar tendon studied by electron microscopy. Cancer 24:948, 1969

302. Mackenzie DH: Clear cell sarcoma of tendon and aponeuroses with melanin production. J Path 114:231, 1974

303. Toe TK, Saw D: Clear cell sarcoma with melanin—report of two cases. Cancer 41:235, 1978

304. Guccion JG, Enzinger FM: Malignant giant cell tumor of soft tissues. Cancer 29:1578, 1972

305. Pratt J, Woodruff JM, Marcove RC: Epithelioid sarcoma: An analysis of 22 cases indicating the prognostic significance of vascular invasion and regional lymph node metastasis. Cancer 41:1472, 1978

306. Bryan RS, Soule EH, Dobyns JH, Pritchard DJ, Linscheid RL: Primary epithelioid sarcoma of the hand and forearm. A review of thirteen cases. J Bone Joint Surg 56-A:458, 1974

307. Enzinger FM: Epithelioid sarcoma. A sarcoma simulating a granuloma or a carcinoma. Cancer 26:1029, 1970

308. Males JL, Lain KC: Epithelioid sarcoma in XO/XX Turner's syndrome. Arch Path 94:214, 1972

309. Moore SW, Wheeler TE, Hefter LG: Epithelioid sarcoma masquerading as Peyronie's Disease. Cancer 35:1706, 1976

310. Santiago H, Feinerman LK, Lattes R: Epithelioid sarcoma. Hum Path 3:133, 1972

311. Gabbiani G, Fu YS, Kaye GI, Lattes R, Majno G: Epithelioid sarcoma. A light and electron microscopic study suggesting a synovial origin. Cancer 30:486, 1972

312. Frable WJ, Kay S, Lawrence W, Schatzki PF: Epithelioid sarcoma: An electron microscopic study. Arch Path 95:8, 1973

313. Bloustein PA, Silverberg SG, Waddell WR: Epithelioid sarcoma. Case report with ultrastructural review, histogenetic discussion and chemotherapeutic data. Cancer 38:2390, 1976

314. Kampmeier OF: Evolution and comparative morphology of the lymphatic system. Springfield (Ill), Thomas, 1969

315. Walsh TS, Tompkins VN: Some observations on the strawberry nevus of infancy. Cancer 9:869, 1956

316. Rhodin JAC: Ultrastructure of mammalian venous capillaries, venules and small collecting veins. J Ultrastruct Res 25:452, 1968

317. Karnovsky MJ: The ultrastructural basis of capillary permeability studied with peroxidase as a tracer. J Cell Biol 35:213, 1967

318. Simionescu N, Simionescu M: The cardiovascular system. In Weiss L, Greep RO (eds): Histology, 4th ed. New York, McGraw-Hill, 1977

319. Harano A, Dembitzer HM, Zimmerman HM: Fenestrated blood vessels in neurilemoma. Lab Invest 27:305, 1972

320. Masson F: Les glomus cutanes de l'homme. Bulletin de la Societe Francaise de Dermatologie et de Syphiligraphie 42:1174, 1935

321. Banner EA, Winkelmann RK: Glomus tumour of the vagina. Report of a case. Obstet Gynecol 9:326, 1957

322. Hrubam Z, Evans W, Humphreys E: An unusual form of a neurovascular hamartoma. Arch Path 69:672, 1960

323. Bindley GV: Glomus tumor of the mediastinum. J Thor Surg 18:417, 1949

324. Allen RA, Dahlin DC: Glomus tumor of the stomach: Report of two cases. Mayo Clin Proc 29:429, 1954

325. Ruding R, Harmsen AE: Glomus tumor of the stomach. Hemangioglomocytoma. Ann Surg 155:221, 1962

326. Kay S, Calahan WP, Murray MR, Randall HT, Stout OP: Glomus tumors of the stomach. Cancer 4:726, 1951

327. Borghard-Erdle AM, Hirsch EF: Glomus tumors of the uterus. Arch Path 65:244, 1958

328. Mackenzie DH: Intraosseous glomus tumors: Report of two cases. J Bone Joint Surg 44-B:648, 1962

329. Murray MR, Stout AP: The glomus tumor: Investigation of its distribution and the identity of its "epithelioid" cell. Am J Path 18:183, 1942

330. Battifra H: Hemangiopericytoma. Ultrastructural study of five cases. Cancer 31:1418, 1973

331. Hahn MJ, Dawson R, Esterly JA, Joseph DJ: He-mangiopericytoma: An ultrastructural study. Cancer 31:255, 1973

332. Harris M: Ultrastructure of a glomus tumor. J Clin Path 25:520, 1971

333. Popoff NA, Malinin TI, Rosomoff HL: Fine structure of intracranial hemangiopericytoma and angiomatous meningioma. Cancer 34:1187, 1974

334. Ramsey HJ: Fine structure of haemangiopericytoma and haemangioendothelioma. Cancer 19:1005, 1966

335. Toker C: Glomangioma: An ultrastructural study. Cancer 23:487, 1969

336. Tarnowski WM, Hashimoto K: Multiple glomus tumors: An ultrastructural study. Cancer 23:487, 1969

337. Mallory FG: The results of the application of special histological methods to the study of tumors. J Exper Med 10:575, 1908

338. Autry JR, Weitzner S: Hemangiosarcoma of spleen with spontaneous rupture. Cancer 35:539, 1975

339. Stutz FH, Tormey DC, Blom J: Hemangiosarcoma and pathologic rupture of the spleen. Cancer 31:1213, 1973

340. Baker H, De C, Pagent GE, Davison J: Haemangioendothelioma (Kupffer-cell sarcoma) of the liver. J Path Bacteriol 72:173, 1956

341. Blumenfeld TA, Fleming ID, Johnson WW: Juvenile hemangioendothelioma of the liver. Cancer 24:853, 1969

342. Unni KK, Ivins JC, Beaubot JW, Dahlin DC: Hemangioma: Hemangiopericytoma and hemangioendothelioma (angiosarcoma) of bone. Cancer 27:1403, 1971

343. Dube VE, Fisher DE: Hemangioendothelioma of the leg following metallic fixation of the tibia. Cancer 30:1260, 1972

344. McCarthy WD, Pack GT: Malignant blood vessel tumors: Report of 56 cases of angiosarcoma and Kaposi's sarcoma. Surg Gynecol Obstet 91:465, 1950

345. Stout AP: Hemangio-endothelioma: A tumor of blood vessels featuring vascular endothelial cells. Ann Surg 118:445, 1943

346. Dunegan LJ, Toben H, Watson CG: Angiosarcoma of the breast: A report of two cases and a review of the literature. Surgery 79:57, 1976

347. Kennedy JC, Fisher JH: Haemangiopericytoma: Its orthopaedic manifestations. J Bone Joint Surg 42-B:80, 1960

348. Stout AP: Tumors featuring pericytes. Lab Invest 5:217, 1956

349. Rewell RE: Haemangiopericytoma of the gum. J Laryngol Otol 82:261, 1968

350. Lidholm SO: Haemangiopericytoma. Acta Path Microbiol Scand 38:186, 1951

351. Greene RR, Gerbie AG, Gerbie MV, Eckman TR: Haemangiopericytomas of the uterus. Am J Obstet Gynecol 106:1020, 1970

352. Seaton D: Primary diaphragmatic haemangiopericytoma. Thorax 29:595, 1975

353. Kaposi M: Idiopathisches multiples pigment sarkom der Haut. Arch Dermat Syph 4:265, 1872

354. Dhana D, Templeton AC, Master SP, Skyalwazi SK: Kaposi's sarcoma of lymph nodes. Br J Cancer 24:464, 1970

355. Masters SP, Taylor JF, Kyalwazi SK, Ziegler JL: Immunological studies in Kaposi's sarcoma in Uganda. Br Med J 1:600, 1970

356. Salvin G, Cameron HM, Forbes C, Mitchell RM: Kaposi's sarcoma in East African children: A report of 51 cases. J Path 100:187, 1970

357. Templeton AC, Bhana D: Prognosis in Kaposi's sarcoma. J Nat Cancer Inst 55:1301, 1975

358. Hashimoto K, Lever WF: Kaposi's Sarcoma: Histochemical and electron microscopic studies. J Invest Derm 43:539, 1964

359. Ramos CV, Taylor HB, Hernandez BA, Tucker EF: Primary Kaposi's sarcoma of lymph nodes. Am J Clin Pathol 66:948, 1976

360. Taylor JF, Iverson OH, Bjerknes R: Growth kinetics of Kaposi's sarcoma. Br J Cancer 35:470, 1977

361. Dayan AD, Lewis PD: Origin of Kaposi's sarcoma from reticuloendothelial system. Nature 213:889, 1967

362. Reynolds WA, Wikleman RK, Soule EH: Kaposi's Sarcoma: A clinicopathologic study with particular reference to its relationship to the reticuloendothelial system. Medicine 44:419, 1965

363. Stewart FW, Treves N: Lymphangiosarcoma in postmastectomy lymphedema. A report of six cases in elephantiasis chirugica. Cancer 1:64, 1948

364. Nelson WR, Morifit HM: Lymphangiosarcoma in the lymphedematous arm after radical mastectomy. Cancer 9:1189, 1956

365. Woodward AH, Ivins JC, Soule EH: Lymphangiosarcoma arising in chronic lymphedematous extremities. Cancer 30:562, 1972

366. Salm R: The nature of the so-called postmastectomy lymphangiosarcoma. J Path 85:445, 1963

367. Silverberg SG, Kay S, Koss LG: Postmastectomy lymphanigosarcoma: Ultrastructural observations. Cancer 27:100, 1971

368. Mackenzie DH: Lymphangiosarcoma arising in chronic congenital and idiopathic lymphedema. J Clin Path 24:524, 1971

369. Finlay-Jones LR: Lymphangiosarcoma of the thigh. Cancer 26:722, 1970

370. Enterline HT, Roberts B: Lymphangiopericytoma. Cancer 8:582, 1955

371. Cornog JL Jr, Enterline HT: Lymphangiomyoma—A benign lesion of chyliferous lymphatics synonymous with lymphangiopericytoma. Cancer 19:1909, 1966

372. Corrin D, Liebow AA, Friedman PJ: Pulmonary lymphangiomyomitosis. Am J Path 79:347, 1975

373. Huggins CB: The formation of bone under influence of epithelium of the urinary tract. Arch Surg 22:377, 1931

374. Binkley JS, Stewart FW: Morphogenesis of extraskeletal osteogenic sarcoma and pseudo-osteosarcoma. Arch Path 29:42, 1940

375. Brookes M: The vascular factors in osteoarthritis. Surg Gynecol Obstet 123:1255, 1966

376. Boneti T: De ventris tumors. In Sepulchretum, sive anatomic practica excadaveribus morbo denatis, vol 3, sect 21, Obs 61. Geneva, Cramer et Parachon, 1700, p 522

377. Fine G, Stout AP: Osteogenic sarcoma of the extraskeletal soft tissue. Cancer 9:1027, 1956

378. Das Gupta TK, Hajdu SI, Foote FW Jr: Extraosseous osteogenic sarcoma. Ann Surg 168:1011, 1968

379. Dahm LJ, Schaefer SD, Carder HM, Vellios F: Osteosarcoma of the soft tissue of the larynx. Report of a case with light and electron microscopic studies. Cancer 42:2343, 1978

380. Rao U, Cheng A, Didolkar S: Extraosseous osteogenic sarcoma: Clinicopathological study of eight cases and review of literature. Cancer 41:1488, 1978

381. Stout AP, Verner EW: Chondrosarcoma of the extraskeletal soft tissue. Cancer 6:581, 1953

382. Enzinger FM, Shiraki M: Extraskeletal myxoid chondrosarcoma. An analysis of 34 cases. Human Path 3:421, 1972

383. Goldenberg RR, Chen P, Steinlauf P: Chondrosarcoma of the extraskeletal soft tissues. J Bone Joint Surg 49-A:1487, 1967

384. Chung EB, Enzinger FM: Chondroma of soft parts. Cancer 41:1414, 1978

385. Angervall L, Enzinger FM: Extraskeletal neoplasm resembling Ewing's sarcoma. Cancer 36:240, 1975

386. Soule EH, Newton W, Moon TE, Tefft M: Extraskeletal Ewing's sarcoma. Cancer 42:259, 1979

387. Abrikossoff A: Uber Myome Ausgehend von der quergestreiften Wilkurlichen Muskulatus. Virchows Arch Path Anat 260:215, 1926

388. Aparicio SR, Lumsdeu CE: Light and electron microscopic studies on the granular cell myoblastoma of the tongue. J Path 97:339, 1969

389. Solbel HJ, Schwarz R, Marquet E: Light and electron microscopic study of the origin of granular cell myoblastoma. J Path 109:101, 1973

390. Pearse AGE: The histogenesis of granular cell myoblastoma. Am J Clin Path 19:522, 1949

391. Garancis JC, Komorowski RA, Kuzma JF: Granular cell myoblastoma. Cancer 25:542, 1970

392. Usui M, Isshii S, Yamawaki S, et al: Malignant granular cell tumor of the radial nerve: An autopsy observation with electron microscopic and tissue culture studies. Cancer 39:1547, 1977

393. Christopherson WM, Foote FW, Stewart FW: Alveolar soft part sarcomas: Structurally characteristic tumors of uncertain histogenesis. Cancer 5:100, 1952

394. Smetana GF, Scott WF Jr: Malignant tumors of the nonchromaffin paraganglia. Milit Surgeon 109: 330, 1951

395. Udekwu FA, Pulvertaft RJV: Studies of an alveolar soft tissue sarcoma. Br J Cancer 19:744, 1966

396. Karnauchow PN, Magner D: The histogenesis of alveolar soft part sarcoma. J Path Bacteriol 86:169, 1963

397. Shipkey FH, Lieberman PH, Foote FW, Stewart FW: Ultrastructure of alveolar soft part sarcoma. Cancer 17:821, 1964

398. Fisher ER, Reidbord H: Electron microscopic evidence suggesting the myogenous derivation of the so-called alveolar soft part sarcoma. Cancer 27:150, 1971

399. Welsh RA, Bray DM, Shipkey FH, Meyer AT: Histogenesis of alveolar soft part sarcoma. Cancer 29:191, 1972

400. Unni KK, Soule EH: Alveolar rhabdomyosarcoma. An electron microscopic study. Mayo Clin Proc 50:59, 1975

401. Cadotte M: Malignant granular-cell myoblastoma. Cancer 33:1417, 1974

402. Hernandez FJ, Fernandez BB: Localized fibrous tumors of pleura: A light and electron microscopic study. Cancer 34:1667, 1974

403. Chan PSF, Balfour TW, Bourke JB, Smith PG: Peritoneal mesothelioma. Br J Surg 62:576, 1975

5
Principles of Clinical Diagnosis and Staging

Tapas K. Das Gupta

The accuracy of clinical diagnoses of soft tissue sarcomas is always questionable. Although lipomas whose margins apparently slip out of the examining finger are classic, occasionally liposarcomas lurk in these seemingly benign tumors. Thus, a blasé attitude is fraught with danger to the patient. It is essential to have a systematic approach to diagnosis and therapy of all soft tissue tumors.

The diagnosis of large ulcerating or fungating tumors (Fig. 5.1) is not difficult; the problem arises with the small, apparently innocuous variety.

History-taking is of utmost importance, and often the clinician is remiss in not obtaining a detailed history of the initial appearance of the tumor and the associated symptoms. These alone often provide a clue to the diagnosis. Several classic examples are described in the following case histories. On the basis of these descriptions it is possible to develop some general guidelines in history-taking for soft tissue tumors.

CASE HISTORIES

Patient 1: A 46-year-old woman had noticed a mass in her right thigh about four to six weeks prior to seeking medical advice. Initially this tumor was thought to be benign; however, she came to us for a second opinion. The relatively soft tumor in the upper anterior aspect of the thigh was found to be a liposarcoma (Fig. 5.2).

Patient 2: A 10-year-old girl was brought to her pediatrician with a small tumor in the right temporal region of several weeks' duration. The pediatric surgeon considered the tumor to be a sebaceous cyst. On excision it was found to be a rhabdomyosarcoma (Fig. 5.3).

Patient 3: A 58-year-old woman was seen with a slowly enlarging tumor in her arm (Fig. 5.4), which had been present for several years without causing any difficulty. The patient had consulted another physician earlier, but since it was a symptomless mass, no further investigation had been undertaken. However, detailed history-taking and clinical examination showed she had some of the stigmata of von Recklinghausen's disease. Because of this association, a biopsy was done and a diagnosis of malignant schwannoma established.

Patient 4: A 51-year-old man complained that he had had perineal pain radiating to the medial aspect of both thighs for about 2 years. A careful urologic examination, including cystoscopy, failed to show any abnormalities in the urethra, prostate, or urinary bladder. A diagnosis of pudendal neuralgia was entertained. However, after two years of this pain, a small tumor in the perineum could be palpated and an x-ray of the pelvis showed complete de-

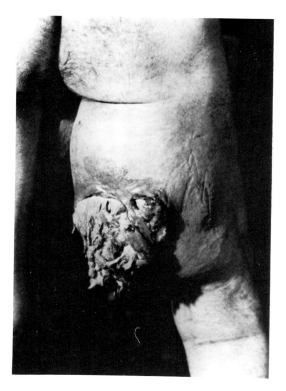

Figure 5.1. Fungating tumor in right posterior thigh of a 55-year-old man. Tumor was subcutaneous for two to three years, then started to grow, but patient did not seek medical attention until the lesion fungated. Microscopic diagnosis of liposarcoma was established.

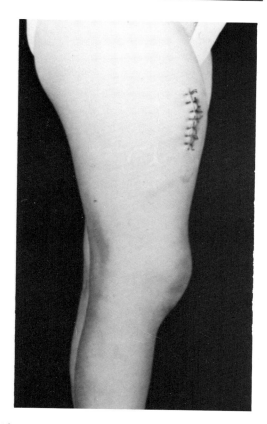

Figure 5.2. Tumor clinically measured 5 × 8 cm, was relatively soft, and appeared to be a benign lipoma. Wedge biopsy showed it to be a liposarcoma.

struction of the inferior pubic ramus of the left side (Fig. 5.5). A wedge specimen was taken and microscopic examination established this tumor as a hemangiopericytoma.

Patient 5: A 21-year-old man was seen by his physician for a tender swelling of the right buttock. He related that several weeks previously he had sustained some kind of trauma while playing basketball. A diagnosis of infected hematoma of the right buttock was made and the patient was treated with antibiotics. When the mass did not subside, it was incised for adequate drainage. Following this procedure the tumor fungated out through the wound and histologic examination established a diagnosis of rhabdomyosarcoma (Fig. 5.6).

Patient 6: A skin tumor was noted in the area of the knee joint of a 41-year-old man. This was considered to be a pyogenic granuloma and

was treated with antibiotics (Fig. 5.7). When the lesion was found to be refractory to conservative treatment, the patient was referred to the University of Illinois Hospital. A wedge biopsy specimen showed this to be a dermatofibrosarcoma protuberans (Fig. 12.9E, Chapter 12).

Patient 7: A 4-month-old male infant was found to have a small tumor in the region of the medial malleolus of the right foot. The tumor was excised elsewhere and a diagnosis of fibrosarcoma was entertained. On the basis of this diagnosis a wide excision or an amputation was contemplated. The parents then sought a second opinion and were referred to the University of Illinois Hospital. They related that the nodule in that area was about 1 cm in diameter when first discovered and had remained mobile for several weeks prior to its relatively rapid

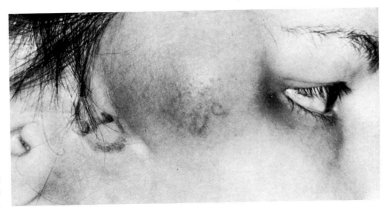

Figure 5.3. Close-up view of tumor in right temple of 10-year-old girl. A glistening of the overlying skin surface can easily be seen. This was found to be a rhabdomyosarcoma.

increase in size. A clinical diagnosis of fibromatosis was made, which was later confirmed by several pathologists. The child was saved an extensive operation, since this type of fibromatosis is self-limiting (Fig. 5.8).

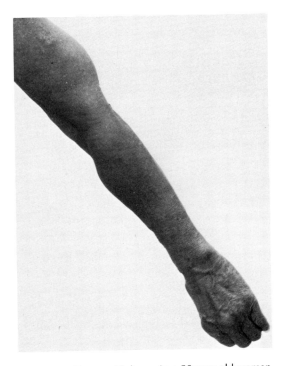

Figure 5.4. Tumor of left arm in a 58-year-old woman. Because of multiple café-au-lait spots on anterior chest wall and posterior trunk, a detailed family history was obtained. Stigmata of von Recklinghausen's disease were found in patient's siblings and parents. Because of this association, a wedge biopsy of the tumor was done, which showed that the tumor was indeed a malignant schwannoma.

These representative case reports illustrate the basic concept that, as in other disease processes, a good clinical history frequently leads to accurate diagnosis. In general, the following points can be used as identifiable clues for the diagnosis of soft tissue sarcomas:

1. A rapid-growing solitary soft tissue tumor in persons in their 40s or older should be considered with suspicion.
2. A tumor of short duration located in the upper aspect of the thigh, especially in a woman, should be considered malignant until proved otherwise.
3. Although exceptions are occasionally seen, the existence of multiple lipomas in general precludes the possiblity of a malignant adipose tissue tumor.
4. Subcutaneous tumors in the head and neck region of a child should be carefully examined to rule out a malignant tumor.
5. All retroperitoneal tumors should be considered sarcomas until proved otherwise.
6. A tumor larger than 10 cm should arouse suspicion of malignancy.
7. An unexplained buttock mass in an adult should be assumed to be a tumor, and injudicious incision and drainage should be avoided even when it resembles an inflammatory mass.
8. Soft tissue sarcomas are frequently associated with certain preneoplastic disease states such as von Recklinghausen's disease, Gardner's syndrome, and several other varieties of neurocutaneous or mucocutaneous syndromes (Table 2.1, Chapter 2).
9. In children, small tumors in the distal ends of the extremities are usually benign and

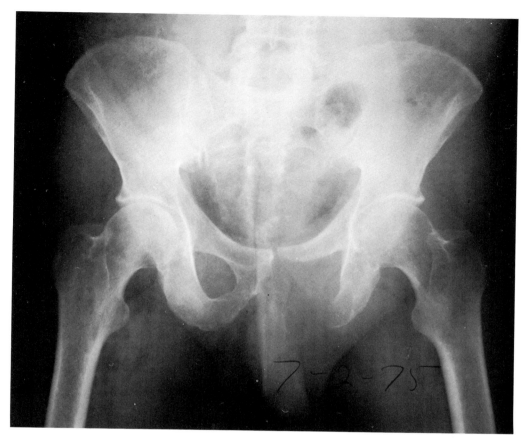

Figure 5.5. Roentgenograph of pelvis showing bony destruction of left inferior ramus of the pubis. This soft tissue mass was revealed on wedge biopsy to be a hemangiopericytoma arising in the perineum.

great caution should be taken before any therapy is undertaken.

10. Almost all angiomatous tumors in children are benign (Fig. 5.9).

11. Long-standing pyogenic granulomas in the extremities should not be treated lightly, as they may be malignant.

12. The persistence of unexplained pain along the course of one or more major peripheral nerves should be viewed with suspicion, since occasionally pain is caused by a malignant tumor pressing on or infiltrating the fibers of a peripheral nerve or a plexus. Malignant schwannomas have frequently been missed because such complaints of pain were not investigated thoroughly. This symptom occurs with all types of cancer and is not produced by soft tissue sarcomas only.

The clinical examination of a patient with a soft tissue tumor likewise must be thorough. A description of systemic examination not directly related to the given tumor is not germane to this chapter and is being excluded; the present discussion will be limited to examination of the primary tumor, the anatomic region in which the tumor is located, and any other associated conditions.

CLINICAL EXAMINATION OF THE PRIMARY TUMOR

Examination of the primary tumor, with a clear, concise, and accurate description of the clinical features, is absolutely essential. Failure to do this frequently results in an incorrect assess-

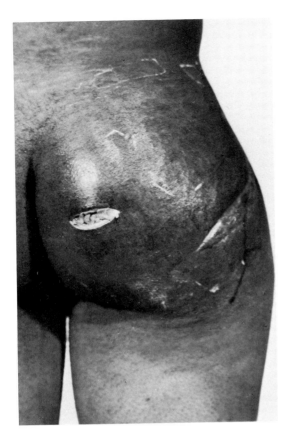

Figure 5.6. Large tumor of right buttock, with diagnosis of an abscess of the buttock. Two incisions were made. Through one of these incisions, the underlying tumor can be seen to protrude. Because the huge fungating tumor was refractory to radiation therapy, the patient underwent a hemipelvectomy, but died two years later with diffuse metastasis.

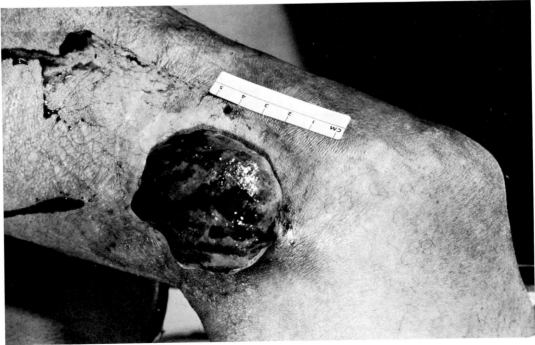

Figure 5.7. Dermatofibrosarcoma protuberans in the region of the knee joint. This was thought to be a pyogenic granuloma.

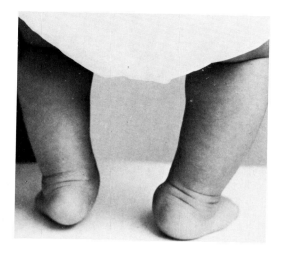

Figure 5.8. Posterior view of ankles of a four-month-old boy. The medial swelling of the right ankle is easily apparent, compared with the left medial aspect. Parents stated that the tumor was discrete at first, then became diffuse.

ment. Often, the microscopic description with accurate histologic diagnosis is missed because the clinician failed to examine the primary tumor thoroughly or record the findings meticulously. Clinical examination of the primary tumor can be performed along the following lines:

Location

The location of the primary tumor should be ascertained. First, determine the broad anatomic location, that is, whether it is in the head and neck region or the trunk or the extremities. Next, determine the specific location in the general anatomic region. A tumor located in the temporal area or in the region of the outer canthus of the eye or along the lateral margin of the nose should arouse suspicion of a rhabdomyosarcoma, especially in a young adult. In contrast, tumors in the scalp are usually benign, although infrequently a liposarcoma or neuro-

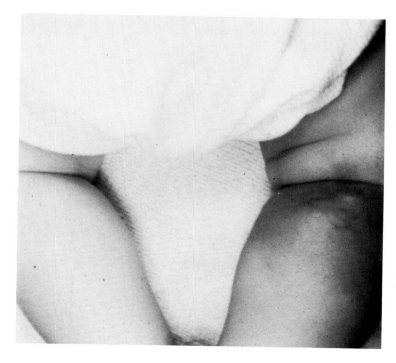

Figure 5.9. A localized cavernous hemangioma of the right leg in an infant six months old. These types of angioma do not need any treatment unless symptomatic.

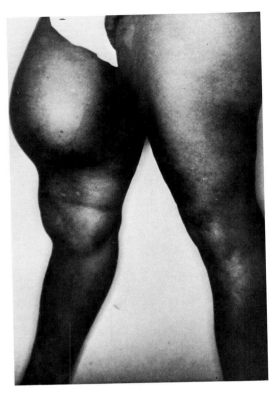

Figure 5.10. Large tumor in the anterolateral aspect of the right thigh. The size itself is an indication of possible malignancy (ie, more than 10 cm). Incision biopsy confirmed diagnosis of liposarcoma. *(Reproduced with permission: Tumors and Tumorlike Conditions of the Adipose Tissue. In Ravitch, MM, et al (eds): Current Problems in Surgery. Copyright 1970 by Year Book Medical Publishers, Inc., Chicago.)*

monly, a large, round subcutaneous mass is either a lipoma or a liposarcoma. A fibrous tissue tumor usually is ovoid.

Size
Although the size of a given primary tumor usually is not an indication of either benignancy or malignancy, an accurate documentation of its size is desirable. If the tumor is malignant, then its size helps in the clinicopathologic staging in a given anatomic location. The size of the primary tumor also indicates the type of primary therapy. For example, a 2-cm liposarcoma located in the upper outer portion of the thigh can be adequately treated with wide soft tissue resection; in contrast, a 15-cm liposarcoma in the same location might require a much larger operation, or radiation, or both. Seldom are malignant soft tissue tumors smaller than 1 cm, and tumors larger than 15 cm frequently are malignant (Fig. 5.10). Within the same histologic type, malignant tumors measuring 5 cm or less carry a better prognosis for the patient.[2–5]

Consistency
The consistency of a primary tumor can frequently lead to a correct clinical assessment. For example, a lipoma is uniformly soft, whereas a liposarcoma can be distinguished by its areas of relatively firm consistency, even though the tumor appears soft on first examination. A uniformly firm or hard soft tissue tumor should be considered malignant, irrespective of its size or location.

fibrosarcoma is encountered. A lesion located in the upper inner aspect of the thigh has a high possibility of being a liposarcoma. Furthermore, especially in the extremities, the prognosis for a patient with a given sarcoma has been linked with whether the tumor is superficial (subcutaneous) or deep (intermuscular or deeper). Generally, the more superficial the tumor, the better the prognosis.[1,2]

Shape
The shape of the primary tumor frequently is indicative of the type of sarcoma. A malignant tumor of a peripheral nerve usually grows in its long axis and frequently appears as a fusiform mass. A lipoma or a liposarcoma, because adipose tissue has more freedom to expand, can assume any shape or size (Fig. 5.10), but com-

Relation to Surrounding Tissues
It is essential that the clinician evaluate the relationship of a primary tumor to the surrounding adipose tissue, muscles, nerves, major vessels, and bones. This information is not only useful in proper staging but also helps the histologist to arrive at a correct microscopic diagnosis. For example, a tumor consisting of spindle-shaped malignant cells may be designated as spindle cell sarcoma. However, if it is known that the tumor arose from a peripheral nerve or was intimately adherent to the nerve, it is highly likely that this tumor is of neural origin. When the ultrastructural findings are added to these data, in most instances an accurate diagnosis can be established. In staging, the relationship of the surrounding structures is used for T-classification. If a tumor invades the major vessels

or the bones, it is classified as T_3, indicating a relatively poor prognosis.

Regional Nodes

Soft tissue sarcomas do not metastasize in large numbers to the regional nodes.[6] However, because some do, it is essential that regional nodes be examined in every case of suspected soft tissue sarcoma.

ASSOCIATED PRENEOPLASTIC OR HAMARTOMATOUS SYNDROMES

Both benign and malignant soft tissue are sometimes associated with preneoplastic or hamartomatous syndromes. For example, a patient with multiple café-au-lait spots presenting with a subcutaneous mass probably has either a benign or malignant neurogenic tumor. An overview of the relationship of these hamartomatous syndromes to soft tissue sarcomas is discussed in the section dealing with epidemiology. The individual syndromes are separately discussed along with those tumors with which they are primarily associated.

Following assessment of the primary tumor and any associated conditions, the overall status of the patient should be evaluated, and this should include all the general physical and laboratory examinations. If the clinicopathologic examination is suggestive of sarcoma, then a complete metastatic workup germane to the histogenetic type of primary tumor should be instituted.

DIAGNOSTIC AIDS IN SOFT TISSUE TUMORS

The following are commonly used in the evaluation of primary soft tissue tumors and can be classified into (1) roentgenologic examinations, (2) radioisotope methods, and (3) biochemical tests.

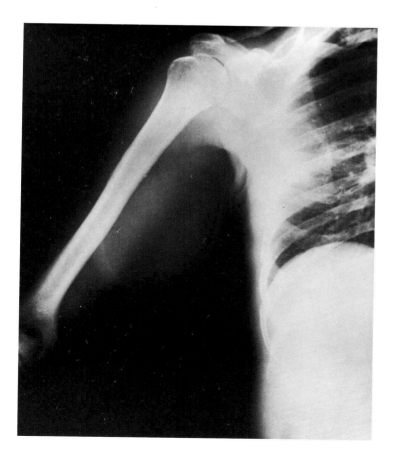

Figure 5.11. Large tumor of the medial aspect of the arm of a 60-year-old man. Roentgenogram of this smooth fatty tumor was suggestive of a lipoma and excision substantiated the diagnosis.

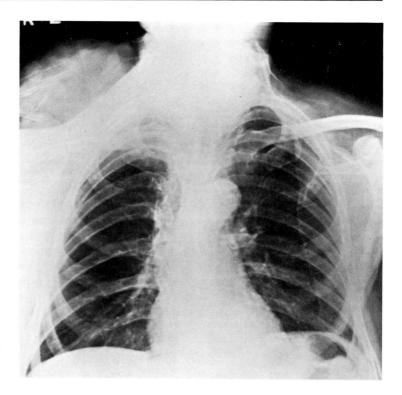

Figure 5.12. Multilobulated tumor in the right side of the neck and the shoulder of a 55-year-old man. Roentgenographic examination suggested a malignant fatty tumor (liposarcoma), later substantiated by a wedge biopsy.

Roentgenologic Examination of Soft Tissue Tumors

Routine X-Rays. Routine biplane x-rays of a common garden variety tumor, eg, a small subcutaneous lipoma, are neither useful nor required. The clinician frequently orders x-rays of such tissue masses more from habit than need. However, in carefully selected patients, roentgenographic examination can solve some of the diagnostic riddles (Figs. 5.11 to 5.13).[7,8] This method of radiography can be extended by use of xeroradiography.

Xeroradiography. Xeroradiography is, in essence, a radiographic method in which a photoconductive (selenium) plate is substituted for conventional radiographs. The contrast and details are far superior. Therefore, when there are indications for a radiographic examination of a given soft somatic tissue tumor, and the facilities exist, the use of xeroradiographs is recommended. It is likely that in some instances a prebiopsy diagnosis of malignancy could be arrived at by judicious use of xeroradiography (Fig. 5.14).

Angiography. The useful role of angiography as a diagnostic aid in soft somatic tissue tumors is unquestionable.

Arteriography. Arteriography for upper and lower extremity soft tissue tumors has been well described by several authors.[9–16] In selected patients with soft tissue sarcoma of an extremity this diagnostic technique can be of some value. In Figures 5.15 and 5.16 its usefulness is apparent. Figure 5.15 shows that sometimes, even in superficially located somatic tumors, arteriographs can be useful and often are diagnostic of malignancy, although no diagnostic method supersedes microscopic examination of the tumor. With the increasing use of infusion or perfusion chemotherapy for extremity sarcomas, preoperative angiography is being used more frequently.

Angiographic studies of cavitary tumors such as retroperitoneal sarcomas are essential. It is axiomatic that no patient with a suspected retroperitoneal tumor should be operated upon without prior angiographic study. Figure 5.17A and 5.17B and Figure 5.18 are arteriograms of selected patients with retroperitoneal tumors; the accompanying case histories in the legends

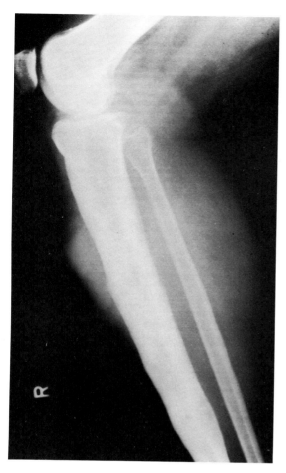

Figure 5.13. Soft tissue mass in the right leg of a 24-year-old man. Roentgenogram showed invasion of the periosteum of the tibia. A clinical diagnosis of sarcoma was made and biopsy examination showed this tumor to be rhabdomyosarcoma.

nostic aids in these uncommon tumors (Fig. 14.20, Chapter 14).

Venography. Venography has a limited role in the diagnosis or management of soft tissue tumors. Contrast studies of the inferior vena cava are of value for the preoperative assessment of retroperitoneal soft tissue tumors (Fig. 5.19). It is noteworthy that the clinician frequently fails to recognize the extent of a retroperitoneal tumor, even after a flush aortogram is obtained. A large retroperitoneal tumor may press on, or be adherent to, the inferior vena cava, with little systemic manifestation in the patient. The extent and severity of the systemic findings are proportional to the interval of time required for the tumor to impinge on the inferior vena cava. Furthermore, the inferior vena cava can occasionally be the site of origin of the retroperitoneal tumor, eg, retroperitoneal leiomyosarcoma.

Venography for intrathoracic tumors is somewhat more useful than arteriography. In anterior mediastinal tumors the diagnosis frequently is made after contrast studies of the superior vena cava. Venography has not been used routinely for extremity neoplasms; however, in patients with an angiomatous malformation or large angiomas, a venogram is sometimes useful.

Lymphangiography. The involvement of regional nodes in patients with soft tissue sarcoma is rare, and clinical examination of the nodes usually is sufficient. Infrequently, however, lymphangiography might be of value in some types of sarcomas in specific locations, eg, in rhabdomyosarcomas of the extremities or of the spermatic cord.

show the need for these angiograms. The need in intrathoracic neoplasms is not as acute as for retroperitoneal neoplasms. The majority of intrathoracic tumors are located in the posterior mediastinum. This usually makes an angiographic study technically difficult. Furthermore, the quality of information that might be obtained does not justify indiscriminate use of an invasive diagnostic test.

Angiography is often useful in certain instances of tumors arising in the carotid body or relatively large tumors of the head and neck region. Intracranial sarcomas are rare; however, as with all other neoplasms of the brain, angiography is one of the most important diag-

Thermography and Echography. Although neither of these methods can be considered radiographic, because of the similarity of techniques they are being described in this section.

The thermogram is a pictorial representation of infrared radiation of the skin. The majority of clinical work with thermography has been in human breast tumors. In this disease there is a true positive rate of 85 to 87 percent.[17] Thermography has been sparingly applied in the diagnosis of soft tissue tumors and in most of these studies the results were unreliable. However, a well-planned study of the application of thermography in soft tissue tumors of the extremities and trunk should be pursued.

Echography is a noninvasive technique for

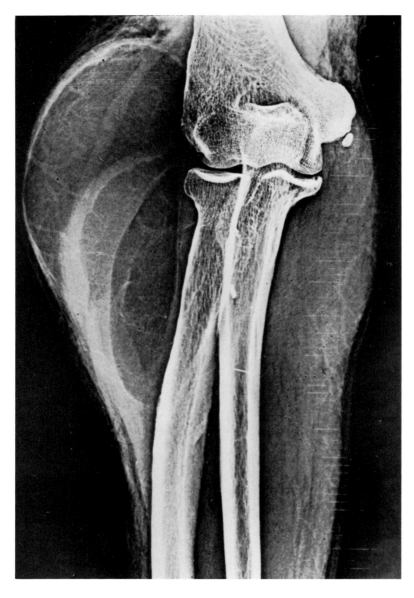

Figure 5.14. A xeroradiograph of a lipoma of forearm. The uniformly smooth, circumscribed, ovoid mass is suggestive of a benign lipomatous tumor.

demonstrating the presence of deep-seated tumors.[18,19] The principle is based on ultrasonics and can be relatively useful in retroperitoneal tumors or cysts (Fig. 5.20). Although the treatment plan should not be altered on the basis of echographic findings alone, echography is a useful additional diagnostic aid for evaluation of retroperitoneal or pelvic tumors.

Computerized Axial Tomography (CAT). The technique is useful both in the diagnosis and in the assessment of the extent of the primary tumor (Fig. 5.21A and 5.21B). The method becomes especially useful for suspected primary tumors of the retroperitoneum, pelvis, or the buttock (Fig. 5.21C). A CAT scan is of immense importance in the assessment of the

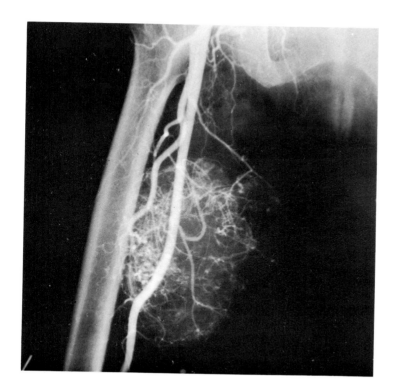

Figure 5.15. Arteriogram of tumor of right thigh. This tumor was discrete and appeared freely mobile. A femoral arteriogram established the prebiopsy diagnosis of a malignant mesenchymal tumor.

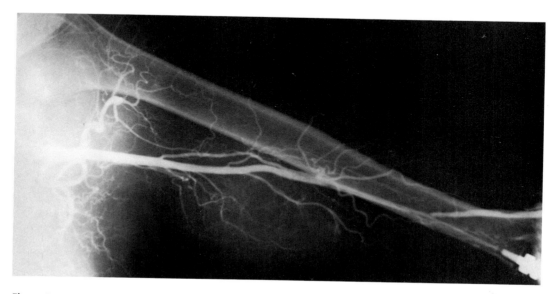

Figure 5.16. Arteriogram of an upper extremity tumor. The neovascularity is strongly indicative of malignancy. Microscopic examination showed this to be alveolar rhabdomyosarcoma.

metastatic status of a patient with sarcoma (vide infra).

Radioisotope Techniques

Radioisotope scintigraphy for the diagnosis of primary soft tissue sarcomas or to determine the extent of metastatic disease has had limited success. Today, no generally accepted radiopharmaceutical drug is available for diagnosis of soft tissue sarcomas. However, certain general radioactive agents that selectively seek out tumors are being increasingly used, among them gallium-67 and phosphorus-32. It is too early to assess the usefulness of these techniques.

In our Division of Surgical Oncology, the applicability of radiolabeled monoclonal antibody to various histologic types of soft tissue sarcomas for imaging of both primary and metastic sarcomas is being investigated. To date, we have used this technique in nine patients and we are optimistic regarding its future usefulness.

Biochemical Tests for Soft Tissue Sarcomas

Biochemical tests for diagnosis of soft tissue tumors or sarcomas are not specific. Unlike for their counterparts, the skeletal malignancies, no specific laboratory test is indicative of either a primary soft tissue sarcoma or a particular type

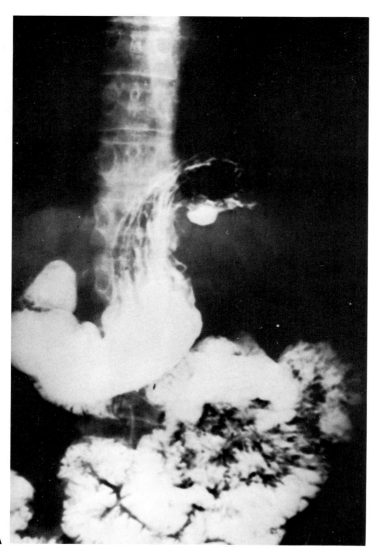

Figure 5.17. (A) Upper gastrointestinal tract series showing the greater curvature of the stomach persistently pushed toward the right, but diagnosis could not be established. Patient was a 45-year-old man with a history of indigestion and vague abdominal discomfort. **(B)** Aortogram showing a tumor of the left retroperitoneum. The neovascularity is suggestive of malignancy.

A

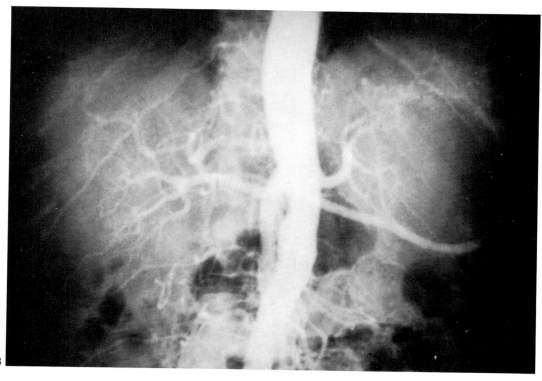

B

Figure 5.17. *Continued*

of sarcoma. In certain sarcomas there appears to be a correlation of local tumor tissue alkaline phosphatase activity and prognosis. Therefore, most of these studies should be geared to a metastatic survey of the patient rather than an attempt to delineate the nature of the primary disease.

Investigations of steroid receptors, fibroblast growth factor, epidermal growth factor, and nerve growth factor in soft tissue tumors are being carried out in several laboratories (details in Chapter 4). It appears that these biologic markers will eventually enter into diagnostic and prognostic assessment of soft tissue tumors.

MORPHOLOGIC DIAGNOSIS OF SOFT TISSUE TUMORS

The most accurate diagnostic method for establishing the identity and nature of a soft tissue tumor is the microscopic examination of either the entire tumor or a representative portion. Undue haste in establishing a pathologic diagnosis not only is unnecessary but on occasion is detrimental to the best interests of the pa-tients. In view of the rarity of soft tissue sarcomas, hasty decisions based on either frozen sections or on an aspiration biopsy are seldom justified, and there is considerable evidence against making such a decision.

The methods used for diagnosis of soft tissue tumors are (1) aspiration biopsy, (2) Silverman needle biopsy, (3) excision biopsy, and (4) incision biopsy.

Aspiration Biopsy

Aspiration biopsy of soft tissue tumors is an accepted diagnostic method in some institutions.[20] The aspiration technique is as follows:

An appropriate area of skin over the tumor is infiltrated with 1 percent plain Xylocaine. Following achievement of local anesthesia, the tumor is held between the index and thumb of one hand and a long, fine aspirating needle with a trochar is introduced. In small tumors the needle is introduced into the center of the tumor, but in larger tumors the site for obtaining the aspirate will depend on the clinician's experience. In general, firm or hard areas should be aspirated. Following placement of the needle

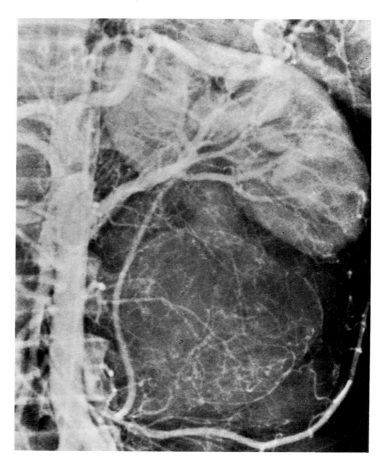

Figure 5.18. Aortogram of palpable abdominal tumors showing a retroperitoneal tumor on the left side. This tumor was found to be a leiomyosarcoma.

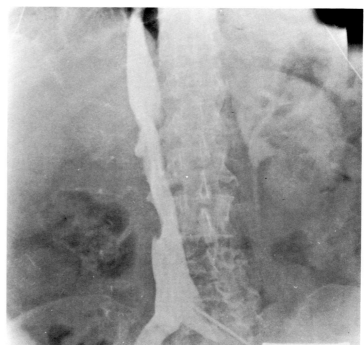

Figure 5.19. Inferior venacavogram of a patient with fibrosarcoma of the retroperitoneum. Note involvement of wall of the vena cava.

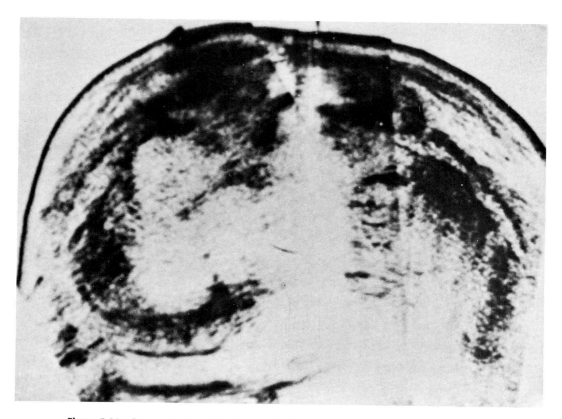

Figure 5.20. Composite view of echogram of a left-sided retroperitoneal leiomyosarcoma.

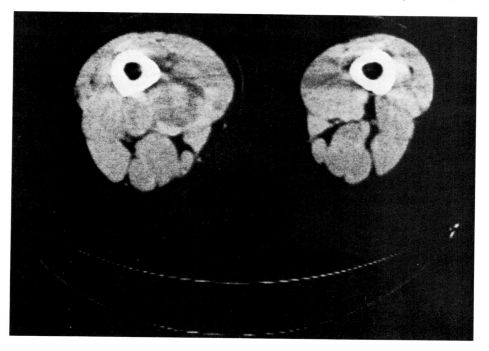

Figure 5.21. (A) CAT scan of a primary soft tissue sarcoma of the thigh. Note the extensive nature of the tumor and adherence to the surrounding muscles.

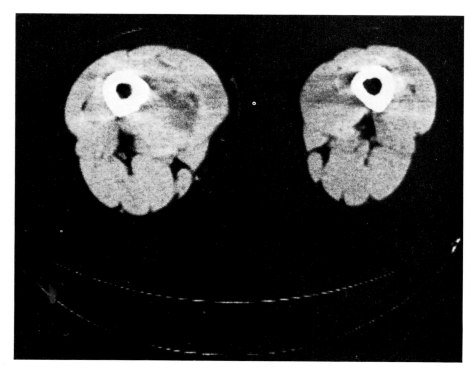

Figure 5.21. (**B**) Same tumor as in (**A**). Another section: observe the involvement of the bone.

in the desired area, the trochar is withdrawn and the needle is attached to a 20-cc syringe. A constant aspiration pressure is then applied for two to three minutes, with minor movement in the depth and direction of the needle. The syringe is then disconnected from the needle and the needle is withdrawn. The needle point is then directed onto a glass slide and either the aspirate is expressed by pushing about 1 cc of air, or the trochar is introduced and a small drop of aspirate is put on the slide. The aspirate is then evenly spread on the slide and processed for cytologic examination. It is essential that the syringe be disconnected prior to the withdrawal of the needle; otherwise the aspirated fluid, which is often less than 1 ml, is drawn into the syringe, making preparation of cytologic slides nearly impossible.

The use of aspiration biopsy in the diagnosis of soft tissue tumors has not found general acceptance in the United States, although in certain European centers it is routinely used.[11]

Silverman Needle Biopsy

The technique of this biopsy is essentially the same as that for aspiration biopsy, the difference being that, instead of an ordinary needle,

either a Vim Silverman or a disposable Menghini needle is used. The cutting trochar is then introduced through the needle, and after a sharp circulatory twist of the cutting trochar, the needle and the trochar are removed. With this method, a slim core of tissue, usually 0.5 cm long and about 1 to 2 mm thick, can be obtained. The tissue is then processed for paraffin-embedding and subsequent histologic examination.

This method of needle biopsy, although used in some centers, is not a commonly accepted method for histologic diagnosis of soft tissue tumors in most places in the United States. The limitations of this method are (1) that only a small piece of tissue is obtained, and it frequently is not a representative area of the tumor; and (2) the relative rarity of these tumors will prevent most pathologists from arriving at a correct diagnosis from this small specimen, even though it may contain the most representative area of a given tumor.

Excision Biopsy

This method of morphologic diagnosis is most commonly used. In relatively small soft tissue tumors, it is appropriate to perform an excision of the tumor with local anesthesia. The detailed

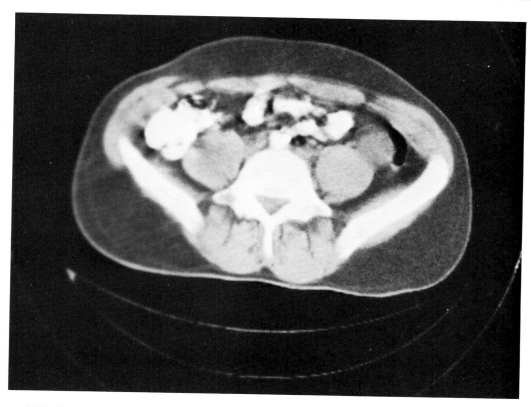

Figure 5.21. (C) A pelvic liposarcoma. The primary tumor, which was located in the mesentery of the sigmoid, was unsuspected until this CAT scan was obtained.

technical aspects are discussed in Chapter 6. It is essential that the surgeon be careful to observe the location of the tumor and its relation to surrounding structures such as muscle, fibrous tissue, vessels, and nerves. All this information is used in the clinicopathologic staging and prognostication, for although the majority of soft tissue tumors are benign (eg, lipomas) and frequently can be diagnosed macroscopically, it is still advisable that the final diagnosis be rendered after microscopic examination of the tissues.

Incision Biopsy

When the tumor is relatively large and there is clinical suspicion that it might be malignant, an incision biopsy is certainly justified. In this method, which is very similar to the method of excision biopsy, an appropriate area of skin overlying the tumor is anesthesized with 1 percent Xylocaine. An incision is made and a representative wedge of the tumor is excised. It is essential that a large wedge of the tumor be removed from the area most likely to yield the

best information. Although this method has the theoretic disadvantage of cutting into the tumor with resultant spillage of tumor cells, no untoward effect has as yet been demonstrated either in terms of longevity, fungation, or local recurrence if definitive therapy is instituted within one to two weeks of biopsy.

The biopsy material obtained by the aspiration technique, although having the distinct advantage of being the least traumatic and possibly providing an immediate diagnosis, has the major disadvantage of being unreliable in most hands. The same criticism is leveled against a needle biopsy of soft tissue sarcomas, albeit this method has found renewed usage in a variety of other tumors. In centers in which there is a concentration of patients with soft tissue sarcomas, it is probable these two methods will find maximum applicability in the future.

The majority of patients with soft tissue tumors, therefore, have either an excisional or an incisional biopsy diagnosis. Once the specimen is obtained, it is sometimes possible to immediately freeze a portion and obtain a histologic diagnosis. Definitive therapy can then be recommended at the same sitting. However, in most instances it is extremely difficult to arrive at an accurate histogenetic diagnosis from examination of the frozen sections. Because of this disadvantage it is recommended that the specimen thus obtained be divided into three parts. The first part is frozen, and cryostat sections are studied to inform the clinician, if possible, whether the tumor is malignant. If the tumor is obviously benign, then appropriate treatment can be immediately instituted. However, if the tumor is malignant, all attempts to arrive at a definitive diagnosis should be avoided until further study. The second part of the specimen should be processed for conventional light microscopy, and the third part for electron microscopy. In most large centers it is possible to obtain an accurate diagnosis within the first seven days of biopsy. However, if such facilities are not available, it is most appropriate to await consultation with other pathologists and oncologists before any therapeutic decision is undertaken. This extra delay of another few days does not jeopardize the patient's condition in any way. In contrast, this masterly delay provides the patient with the maximum therapeutic advantage.

Once a diagnosis of sarcoma is made, it is essential that the patient be assessed for metastatic status before recommending definitive therapy for the primary tumor.

Evaluation of the metastatic status depends on the natural history of the specific sarcoma. The majority of sarcomas have similar patterns of metastatic spread; however, there are some with specific characteristics. The general workup to determine metastases will be described in this section; the detailed points regarding specific sarcomas will be discussed in chapters dealing with individual types of tumor.

GENERAL WORKUP TO DETERMINE METASTASES

Whole-Lung Tomograms

The lung is the most common site of metastases from any sarcoma, and the presence of pulmonary metastases must be excluded prior to any therapy. Small metastatic nodules are often missed in a normal chest x-ray, and therefore bilateral whole-lung tomograms are strongly recommended prior to planning any definitive therapy.

Other Radiographic Examinations

Few radiographic examinations are of any value in the metastatic workup of a sarcoma patient. In exceptional cases, however, the use of angiography or lymphangiography can be of value. For example, in neuroblastoma, hepatic angiograms might be of value in assessing the status of the liver; in rhabdomyosarcoma, regional lymphangiography might be used to ascertain the status of metastatic involvement of either the regional or the extraregional nodes.

Computerized Axial Tomography (CAT)

This method of computerized tomography is of immense value in ascertaining the overall metastatic status of a patient with a sarcoma. A CAT scan of the chest will demonstrate the presence of pleural metastases that otherwise would have been missed. Similarly small otherwise occult metastatic deposits in other areas can also be diagnosed by this method (Fig. 5.22).

Biochemical Tests

There is no specific biochemical test for ascertaining the metastatic status of a sarcoma patient. However, since in some instances metastasis to the liver occurs, liver function studies should be performed prior to therapy for the primary tumor.

Scintigraphy

Investigation with scintigraphy is indicated for evaluation of the liver, the brain, and the skeletal system. These anatomic locations, however, are infrequent sites of metastases except in relatively advanced neoplasms. Furthermore, with the increasing use of computerized axial tomography, the role of scintigraphy in soft tissue sarcomas is diminishing. However, it appears that in the future, the method of imaging with radiolabeled monoclonal antibody in detecting occult metastases will become of value.

Soft somatic tissue tumors, once they are apparent, can be classified as benign or malignant, and the histogenetic type can be properly ascertained in most instances. After the histologic diagnosis is made and the patient adequately evaluated for evidence of metastatic disease, the tumor should be staged.

STAGING OF SARCOMAS

Soft tissue sarcomas and all the variants thereof should be staged clinicopathologically for ade-

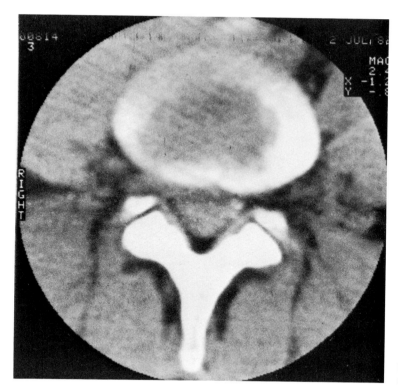

Figure 5.22. Liposarcoma metastatic to the dura of the spinal cord.

quate assessment of the mode of treatment, as well as for reporting the end result. The staging methods have been varied over the years. Recently the American Joint Committee for Cancer Staging and End Result Reporting[3] published a minimally acceptable staging method. Although open to considerable criticism it still is a guideline for staging soft tissue sarcomas. This staging system is described in the following paragraphs.

Primary Site
The exact location of the tumor, its depth from the skin surface, its size, and its relation to the surrounding structures require accurate estimates. This information constitutes the T-classification.

Regional Nodes
The lymph node basin relates to the site of origin of the sarcoma, and any of the major lymph node compartments may be at risk (N-classification).

Metastatic Site
The lung is the most common metastatic site of involvement, but a large variety of other viscera may also be invaded, such as bone, liver, brain, etc. (M-classification).

Histologic Classification[3]
Determination of the histogenesis of a given tumor (Table 3.1, Chapter 3) is of primary importance. Once the histologic type is established, the tumor should be graded according to the accepted criteria for malignancy, including cellularity, cellular pleomorphism, and mitotic activity (Fig. 5.23A to 5.23D). The tumor grades (G-classification) are expressed as follows:

G_1	Well-differentiated
G_2	Moderately well-differentiated
G_3 to G_4	Poorly to very poorly differentiated (undifferentiated)

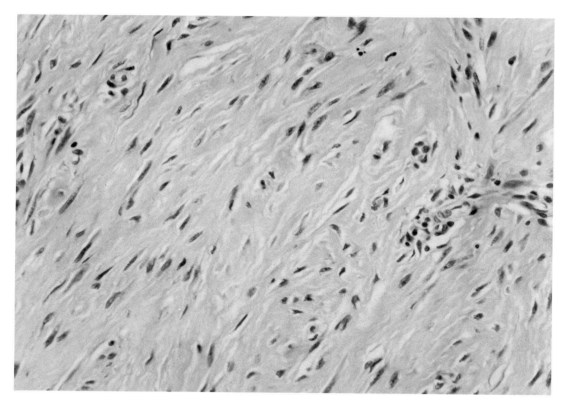

Figure 5.23. (A) Well-differentiated fibrosarcoma (G₁). (H&E. Original magnification × 250.)

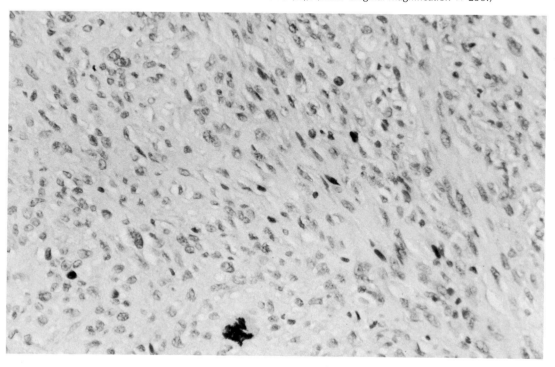

Figure 5.23. (B) Moderately well-differentiated fibrosarcoma (G₂). (H&E. Original magnification × 250.)

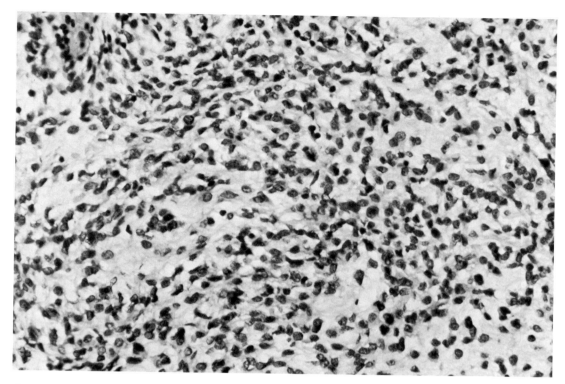

Figure 5.23. (C) Poorly differentiated or undifferentiated fibrosarcoma (G_3 or G_4). (H&E. Original magnification × 250.)

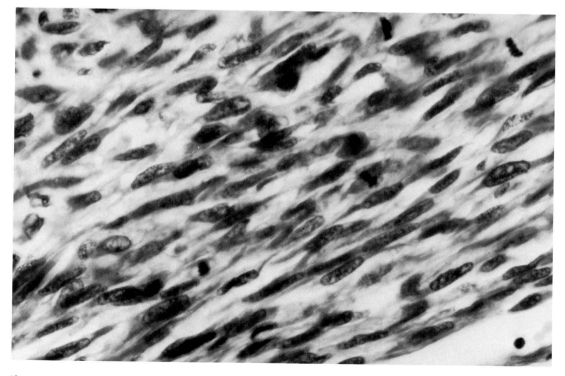

Figure 5.23. (D) Higher-power magnification of a poorly differentiated fibrosarcoma. (H&E. Original magnification × 375.) The distinction between G_3 and G_4 is sometimes difficult.

Some tumors are highly malignant, regardless of their cellular differentiation, and should be classified as G_3; for example, rhabdomyosarcoma in adults, certain types of angiosarcoma, and synovial sarcoma.

The TNM classification is as follows:

Primary Tumor (T)

T_X	Minimum requirements cannot be met
T_0	No demonstrable tumor(s)
T_1	Less than 5 cm in maximum diameter
T_2	Tumor 5 cm or greater in diameter
T_3	Tumor showing macroscopic invasion of the surrounding bone, major vessels, or major nerves

Nodal status (N)

N_X	Minimum requirements cannot be met
N_0	No histologically verified metastases to regional nodes
N_1	Histologically verified regional node metastases

Distant Metastases (M)

M_X	Not assessed
M_0	No known distant metastases
M_1	Distant metastases present (specific site)

Specific site according to the following notation:

Lung	PUL
Osseous	OSS
Hepatic	HEP
Brain	BRA
Lymph nodes	LYM
Bone marrow	MAR
Pleura	PLE
Skin	SKI
Eye	EYE
Other	OTH

Following therapeutic excision of the primary tumor a postsurgical residual tumor R-classification is also indicated.

R_0	No residual tumor
R_1	Microscopic residual tumor
R_2	Macroscopic residual tumor

The clinicopathologic information described above helps in staging soft tissue sarcomas. The proposed staging is shown below:

Stage Grouping.

Stage   I: I_A G_1 T_1 N_0 M_0
Grade 1 tumor, less than 5 cm in diameter with no regional lymph nodal or distant metastases
I_B G_1 T_2 N_0 M_0
Grade 1 tumor, 5 cm or greater in diameter with no regional lymph nodal or distant metastases

Stage II: II_A G_2 T_1 N_0 M_0
Grade 2 tumor, less than 5 cm in diameter with no regional lymph nodal or distant metastases
II_B G_2 T_2 N_0 M_0
Grade 2 tumor, 5 cm or greater in diameter with no regional lymph nodal or distant metastases

Stage III: III_A G_3 T_1 N_0 M_0
Grade 3 tumor, less than 5 cm in diameter with no regional lymph nodal or distant metastases
III_B G_3 T_2 N_0 M_0
Grade 3 tumor, 5 cm or greater in diameter with no regional lymph nodal or distant metastases
III_C Any G $T_{1,2}$ N_1 M_0
Tumor of any histologic grade or size (no invasion), with regional lymph node metastases but without distant metastases

Stage IV: IV_A Any G T_3 Any N M_0
Tumor of any histologic grade of malignancy that grossly invades bone, major vessels, or major nerves with or without regional lymph node metastases but without distant metastases
IV_B Any G Any T Any N M_1
Tumor with distant metastases

It is obvious that the staging system described above is cumbersome. However, it should form the basis for a more practical staging system classifying the primary tumors, local extension, histologic type, grade, and regional and extra-regional metastatic status. It appears that if all patients with soft tissue sarcomas are assessed accordingly, the end result reporting following one or the other form of treatment program can be properly evaluated between the various groups reporting on the end results.

Following the diagnosis and staging of soft tissue tumors, treatment planning should begin. There are three main modes of treatment: surgery, radiation therapy, and chemotherapy. Currently, the role of immunotherapy is being extensively investigated. In Chapters 6 to 8 the general principles of these three modalities will be discussed, Chapter 9 will deal with the immunobiology and therapy of these tumors, and Chapter 10 discusses the general principles of rehabilitation.

REFERENCES

1. Soule EH, Geitz M, Henderson ED: Embryonal rhabdomyosarcoma of the limbs and limb girdles. Cancer 23:1336, 1969
2. Pritchard RF, Soule EH, Taylor WF, et al: Fibrosarcoma: A clinicopathologic and statistical study of 199 tumors of soft tissue of the extremities and trunk. Cancer 33:888, 1976
3. Manual for Staging of Cancer. Chicago, American Joint Committee for Cancer Staging and End Result Reporting, 1978
4. Suit HD, Russell WD: Soft part tumors. Cancer 39:830, 1977
5. Suit HD, Russell WD, Martin RG: Sarcoma of soft tissue: Clinical and histopathological parameters and response to treatment. Cancer 35:1478, 1975
6. Weingrad DN, Rosenberg SA: Early lymphatic spread of osteogenic and soft tissue sarcoma. Surgery 84:231, 1978
7. Bowden L: The diagnosis and treatment of soft part sarcomas. Virginia Med Monthly 81:463, 1954
8. Jenkins HP, Delaney PA: Benign angiomatous tumors of skeletal muscles. Surg Gynecol Obstet 55:464, 1932
9. Lester J, Rosenklint A, Rovsing TH, Stephensen N, Struve-Christensen E: Angiography in tumors of the extremities. Acta Orthop Scandinav 42:152, 1971
10. Cockshott P, Evans KT: The place of soft tissue arteriography. Br J Radiol 37:367, 1964
11. Diethelm L, Fischer W, Habighorst LV, Schweikert CH, Wessinghage D: Angiographische und szintigraphishe untersuchungen an eingen seltenen knochentumoren. Radiologie 9:311, 1969
12. Lagergren C, Lindbom A, Soderberg G: Vascularization of fibromatous and fibrosarcomatous tumors. Acta Radiol 53:1, 1960
13. Lagergren C, Lindbom A, Soderberg G: The blood vessels of osteogenic sarcomas. Acta Radiol 55:161, 1961
14. Lagergren C, Lindbom A, Soderberg G: The blood vessels of chondrosarcomas. Acta Radiol 55:321, 1961
15. Templeton AW, Stevens E, Jansen C: Arteriographic evaluation of soft tissue masses. South Med J 59:1255, 1966
16. Margulis AR, Murphy TO: Arteriography in neoplasms of extremities. Am J Roentgenol 80:330, 1958
17. Dodd GD, Goldman AM: Mammography, xeroradiography and thermography in the diagnosis of breast cancer. In Holland JF and Fice E III (eds): Cancer Medicine. Philadelphia, Lea & Febiger, 1973
18. Spencer WH III, Peter RH, Orgain ES: Detection of a left atrial myxoma by echocardiography. Arch Intern Med 128:787, 1971
19. Weiss L, Holyoke ED: Detection of tumors in soft tissues by ultrasonic holography. Surg Gynecol Obstet 128:5:953, 1969
20. Koss LG, Durfee GR: Diagnostic Cytology and Its Histopathologic Bases. Philadelphia, Lippincott, 1961

SECTION TWO: General Principles of Treatment

6

Surgical Treatment

Tapas K. Das Gupta

The spectrum of surgical techniques used in treating primary soft somatic tissue tumors ranges from simple excision of a benign lipoma to the most challenging of radical excisions, such as a quarterectomy. In any given sarcoma, the surgeon, before making a decision to operate, must take into consideration such factors as the histologic type and grade, the anatomic location, the fixity to or mobility from the surrounding tissue, the presence of regional or distant metastases, and, finally, his or her own experience and familiarity with sarcomas in general.

The technical aspects of excision of a benign tumor such as a lipoma are simple, and usually the local excison methods to be described herein cover the principles of management of other benign tumors. However, in some specific instances, modifications in the techniques of local excision are required—for example, excision of a palmar or plantar fibromatosis.

The purpose of surgical treatment is eradication of the primary tumor. Unless an initial aggressive approach is undertaken, the therapy program will ultimately fail in a majority of patients. Thus, on balance, comes the realization that a major operation might be the only opportunity a patient has for living, and the surgeon cannot deny the patient that opportunity. With the utilization of multimodality therapy, however, the need and indications for major ablative procedures are becoming less and less. No patient should be denied the ideal therapy on the basis of chronologic age alone. For example, a total cystectomy should be performed in an infant with rhabdomyosarcoma of the urinary bladder, if indicated. Similarly, an elderly patient with a sarcoma arising in an extremity should have appropriate resection. Once all the facts are provided, the patient (or parents) should have the opportunity to make the final decision. A scrutiny of the results of treatment of soft tissue sarcomas shows that in the majority of instances the incidence of local recurrence is directly proportional to the inadequacy of treatment of the primary.[1-6] Therefore, unless there is a systemic contraindication that might in itself be life-threatening, the patient should have the opportunity for appropriate resection.

The following general guidelines have been developed in defining contraindications to a major operation, including amputation:

1. Associated unrelated systemic disease of such severity that an operation of any magnitude might endanger life: for example, severe bilateral emphysema or extensive myocardial disease, end-stage renal disease treated by dialysis, or life-threatening asthma.
2. In most instances, the presence of synchronous metastases constitutes a contraindication for a major operation.

3. Inability of the patient to cope psychologically with a major operation, especially an amputation. However, in our experience, when an in-depth discussion is carried on, the majority of patients recognize the need for the operation and accept it. The clinician must not try to "sell" any form of therapy to a patient; rather, it is his or her responsibility to provide the patient with all the pertinent facts and allow the patient to make the decision.

4. Finally, in an unusual instance in which the rehabilitation of a patient, either psychological, social, or functional, poses an enormous problem, a major operation is preferably avoided. However, this is applicable only when a suitable alternative is available and the patient or the family is aware of that alternative.

After careful assessment of the type of excision or amputation necessary, the surgeon must proceed with the most optimum type of operation, without compromise for cosmetic or emotional reasons. It cannot be overemphasized that initial inadequate excision increases the incidence of local recurrence. Most clinicians have observed that a locally recurrent sarcoma is more aggressive than the primary tumor and carries a graver prognosis for the patient. The old adage that the first surgeon has the best opportunity for cure is substantially true.

INDICATIONS AND TECHNIQUES FOR LOCAL EXCISION

Limited Local Excision

This method is used in the management of the majority of benign soft tissue sarcomas. It is also a means of obtaining biopsy material from tumors clinically suggestive of malignancy.

Technique. The excision can be performed under local, regional, or general endotracheal anesthesia, depending upon the age of the patient and the location and size of the tumor.

After the patient is anesthetized and properly positioned, an elliptical skin incision is made over the prominent part of the tumor (Fig. 6.1A, inset). The skin is elevated on both sides of the tumor, delineating its extent (Fig. 6.1A, right). The tumor is then dissected from the surrounding muscles or other structures (Fig. 6.1B) and

delivered out of the wound (Fig. 6.1C). Following removal of the tumor and after adequate hemostasis, the wound is closed in layers (Fig. 6.1D).

It is not generally recognized that almost all soft tissue sarcomas have a pseudocapsule and enucleation will leave the peripheral part of the tumor behind. Although lipomas are usually enucleated, as a general principle it is judicious to avoid enucleation of any other soft tissue tumor, even if it appears benign.

If there is any question in the mind of the surgeon as to the benignity of the tumor, a frozen section diagnosis should be obtained to determine whether the tumor represents a sarcoma. If the tumor is found to be malignant, then it is certainly appropriate to delay the definitive therapy until all relevant data are in hand. However, with a proper index of suspicion and the increasing use of diagnostic aids such as xeroradiography, angiography, and computerized axial tomography, instances of such unpleasant surprises are becoming rare.

Limited local excision of sarcomas is seldom indicated. Therefore the method of local excision described above should be reserved for benign tumors, for example, lipomas or neurofibromas. For all practical purposes this method can also be used as a diagnostic method in a suspected sarcoma of relatively small dimensions. But if the tumor is large, a wedge biopsy is certainly indicated to obtain a correct microscopic diagnosis.

Wide Local Excision

Wide local excision, if adequate, has a definite place in the management of soft tissue sarcomas. The definition of wide excision is somewhat confusing and frequently is misinterpreted by a clinician not familiar with the management of soft tissue sarcomas.

The term "wide excision" means a three-dimensional excision of the tumor. It is frequently a conceptual problem, and often it is not recognized that a soft tissue tumor grows in all directions (Fig. 6.2) and that the deeper extensions must be determined prior to planning the excision. The extent of the lateral excision of the surrounding tissues depends on the type of tumor, although a 5- to 6-cm margin on all sides usually is adequate. Furthermore, a skin incision to encompass the entire extent of the tumor frequently requires an imaginative approach with due consideration to function and cosmesis, since an unconventional scar frequently results.

In such a complicated and rare neoplastic problem as soft tissue sarcoma, a cookbook list of indications or contraindications for operations cannot be given. Frequently the decision for a specific operation in a given patient will be guided by the surgeon's knowledge and experience with the tumor, as well as by the procedure itself. However, there are some guidelines that will help in making the decision.

Indications.

1. Low-grade, well-differentiated fibrous tissue tumors, eg, dermatofibrosarcoma protuberans, and aggressive fibromatoses in certain anatomic locations
2. Low-grade, well-differentiated liposarcomas
3. Certain embryonal types of rhabdomyosarcoma, especially those arising in the head and neck region of children
4. Low-grade synovial cell sarcoma, malignant granular cell myoblastoma, solitary malignant schwannoma, and other sundry tumors of low-grade malignancy
5. With the increasing use of adjuvant radiotherapy and chemotherapy, some of the high-grade sarcomas can now be treated by wide local excision or variants thereof
6. All other benign tumors not amenable to limited local excision as described earlier, the prime examples being intermuscular or intramuscular lipomas and angiolipomas

Contraindications.

1. Wide local excision is generally not indicated in the management of high-grade or anaplastic sarcomas of most histologic types. These tumors should be managed by aggressive surgical therapy.
2. Wide local excision is not usually indicated for sarcomas arising in an extremity when a basic defect in the extremity is the cause of development of the sarcoma; for example, lymphangiosarcoma arising in an arm with postmastectomy or congenital edema. Similarly, in patients with neurofibromatosis, a malignant schwannoma arising in an extremity is usually associated with plexiform neuromas of the major nerve bundles. In such instances an elective major amputation is the treatment of choice.

Technique of Wide Local Excision. This operation should be performed under general endotracheal anesthesia. An adequate supply of blood should be kept available in case blood transfusion is found necessary during the operation. Additionally, in large tumors, provision must be made for a split-thickness skin graft if such becomes necessary.

The skin incision is made in an elliptical manner over the protruding part of the tumor (Fig. 6.2), excising the redundant skin along with the tumor. The incision is deepened through the subcutaneous tissue and flaps are raised on Fall sides to delineate the boundaries of the tumor (Fig. 6.3A). The dissection, with adequate margins on all sides, is then carried deep to the tumor. In a subcutaneous tumor the deeper excision line extends beneath the deep fascia. Sometimes, when the tumor is attached to a muscle (Fig. 6.3B), the muscle must be included in the dissection. Following such a three-dimensional dissection, the tumor and the surrounding normal tissues are removed (Fig. 6.3C). The wound margins should be checked for residual tumor by means of frozen sections when indicated. The wound is then closed with suction catheters in place to drain serous fluid collection. In patients in whom the overlying skin needs larger excision, the defect is covered with a split-thickness skin graft (Fig. 6.3D).

The postoperative course after such an operation is usually smooth and very little extra care is required. In case a skin graft is used, the postoperative management is similar to that for any other wound requiring a split-thickness skin graft.

Wide local excision has several variants, and although these are termed differently, the basic concepts in the treatment, being the same, will be included in this section on wide local excision. They are as follows:

1. Muscle group excision
2. Minor amputation of either the upper or lower extremities
3. Subtotal scapulectomy
4. Tikhor-Lindberg operation
5. Chest wall resection
6. Abdominal wall resection
7. Excision of retroperitoneal tumors
8. Excision of intrathoracic tumors

Muscle Group Excision
Excision of the group of muscles surrounding and underlying a soft tissue tumor is increas-

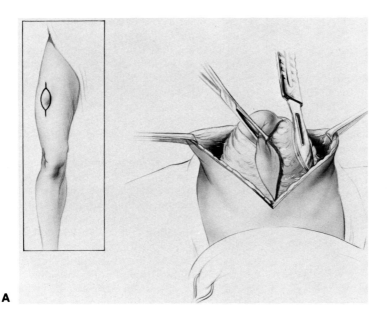

A

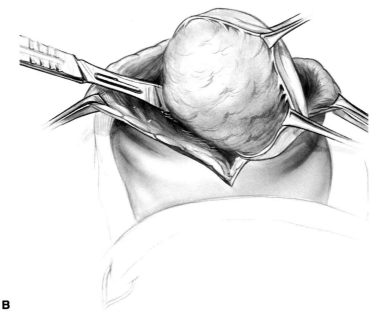

B

Figure 6.1. (A) *Inset:* Elliptical skin incision over a tumor of the thigh. The dimensions of the ellipse and the skin to be removed vary with the size of the tumor. For a tumor less than 3 cm in diameter skin excision frequently is not required. *Right:* Skin flaps are being raised for a proposed limited excision. **(B)** A benign tumor is being dissected. Underlying muscles are free of any invasion. Occasionally some of these tumors infiltrate the muscles (intermuscular lipoma), requiring excision of parts of the muscle as well. **(C)** A benign subcutaneous lipoma is being removed. Note the tumor is free of any attachment to the underlying muscle bed. **(D)** The wound has been closed in layers.

ingly becoming the method of choice in the treatment of a large number of sarcomas located in the extremities. This operation takes into consideration the fact that all soft tissue sarcomas spread locally along the muscle bundles or the tissue planes. Probably it is more appropriate to use the term "major soft tissue resection,"

since in a number of instances the excised specimen consists of more than one group of muscles, either in their entirety or in parts.

Indications. The indications for muscle group excision or major soft tissue resection are as follows:

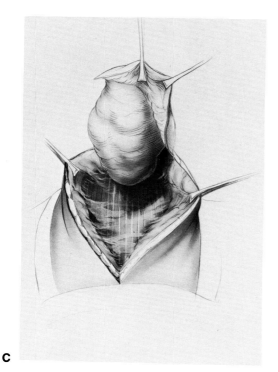

C

D

Figure 6.1. *Continued*

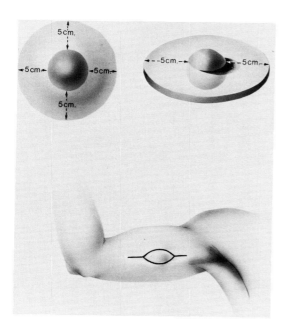

Figure 6.2. *Above, left:* Conceptual rendition of the extent of three-dimensional extension of a spheroidal tumor. Although most tumors of the soft tissues are oblate spheroids, for artistic clarity the tumor is sketched as a perfect spheroid. *Right:* The deeper extension of the tumor is comprehensible. *Below:* An elliptical skin incision is made over a subcutaneous tumor of the arm, with consideration of the extension.

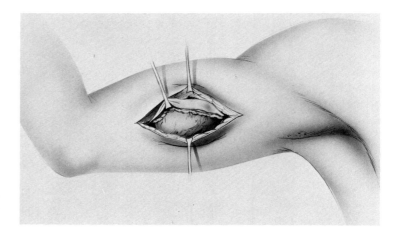

Figure 6.3. (A) The skin flaps are being raised, delineating the margins of the tumor.

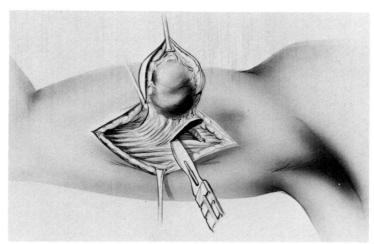

Figure 6.3. (B) The deeper extent of the tumor is being dissected.

1. Differentiated liposarcoma, rhabdomyosarcoma, leiomyosarcoma, malignant fibrous tissue, and synovial and angiomatous tissue tumors arising in a location where the muscle groups can be excised and a cure can be achieved, eg, in the buttocks, the lateral or medial compartments of the thigh, and the lateral and medial aspects of the arm.
2. Malignant schwannomas either in the lateral compartment of the thigh or the lateral aspect of the arm, when arising in a cutaneous nerve at this region. This is because, in these instances, the proximal end of the nerve can be excised.

Contraindications. The location of the tumor, however well-differentiated it might be, may preclude a proper muscle group excision; for example, sarcomas located distal to the elbow or the knee cannot be adequately treated by this procedure, nor can tumors located in the groin or axilla. In essence, if there is any doubt because of the anatomic location of the tumor, the operation should not be attempted.

In all high-grade sarcomas in which the incidence of recurrence and metastases is high, muscle group excision alone should be avoided. However, it can be resorted to if the use of multimodal therapy is indicated.

Technique of Muscle Group (Major Soft Tissue) Resection.

Anesthesia. In our experience, this operation is best performed when the patient is under general anesthesia. The operation can be time-consuming and might require blood transfusion, so adequate preparation should be made.

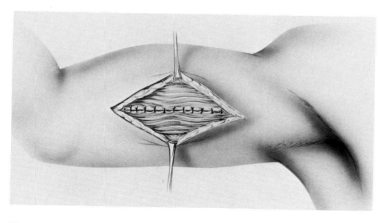

Figure 6.3. (C) The tumor has been excised and the muscle bed is sutured.

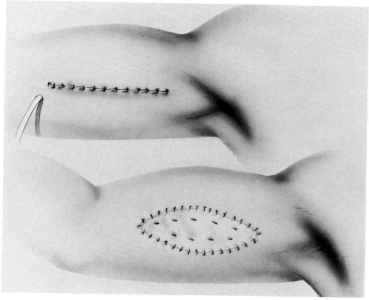

Figure 6.3. (D) The skin margins can be closed primarily or can be covered with a split-thickness skin graft.

Position of Patient. The position should be that which provides the best access and exposure of the group of muscles requiring excision. For example, excision of the gluteal muscles requires that the patient be in the prone position; excision of the lateral compartment muscles of the right thigh requires that the patient be positioned on a semi-left lateral decubitus.

Steps of the Operation. An elliptical incision is made, encompassing the tumor and extending vertically along the entire course of attachment of the muscles to be excised (Fig. 6.4A). The incision is deepened to include the subcutaneous tissue, and skin flaps are raised on both sides (Fig. 6.4B). The dissection is then started on the proximal aspect of the excision.

The medial attachment of the muscle group is dissected and the dissection carried out from the proximal to the distal attachments (Fig. 6.4B). This stage of the operation provides the first opportunity for inspection and evaluation of the undersurface of the tumor. If the deep border of the tumor is found free of any attachments or extension, the operation proceeds and the lateral line of attachment of the muscle group is excised (Fig. 6.4C). Ideally, one should be able to remove the entire muscle group containing the tumor without handling the tumor (Fig. 6.4D), but if the tumor is found infiltrating bones or structures that cannot be properly included in this type of operation, the attempt should be terminated. The resected ends of the muscles

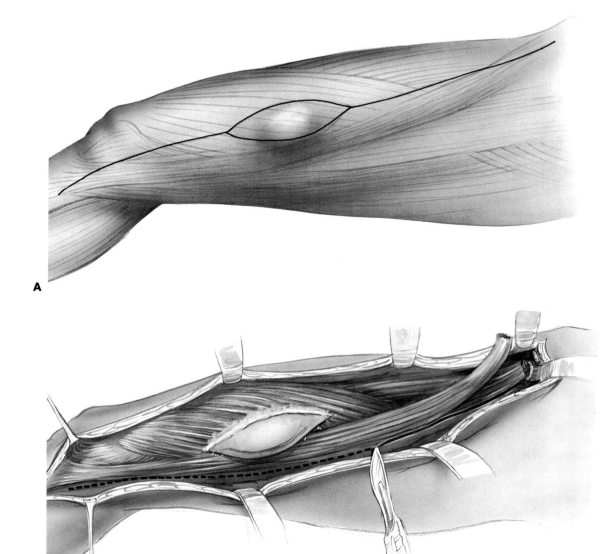

A

B

are attached to the surrounding muscles with intact nerve supply. The wound is then closed in layers. Suction catheters are placed to avoid collection of any serum (Fig. 6.4E). If the ellipse of skin included in the operation is large, the defect can be covered by a split-thickness skin graft.

When the general principles of good surgical technique are applied, the postoperative course is smooth and the patients may not require any special type of management. Although initially it seems they will be unable to either walk or move their arms, within a few weeks most patients, with proper physical therapy, can return to normal activity. The residual deformity, if any, is so minimal that frequently an untrained observer fails to recognize it. The fibrosarcoma shown in Figure 6.4F was re-

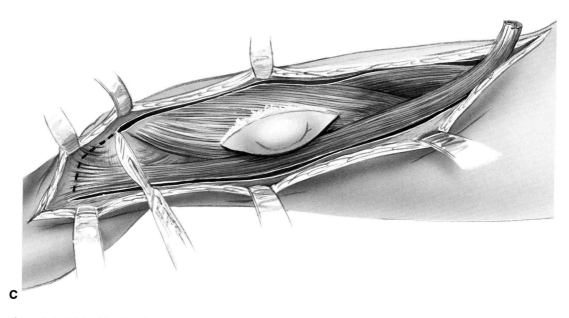

C

Figure 6.4. **(A)** Incision line for a proposed muscle group excision of the anteromedial aspect of the thigh. An ellipse is designed at the most prominent part of the tumor. **(B)** The skin flaps on both sides have been raised. The proximal attachment of the sartorius muscle is resected. The dotted line shows the medial margin of the resection. Resection is continued from the proximal to the distal end. **(C)** The lateral margin of resection has been defined and the muscles are being resected at the distal end.

moved from a 61-year-old woman who was able to resume all her preoperative activities within six months and has remained well for more than six years. Thus, from a rehabilitation standpoint, this type of operation, whenever feasible, constitutes one of the ideal forms of treatment of soft tissue sarcomas of the extremities.

Planning the exact technique to be applied in excising different groups of muscles for a malignant tumor at any given anatomic site requires a thorough orientation with the regional anatomy and the ability to modify the surgical technique in accordance with the principles of operation discussed above. One such modification is the technique of excision of the gluteal group of muscles for sarcomas of the buttocks.[7] Because of the specific modifications, the operative technique is described in detail.

Radical Excision of the Buttock (Gluteal Group Excision)

Indications. This operation is indicated in all well-differentiated sarcomas of the buttock area that are well circumscribed and can be extirpated by excising the gluteal group of muscles.

It is advisable to discuss the limits of this operation in detail with the patient, since in some instances the tumor will be found to be more extensive than originally assessed clinically, requiring a hemipelvectomy or excision of part of the sacrum, coccyx, and the iliac crest. Before operating, the surgeon should obtain permission to extend the operation if necessary.

Contraindications. This operation is not recommended if the tumor extends into the pelvis through the sciatic foramen (dumbell-shaped tumors), or if there is extensive local recurrence.

Technique.

Position of the Patient. Frequently the vascularity of the tumors requires ligation of the internal iliac vessels; thus, initially the patient should be in the supine position, then in the prone position.

Steps of Operation. It is our practice to perform an initial exploratory laparotomy and evaluate the stage of the tumor, the status of the liver and other intra-abdominal viscera, and the

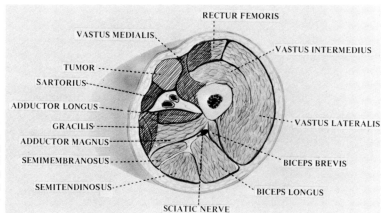

Figure 6.4. (D) A transverse section through the middle of the thigh, showing relation of the tumor to the surrounding muscles. The shaded muscles, along with the tumor, are being resected. If such a margin is adhered to, the chances of handling the tumor are minimized.

RECTUR FEMORIS

VASTUS MEDIALIS

VASTUS INTERMEDIUS

TUMOR

SARTORIUS

VASTUS LATERALIS

ADDUCTOR LONGUS

GRACILIS

ADDUCTOR MAGNUS

SEMIMEMBRANOSUS

BICEPS BREVIS

SEMITENDINOSUS

BICEPS LONGUS

SCIATIC NERVE

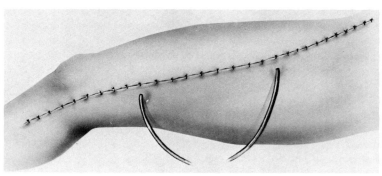

Figure 6.4. (E) The wound is closed with a suction catheter in place. Although a large muscle mass was removed, there is no impairment of activity. All our patients have been able to resume their preoperative activities within four to six months after the operation.

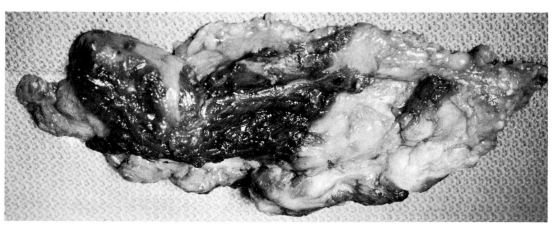

Figure 6.4. (F) The resected specimen of a muscle group excision of the thigh. This was a low-grade fibrosarcoma in a 61-year-old woman. She resumed all her preoperative activities within six months and has remained disease-free for the last six years.

pelvic and retroperitoneal nodes (especially in cases of rhabdomyosarcoma and synovial sarcoma of the buttock). If no contraindication is found, then the internal iliac vessels are ligated. The ligature should be applied above the superior gluteal branch of the artery; otherwise the bleeding is not curtailed and this step becomes a technical exercise without any benefit (Fig. 6.5A, inset). Although both internal iliac vessels are usually tied, in smaller tumors that are strictly localized to one side, unilateral ligation might suffice. Following this step the lap-

arotomy wound is closed and the patient is placed in the prone position. The patient is then prepared and the operative field so draped that the entire buttock, most of the posterior thigh, and part of the lateral and medial aspects of the body are within the operative field.

A generous elliptical skin incision is made, with the tumor in the central position (Fig. 6.5A, right). The skin flaps are raised on both sides (Fig. 6.5B). The proximal attachment of the gluteus maximus muscle from the lateral edge of the sacrum and coccyx and from the posterior

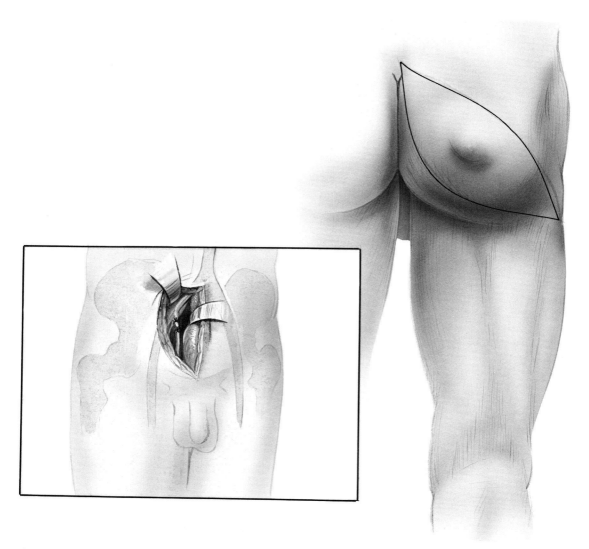

Figure 6.5. (A) *Inset:* Preliminary exploratory celiotomy with ligation of internal iliac artery is a helpful initial step prior to excision of a buttock tumor. *Right:* Elliptical skin incision is shown. The width of the skin ellipse to be removed depends on the size of the primary tumor and the histologic diagnosis.

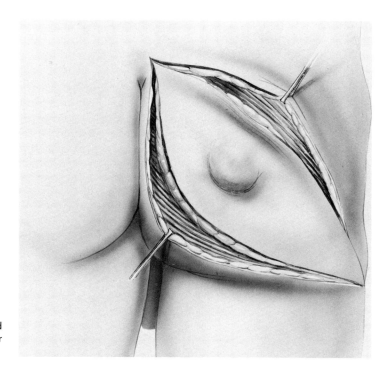

Figure 6.5. **(B)** Skin flaps are raised on both sides in the same manner as for radical mastectomy.

portion of the iliac crest is exposed medially (Fig. 6.5C) and its distal attachment into the greater trochanter of the femur and into the ileotibial band is exposed laterally (Fig. 6.5D). A vertical incision is then made through the distal attachment of the gluteus maximus muscle and the muscle is lifted medially (Fig. 6.5E). This exposes the underlying piriformis muscle, and the sciatic nerve is seen emerging from the sciatic foramen underneath the inferior margin of the muscle. The inferior gluteal vessels are identified, ligated, and resected (Fig. 6.5E). At this stage of the operation the extent of the tumor is reassessed and, if indicated, excision of the gluteus maximus muscle alone might be resorted to. In most instances, however, we have found that, to accomplish an adequate margin, the gluteus medius and piriformis muscles must be excised. Therefore, the tendinous distal attachment of the piriformis is then resected and the incision carried superiorly to include the distal attachment of the gluteus medius muscle to the trochanter of the femur (Fig. 6.5E and 6.5F). By exploring underneath these muscles the deeper extension of the tumor is reassessed, and if the deeper margin is free of any tumor extension, then the entire muscle mass is re-

tracted medially and the proximal attachments of these muscles are excised (Fig. 6.5G). Following removal of the muscles along with the tumor, proper hemostasis is obtained.

This operation naturally leaves a large operative defect, which can be closed either by approximating the skin margins, by rotation of a flap, or by a split-thickness skin graft. Although it is preferable to attempt either a primary closure (Fig. 6.5H) or rotation of a flap, split-thickness skin grafts over this area, even immediately over the sciatic nerve, are reasonably well tolerated and we have used them in several instances.

In some cases, this operation can be extended medially and proximally to incorporate the coccyx, part of the outer table of the sacrum, and the posterior lip of the iliac crest (Fig. 6.6) laterally and distally to include the proximal portions of the muscles of the posterior thigh. The decision to extend the limits of this operation lies largely in the experience of the surgeon and his or her familiarity with sarcomas. To develop general guidelines is neither possible nor desirable. However, if the tumor is found to be infiltrating the sciatic nerve or the bones, and in the opinion of the surgeon re-

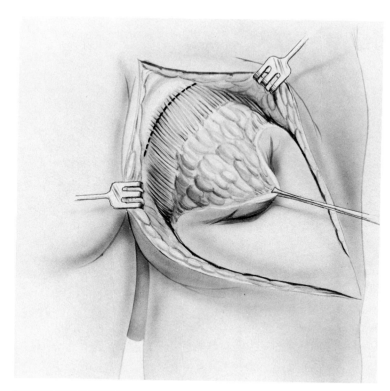

Figure 6.5. **(C)** Medial proximal attachment of gluteus maximus muscle is exposed. Dotted line represents the future line of resection of the muscle.

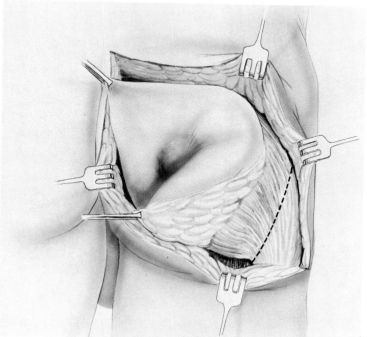

Figure 6.5. **(D)** Distal attachment of gluteus maximus muscle with the proposed line of resection.

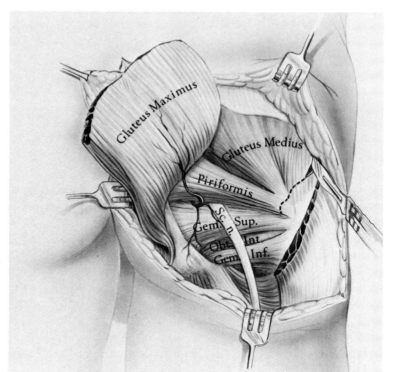

Figure 6.5. (E) Distal attachment of the gluteus maximus muscle resected and retracted proximally. The piriformis muscle, sciatic nerve, inferior gluteal vessels, and gluteus medius muscles are seen. The dotted line represents the line of resection of the gluteus medius and pyriformis muscles.

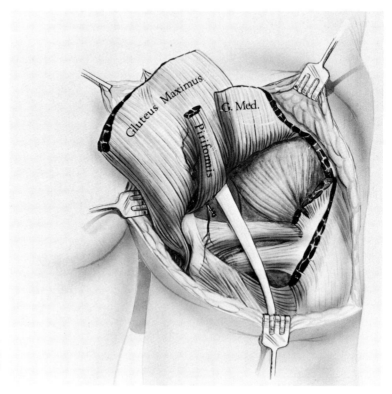

Figure 6.5. (F) The distal attachments of the piriformis and gluteus medius muscles are resected and retracted proximally.

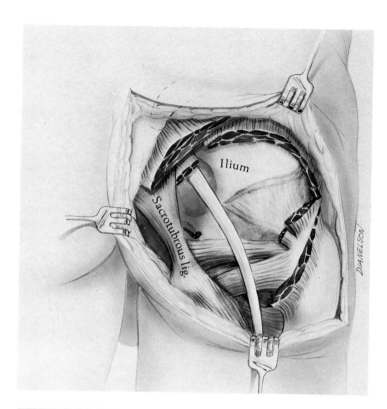

Figure 6.5. (G) The muscles have been resected proximally and the specimen removed. The cut margins of the glutei and the piriformis are easily discernible.

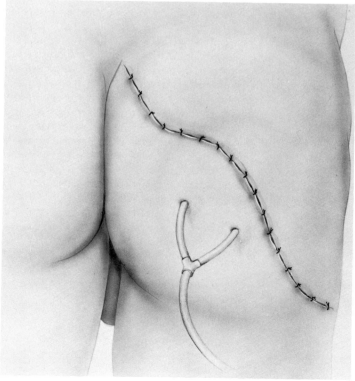

Figure 6.5. (H) Appearance of the operative site following a primary closure. Suction catheters are attached to wall suction.

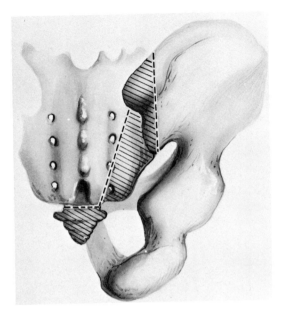

Figure 6.6. Diagram of pelvic skeleton from the back. The dotted lines show the extent to which bones can be excised along with this operation without creating any appreciable deformity.

section will not result in cure, the operation should be abandoned in favor of a hemipelvectomy.

A resection of the buttock is well tolerated by the patient and, in spite of resection of these muscles, he or she is able to walk, the only deformity being a Trendelenberg gait, which frequently is not noticeable to an inexperienced observer.

Conservative Amputation

The minor and conservative amputations to be discussed herein must be considered as variants of the wide local excision already described. A minor amputation is resorted to only when the sarcoma is well differentiated and is located in an area in the extremity where a conservative amputation is feasible.

Minor Amputations of the Upper Extremities

In conservative amputations of the hand it is essential to bear in mind that retention of any of the fingers will be most rewarding to the patient. Even if the thumb and only one other finger are preserved, the patient will have a functioning hand.

Amputations at the level of the wrist, midforearm, or below the elbow, are seldom indicated in the management of soft tissue sarcomas. With the increasing use of adjuvant chemotherapy and radiation therapy, the indications for minor amputations, especially of the upper extremities, have become rarer still. The technical considerations for these operations are standard and will not be discussed.

There are, however, two types of conservative amputations in the upper extremities that are sometimes used in the management of soft tissue sarcomas. These are subtotal scapulectomy and en bloc resection of the shoulder girdle (Tikhor-Linberg operation). Although the indications for such operations are few, it is appropriate to discuss the indications and techniques of these two unusual operations.

Subtotal Scapulectomy. A procedure for removal of tumors in the scapular region was originally described by Syme[8] in 1864. In his monograph he described three patients in whom he had performed this operation, showing it to be feasible and practical. However, de Nancrede,[9] in his presidential address to the American Surgical Association in 1909, categorically stated that scapulectomy was an inferior operation. Thereafter it fell into disrepute, and only occasional reports of results with this operation were published. Pack and Ariel[10] mentioned this procedure in 1958 but did not elaborate either in favor of or against it. It is thus apparent that the indications for scapulectomy have never been clearly defined; consequently, the end results sometimes have been unsatisfactory. Scapulectomy has a limited role in surgery for neoplastic disease, and strict criteria must be set up for its performance; otherwise, a perfectly suitable operative procedure will not be properly used.[11]

Indications. Scapulectomy is indicated in the following types of tumors:
Soft tissue sarcomas
Low-grade fibrosarcoma invading the scapular muscles
Aggressive fibromatoses (desmoids) infiltrating the scapular muscles
Liposarcoma arising from the adipose tissue in the scapular region, with local infiltration
Bone tumors
Primary malignant bone tumors arising in the scapula (this is rare); however, scapulectomy may be useful in unusual cases of

a low-grade chondrosarcoma or giant cell tumor of the scapula

Contraindications. Scapulectomy is definitely contraindicated if the sarcoma is located in the superior pole of the scapula, or if the tumor extends beyond the scapula and the muscles immediately attached to the scapula. It cannot be overemphasized that indications for scapulectomy are few and far between.

Technique of Subtotal Scapulectomy.

POSITION OF PATIENT. The patient is placed in the prone position with the arm resting in a 90-degree abduction on an arm board. The arm should be draped so that an assistant can move the arm as required during the operation (Fig. 6.7A).

An elliptical skin incision is then made, encompassing the tumor and extending from the tip of the acromion superolaterally to the paravertebral region inferomedially. The lower end of the incision can be extended to cross the midline if the tumor is so large as to make this necessary (Fig. 6.7A).

The medial and lateral skin flaps are raised and the superficial dorsal muscular attachment of the scapula is identified. The attachment of the trapezius muscle to the scapula is identified and resected. Reflection of the trapezius muscle exposes the supraspinatous muscle superiorly and rhomboid major inferiorly (Fig. 6.7B). The attachment of the deltoid muscle to the lateral tip of the scapular spine is similarly resected and retracted superomedially, exposing the remainder of the supraspinatus muscle. At this stage the rhomboid major muscle at the vertebral border, the latissimus dorsi inferiorly, the teres major and minor muscles laterally, and the infraspinous muscle can be easily identified.

The insertion of the latissimus dorsi muscle at the tip of the scapula is then excised and the muscle is retracted downward, exposing the tip of the scapula (Fig. 6.7C). The tip is then held by an assistant with a straight clamp and pulled inferolaterally. This provides traction to the muscles at the vertebral border and excision of their scapular attachment is made simple (Fig. 6.7C).

The muscular attachments in the superior angle of the scapula are then resected along the vertebral border of the scapula. The levator scapulae and the rhomboids, easily delineated, are then cut. This maneuver can be quite simple if the assistant maintains constant traction at the tip of the scapula. The inferior tip of the scapula

is then rotated and a medial pull is applied while the arm is abducted (Fig. 6.7D). The lateral muscles, teres major and minor, and the long head of the triceps (Fig. 6.7B) are then resected, protecting the axillary neurovascular bundle. Next, the supraspinatus tendons and the attachment of serratus anterior muscles are cut (Fig. 6.7D). The shoulder joint is then exposed and identified, and the spine is cut near the acromion process by use of an osteotome. Thus the acromioclavicular joint is kept intact. The only muscle remaining attached to the scapula, humerus, and shoulder joint is the subscapular, which is resected under the guidance of the operator's finger (Fig. 6.7E. Part I).

A Gigli saw is then passed around the neck of the scapula, avoiding the glenohumeral joint. The scapula is resected and the specimen removed, care being taken to avoid injury to the glenohumeral joint (Fig. 6.7E. Part II).

After proper hemostasis is achieved, the cut edge of the trapezius muscle is sutured to the deltoid muscle at the line of the previous position of the spine of the scapula (Fig. 6.7F). The lateral margins of these muscular stitches incorporate the remnant of the acromion process. The teres major and minor muscles are sutured to the chest wall (Fig. 6.7F).

The suction catheter beneath each skin flap is then brought out through normal skin, the wound is closed by interrupted subcutaneous chromic catgut sutures, and the skin margins are apposed by interrupted 3-0 nylon stitches. A firm pressure dressing is applied and the arm is placed in a Velpeau dressing. The long-term result of thi〉 operation is satisfactory (Fig. 6.7G).

En Bloc Resection of the Shoulder Girdle (Tikhor-Linberg Operation). This operation encompasses total scapulectomy, partial or complete excision of the clavicle, and resection of the head and neck of the humerus with preservation of the arm, brachial plexus, and subclavian vessels.

The operation was first planned by Tikhor[12] in 1900 under the name "resectointerscapulothoracica" as an alternative to forequarter amputation. However, Linberg[13] first described the technique of the operation, while discussing the management of malignant tumors of the shoulder girdle. Pack and Baldwin[14] discussed indications for the operation and described one patient on whom they operated.

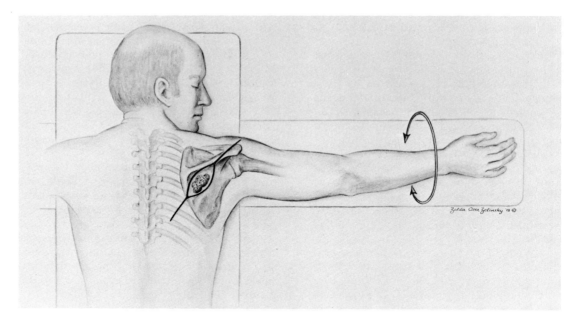

Figure 6.7. (A) The position of the patient and the incision for a tumor located in the center of the scapular region are shown. The arm should be draped in such a way that an assistant can freely move the arm to facilitate excision of muscular attachments.

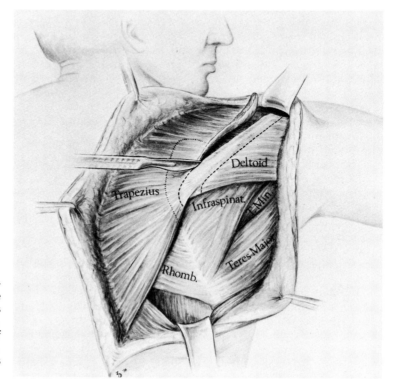

Figure 6.7. (B) The scapular muscles are exposed after raising the skin flaps. The trapezius muscle is then resected at the scapular spine. The dotted line shows the site of excision of the deltoid attachment. Reflection of the trapezius exposes the supraspinatus muscle.

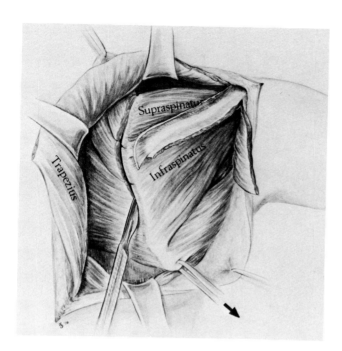

Figure 6.7. **(C)** Trapezius and deltoid muscles are reflected and the latissimus dorsi retracted downward. An assistant is pulling the tip laterally (arrow). This maneuver makes resection of the muscle attached to the vertebral border quite simple.

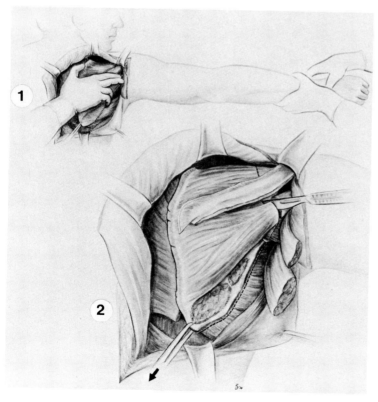

Figure 6.7. **(D) Part 1:** Palpation of the axillary contents. **Part 2:** The tip of the scapula is now pulled inferomedially and the lateral muscles are cut. The dotted line shows the line of resection of the supraspinatus, infraspinatus, and the serratus anterior muscles.

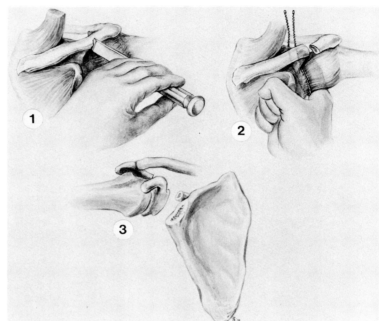

Figure 6.7. (E) Part 1: The scapular spine is cut with an osteotome. The subscapular muscle is cut under the guidance of the operator's finger. **Part 2:** A Gigli saw is then passed around the neck of the scapula (any other saw can also be used). **Part 3:** The specimen is removed.

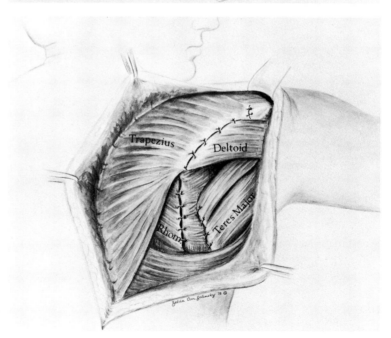

Figure 6.7. (F) Suture line between deltoid and trapezius muscles. The acromion process is shown at the top. The teres major and minor muscles are attached to the rib cage.

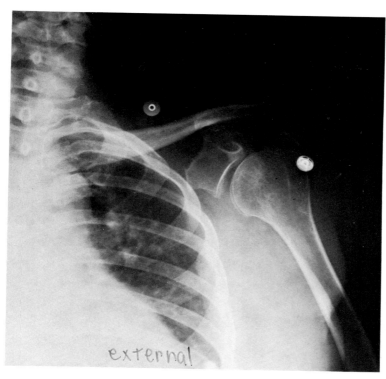

external

Figure 6.7. (G) Roentgenogram showing the shoulder joint *(left)* in patient who underwent subtotal scapulectomy three years ago. Patient has good use of her arm.

Indications.

1. Low-grade fibrosarcoma or well-differentiated liposarcoma located in the superior pole of the scapula or in the region of the lateral third of the clavicle.
2. Localized chondrosarcoma of the scapula or clavicle, not infiltrating the surrounding muscles.

Contraindications.

1. This operation is not indicated in any high-grade sarcoma of this region.
2. Any patient with sarcoma of the scapula that infiltrates the subscapularis muscle is not a candidate for this operation.

One of the most important accomplishments of this operation is the preservation of a relatively useful forearm and hand.

Technique of Operation.

POSITION OF PATIENT. The patient lies on the unaffected side in a modified lateral position. The arm is prepared and draped so as to be included in the operative field and is positioned so that the assistant can manipulate it during the operation.

STEPS OF OPERATION. A racquet incision is made along the anterior surface of the clavicle and is extended laterally over the deltoid about 5 cm below the acromion process (Fig. 6.8A). The second part of the incision is usually begun at the midclavicular line anteriorly and is extended posteriorly over the neck, near the medial border and around the inferior tip of the scapula, to be connected with the distal arm of the racquet (inset, Fig. 6.8D).

Following this outlining of the skin incision, the dissection is started anteriorly along the anterior border of the clavicle and extended laterally, exposing the deltoid muscle (Fig. 6.8A). The clavicle is then resected at the junction of the medial third and lateral two thirds by means of a Gigli saw. The pectoralis major muscle, including the clavicular head anteriorly and the deltoid laterally, are resected, exposing the coracoid process. The resected medial and lateral parts of the clavicle are retracted from the operative field. The pectoralis minor muscle attached to the coracoid process is exposed and resected (Fig. 6.8B). With the resection of the pectoralis minor near the tip of the coracoid process, access is gained to the axillary contents (Fig. 6.8C). The anterior circumflex humeral artery and subscapular vessels are defined, li-

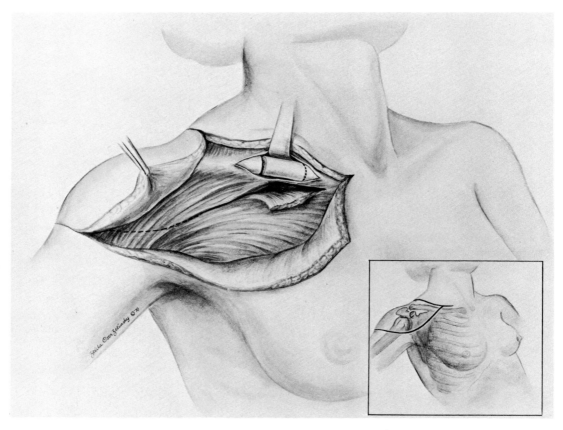

Figure 6.8. (A) With the patient in a modified lateral position, the incision is started on the anterior surface of the clavicle. The lateral handle of the racquet is extended along the clavicle laterally over the deltoid 5 cm below the acromion process, the medial handle over the neck to the back *(inset)*, and then along the medial border to the tip of the scapula, and there laterally to meet the lateral handle of the racquet over the lateral aspect of the arm *(see inset, Fig. 6.8D)*. Anterior incision is deepened. The clavicle is resected at the junction of the lateral two thirds and medial third. Dotted line is the line of resection of the muscles.

gated, and resected. The resected lateral part of the clavicle is retracted laterally, further exposing the brachial plexus (Fig. 6.8C). The incision is then carried along the vertebral border of the scapula and the muscles are resected in a manner identical to that shown for the technique of scapulectomy (Fig. 6.8D and 6.8E). The posterior incision is then connected with the lateral arm of the racquet, and the remaining portion of the deltoid, the long head of the triceps, and the teres major are divided (Fig. 6.8F). The surgical neck of the humerus is then exposed and, after ensuring the safety of the radial nerve, is resected and the specimen removed (Fig. 6.8F, inset).

The humerus is then suspended by ligatures to the remaining trapezius muscle or to a

rib (Fig. 6.8G). The trapezius and deltoid muscles are then sutured together, covering the defect (Fig. 6.8H). The skin is closed with suction catheters in place (Fig. 6.8I).

At the completion of the operation, the arm, forearm, and hand are intact. The functions of the forearm and hand are retained but the shoulder and upper arm movements are no longer possible. With appropriate physiotherapy and training the patient will have reasonable use of the forearm and the hand (Fig. 6.9).

Minor or Conservative Amputations of the Lower Extremities. In considering limited amputations of the foot, one must bear in mind that a retention arch will permit utilization of the foot. If possible, a transmetatarsal ampu-

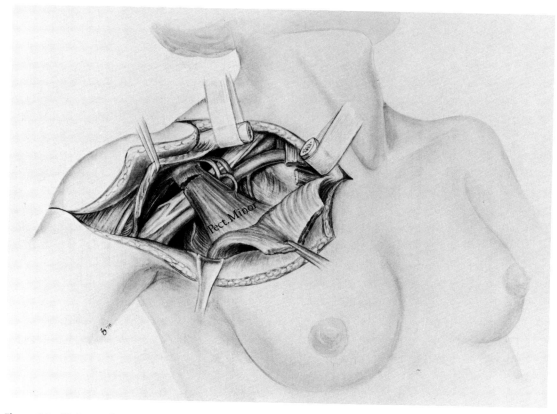

Figure 6.8. (B) Pectoralis major muscle anteriorly and the deltoid laterally are resected, exposing the coracoid process and the pectoralis minor muscle. The pectoralis minor muscle at its attachment to the coracoid process is then excised.

tation is satisfactory insofar as a functional foot is concerned. Of the variety of other conservative amputations practiced and described, few, if any, are applicable to the management of soft tissue sarcomas. A below-the-knee amputation has occasional applicability. The technique is standard and can be found in any textbook of orthopedic surgery.

Chest Wall Resection. Resection of a part of the anterior, lateral, or posterior part of the thoracic cage occasionally is required for tumors arising in these sites. The basic surgical concept is the same as that for an adequate wide excision, the only modification being that necessitated by the location of the tumor.

Indications.
1. All soft tissue sarcomas, osteosarcomas, and chondrosarcomas arising from the tissues of the chest wall

2. Locally recurrent skin cancers invading the ribs or the perichondrium

Contraindications. There are relatively few contraindications for a chest wall resection in the management of soft tissue sarcomas of the thoracic cage. In some highly malignant tumors to which judicious radiotherapy can be applied without injuring the underlying lung and pleura, a massive resection of the thoracic cage should be avoided; for example, rhabdomyosarcoma located in the chest wall.

Steps of the Operation. The technical aspects of the chest wall resection are simple. After assessing the resectability of a given tumor, the extent of the resection is outlined and the appropriate number of ribs on either side of the tumor is resected (Figs. 6.10A to 6.10C). The resected segment of the ribs must be adequate in length; otherwise, extension of the tumor along the marrow of the ribs will be overlooked, resulting in an inadequate operation. We perform

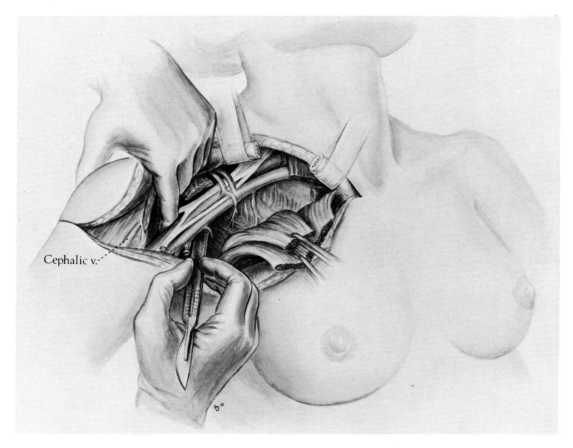

Cephalic v.

Figure 6.8. (C) Resection of anterior muscle attachments is completed, exposing the axillary contents and the brachial plexus.

intrapleural chest wall resections rather than extrapleural, since on several occasions we have found the undersurface of the tumors in intimate contact with the pleura.

The reconstruction following chest wall resection, however, is laden with diverse ideas and techniques. The major area of discord has been in the type of material to be used for replacing the lost chest wall. We use bovine fascia lata (Fig. 6.10D) for reconstruction and have found it to be satisfactory. The end result after these repairs is excellent and our patients have been able to resume normal activity (Fig. 6.11A and 6.11B). Lately in selected instances we are using various types of myocutaneous flaps with improved cosmetic and functional results.

Abdominal Wall Resection. The anterior abdomen is often the site of several types of tu-

mors. Most notable among these are the abdominal wall desmoids (aggressive fibromatosis). Frequently it is stated that in this anatomic location the incidence of local recurrence following excision is very high. A fatalistic attitude of acceptance of local recurrence by most authors reporting on this subject is commonly found in the literature.[15] The recurrence rate can be reduced to a minimum, however, if the proper concept of wide excision is applied. To accomplish this, the anterior abdominal wall must be excised totally, including the underlying peritoneum. A 3- to 5-cm margin on all sides of the primary tumor should be mapped out and a block of tissue containing skin, fascia, anterior abdominal wall musculature, and the underlying peritoneum must be resected (Fig. 6.12A and 6.12B). The defect is closed either by using synthetic material or by bovine fascia lata (Fig.

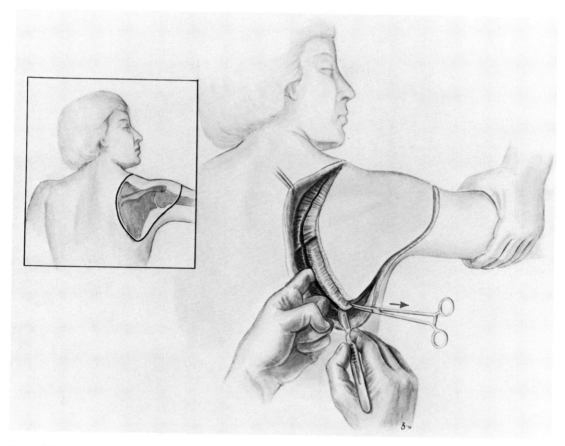

Figure 6.8. (D) The posterior incision is deepened and vertebral attachments of the scapula are severed. The inset shows the posterolateral part of the incision.

6.12C). The skin is closed with interrupted sutures. In our hands, application of this principle has lowered the incidence of recurrence to a minimum, and there is no functional handicap after this operation (Fig. 6.13). Similarly in some patients abdominal wall defects can be effectively closed by myocutaneous flaps.

Excision of Retroperitoneal Tumors. Retroperitoneal sarcomas are indeed difficult to operate upon. The boundaries of the retroperitoneum are varied and the surgeon may be confronted with a sarcoma of immense size. Therefore, it is not possible to describe the steps of the operation. The surgeon should plan the extent of the operation after a preliminary exploration of the abdominal cavity and assessment of the situation. We try to ascertain the extent of the tumor and its relation to the aorta and inferior vena cava by extensive use of preoperative investigative techniques (Chapter 5). Adequate exposure is always the key to the excision of these retroperitoneal tumors. Figure 6.14 shows the incisions that have been found useful in our hands. Multiple variations of these basic incisions can be adopted as the situation dictates. During the operation, adherence to surrounding organs is ascertained and a plan for resection outlined. Frequently, whole or part of several viscera must be excised.

The recurrence rate of these tumors is high, and some patients need multiple operations. One of our patients with a retroperitoneal liposarcoma required 11 procedures. At the time of this writing, six years after the date of initial operation, she is living apparently disease-free.

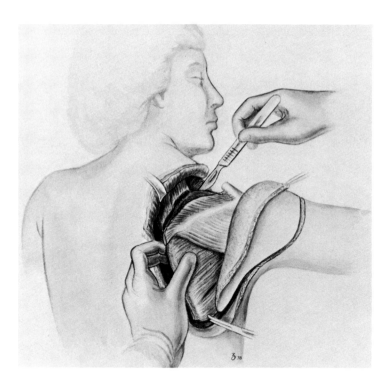

Figure 6.8. (E) All the posterior muscles have been resected, including the trapezius muscle; the tip of the scapula is pulled inferolaterally.

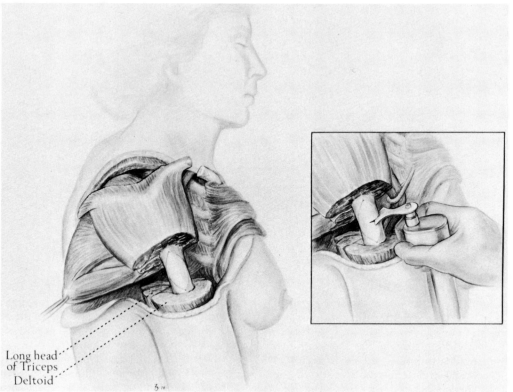

Long head of Triceps
Deltoid

Figure 6.8. (F) The distal part of the deltoid and long head of the triceps are cut and the surgical neck of the humerus exposed. The *inset* shows the line of resection of the humerus, following which the specimen is removed.

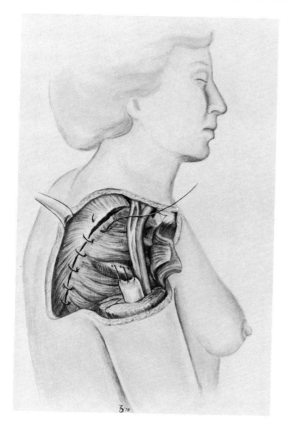

Figure 6.8. (G) The distal humerus is anchored to the lateral chest wall with several monofilament sutures.

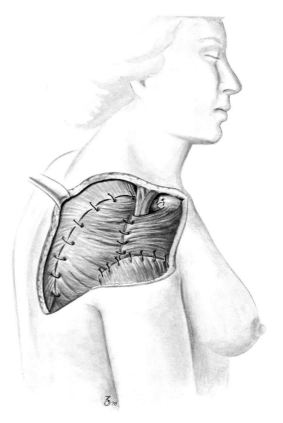

Figure 6.8. (H) The ends of the muscles are approximated with interrupted absorbable sutures covering the brachial plexus and the vessels.

Excision of Intrathoracic Tumors. Mediastinal soft tissue tumors are less common, and, unlike in their retroperitoneal counterpart, surgical management is relatively simple. Once a mediastinal tumor is diagnosed and the patient properly assessed, an exploratory thoracotomy is performed, and the tumor is approached. If it is truly a soft tissue tumor, it is excised. With today's advances in anesthesia and postoperative management techniques, the results of the operation are usually excellent.

Wide Excision and In-continuity Node Dissection. The well-known concept of excision of the primary tumor and simultaneous dissection of the regional node-bearing area, as proposed by Halstead[16] for cancer of the breast, is seldom required for the management of soft tissue sar-

comas. Rarely do these tumors metastasize to the regional nodes of the neck, axillae, or groin. However, in some instances of high-grade synovial sarcoma, rhabdomyosarcoma (all types), and other sundry sarcomas, regional node metastases may occur (details are described under each type elsewhere in this book). Therefore, the concept of wide excision with in-continuity regional node dissection should be kept in mind.

The procedure to be applied must be tailored to a given patient, and it must be planned with the concept of wide excision of the primary sarcoma, as described earlier, with extension of the excision in-continuity to include the regional node-bearing area. Because of the location of the primary tumor, bizarre types of incision lines often will result, but this should not deter the surgeon from undertaking these operations.

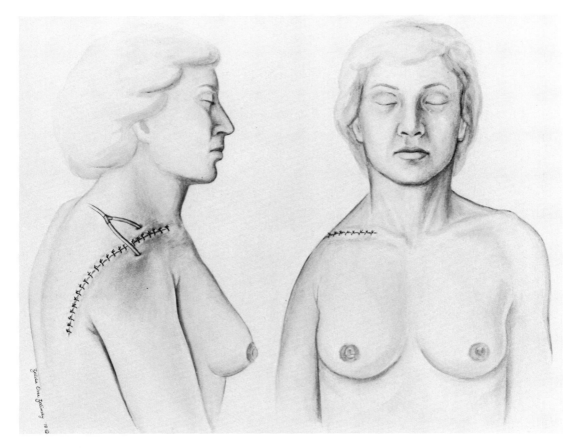

Figure 6.8. (I) The wound is closed with interrupted nylon sutures, and suction catheters are placed. The appearance of the shoulder after this resection is cosmetically tolerable.

INDICATIONS AND TECHNIQUES FOR RADICAL AMPUTATION

The principles governing the choice of a radical amputation of an extremity are varied. Probably the single most important factor is the clinical experience of the surgeon treating the patient. However, when all the available information is considered, it is possible to develop certain guidelines for application in planning amputations for sarcomas. These are as follows:

1. Many sarcomas extend imperceptibly proximally along the muscular or fascial planes, sometimes making it difficult to assess the extent of the disease.
2. Fibrosarcomas extend along the fascial plane, and along all the fascial attachments proximally, distally, and deep to the tumor.

3. Malignant schwannomas extend along the nerve sheath, and with the coexistent beading of the nerves commonly seen in plexiform neuroma, it is often difficult to be certain of the level of excision, even with appropriate use of rapid histologic techniques for examination of the margins of the resected specimens.
4. Invasion of a soft tissue sarcoma to the underlying bone or blood vessels and nerves usually requires an amputation.
5. Sarcomas of any histologic type that persistently recur after primary therapy: the need for a major amputation becomes more acute after a number of local recurrences.

Based on the five points above, the general principles to be applied in making a decision for or against an amputation can be made. How-

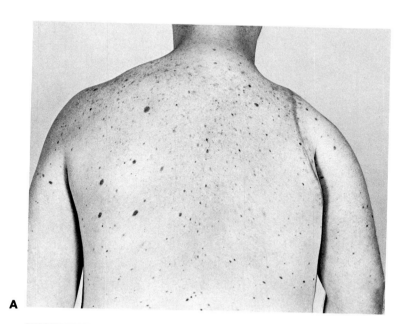

A

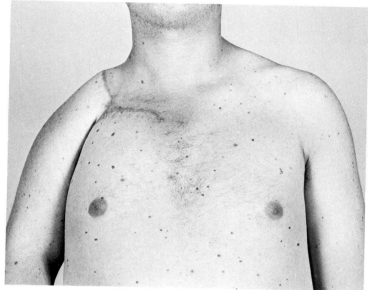

B

Figure 6.9. (**A**) Anterior and (**B**) posterior views of a patient who underwent an en bloc resection of the shoulder girdle. The functions of hand and forearm are intact.

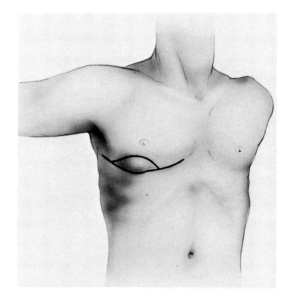

Figure 6.10. (A) A tumor in the anterior chest wall. The proposed incision is shown.

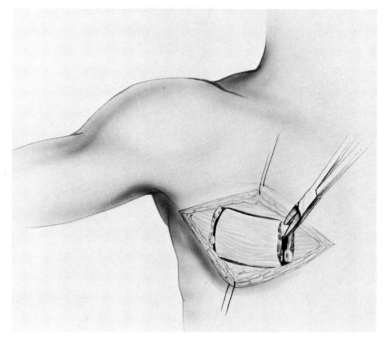

Figure 6.10. (B) The skin flaps have been raised, the resectability assessed, and the ribs are being resected.

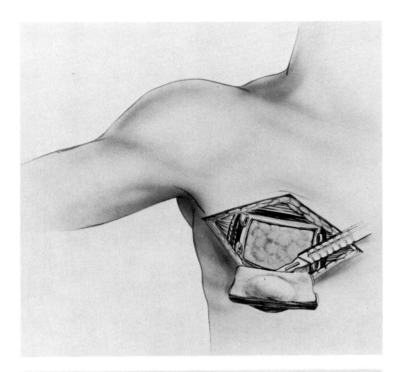

Figure 6.10. (C) Segment of the chest wall being removed. Unaffected lung can be seen underneath.

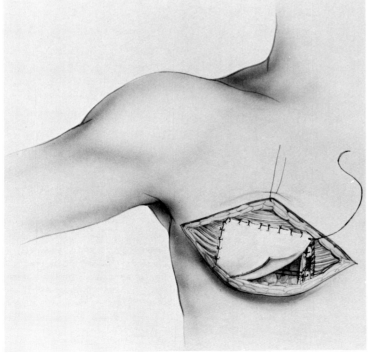

Figure 6.10. (D) Chest wall being repaired by a strip of bovine fascia lata.

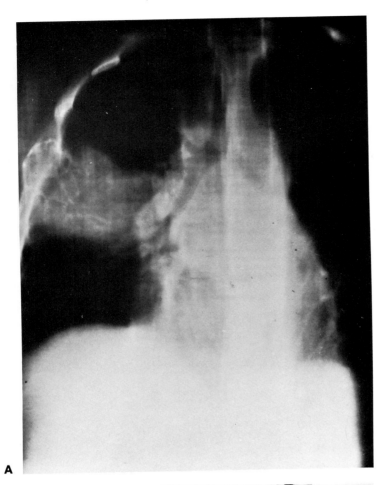

A

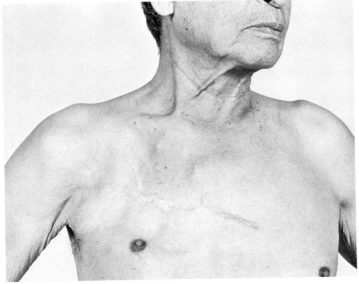

B

Figure 6.11. **(A)** Roentgenogram of chest showing a fibrosarcoma tumor of the chest wall in a 9-year-old girl. Following chest wall resection she has remained well for 10 years. **(B)** Another patient, a 56-year-old man, two years after chest wall resection and repair with bovine fascia lata for a myxoid liposarcoma of the pectoral region.

ever, before making the decision, all other options for therapy must be evaluated.

The surgeon performing amputations for soft tissue sarcomas does not have wide latitude in selecting the site of amputation, as in the management of trauma or peripheral vascular disorders. This does not imply that a thorough consideration of a good functional prosthesis is not advocated, but rather that prosthetic considerations should not interfere with the potential cure. We have seen a number of patients in whom, for the sake of a better prosthesis, inadequate amputations have been performed with resultant local recurrences in the stump. Local recurrence after a major amputation is indeed a failure of treatment, and every attempt should be made to avoid it.

With the combination of radiation therapy and chemotherapy the need for radical amputation is decreased in some sarcomas, and the patients can be well treated with wide soft tissue resections and adjuvant chemotherapy or irradiation, or both. The types of tumors and the kind of patients in whom such multimodality therapy is possible have been described in the chapters dealing with specific tumor types.

Preoperative Care for Patients Undergoing Radical Amputations

Preoperative preparation of patients who will undergo radical amputation is essentially the same as that for any other major operation. There are excellent monographs dealing with this subject alone and the reader is urged to consult them. Suffice it to point out that all major limb ablative procedures are operations of major magnitude and the patient must be adequately evaluated regarding cardiopulmonary and renal status, blood volume, underlying infection, and any other concomitant feature that might produce postoperative complications.

We advocate an in-depth discussion with the patient and his or her spouse, or with appropriate relatives or friends, of the indications for and against the proposed amputation. We have found that a well-informed patient always adjusts better to the deformity and has fewer associated symptoms, for example, the phantom limb syndrome or similar complaints. This discussion results in less hostility and in a useful member of society. We strongly recommend that a major amputation not be "sold" to a patient, and if he or she has any doubt, then such an

operation should be abandoned. The objective of the surgeon is to provide all the necessary information, then let the patient make the final decision.

We perform a preliminary exploratory laparotomy in a large number of our patients undergoing major amputation, and we take all precautions for a patient undergoing a major intra-abdominal operation. For patients who require hip joint disarticulation or hemipelvectomy, we routinely use preoperative cleansing of the colon, evaluate the urinary bladder, and in male patients, the prostate as well.

Radical Amputations of the Upper Extremity

Mid-Arm Amputation. There are few indications for mid-arm amputation. This operation is indicated when the tumor is located in the forearm and amputation must be above the common flexor or extensor attachments in the lower end of the humerus. Occasionally, in cases of tumors of the hand and forearm in which there are palpable nodes in the axilla, a mid-arm amputation with axillary dissection can be resorted to instead of a forequarter amputation (Fig. 6.15). The technique is standard, and will not be repeated here.

Shoulder Joint Disarticulation. Shoulder joint disarticulation has little or no value in the management of soft tissue sarcomas. We have never had occasion to use this operation for the management of any of our patients. Although we can conceive of an occasional application of this technique, we think in most of these patients the better operation would be a forequarter amputation. For this reason, the technical aspects of the operation will not be described.

Interscapulothoracic Amputation (Forequarter Amputation or Berger's Amputation). In this operation the entire upper extremity and the shoulder girdle and its muscular attachments are removed. The first interscapulothoracic amputation for cancer was performed by Crosby[17] in 1836 for removal of an osteosarcoma. The technique of the operation, however, was standardized by Berger[18] in 1887. This classic operation still bears his name. Since the turn of the century it has been increasingly used for the management of sarcomas of the upper extrem-

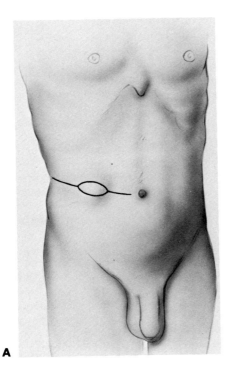

A

Figure 6.12. (A) Proposed skin incision for an anterior abdominal wall tumor. **(B)** Skin flaps have been raised, the line of resection is outlined, and the resection is begun in the medial end. Extent of resection is shown by the dotted line. **(C)** Specimen has been removed, including the parietal peritoneum. Small intestine can easily be seen. Defect is being closed with bovine fascia lata. Following this repair, we have not come across any abdominal wall hernia in an otherwise healthy person.

ities. Pack and associates[19] published an elegant review of the operation in 1942 and reported on their series of 31 patients so treated at Memorial Sloan-Kettering Cancer Center. Subsequently, Moseley[20] published a review on forequarter amputateions. Interested readers should review these classic works. With the development of better anesthesia and blood transfusion methods, this operation has become less of a technical feat than it used to be.[21-23]

Indications.
1. All malignant tumors of the upper arm, axilla, and the shoulder region
2. Bone sarcomas proximal to the elbow, particularly those involving the upper end of the humerus or those extending into the medullary cavity or to the surrounding soft tissues
3. All malignant tumors infiltrating the capsule of the shoulder joint, the deltoid, subscapularis, and the pectoral muscles
4. Tumors of the shoulder girdle for which an attempted Tikhor-Linberg operation or a scapulectomy procedure has been deemed unsuitable
5. Aggressive fibromatoses of the upper arm

that are symptomatic, especially those infiltrating the brachial plexus or the periosteum of the humerus

Contraindications. The usual contraindications to any major surgical procedure because of systemic disease apply. Additionally, sarcomas that are deemed sensitive to chemotherapy and radiation therapy should not be treated by this operation. Patients with such tumors in an upper extremity should be treated with regional chemotherapy, wide soft tissue resection, and adjuvant radiation therapy and chemotherapy, or both. We think that adoption of this policy will further reduce the need for forequarter amputation in the management of soft tissue sarcomas of the upper extremities.

Technique of Operation.

ANESTHESIA. Standard endotracheal anesthesia is generally used. In some patients with large tumors in whom there is a possibility of major bleeding, the use of hypotensive anesthesia might be of value.

POSITION OF PATIENT. The patient is placed on his or her back with the affected shoulder elevated so that the skin of the upper arm, axilla, and the skin of both the anterior and pos-

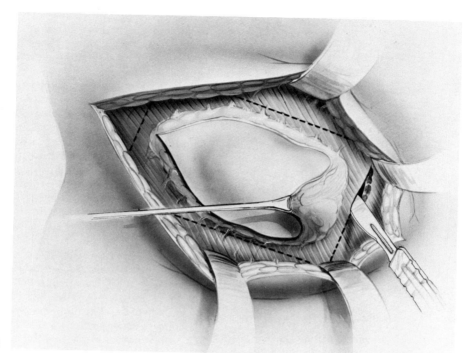

B

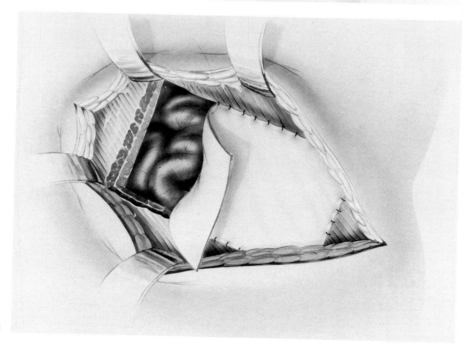

C

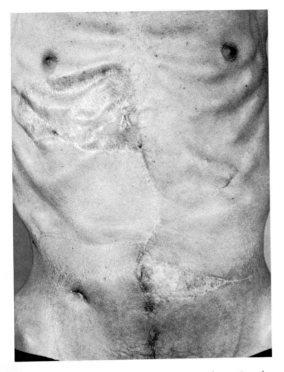

Figure 6.13. Three years after resection of anterior abdominal wall for hemangiopericytoma. Patient had no disability.

terior chest wall up to the midline can be prepared and draped to be included in the operative site.

STEPS OF OPERATION. A linear incision is first made over the medial third of the clavicle (Fig. 6.16A). This incision is deepened to the periosteum, and the periosteum is elevated by means of a periosteal elevator. The clavicle is resected with the Gigli saw (Fig. 6.16B). Through this window the subclavian vessels are exposed, with the artery lying deeper than the vein (Fig. 6.16C). The subclavian vessels are then individually ligated and resected. It is our practice to double-ligate the proximal end of these structures using 2-0 silk and do the suture ligature with 3-0 silk (Fig. 6.16D). Ligation of the superficial cervical and descending scapular arteries along with the transverse cervical vessels will prevent excessive blood loss during the rest of the operation. After ligating the vessels, the skin incision is extended laterally to the tip of the acromion process, then downwards anteriorly toward the axilla (Fig. 6.16D). The arm is then drawn across the body and the posterior flap is outlined by an incision of the skin along the vertebral border of the scapula, which unites with the inferior tip of the anterior incision at the lateral margin of the axillary fold (Fig. 6.16E).

Figure 6.14. Three types of incision are shown. The transverse incision usually is best for most retroperitoneal structures. However, the lateral might be of value in tumors of the renal region with a need for entry into the thoracic cavity in situations in which the tumors are located in association with the adrenal, or behind the liver bed.

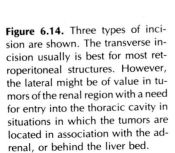

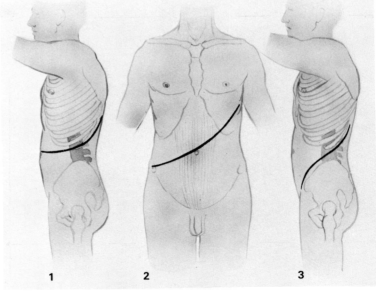

1   2   3

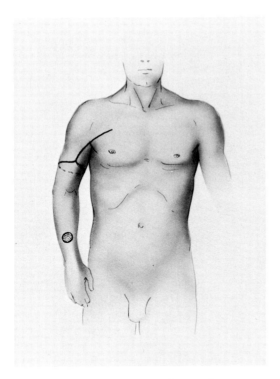

Figure 6.15. Suggested incision for a mid-arm amputation with incontinuity axillary node dissection for a tumor of the forearm.

The arm is then brought back to its original position and the anterior incision is deepened up to the pectoral muscles. Resection of the pectoralis major and minor muscles gives an excellent exposure of the brachial plexus (Fig. 6.16F). The brachial plexus is then resected as proximally as possible. The arm is brought forward again and the patient is rotated anterolaterally. The posterior incision is then deepened, exposing the trapezius muscle, and the muscles attached to the vertebral border of the scapula are sequentially resected (Fig. 6.16G and 6.16H). This step of the operation is similar to that described for subtotal scapulectomy. With detachment of the scapula the amputation is complete and the extremity is removed (Fig. 6.16I). After proper hemostasis the wound is closed, using absorbable sutures for muscle and subcutaneous tissue and interrupted 3-0 nylon sutures for skin. The Hemovac suction catheters are left behind (Fig. 6.16J).

The exposure of the subclavian vessels through the window described above sometimes becomes difficult. In such cases, following resection of the clavicle the ligation of the vessels is postponed until the anterior incision is carried through the pectoral muscles into the axilla. With this dissection the axillary vein and artery come into view and ligation of the vessels becomes relatively simple. The rest of the operative steps are the same as above.

Occasionally, an unusual location of the primary tumor, for example, over the superior aspect of the shoulder, will prevent adequate exposure of the subclavian vessels by the method described above. For such cases, Nadler and Phelan[21] have described a posterior method for approaching the subclavian vessels as well as for assessing the resectability of the tumor. In these patients, the posterior skin incision is first deepened and the pleural cavity entered through the bed of the second rib. If the lesion is resectable, the subclavian vessels are identified and ligated within the chest cavity. Care should be taken to avoid injury to the innominate vessels on the right side, and the vagus and phrenic nerves on both sides. The chest wall defect is closed with fascia, as described in chest wall resection.

Bowden[22] described a method of extending forequarter amputation to include an ipsilateral neck dissection (Fig. 6.16A). This extension of the operation is useful in tumors of the axilla or shoulder that could metastasize to neck nodes, for example, some cases of rhabdomyosarcoma or synovial cell sarcoma.

In a number of patients the operation can be extended to include resection of the chest wall, radical mastectomy, excision of part of the intrathoracic viscus, etc. All these modifications are applied whenever indicated, and in our hands these extended operations have been useful in selected patients (Fig. 2.1, Chapter 2).

Although the operation is dramatic and mutilating, in properly selected patients operative complications or problems are minimal. Blood loss is usually less than one liter and in patients in whom hypotensive anesthesia is used, it is still less. The incidence of traumatic neuroma is high following an interscapulothoracic amputation.[24] In our hands, the only satisfactory method for reduction of the incidence has been sharp excision of the plexi at the most proximal point. This allows the individual roots to retract without getting encased in the fibrous

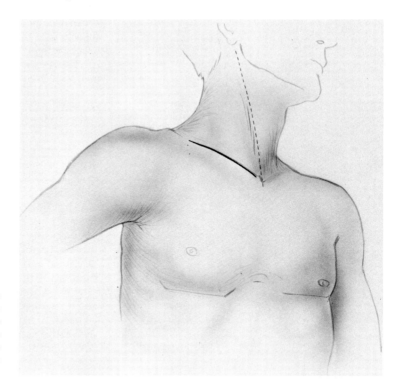

Figure 6.16. **(A)** The deep line represents the first step of the incision in forequarter amputation. The dotted line in the neck shows the incision that can be used for a concomitant neck dissection when indicated.

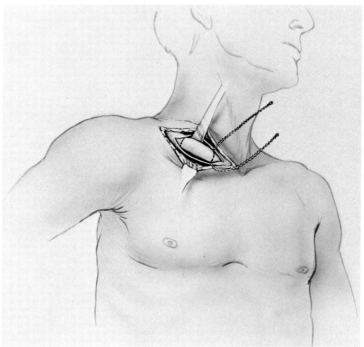

Figure 6.16. **(B)** Incision has been deepened. The clavicle is exposed, clavicular periosteum is incised, and the clavicle resected with a Gigli saw.

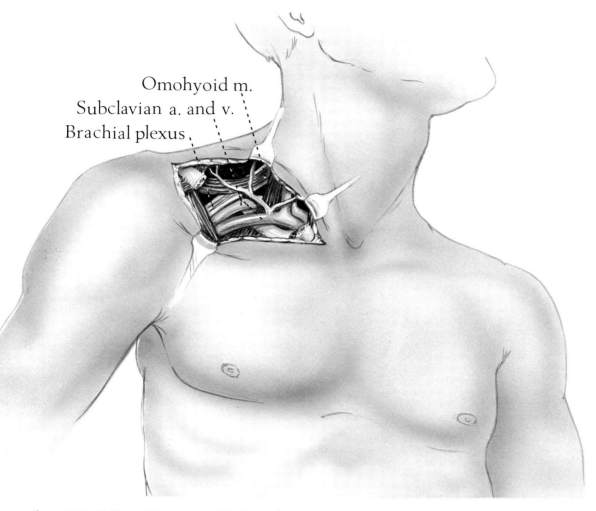

Omohyoid m.
Subclavian a. and v.
Brachial plexus,

Figure 6.16. **(C)** The middle segment of the clavicle has been removed. The subclavian vessels (artery and vein) and the brachial plexus can be seen.

scar of the incision. Sometimes reexcision of these painful neuromas becomes necessary.

The postoperative course is usually smooth. The patient is ambulatory the day after the amputation and in uncomplicated cases can be discharged within seven to nine days. Patients adjust to this operation well and continue to function as useful members of society (Fig. 6.17).

A forequarter operation becomes complicated, however, in patients with recurrent tumors who have been previously irradiated to the maximum tolerable dose. In such instances, the major problem is postoperative wound healing, since in a number of patients the skin flaps necrose, leaving a large defect. Frequently, the

closure of these defects taxes the imagination of the best of plastic surgeons.

Radical Amputations of the Lower Extremities

Above-the-Knee or Mid-Thigh Amputations.
Amputations above the knee joint for soft tissue sarcomas arising in the foot or in the leg have a definite place in the armamentarium of surgical treatment. The usual indications for such an operation are fibrosarcomas, synovial sarcomas, rhabdomyosarcomas, and liposarcomas arising in the leg. The technical aspects of a mid-thigh amputation are well known and will not

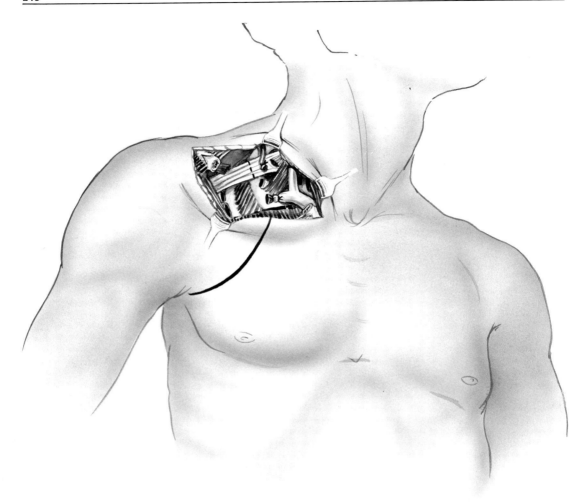

Figure 6.16. (D) The vessels are ligated and resected. Dotted line shows the proposed line of resection of the brachial plexus and the dark line shows the skin incision to the axilla. The anterior skin incision is sometimes extended to the axilla prior to ligation of the vascular bundle.

be repeated. In certain instances, eg, in rhabdomyosarcomas and synovial sarcomas, above-the-knee amputation is combined with a radical groin dissection (Fig. 6.18).[25] The technique of groin dissection is described in detail in combination with hip joint disarticulation (see below).

Hip Joint Disarticulation. Amputation of a lower extremity through the hip joint is a formidable procedure and should be undertaken only when the indications for this operation are unassailable.

Hip joint disarticulation apparently was first performed by Walter Bonchear of Bardstown, Kentucky in August of 1806, but an account was never published. Frank[26] described Bonchear's performance of this operation, without anesthesia, in a 17-year-old boy with a comminuted multiple fracture of the femur. The earliest recorded instance of an anatomically well-conceived hip joint disarticulation was that of Sir Astley Cooper.[27] The operation was performed at Guy's Hospital on January 16, 1824, on a 40-year-old man, again without anesthesia. The patient did well and was free of disease one year after the operation. The courage, imagination, and perseverance of the patients, as well

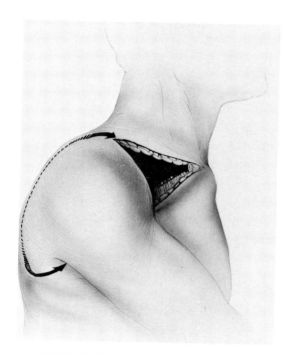

Figure 6.16. (E) Artistic rendition of the incision in the back along the vertebral border of the scapula. This incision, bound by arrows, is extended from the acromion process, and, encircling the tip of the scapula, reaches the anterior axillary incision, as seen in Figure 6.16D.

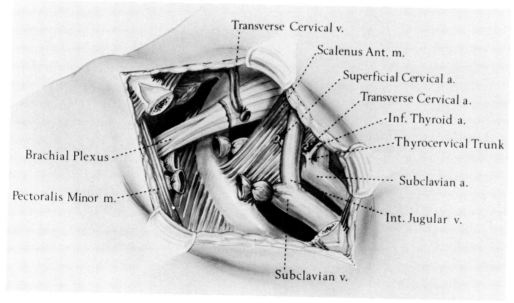

Transverse Cervical v.

Scalenus Ant. m.

Superficial Cervical a.

Transverse Cervical a.

Inf. Thyroid a.

Thyrocervical Trunk

Brachial Plexus

Subclavian a.

Pectoralis Minor m.

Int. Jugular v.

Subclavian v.

Figure 6.16. (F) Anterior view of the completed axillary resection. Vessels are resected, brachial plexus is being cut. All the anterior structures are resected, completing the anterior separation of the extremity.

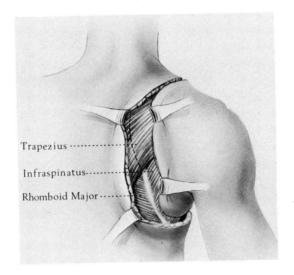

Figure 6.16. (G) Posterior excision is begun. First layers of the muscles are exposed and resected.

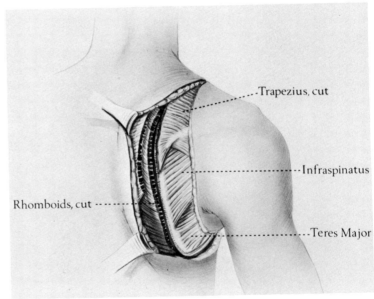

Figure 6.16. (H) The deeper muscles attached to the vertebral border of the scapula are sequentially resected.

as of the surgeons, in those earlier days of extended surgery is indeed unimaginable in the latter half of the twentieth century. Today, with the advances in anesthesia and transfusion, the operation of hip joint disarticulation has become a relatively routine procedure. Most of the credit for application of this operation to the management of soft tissue sarcomas should go to the late George T. Pack and his colleagues at Memorial Sloan-Kettering Cancer Center.[1,4,10]

Indications. Patients with malignant tumors of the soft somatic tissues of the thigh which cannot be removed adequately either by a muscle group excision or a mid-thigh amputation are candidates for hip joint disarticulation. However, those tumors that are sensitive to chemotherapy and radiation therapy should not be treated by hip joint disarticulation unless all other measures fail.

Preliminary exploratory celiotomy through

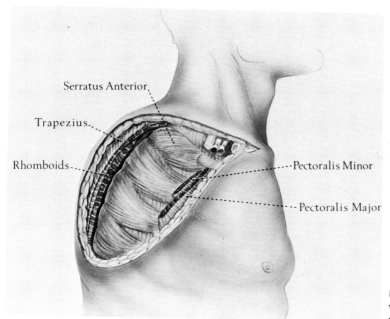

Serratus Anterior

Trapezius

Rhomboids

Pectoralis Minor

Pectoralis Major

Figure 6.16. **(I)** Appearance of the wound after the extremity has been separated.

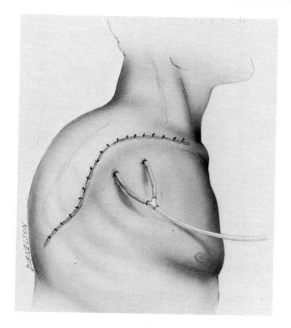

Figure 6.16. **(J)** Wound closed, with suction drainage.

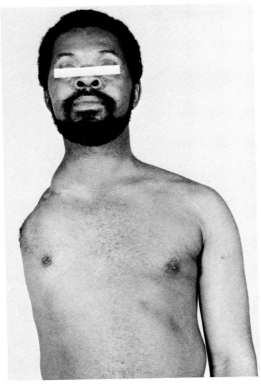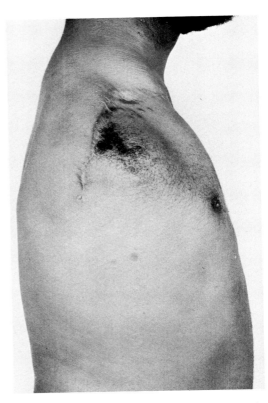

Figure 6.17. Anterior and lateral views of a 31-year-old man who underwent a forequarter amputation for a low-grade fibrosarcoma five years ago. He has remained well and active.

an upper lateral incision is always the first step in our hands. Before undertaking any major amputation, it is essential that all steps be taken to eliminate any possibility of an unnecessary operation. To perform an exploratory procedure at this stage requires little additional time. If the findings are negative for metastatic disease, the peritoneum is closed and the steps of the amputation begun.

Steps of Operation. An anterior racquet incision is most suitable (Fig. 6.19A, inset [left hip]). The vertical part of the incision is carried downward and outward across the anterior aspect of the thigh, coursing just above the greater trochanter. The medial incision is similarly carried across the thigh about 4 cm below the genitofemoral fold. The two incisions join posteriorly at the infragluteal fold. Although an attempt is always made to adhere to this classic racquet incision, deciding the amount of skin to be sacrificed depends on the location of the tumor. Frequently, this decision results in several modifications of the standard skin incision.

A detailed description of the subsequent steps of the operation will be found in the following section dealing with hip joint disarticulation and radical groin dissection. The minor differences in steps between these two operations will be pointed out as they occur.

Hip Joint Disarticulation and Radical Groin Dissection.

Indications. Rhabdomyosarcomas, synovial cell sarcomas, malignant fibrous histiocytomas, and certain other highly anaplastic sarcomas that have a tendency to metastasize to the regional nodes should be treated by combined hip joint disarticulation and radical groin dissection.

Technique of Operation. The choice of anesthesia and the method of positioning the patient are the same as for the standard hip joint disarticulation described above.

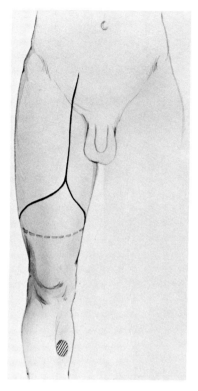

Figure 6.18. Incision for mid-thigh amputation and radical groin dissection. For indications of this type of composite operation, see text.

Steps of Operation. The vertical incision extends from the subcostal region inferiorly on a straight line crossing the midpoint of the inguinal ligament and is continued about 4 cm below, on the skin of the thigh. The lateral arm of the incision is carried laterally, just above the greater trochanter. The medial incision is similarly carried across the medial aspect of the thigh about 4 cm below the inguinal fold (Fig. 6.19A, inset [right hip]). As before, the skin incision in the thigh might require modification, depending on the amount of skin to be excised in a given patient.

The vertical incision on the anterior abdominal wall is deepened up to the mid-inguinal point. The anterior abdominal wall muscles and the peritoneum are incised along the same line as the skin incision (Fig. 6.19A). The peritoneal cavity is explored (Fig. 6.19B) and if necessary, questionable areas in the liver or other viscera and the para-aortic nodes are examined by means

of frozen section. If there is any evidence of intra-abdominal metastases, the proposed hip joint disarticulation is not carried out. Upon completion of the exploration, the peritoneum is closed (Fig. 6.19B). Next, the retroperitoneal area is exposed by pushing the peritoneal contents medially with a sponge stick, which can be accomplished with relative ease and without any blood loss (Fig. 6.19C). This method will expose the bifurcation of the aorta and the formation of the inferior vena cava proximally to the iliac vessels distally. The ureter will be seen reflected along with the posterior peritoneum medially.

The deep part of the groin dissection is then begun about 2 cm above the bifurcation of the aorta and carried distally to include the iliac and obturator group of nodes. The most proximal part is marked with metal clips and the areolar tissue containing the nodes is dissected distally (Fig. 6.19D). The dissection includes the adventitial layer of both the external iliac artery and vein distally from the bifurcation of the common iliac vessels. These vessels are ligated and resected about two centimeters from the bifurcation. The resected blood vessels and their areolar envelope, along with the nodes, are dissected distally. The obturator contents are dissected out from the obturator fossa and the perivesical fat (Fig. 6.19E). In contrast to the conventional radical groin dissection described earlier,[25] the dissection is not carried to the femoral triangle, since that part is included when the limb is removed at the level of the hip joint.

Following the deep node dissection, the hip joint disarticulation is begun. Both the external iliac artery and vein have been previously ligated and resected. The inguinal ligament and the femoral nerves are then resected. The medial and lateral incisions of the thigh are deepened, and thick flaps are developed both medially up to the pubis and laterally to the greater trochanter. The anterior compartment muscles are then resected. The limb is abducted by an assistant and the medial compartment muscles are then resected at their point of proximal attachment (Fig. 6.19F). The limb is then adducted and the tensor fascia lata resected. This completes the dissection of the anterior aspects of the hip joint. The limb is then adducted and internally rotated. As a result, the greater trochanter comes into view and the lateral muscles attached to the greater trochanter are resected.

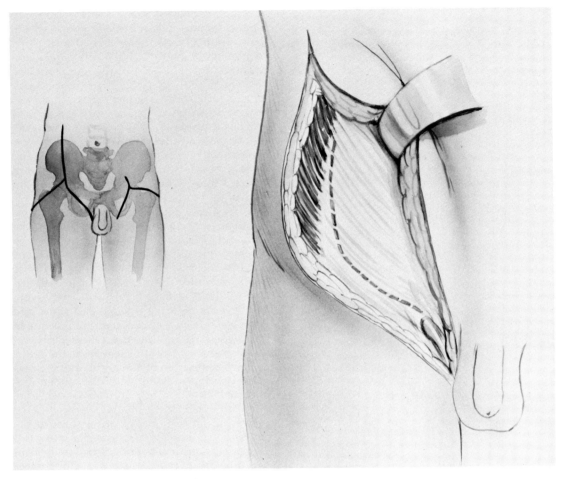

Figure 6.19. (A) *Inset:* Outline of incision for a hip joint disarticulation and ipsilateral radical groin dissection. Incision for a standard hip joint disarticulation is shown on left. *Right:* Upper abdominal incision used for exploratory celiotomy.

After this, the limb is rotated and the gluteal group of muscles is resected. The capsule of the hip joint is exposed and incised. The ligamentum teres is then exposed and resected, and the head of the femur is delivered out of the acetabulum (Fig. 6.19G). The limb is now attached only posteriorly by the sciatic nerve and the hamstring muscles. These are resected and the limb removed.

Following removal of the specimen, the bleeding points are caught and ligated. Any extra muscles or fat is trimmed. The acetabular cavity is curetted to remove as much of the synovial surface as possible; otherwise, the membrane secretes synovial fluid for a prolonged period. The wound is then closed, with an ad-

equate drain (Fig. 6.19H), and a firm pressure dressing is applied.

If node dissection is not indicated, the superior limit of the incision is initially deepened to expose the inguinal ligament, which is resected. Following this, femoral vessels are dissected, isolated, and individually ligated and resected. The femoral nerve is then divided. The technique of severing the limb is the same as described above.

Sometimes it is possible to cut the anterior muscles lower than the contemplated line of resection. In such instances these muscles can be used to plug the acetabular cavity. This step, although desirable, is not essential and should not be performed at the risk of jeopardizing a

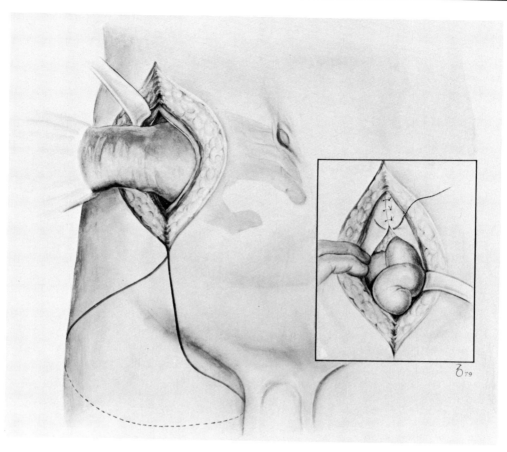

Figure 6.19. (B) *Left:* The peritoneal cavity is entered through the upper part of the incision. Exploratory laparotomy constitutes examination of the intra-abdominal viscera and para-aortic nodes. The entire incision, including the posterior extent in the back of the thigh, is outlined. The inset *(right)* shows the peritoneum being closed.

good cancer operation. The operative blood loss seldom is more than one liter.

The postoperative course of these patients is relatively smooth. Usually they are up and about by the second day. With physiotherapy, the patients shortly can be taught to use a crutch, and can be discharged within 8 to 10 days. Wound healing is not a problem in nonirradiated patients. The problem of phantom pain is similar to that in other major amputations and is infrequently a physiologic or rehabilitational problem.

Hemipelvectomy (Sacroiliac Disarticulation or Hindquarter Amputation).

Historical Background. The operation was first performed by Girard[28,29] in 1895. The principles of the surgical procedure were laid down by J.

Hogarth Pringle[30] in 1916. Pringle reviewed the literature and described his own two cases. Subsequently the literature was reviewed by Judin[31] in 1926, by Gordon-Taylor and Wiles[32] in 1935, by Sugarbaker and Ackerman[33] in 1945, and again by Gordon-Taylor and Paley[34] in 1946. In 1952, Gordon-Taylor and Monroe[35] described the technique used in their 64 cases. Pack and Ehrlich,[36] in 1946, and Pack,[37] in 1956, reviewed both the technical and the end result experience at Memorial Sloan-Kettering Cancer Center. These reports provide an insight into the development of this operation.

During the past 65 years, the operative mortality has been reduced from approximately 45 percent to an acceptable level of 5 percent in most of the centers engaged in this type of radical amputation.

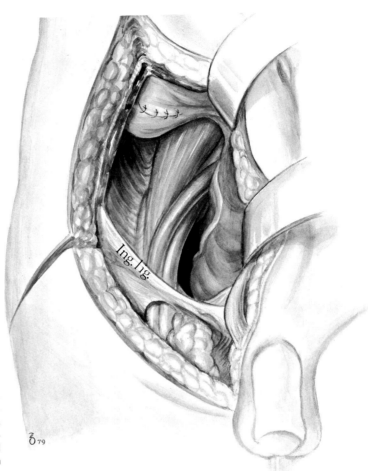

Figure 6.19. (C) The peritoneum, with its contents, has been pushed medially. On the upper part of the diagram the recently sutured peritoneum is seen. The ureter can be observed to be adherent to the posterior peritoneum retracted medially. The external iliac vessels, psoas major, and iliacus muscles are apparent. The femoral vessels distal to the inguinal ligament can be seen at the lower part of the diagram.

A radical procedure such as hemipelvectomy should be used only when the indications are clearly defined and standardized. In its evolutionary phase the operation was either performed with bravado by some surgeons, or abandoned out of fear by others. As a result, the proper place for this operation in the therapeutic armamentarium of the cancer surgeon was never defined. In recent years, however, hemipelvectomy as an operative technique has become reasonably standardized and is being performed in several centers in the United States and elsewhere with decreasing morbidity and mortality. The novelty of a "big operation" has now worn off and the extent of the operation and the indications and contraindications can be adequately defined. In properly selected cases this operation provides a good end result.

Definition. The term hemipelvectomy means removal of one side of the pelvis along with the buttock and the entire lower extremity. The operative limit in the pelvis usually is through the sacroiliac synchondrosis and pubic symphysis. However, this operation can be extended and can be performed by cutting through the sacrum and lumbar vertebrae, or can be modified by resecting through the innominate bone.

Other names that have been used to describe this operation are sacroilial disarticulation, and interinnomino-abdominal, hindquarter, and interpelvic-abdominal amputation.

Indications. Hemipelvectomy as a curative operation is indicated in the following clinical settings:

1. A well-differentiated soft tissue sarcoma located in the upper part of the thigh, extend-

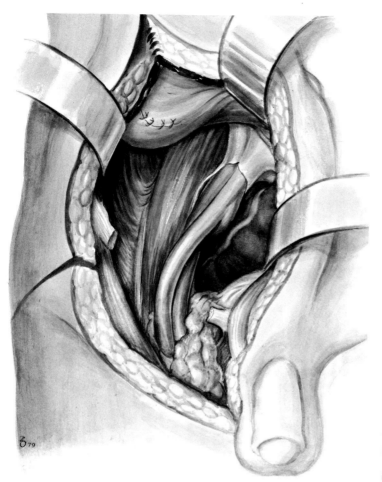

Figure 6.19. (D) Dissection is initiated at the bifurcation of the aorta or the formation of the inferior vena cava. The dissection includes the adventital layer of the external iliac vessels, along with the nodes. In this diagram the inguinal ligament is resected medially, exposing the obturator fat pad at the lower end. The spermatic cord and the urinary bladder are retracted medially. The internal iliac artery is seen curving into the pelvic cavity.

ing to the inguinal ligament or to the pubic symphysis, a situation in which a clear proximal margin of the resection cannot be accomplished without resorting to this operation, for example, a low-grade fibrosarcoma that has infiltrated the areas mentioned above, or the adjacent femur or the major blood vessels and nerves. Hemangiopericytoma, malignant schwannoma, and similar tumors in this region might also require a hemipelvectomy.

2. Primary malignant osseous and periosteal tumors of the upper femur, if the tumor has extended to or through the hip joint; and similar neoplasms of the innominate bones.

3. Primary soft tissue sarcomas of the iliac fossa or upper thigh, extending through the obturator foramen.

4. Soft tissue sarcomas of the buttock, extending to the pelvis through the sciatic notch, which cannot be extirpated by excision of the buttocks.

   Contraindications.

1. In any soft tissue sarcoma that can be treated by either muscle group excision or hip joint disarticulation, alone or in conjunction with node dissection.

2. In those soft tissue sarcomas that are known to respond well to chemotherapy (Tables 8.11 and 8.14, Chapter 8). Patients with these tumors can be treated with a multimodal program and any form of major amputation can usually be avoided.

3. With judicious use of advanced techniques in radiation therapy, a number of various

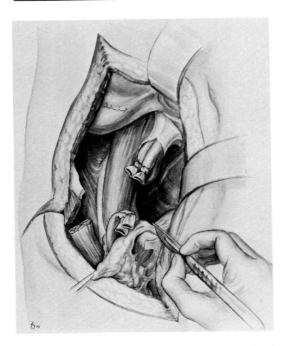

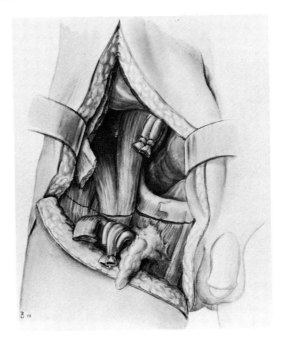

Figure 6.19. **(E)** The external iliac vessels are ligated and resected. The areolar tissue and the nodes, along with the vessels, are pushed distally towards the inguinal ligament. The obturator contents are identified and dissected free from the adherent perivesical fat. The femoral nerve is seen emerging lateral to the psoas major muscle. It is resected at this level. The sartorius muscle is already resected. The outline of the ureter attached to the posterior wall of the peritoneum should always be visible during the dissection.

Figure 6.19. **(F)** The obturator dissection is completed. The anterior and the lateral muscles are resected, with patient in supine position. The extremity is then abducted and the medial compartment muscles are resected. The cut ends of the vessels and femoral nerve are seen in the lower end of the diagram.

types of soft tissue sarcomas can be managed by lesser operations, for example, myxoid liposarcoma or embryonal rhabdomyosarcoma. In these tumors every attempt should be made to preserve the limb.

4. In some instances of highly anaplastic soft tissue sarcomas in which there is minimal life expectancy, for example, in highly anaplastic fibrosarcoma. In these patients the operation neither cures nor serves as an effective measure of palliation.

5. Hemipelvectomy is not an optimum operation for patients with psychological disorders, even though the tumor can be eradicated.

Preoperative Preparation. The general principles of preoperative preparation have been described earlier. We recommend preparation of the colon as though the patient were undergoing a colon resection. An intravenous pyelogram and cystoscopic evaluation of the urinary bladder are also indicated. In female patients, antibiotic vaginal suppositories are used for three to five days prior to the operation.

Technique of Operation.

ANESTHESIA. General endotracheal anesthesia is usually employed in our hospitals. Our anesthesiologists utilize controlled hypotension whenever feasible, and this has made the operation easier and usually less time-consuming.

POSITIONING OF THE PATIENT. The patient is placed on the table, lying on the side opposite to the lesion, and is turned slightly onto the back (45 degree angle). The position is maintained by a support against the lower ribs and dorsal spine, well clear of the iliac crest. The limb is kept free and is prepared and draped within the operative field. The ipsilateral arm is supported at the ether screen. Care should be taken to avoid sustained pressure on the brachial plexus on the contralateral side. The table

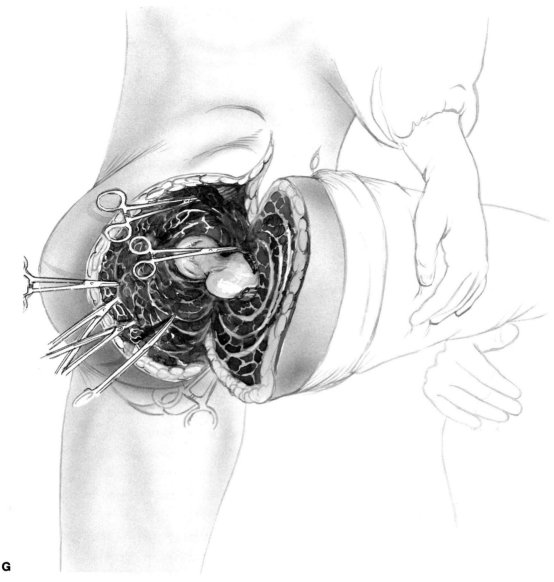

G

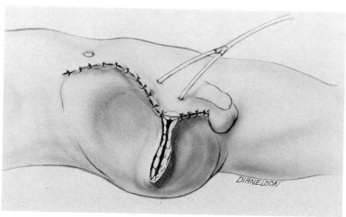

H

Figure 6.19. (G) The extremity is adducted and internally rotated. All the lateral muscles to the greater trochanter are being cut, then the gluteal muscles are resected. The femoral head is delivered out of the acetabular cavity. Ligamentum teres, clearly seen in this diagram, is cut. The limb is now attached posteriorly by the sciatic nerve and hamstring muscles; these are cut and the extremity removed. **(H)** The Y-shaped wound closure. Once the wound heals, a prosthesis can easily be fitted.

259

is then rotated toward the surgeon's side to about 20 degrees, allowing easier access to the anterior abdominal wall. An indwelling urinary catheter is attached to a urinal. In male patients the scrotum is either sutured or taped to the opposite thigh. Meticulous preparation and draping of the entire side are essential; otherwise, movement of the limb during the operation can contaminate the operative field.

STEPS OF OPERATION. The preliminary incision is lateral and vertical, extending from the subcostal margin down about 4 to 5 cm laterally to the level of the umbilicus. The medial arm of the incision is then carried medially 3 cm higher and parallel to the inguinal ligament up to the pubic tubercle. The posterolateral limb of the incision extends to the greater trochanter and along the infragluteal groove to the perineum. It is then joined with the medial end of the anterior incision at the superior border of the symphysis pubis (Fig. 6.20A). The incision described above is the standard one we use whenever feasible. In some instances, however, the skin incision must be modified because of the size, location, and concomitant fungation of the tumor, or because of the effects of previous irradiation of the area. These modifications might include a large anterior flap or a large gluteal flap. The decision as to the type of modification best suited for a given patient depends mostly on the experience of the operating surgeon.

The upper part of the vertical incision in the lateral abdominal wall is deepened and the peritoneal cavity is entered. Following adequate exploration of the abdomen, if no contraindication to hemipelvectomy is found, the operation proceeds. The peritoneum is closed with 2-0 chromic catgut suture. The lower part of the skin incision is then deepened and the anterior abdominal wall muscles are cut along the line of the incision. The rectus abdominis muscle is resected at its attachment to the pubis and the inguinal ligament at the iliac crest and pubic tubercle (Fig. 6.20B). This results in detaching the anterior abdominal wall from the bony pelvis, forming the anterior flap. The peritoneal cavity is then pushed medially by means of sponge sticks. In male patients the spermatic cord is preserved carefully. By placing packs and using retractors, the entire lateral wall of the pelvis from the sacroiliac synchondrosis to the pubic symphysis is brought into view. The intestines are held medially and upward and the urinary bladder is held medially and downward, care being taken not to injure the ureter. The common iliac vessels are dissected out and 1-0 silk ties are placed around all these vessels (Fig. 6.20C). For purposes of orientation, an anatomic diagram is included (Fig. 6.20D). This shows the bifurcation of the aorta, formation of the inferior vena cava proximally, and the contents of the lateral wall of the pelvis up to the symphysis pubis distally. It is better not to ligate the vessels at this stage, since once they are ligated the surgeon is committed to perform the operation. We advocate a thorough reassessment of the resectability of the tumor at this stage of the operation, and if no contraindica-

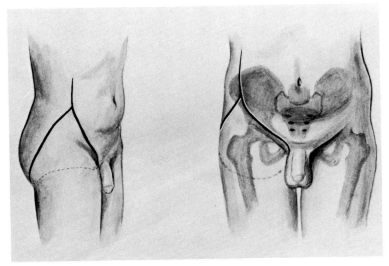

Figure 6.20. (A) Anterolateral and anterior views of incision for a conventional hemipelvectomy.

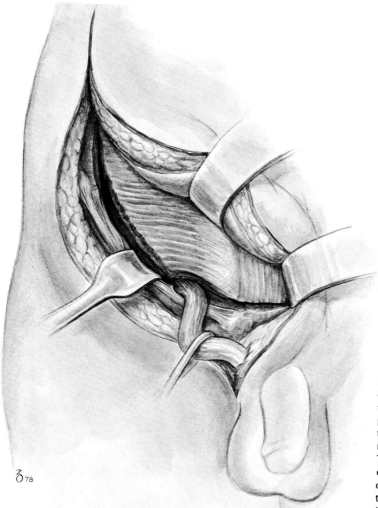

Figure 6.20. (B) The anterior abdominal wall muscles are cut along the line of the skin incision. In male patients the spermatic cord is identified and protected. The rectus muscle is detached from the pubis. The spermatic cord is retracted laterally to show the line of resection of the rectus abdominis muscle. In this diagram the inguinal ligament is still in place.

tions for a hemipelvectomy are found, then to proceed to the next stage of the operation.

In this stage, the pubic symphysis is exposed, skeletonized, and divided (Fig. 6.20E). This is easily accomplished by using the scalpel; seldom is there a need for a Gigli saw or a chisel. Care must be taken to protect the urethra below, and it is advisable to put a narrow malleable retractor immediately below the symphysis. Following separation of the pubic symphysis, the incision is deepened inferiorly along the previously outlined skin incision at the inner aspect of the thigh (Fig. 6.20E). At this stage some bleeding might be incurred, especially in male patients, due to cutting of the vascular erectile tissue. We advocate that the resectabil-

ity of the tumor be reassessed for the second time. Even if the tumor is found to be unresectable for cure it is possible to close the wound by wiring the pubic symphysis, and the patient can be rehabilitated insofar as the use of the limb is concerned. However, if there are no contraindications for a curative hemipelvectomy, the surgeon should proceed with the third stage of the operation.

The iliac vessels are then ligated. Both the common iliac, the external iliac, and the internal iliac vessels are doubly ligated and resected in the same locations where the original ties were placed (Fig. 6.20F). The femoral nerve trunk located laterally to the vessels is also resected at this stage.

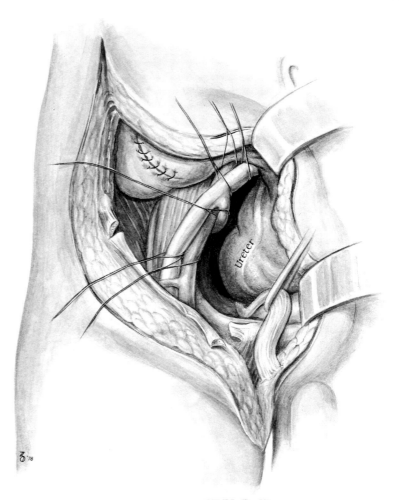

Figure 6.20. (C) Exploratory celiotomy has been completed and the anterior abdominal wall muscles are cut laterally and at the pubic symphysis. In male patients the spermatic cord is moved out of harm's way. The retroperitoneal space is seen. Ureter is seen adherent to the posterior peritoneum. Silk sutures are placed around the iliac vessels. If the operation becomes feasible these sutures will be tied and the vessels resected. In this diagram, the inguinal ligament has been resected.

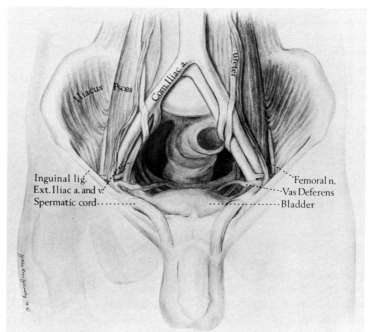

Figure 6.20. (D) Anterior view of the pelvic contents for orientation.

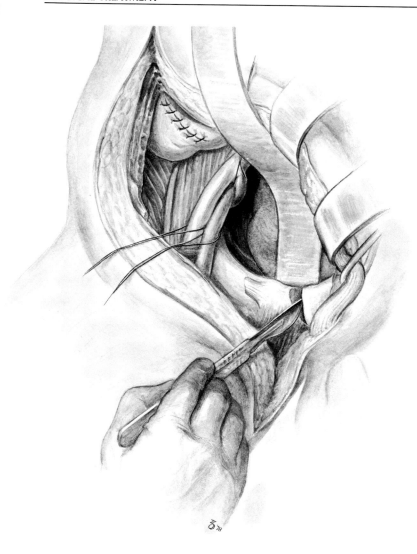

Figure 6.20. (E) Pubic symphysis has been exposed and skeletonized. In most instances the symphysis can be cut with a scalpel. Care should be taken to avoid injury to the urethra. A small malleable metallic retractor can be used for this purpose. The muscles of the inner aspect of the thigh can be resected at this stage by moderate abduction of the extremity.

The anterior dissection is then continued. The crest of the ileum is skeletonized, including resection of the attachment of the quadratus lumborum muscle. The iliopsoas muscles are transected high. The assistant then flexes the knee and pushes it down to the surface of the table, exposing the piriformis and levator ani muscles. These are resected as high as possible (Fig. 6.20F), care being taken to avoid injury to the rectum or bladder. This completes the anterior dissection, and the sacroiliac synchondrosis is then exposed. All the major bleeding points are caught and ligated. A packing is placed in the pelvic space.

The posterior flap is then raised, first by extending the skin incision as far back as the sacrum (Fig. 6.20G). The table is then tilted to the opposite direction, making the patient lie on the lateral decubitus. With the extremity held in extreme adduction, the posterior attachments of the gluteal muscles are then divided and the remainder of the posterior dissection is completed (Fig. 6.20G). The limb is then flexed and abducted sharply, and all the remaining medial muscle attachments are cut.

At this stage the limb is attached only at the sacroiliac synchondrosis. We consider severance of this synchondrosis as the penultimate

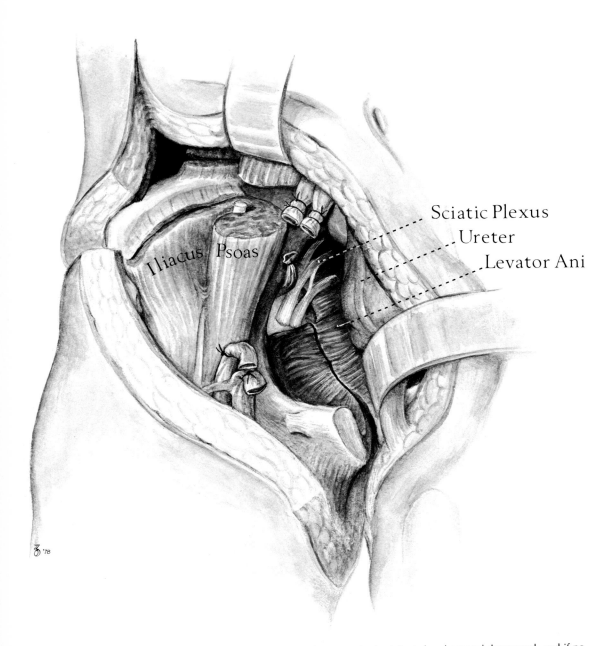

Figure 6.20. (F) With separation of the pubic symphysis, the extremity is abducted and pressed downward, and if no contraindication to hemipelvectomy is found, the iliac vessels are ligated and resected. The perineal muscles are cut along the line shown. Injury to the rectum is avoided by reflecting it away from the operative field. The iliac crest is also skeletonized at this juncture.

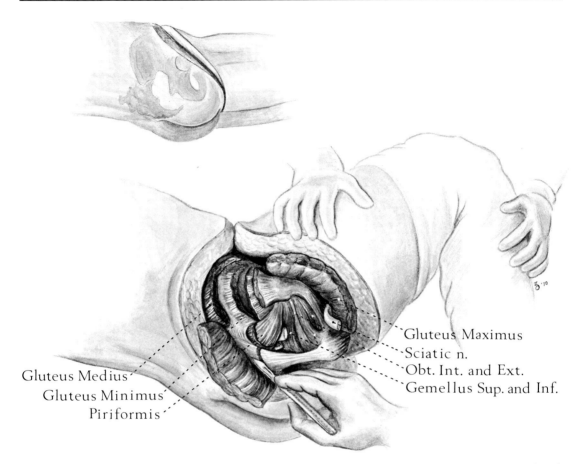

Figure 6.20. (G) The posterior flap, as shown in the inset, is then raised. The posterior attachments of the gluteal muscles are resected with the leg held in extreme adduction. The remaining posterior muscles and sciatic nerve are cut. Following completion of the entire posterior dissection, the extremity is held in extreme abduction and all the remaining attachments of the medial muscles of the thigh are severed.

phase of the operation. The limb, as before, is flexed and moved by the assistant so that the surgeon can find the uppermost part of the synchondrosis. Once the scalpel is in this space, the assistant sharply abducts the limb. The surgeon, by placing the blade of the scalpel at an angle of 45 degrees, can easily cut through the synchondrosis (Fig. 6.20H). We have seldom found the need for use of chisels, saws, or any other bone-cutting instruments.

The limb is now attached to the patient by the ligaments of the sacrum. These are resected, the gluteal arteries are caught, ligated, and resected, and the specimen is removed (Fig. 6.20I). Dry packs are placed on the exposed surface.

After removal of the limb, meticulous care is taken to obtain perfect hemostasis. If the patient is under hypotensive anesthesia, blood pressure is raised and the status of hemostasis reassessed. It is essential that all the nerve trunks are cut sharply and allowed to retract. This reduces the incidence of traumatic neuromas. We have found that use of local anesthetic in the proximal end of the nerve trunk invariably reduces the incidence of postoperative pain and occasionally reduces the intensity of the phantom limb syndrome as well.

The anterior abdominal wall is closed with a Penrose drain in the retroperitoneal space and the skin incision is closed, using suction cath-

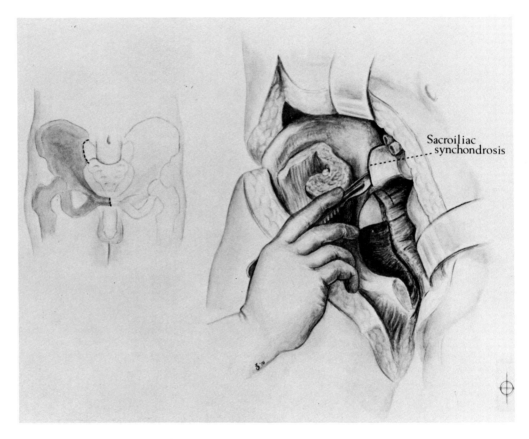

Figure 6.20. (H) The only major attachment is the sacroiliac synchondrosis. The space is being entered at the superior end by means of a scalpel. If the scalpel is now maneuvered at an angle of 45 degrees, the synchondrosis can be cut. We seldom use any bone-cutting instruments. The inset shows the line of sacroiliac joint; pubic symphysis and shaded part of the pelvic skeleton constitute the upper part of the specimen.

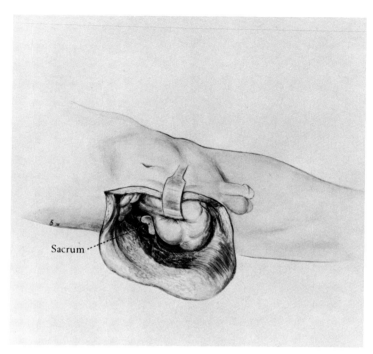

Figure 6.20. (I) The wound after removal of the extremity. The sacrum and the peritoneal contents can be seen.

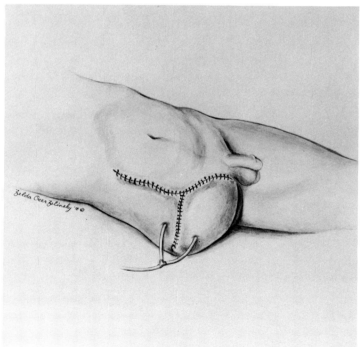

Figure 6.20. (J) Appearance after wound closure.

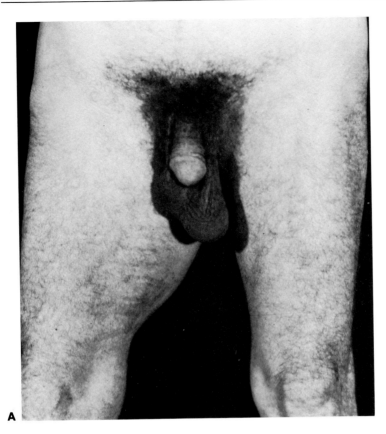

A

Figure 6.21. **(A)** Fifty-year-old man with extensive liposarcoma of the thigh. **(B)** Appearance six months later. Note the excellent wound-healing process.

eters (Fig. 6.20J). An Ace bandage pressure dressing is kept in place for about five to six days postoperatively.

POSTOPERATIVE MANAGEMENT. It is expected that the blood volume loss will be corrected either during the operation or within two to three hours thereafter. Following this immediate management, care is taken to record blood pressure, urinary output, wound drainage, and hematocrit. Based on these, the intravenous administration of fluids and blood is monitored. The patients should have nasogastric suction until the bowel sounds appear. Frequently, the urinary bladder develops some paresis. The Foley catheter should be kept in place until the patient regains bladder control. Excluding these usual problems, seldom in well-selected cases are there any major complications. Phantom limb pain or development of neuromas are accepted problems associated with any radical amputation and we think there is no higher incidence with hemi-

pelvectomy. Proper physiotherapy often reduces these problems.

Wound healing can sometimes be complicated by skin flap necrosis. This is more common in patients with a large tumor or in those who have had prior irradiation. It has been our experience that these problems of skin flap necrosis, although annoying, have never been unmanageable. Patients should be encouraged by the seventh day to use crutches and move about. Usually a well-motivated patient can maneuver on a plane surface by the end of two weeks. A cooperative and competent physiotherapist with a good program can make a patient self-reliant within four weeks (Fig. 6.21A and 6.21B). Although the use of a prosthesis after hemipelvectomy is not always as satisfactory as in cases of amputations performed at lower levels, some excellent prosthetic results are still possible.

The operation of hemipelvectomy can be extended by including part of the sacrum or

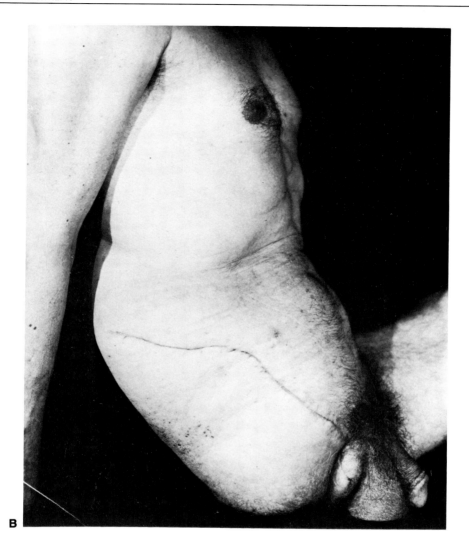

B

parts of the vertebrae. These types of extension are seldom required, but when indicated can be accomplished without any associated increase in morbidity. However, care must be taken to avoid injury to the spinal dura, thereby incurring spinal fluid leak.

A modified and limited type of hemipelvectomy was first described by Sherman and Duthie[38] in 1960. This essentially consists of excising the innominate bone and not separating the extremity at the sacroiliac synchondrosis. The level of excision of the innominate bone depends on the type and location of the tumors. If feasible, the presence of the iliac crest and a relatively stable sacroiliac joint provides a better prosthesis and better rehabilitation.

REFERENCES

1. Pack GT: The definition of inoperability of cancer. Ann Surg 127:1105, 1948
2. Pack GT, Anglem TJ: Tumors of the soft somatic tissues in infancy and childhood. J Pediat 15:372, 1939
3. Stout AP: Sarcomas of the soft parts. J Missouri State Med Assoc 44:329, 1947
4. Pack GT: Argument for radicalism in cancer surgery. Am Surg 17:271, 1951

5. Barber JR, Coventry MD, McDonald JR: The spread of soft tissue sarcomata of the extremities along peripheral nerve trunks. J Bone Joint Surg 39-A:534, 1957

6. Bowden L, Booher RF: The principles and technique of resection of soft part sarcoma. Surgery 44:963, 1958

7. Bowden L, Booher R: Surgical consideration in the treatment of sarcomas of the buttock. Cancer 6:89, 1953

8. Syme J: Excision of the scapula. (Monograph). Edinburgh, Edmonstom and Douglas, 1864

9. de Nancrede CBG: The end results after total excision of the scapula for sarcoma. Ann Surg 50:1, 1909

10. Pack GT, Ariel IR: Tumors of the Soft Somatic Tissues. New York, Hoeber, 1958

11. Das Gupta TK: Scapulectomy: Indications and technique. Surgery 67:601, 1970

12. Tikhor PT: Tumor Studies. Russia, 1900

13. Linberg BE: Interscapulo-thoracic resection for malignant tumors of the shoulder joint region. J Bone Joint Surg 10-A:344, 1928

14. Pack GT, Baldwin JC: The Tikhor-Linberg resection of shoulder girdle—Case report. Surgery 38:753, 1955

15. Brasfield RD, Das Gupta TK: Desmoids of the anterior abdominal wall. Surgery 65:241, 1969

16. Halstead WS: The results of radical operation for the cure of cancer of the breast. Ann Surg 46:80, 1907

17. Crosby AB: The first operation on record for removal of the entire arm, scapula, and three fourths of the clavicle by Dixie Crosby. Concord NH, Republican Press Assoc, 1875; Med Rec 10:753, 1875

18. Berger P: L'amputation du membre superieur dans la contiguite du tronc (amputation interscapulothoracique). Paris, G. Masson, 1887

19. Pack GT, McNeer G, Coley BL: Interscapulothoracic amputation for malignant tumors of the upper extremity: A report of 31 consecutive cases. Surg Gynecol Obstet 74:171, 1942

20. Moseley HF: The Forequarter Amputation. Edinburgh, Livingston, 1957

21. Nadler SJ, Phelan JT: A technique of interscapulothoracic amputation. Surg Gynecol Obstet 122:359, 1966

22. Bowden L: A more thorough incontinuity neck and axillary dissection. Ann Surg 141:481, 1956

23. Fanus N, Didolkar MS, Hoyoke ED, Elias EG: Evaluation of forequarter amputation in malignant diseases. Surg Gynecol Obstet 142:381, 1976

24. Das Gupta TK, Brasfield RD: Amputation neuromas in cancer patients. NY State J Med 69:2129, 1969

25. Das Gupta TK: Radical groin dissection. Surg Gynecol Obstet 129:1275, 1969

26. Frank L: Lest we forget. Am J Surg 20:160, 1933

27. Eckoff N: An account of Sir Astley Cooper's first case of amputation at the hip joint, January 16, 1824. Guy's Hospital Reports 89:9, 1939

28. Girard C: Sur la desarticulation interilio-abdominale. Congres Francais de Chir, 9:823, 1895

29. Girard C: Sur la desarticulation interilio-abdominal. Rev de Chir (Paris) 18:1141, 1898

30. Pringle JH: The interpelvic-abdominal amputation with notes on two cases. Br J Surg 4:283, 1916

31. Judin SS: Ilioabdominal amputation in a case of sarcoma; recovery, pregnancy, and birth of a living child. Surg Gynecol Obstet 43:668, 1926

32. Gordon-Taylor G, Wiles P: Interinnominoabdominal (hindquarter) amputation. Br J Surg 22:671, 1935

33. Sugarbaker ED, Ackerman L: Disarticulation of the innominate bone for malignant tumor of the pelvic parietes and upper thigh. Surg Gynecol Obstet 81:36, 1943

34. Gordon-Taylor G, Paley D: A further review of the interinnomino-abdominal operation based on 21 personal cases. Br J Surg 34:61, 1946

35. Gordon-Taylor G, Monroe R: The technique and management of hindquarter amputation. Br J Surg 39:536, 1952

36. Pack GT, Ehrlich HE: Exarticulation of the lower extremities for malignant tumor: hip joint disarticulation (with or without deep iliac dissection) and sacroiliac disarticulation (hemipelvectomy). Ann Surg 124:1, 1946

37. Pack GT: Major exarticulations for malignant neoplasms of the extremities; interscapulothoracic amputation, hip joint disarticulation, and interilio-abdominal amputation: A report of end results in 228 cases. J Bone Joint Surg 38-A:249, 1956

38. Sherman CD Jr, Duthie RB: Modified hemipelvectomy. Cancer 13:51, 1960

7

Radiation Therapy

Edwin J. Liebner

In the past, a generally pessimistic attitude prevailed among clinicians concerning the radioresponsiveness and radiocurability of soft tissue sarcomas. Much of this pessimism was due to experiences in the premegavoltage period when patients who received radiation therapy had troublesome skin reactions and no appreciable beneficial effects. Often, the patients referred for radiation therapy had advanced sarcoma, and the results of radiation therapy could not be properly assessed. Therefore, the tumor was often judged to be radioresistant. It was not appreciated that the slow response was not necessarily a lack of radioresponsiveness.[1,2] Additional difficulties in studying soft tissue sarcomas have been the lack of any cohesive effort to assess their response to radiation therapy as related to the histologic type and size of the primary tumor, and the continuing problem of identifying specific histogenetic tumor types. A detailed discussion of the need and the methods for accurate histogenetic diagnosis is found in Chapters 3 and 4. With the advent of megavoltage equipment, a sufficient number of patients with soft tissue sarcomas have been treated with encouraging results to change the previous pessimistic attitude to one of cautious optimism in respect to curative radiation therapy for certain histologic types of primary soft tissue sarcomas.[3] Some of the radiobiologic investigations

in soft tissue sarcomas in regard to the role of radiation therapy, with (or without) radiation-sensitizing agents,[4] chemotherapeutic agents,[5,6] different methods of producing hypoxic tumor cells,[7,8] and various fractionation schedules,[9] are still being pursued; but there is now adequate clinical experience to state that radiation therapy controls certain forms of primary soft tissue sarcoma.[10-13] It is suggested that preoperative irradiation exerts a direct effect on the tumor by sterilizing peripheral well-oxygenated cells, thereby rendering the tumors more amenable to conservative excision.[10,14-16] A combination of conservative surgery and radiation therapy based upon radical dose levels can control certain sarcomas and avoid deformity or loss of limb.[12]

The concept has evolved that in soft tissue sarcomas microscopic disease is controlled with doses of radiation that allow good cosmetic and functional results, thereby avoiding disabling operations. This is consistent with biologic concepts of greater "log kill" of well-oxygenated microscopic tumor extensions with a moderate radiation dose such as 4,500 to 5,000 rads, and apparently circumvents the problem of hypoxia. The appropriateness of this has already been demonstrated in other sites (breast, salivary gland, neck nodes, etc).

Although different histologic subtypes have different natural histories, within a specific tumor type the major determinants of local control (and survival) are grade, location, and size.

The beneficial role of radiation therapy in the palliative management of patients with soft tissue sarcoma has been adequately demonstrated and this type of therapy is now in general use.

In the following sections of this chapter the effect of radiation therapy on specific histologic types of sarcoma is discussed.

LIPOSARCOMA

McNeer and associates[10] provided historical background for the treatment of liposarcomas. Radiation was the sole method of treatment in four of their patients who survived five years. The tumor doses were 2,500, 3,000, 3,500, and 5,000 rads, respectively. Although these results were interesting, they probably did not reflect an adequate dose trial. Perry and Chu[17] found that all their patients responded to irradiation when a dose of 3,000 rads or higher was given. The beneficial effects lasted for an average of 10.7 months, with the myxoid variety showing a favorable response more frequently than other types. Friedman and Egan[18] reported that, in their experience, a dosage of 9,000 rads in 30 to 50 days was required. These large doses to the lower extremities resulted in a high incidence of radiation injury. For this reason Moss and associates,[19] whenever practical, favored radical surgery from the start.

Edland[20] reviewed his data and concluded that, although a dose of 5,000 to 6,000 rads could at times ablate a tumor, the incidence of local control of bulky tumors with radiation therapy alone was low. Reszel and co-workers[21] found that radiation therapy was useful as an adjuvant to local excision in some of the more undifferentiated types of tumors. Brasfield and Das Gupta[22] reported that preoperative radiation therapy reduced the size of the tumors, with spectacular results achieved in the myxoid type. A similar observation of response to radiation therapy in the myxoid types was made by Enterline et al.[23]

Suit and co-workers,[12,24] using cobalt teletherapy or the betatron electron beam, treated 100 patients with soft tissue sarcoma. These patients had had limited excision of the primary tumor. The disease was locally controlled in eleven patients with liposarcoma. Eight of the

11 had tumors larger than 5 cm, graded as 1 to 1.5 in three, and from 2 to 2.5 in the remaining five. Lindberg and associates[25] reviewed the treatment results in 41 patients with liposarcoma following conservative surgery and radical dose radiation therapy. In their series, the five-year disease-free survival was 81 percent and the incidence of local recurrence was only 12 percent.

It appears that radiation therapy as an adjuvant to limited local excision is most useful in tumors located in the distal extremities and in the retroperitoneum.

Radiation therapy for palliation of liposarcoma is generally accepted.[17] Localized radiation with 3,000 to 4,000 rads in 20 to 30 days[17,18] has been found useful. Higher doses have also been tried with beneficial results.

FIBROSARCOMA

Cade[26] reported that four of six fibrosarcoma patients treated by irradiation alone were free of disease for five years or longer. Windeyer and co-workers[13] treated 22 fibrosarcomas (11 primary tumors and 11 postsurgical recurrences) by radical-dose radiation therapy (6,000 to 8,000 rads in five to nine weeks). Nine of these patients (41 percent) survived free of disease for between two and five years. Suit and associates[12,24] treated nine fibrosarcoma patients by simple excision followed by radical-dose radiation therapy: 6,300 to 7,000 rads given over a period of six and one half to seven and one half weeks on the basis of 200 rads per day for five days per week. These patients, and others with sarcoma of the soft tissues of the extremities, were evaluated for local recurrence and disease-free survival time. Correlation was made also with the histopathologic type and grade, and the size of the tumor (whether it was less or greater than 5 cm). Of their nine patients, only one had local recurrence; five survived disease-free for at least 24 months. In this small number of fibrosarcomas, the correlation with grade was not significant. Lindberg and associates,[25] using the same technique for management of 41 fibrosarcomas of all histologic grades and stages, found a local recurrence rate of 12 percent and absolute five-year disease-free survival of 86 percent. Our own experience in treating primary fibrosarcomas with radiation therapy is limited, since only 11 patients with fibrosarcoma have been so treated in our department. Four of these patients received radiation therapy as an adjuvant to excision of the primary tumor. Two of the four had wide local excision and were irradiated with doses of 6,000 to 8,000 rads in five to nine weeks. They are still well at two and nine years, respectively. The remaining two had preoperative radiation therapy: 2,000 rads in five fractions, followed by hemipelvectomy. They are still disease-free at 11 and 12 years, respectively. The remaining seven patients had disseminated disease and radiation therapy was used for palliation only.

Analysis of a much larger series of 199 patients with fibrosarcoma by Pritchard and associates[27] at the Mayo Clinic, and the clinical data reported in Chapter 12 confirm that the histologic grading of fibrosarcomas plays an important role in the ultimate prognosis for these patients. Pritchard and co-workers[27] found that, in general, radical excision is the best method of treatment. We support their overall conclusions; however, the role of adjuvant radiation therapy in fibrosarcomas has not been evaluated in a prospective manner.

MALIGNANT FIBROUS HISTIOCYTOMA (MFH)

Suit and co-workers[12] described their experience with 18 patients with malignant fibrous histiocytoma, all of whom were treated with limited surgery and radical-dose radiation therapy. Two-year followup data were available. Within this time period, 5 of the 18 (28 percent) had local recurrence and 10 (55.5 percent) were living disease-free. Lindberg and co-workers[25] described their experience at M.D. Anderson Hospital with 300 soft tissue sarcomas in adults, including 60 cases of MFH. All patients received conservative excision followed by postoperative radiotherapy to a dose of 6,000 to 7,500 rads administered in six to seven and one half weeks. Nineteen (31.6 percent) of the 60 patients treated had local recurrence. Two- and five-year disease-free survival rates of 65 percent and 56 percent, respectively, were achieved. Our experience with this disease is limited; however, even in a small series we have found radiation therapy to be useful (Fig. 7.1A and 7.1B). In general, adjuvant radiation therapy is recommended for all patients with MFH located in the trunk or retroperitoneum, and for those with deep infiltration of fascia and skeletal muscle.

AGGRESSIVE FIBROMATOSIS

Low-grade nonmetastasizing tumors (such as desmoids), if not amenable to resection, occasionally can be treated by properly administered high doses of radiation.[28-30]

Suit and Russell[30] used radiation therapy for six patients with nonresectable extra-abdominal desmoids and had followup data ranging from two and one half to eight and one half years. One patient, who was still well after eight and one half years, had received 7,500 rads to the left cervico-supraclavicular region in 54 fractions over a period of 78 days. Benninghoff and Robbins[28] treated four patients with inoperable or incompletely resected desmoids (inguinal, neck, mediastinum, and arm) to a dose range of 2,000 rads in three weeks to 4,000 rads in four weeks. There was one recurrence (inguinal) after 3,000 rads, but the other three patients were still free of disease more than two years later. Hill and associates[29] achieved complete regression of desmoids (neck, shoulder, and sacrum) treated with 5,000 to 6,000 rads over a period of six to seven weeks and followed up for at least two years. Suit and his co-workers[2] emphasized that following radiation therapy the rate of regression is extremely slow and complete disappearance of the tumor takes a long time. These authors recommended that, if and when these lesions are irradiated, they receive 6,000 rads in seven to eight weeks.

We believe that the ideal treatment of aggressive fibromatosis is wide excision (Chapter 12). However, in certain instances in which resection is technically or functionally hazardous, radiation therapy can be successfully utilized.

JUVENILE NASOPHARYNGEAL ANGIOFIBROMA

The general course of this tumor is benign, and it usually regresses after sexual maturity. Frequent episodes of severe epistaxis are the main presenting clinical feature. Local erosion and destruction of the surrounding tissue occasionally are encountered. It is generally accepted that the best treatment is excision (Chapter 12).

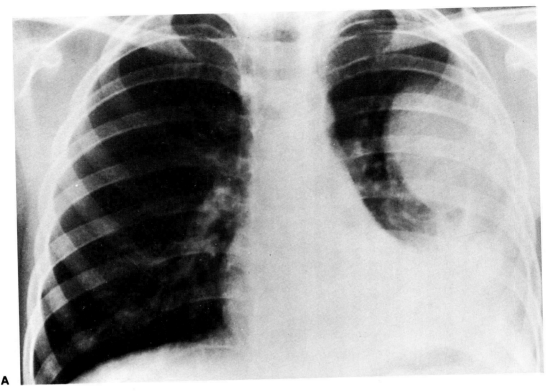

A

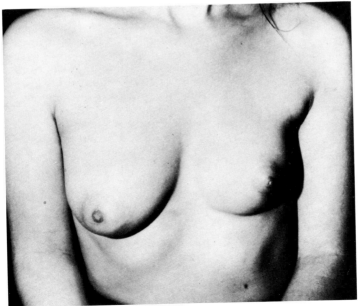

B

Figure 7.1. (A) Posterior-anterior roentgenogram of chest of 8-year-old girl. A large tumor (MFH) can be seen involving the left upper inner chest wall, pleura, and adjacent lung. The child was treated with 5000 rads. (B) Clinical photograph of the anterior chest of the patient 10 years after irradiation treatment. The asymmetry of the left breast is not marked.

However, in rare instances the degree of local involvement and the extension of disease might require use of radiation therapy. In all, we have treated three such patients with irradiation. In recent years we have had only one patient who required radiation therapy. This young man, 19 years old, was sent to us because of a recurrent large fungating and bleeding tumor not amenable to excision. He was treated with external cobalt therapy: 5,000 rads to the nasopharynx in 25 fractions. Two lateral portals and one anterior portal were used. The tumor shrank within six months, and five years later there was no evidence of local tumor. Our experience in these three patients leads us to suggest that a dose of 5,000 to 6,000 rads in five to six weeks is necessary to produce best results. However, such a cancericidal dose of irradiation should not be used *ab initio* for a benign lesion. Only in rare instances in which excisional treatment fails should radiation therapy be used. Massoud and Awwad[31] irradiated seven patients with extensive lesions, causing local bone destruction. They noted disappearance of the mass in three patients and regression in two after doses of 4,000 rads in five weeks.

LEIOMYOSARCOMA

Leiomyosarcomas have not been adequately tested for radiocurability. McNeer et al.[10] reviewed the Memorial Sloan-Kettering Cancer Center series of 653 soft tissue sarcomas and found only one patient with leiomyosarcoma, and this patient had been operated upon. Lindberg et al.[32] reviewed the end results in 100 soft tissue sarcoma patients from the M. D. Anderson Hospital who were treated with conservative local surgery and radiation therapy. Of the four leiomyosarcomas in the group, one (25 percent) recurred locally. Suit and co-workers,[12] in the same year, published a report of 100 patients with soft tissue sarcoma from the same institution and found that of three leiomyosarcoma patients treated with radical radiation therapy, none showed any evidence of local failure; however, all three patients died within two years of treatment of the primary tumor. Lindberg and co-workers[25] recently updated the M.D. Anderson experience. They found that local recurrence developed in six out of 16 patients (37 percent). Four of these six patients had intra-

abdominal leiomyosarcoma. Only five of the 16 patients were eligible for five-year analysis and only two were still disease-free. Our experience in treating primary leiomyosarcoma by means of radiation therapy alone is limited as well: A patient with retroperitoneal leiomyosarcoma, deemed unresectable after an exploratory laparotomy, was treated with a dose of 4,000 rads over a period of four weeks. The patient was palliated for two years (Fig. 7.2A and 7.2B). In our recent group, three patients have been treated with our ongoing protocol of wide soft tissue resection and postoperative radiation therapy. All three are presently living disease-free at 16, 28, and 32 months, respectively, following treatment.

RHABDOMYOSARCOMA

Rhabdomyosarcoma is the most frequently diagnosed soft tissue sarcoma in children. The improvement in end results in this type of sarcoma probably represents one of the most fascinating and rewarding experiences in the field of oncology. The dramatic improvement in the last ten years, resulting from judicious use of conservative surgery, radiation therapy, and chemotherapy, constitutes one of the cornerstones of a multimodality treatment program for all soft tissue sarcomas.

Rhabdomyosarcomas are classified into various clinical and cytologic subgroups, depending on their histologic features, natural history, and anatomic location. These have been discussed in detail in Chapters 4 and 13. In this section the major emphasis will be on the role of radiation therapy in the management of these tumors, whether primary or metastatic. They have been divided into two groups: those in the head and neck region, and those in other sites.

Head and Neck Region
Embryonal rhabdomyosarcomas, after lymphomas, are the most common tumors of the head and neck region. They can be classified into three subgroups according to the site of origin of the primary tumor: (1) those located in the orbit, (2) those located in the soft tissue of the face, and (3) those in miscellaneous sites in the head and neck region (Fig. 7.3). Sutow[33] described the primary sites of head and neck rhabdomyosarcoma in 36 children. The data from

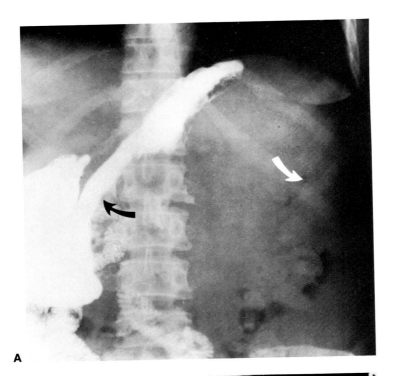

A

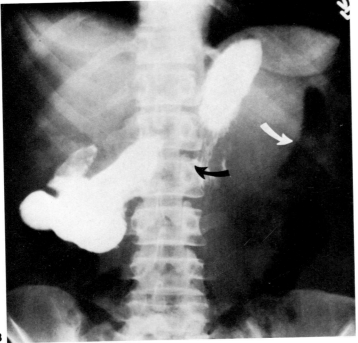

B

Figure 7.2. (A) Anterior-posterior roentgenogram of the abdomen of a 51-year-old woman following a barium meal. Black arrow shows marked displacement of the stomach medially, and white arrow shows displacement of the colon laterally due to a large retroperitoneal leiomyosarcoma. Diagnosis was established by celiotomy. (B) A similar anterior-posterior roentgenogram of the abdomen four months after a radiation tumor dose of 4,000 rads. Marked reduction in size of the sarcoma is evident. The arrows provide the coordinates for measurement of relative size. She lived for two years following radiation therapy alone.

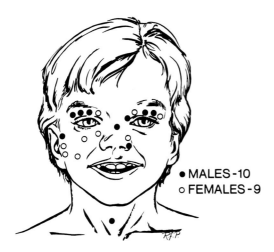

● MALES -10
○ FEMALES -9

Figure 7.3. Schematic drawing showing the site in 19 consecutive cases of childhood head and neck rhabdomyosarcomas. *(Courtesy of Cancer 37:1777-1786, 1976.)* Since the publication of our data, three additional cases of orbital rhabdomyosarcoma have been treated (Tables 7.1 and 7.2).

that study, and from our own material consisting of 26 patients, are shown in Table 7.1.[34] From this combined series it appears that the orbit is the commonest anatomic site in the entire head and neck region (Fig. 7.3).

Orbit. We have treated 12 rhabdomyosarcomas of the orbit. Eleven patients were between the ages of 2.5 and 17 years, with a mean age of 8.9 years, and one was an adult. A brief resumé

TABLE 7.1. ANATOMIC DISTRIBUTION OF HEAD AND NECK RHABDOMYOSARCOMAS IN CHILDREN IN TWO SERIES OF CASES

Primary Site	Sutow*[33] (1964)	Liebner†[34] (1981)
Orbit	14	12
Face	8	5
Nasopharynx	7	2
Larynx	1	1
Palate	3	0
Temporal bone	0	3
Paranasal sinuses	3	1
Neck	0	2
Total	36	26

*M.D. Anderson Hospital and Tumor Institute (1964).
†University of Illinois Hospital (1976).

of the clinical features of these 12 cases is given in Table 7.2. The first patient is of historical interest since, in 1960, she was the first patient with orbital rhabdomyosarcoma to be primarily treated with electron beam therapy at the University of Illinois Hospital. She is still free of any evidence of disease 22 years after the completion of all therapy (Fig. 7.4A and 7.4B).

Satisfactory local control of the disease is possible with a 5,000 to 6,000 rad dose level (or 1,650 to 1,750 rets) (Table 7.2). The expression *rets* represents rad equivalent therapy and is calculated according to Ellis's[35] formula for a nominal standard dose (NSD). This concept takes into consideration not only the total dose the patient receives, but the number of fractions required to attain the total dose and over what period of time it was administered. However, the major objective in any form of therapy in this region is not only to locally control the tumor but also to preserve vision. Our first attempt at an eye-saving technique was made in 1962 (Patient 4, Fig. 7.5A to 7.5D). Since then we have treated five additional children with orbital lesions who had only incisional biopsy to establish the diagnosis and were treated by radiation therapy and chemotherapy. All but one have retained excellent vision. The only long-term sequela of radiation therapy has been minor asymmetry of the ipsilateral orbit with some hair loss over the eyebrow (Fig. 7.5). Cassady and associates[36] and Sagerman et al.[11] reported similar end results.

A review of the published data[11,36,37] and our own experience with orbital rhabdomyosarcoma demonstrates the increasing importance of radiation therapy in local control and in the preservation of a useful eye. The paucity of periorbital lymphatics probably keeps the rhabdomyosarcoma localized for a relatively long period, allowing time for control of the local disease by radiation therapy. Early in the evolution of management of these neoplasms at the University of Illinois, exenteration was the procedure of choice. As a rule, radiation therapy was used only after postoperative recurrence. Three children with recurrent tumor following excision of the orbital contents were treated with high doses of irradiation with excellent results (Table 7.2). Today, irradiation has become the therapy of choice in the primary treatment of localized orbital rhabdomyosarcoma. In 1968, Cassady and co-workers[36] published 17 case reports of orbital rhabdomyosarcoma in children.

TABLE 7.2. SUMMARY OF DATA ON TWELVE CONSECUTIVE ORBITAL RHABDOMYOSARCOMAS IRRADIATED AT UNIVERSITY OF ILLINOIS

Patient No.	Age (yr)/ Sex	Stage	Histologic Diagnosis	Surgery	Radiation*	Chemotherapy	Comment
1	13/F	T_2N_0	Undifferentiated rhabdomyosarcoma, R orbit	Enucleation, R eye; local excision of R eyelids 22 mo later	6,400 rads electron beam, 36 fractions, (1,750 rets)	None	12/3/60, no tumor found in specimen; 22-yr cure, alive and well
2	10/M	T_2N_0	Embryonal rhabdomyosarcoma, R orbit	Exenteration R orbit; biopsy of recurrence	6,200 rads electron beam, 33 fractions, (1,750 rets)	Actinomycin D first and last weeks of radiation treatments	Recurrence with orbit involvement; 16-yr cure, alive and well
3	8/M	T_2N_0M	Poorly differentiated sarcoma, L orbit	Incisional biopsy only	6,200 rads electron beam, 36 fractions, (1,650 rets)	Actinomycin D and Cytoxan	Died 16 mo later; autopsy showed no local tumor in orbit; lung and skeletal metastases
4	3/M	T_3N_0	Undifferentiated sarcoma, L orbit	Biopsy, left orbital tumor	5,100 rads electron beam, 22 fractions (1,660 rets)	Cytoxan maintained 1 yr	Osseous orbit involved; 15-yr cure, alive and well (Fig. 7.5A to 7.5D)
5	8/M	T_1N_0	Undifferentiated sarcoma, L orbit	Excision of L eyelid mass; left orbital exenteration 1 mo later	5,200 rads 4-mm Cu, H.V.L. 22 fractions (1,910 rets)	Actinomycin D, 1 course	11-yr cure; alive and well
6	4/M	T_1N_0	Embryonal rhabdomyosarcoma, R upper eyelid	Excisional biopsy of R upper eyelid mass	6,100 rads betatron, 21 meV and 300 kV, 4-mm H.V.L. 34 fractions (1,750 rets)	Actinomycin D, 1 course	Excellent vision right eye; 9½-yr cure, alive and well

7	2½/M	Rhabdomyosarcoma, R upper eyelid	Biopsy only	5,000 rads, 4-mm Cu H.V.L. 300 kV 23 fractions (1,790 rets)	Actinomycin D, first and last weeks of irradiation	Good functional vision; 9-yr cure, alive and well
8	17/F	Undifferentiated sarcoma, R orbit	March 1968, orbital exenteration and maxillectomy	Recurrence; irradiated orbit, betatron x-ray, 21 fractions, 5,600 rads; 21 fractions, radium mold (2,260 rets)	Actinomycin D 1 course	Therapeutic abortion at time of recurrence; osseous involvement; 9-yr cure, alive and well, normal 3-yr-old son
9	8/F	Embryonal rhabdomyosarcoma, L upper eyelid	Incisional biopsy only	Cobalt, 5,600 rads 28 fractions (1,680 rets)	Actinomycin-vincristine-Cytoxan, long maintenance	Initial diagnosis pseudotumor of orbit; 2-yr, alive and well, then recurrence followed by exenteration and cesium mold therapy
10	41/F	Alveolar rhabdomyosarcoma, R lower eyelid	Incisional biopsy	Cobalt 5,600 rads, 28 fractions (1,680 rets)	Actinomycin D	Died of pulmonary metastases
11	6/F	Embryonal rhabdomyosarcoma, L lower eyelid	Biopsy only	5,600 rads, 29 fractions (1,655 rets)	Actinomycin D and 2-yr VAC maintenance	3 yr N.E.D.† Vision in L eye, 20/40
12	5/F	Embryonal rhabdomyosarcoma, L upper eyelid	Biopsy only	6,040 rads, 32 fractions	Actinomycin D and VAC maintenance (1 year)	N.E.D., vision in L eye, 20/30

*The expression "rets" represents rads equivalent therapy and is calculated by the formula of normal standard dose (NSD). The equation is $NSD (rets) = Dose (rads) \times N^{-0.24} \times T^{-0.11}$. For example, a treatment program of 30 fractions of 200 rads for 5 days a week over a period of 39 days, giving a total of 6,000 rads, can be converted to 6,000 rads $\times 30^{-0.24} \times 39^{-0.11} = 1,773$ rets (NSD).

†No evidence of disease.

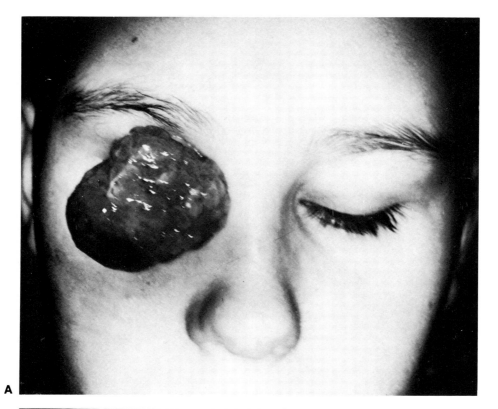

A

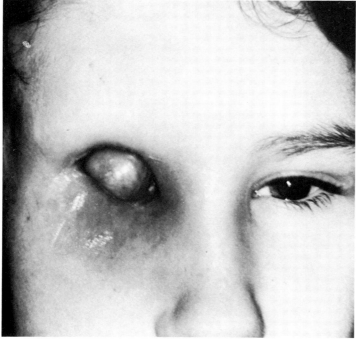

B

Figure 7.4. (A) Thirteen-year-old girl with recurrent rhabdomyosarcoma one and one half years after surgery (Table 7.2, Patient 1). **(B)** Appearance of patient after completion of 6,400-rad electron beam therapy.

Later, Sagerman et al.[11] reported 14 additional cases and were able to present the results of irradiation as the primary treatment for rhabdomyosarcoma of the orbit in 31 children. The data presented by Cassady and Sagerman and their co-workers, together with the author's personal experience, indicate that local control can be achieved by irradiation in about 90 percent of orbital rhabdomyosarcomas. This mode of primary therapy provided a five-year disease-free survival in about 70 percent of the patients.[11,34,36,37] In Chapter 13, Table 13.9, Das Gupta has summarized an additional eight patients. The end result data clearly indicate that radiation therapy should be the primary mode of treatment of orbital rhabdomyosarcomas (Fig. 7.6A and 7.6B).

In treating tumors of the head and neck region, head and neck casts must be used for older children, and head, neck, and body casts for infants and young children.* Other than the occasional use of sedation for the first visit to make the cast, measurements, and shields, all treatment can be administered without anesthesia or sedation. After therapy has been initiated and established, the majority of therapy fractions can be given on an outpatient basis. When the tumor is predominantly retrobulbar, greater emphasis should be given to the lateral portal. At times the dose to the depth of the orbit is divided between an anterior and posterior portal.

Facial Soft Tissue Rhabdomyosarcoma. Cassady and associates[36] concluded that localized forms of the embryonal, alveolar, and pleomorphic varieties of rhabdomyosarcoma that occur in sites other than the orbit are also potentially radiocurable. The author has treated five such patients; their clinical summaries are presented in Table 7.3. In this group of five, the longest survivor is a child who was nine years old when first treated (Patient 1) and who has now been disease-free for 17 years (Fig. 7.7A to 7.7C).

The incidence of regional node metastasis in facial rhabdomyosarcomas is higher than in the orbital variety, and treatment planning must include the regional lymph nodes.

Four of the five children in our group are alive and well (Table 7.3). The control of the primary tumor and neck nodes in our series was obtained by an NSD range of 1,610 to 1,700 rets. Masson and Soule[37] reported seven cases of embryonal rhabdomyosarcoma in this location, but only one patient, a nine-year-old girl, was alive and well eight years after radiation therapy for the primary tumor. Donaldson and co-workers[38] described a patient with a T_1N_0 cheek sarcoma who was alive and well two years after combined treatment with 6,000 rads in five weeks and chemotherapy. Heyn and associates[39] described two additional cases of cheek sarcoma treated with a combination of the two modalities; one of the two survived for 43 months. Recently Fernandez and co-workers[40] retrospectively analyzed 69 cases of rhabdomyosarcoma in children. Seven of these were facial, but because of the paucity of data, an adequate assessment of the end results was not possible. Our most recent case of facial soft tissue rhabdomyosarcoma was encountered in a five-year-old girl who also had ipsilateral neck node metastases. Both the primary tumor and the neck metastases were treated with 5,500 rads (1,670 rets) (Patient 5, Table 7.3). It is of interest that our only fatality in childhood facial soft tissue sarcoma was Patient 4, who received the minimum dose of radiation; the nominal standard dose (NSD) in this patient was 1,383 rets.

We have had limited experience in the management of rhabdomyosarcomas located in the head and neck region of adults. One man with a facial rhabdomyosarcoma was treated by adjuvant radiation therapy following an extensive resection. The patient died with metastatic disease four years later.

In Tables 13.10 and 13.11, found in Chapter 13, Das Gupta has summarized his experience with 23 cases of soft tissue rhabdomyosarcoma of the head and neck region, excluding the orbit. This group of 23 patients includes both adults and children. Our combined experience shows that most of the head and neck rhabdomyosarcomas in children are curable, with radiation therapy providing the most effective means of local control.

Miscellaneous Sites of the Head and Neck. Although rhabdomyosarcoma is the most commonly observed sarcoma of the head and neck region in children, only rarely is it encountered in such sites as the larynx, neck, sinus, nasopharynx, or middle ear, to name a few unusual

---

*The technique and philosophy of immobilization of pediatric radiotherapy patients at the University of Illinois Hospital are summarized in Liebner EJ, Haas RE, DeSio, V. Immobilization of pediatric radiotherapy patients. Applied Radiology 9(4):40, July/August 1980.

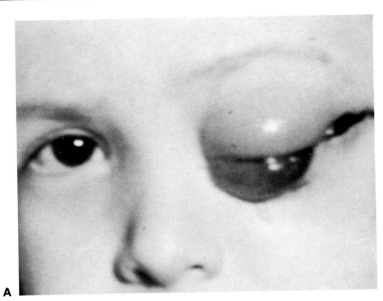

A

Figure 7.5. (**A**) Left eye of a 3-year-old boy before initiation of radiation therapy (Table 7.2, Patient 4). (**B**) Roentgenogram of the orbit shows extension of the tumor. The arrows point out the destruction of the posterior and lateral walls of the orbit.

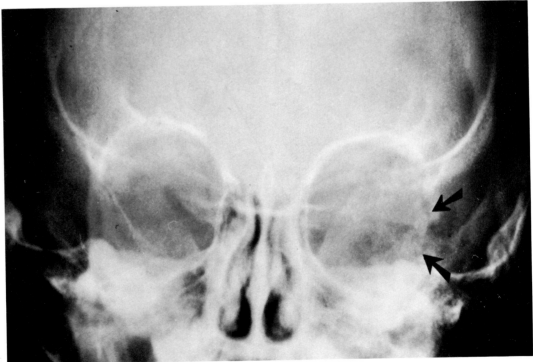

B

anatomic locations. Over the years we have treated nine childhood head and neck rhabdomyosarcomas arising in unusual locations. Table 7.4 summarizes the treatment and clinical data.

Rhabdomyosarcoma of the Larynx. This tumor comprises less than 1 percent of all laryngeal malignancies.[41] Harris[41] found three cases of fibrosarcoma, one lymphosarcoma, and one rhabdomyosarcoma in a series of some 300 cases of malignancies of the larynx. Table 7.5 summarizes the clinical features of 11 published cases of rhabdomyosarcoma of the larynx.[34,39,41-47] Two of the 11 cases (Patients 5 and 8) were treated

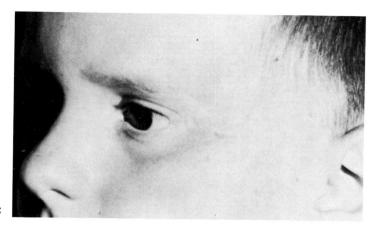

C

Figure 7.5. (C) Left eye five years after treatment with 5,100 rads of electron beam therapy. NSD was 1,600 rets. Useful vision reported as 20/100. Note well-preserved eyelashes. **(D)** Anterior-posterior roentgenogram of orbit of the patient 5 years later. Arrows show reossification of the previously destroyed lateral wall of the orbit. Left orbit is now smaller than the right. *(Courtesy of Cancer 37:1777, 1976.)*

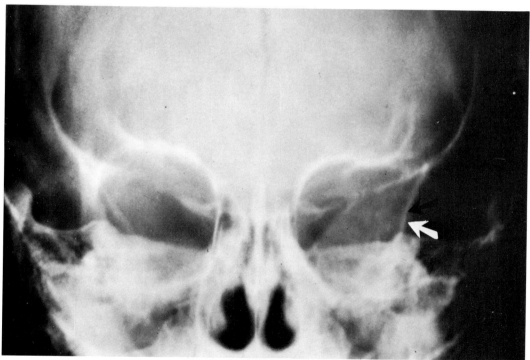

D

primarily by radiation therapy. One, a 7-year-old boy, was alive and well seven and one half years following his radiation treatments. The second, a 2½-year-old girl, received 6,000 rads during a period of four weeks, but died from osseous and lung metastases eight months after initial diagnosis. Heyn and associates[39] treated two children (Patients 9 and 10, Table 7.5) with adjuvant radiation therapy in their combined chemotherapy trial study. However, in Patient 9 the histologic type of the sarcoma was not determined. Nevertheless, he received 4,000 rads after surgery and was alive and well 70 months later. Our patient (Table 7.5, No. 11) was treated for a postlaryngectomy recurrence with radiation and chemotherapy and is still disease-free 17 years later (Fig. 7.8A and 7.8B). From this limited experience it appears that there is a definite role for radiation therapy in the treatment of laryngeal rhabdomyosarcoma.

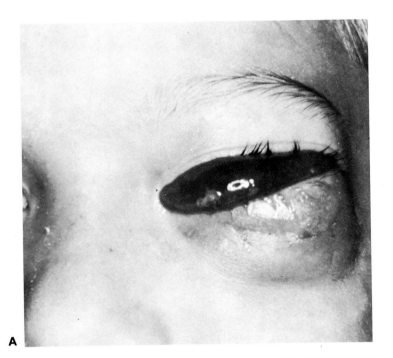

A

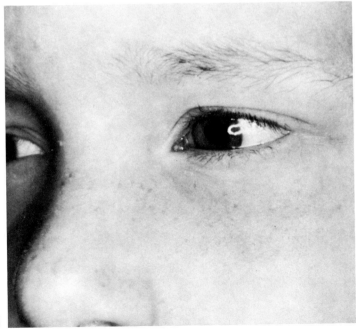

B

Figure 7.6. **(A)** Six-year-old girl with embryonal rhabdomyosarcoma of left eyelid (Table 7.2, Patient 11). **(B)** Same patient three years after treatment with 5,600 rads (1,655 rets). She is still well and has 20/40 vision in left eye. Photographic light artifact present over iris.

TABLE 7.3. SUMMARY OF DATA ON CHILDHOOD FACIAL SOFT TISSUE RHABDOMYOSARCOMA (UNIVERSITY OF ILLINOIS)

Patient No.	Age (yr)/ Sex	Stage	Histologic Diagnosis	Surgery	Radiation	Chemotherapy	Comment
1	9/F	T_2N_1	Embryonal rhabdomyosarcoma, right cheek and submandibular node	Biopsy only	5,200 rads, 300 kV H.V.L. 4-mm Cu, 32 fractions (1,620 rets)	Actinomycin D first and last weeks of irradiation	17-yr cure, alive and well (Figs. 7.4 and 7.5)
2	8/M	T_2N_0	Rhabdomyosarcoma, left nasobuccal area	Biopsy only	4,900 rads 300 kV H.V.L. 4-mm Cu, 20 fractions (1,610 rets)	Actinomycin D first and last weeks of irradiation	13-yr cure, alive and well
3	$3\frac{1}{2}$/F	T_2N_1	Rhabdomyosarcoma, right infraorbital nasal region	Biopsy only	5,000 rads, cobalt, 27 fractions (1,380 rets)	Actinomycin D-vincristine-Cytoxan	Lung and metastases during therapy; died in 9 mo
4	10 mo/F	T_2N_0	Rhabdomyosarcoma, right infraorbital nasal region	Biopsy only	5,560 rads cobalt 27 fractions (1,700 rets)	Actinomycin D-vincristine-Cytoxan	$3\frac{1}{2}$-yr cure, alive and well
5	5/F	T_2N_1	Rhabdomyosarcoma, left submandibular node	Biopsy only	5,500 rads cobalt, 28 fractions, (1,680 rets)	Actinomycin D-vincristine,	1 yr, alive and well

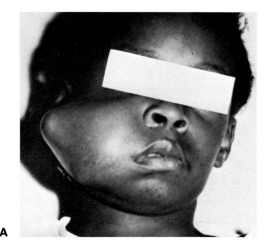

A

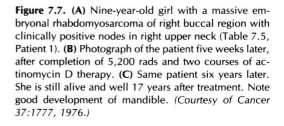

Figure 7.7. (A) Nine-year-old girl with a massive embryonal rhabdomyosarcoma of right buccal region with clinically positive nodes in right upper neck (Table 7.5, Patient 1). **(B)** Photograph of the patient five weeks later, after completion of 5,200 rads and two courses of actinomycin D therapy. **(C)** Same patient six years later. She is still alive and well 17 years after treatment. Note good development of mandible. *(Courtesy of Cancer 37:1777, 1976.)*

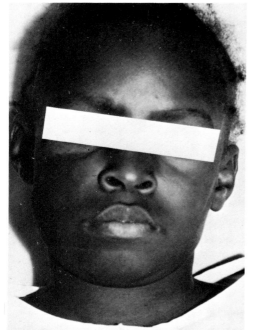

B

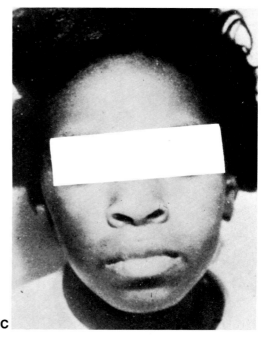

C

Two children had a primary rhabdomyosarcoma in the soft tissues of the neck (Patients 7 and 8, Table 7.4). Both are alive and well four years and five years, respectively, after surgery, irradiation, and adjuvant chemotherapy.

Nasopharyngeal Rhabdomyosarcoma. Although we have encountered only two such cases (Patients 2 and 6, Table 7.4), the nasopharynx is not as uncommon a location as, for example, the larynx, for rhabdomyosarcoma to occur.[37,39,48-51] One of our patients was a 3 1/2-year-old boy with nasopharyngeal rhabdomyosarcoma who had a partial resection elsewhere, following which he had received 5,000 rads over a period of 52 days in 30 fractions (1,420 rets). A month later he was referred to the University

TABLE 7.4. SUMMARY OF DATA ON CHILDHOOD RHABDOMYOSARCOMA IN UNUSUAL SITES: LARYNX, NECK, NASOPHARYNX, SINUS, AND MIDDLE EAR (UNIVERSITY OF ILLINOIS)

Patient	Age/Sex	Stage	Site	Surgery	Radiation	Chemotherapy	Comment
1	7 yr/M	T_2N_0	Larynx	Laryngectomy	6,200 rads electron beam, 36 fractions (1,730 rets)	Actinomycin D first and last weeks of irradiation	Recurred in 10 mo; 17-yr, alive and well
2	3½ yr/M	T_3N_2M	Nasopharynx	Partial resection	Received 5,100 rads at another hospital, 34 fractions (1,420 rets)	Actinomycin D, vincristine	1,500 rads, palliative; died 3/27/65; autopsy showed primary not controlled, involvement of base of skull, brain, and lungs
3	5 yr/M	T_3N_1	Right petrous bone and ear canal	Biopsy only	6,000 rads betatron x-rays, 34 fractions (1,700 rets)	Actinomycin D, vincristine	Presented with multiple cranial nerve paralysis, marked destruction of right petrous bone; died six months later; autopsy showed no evidence of tumor locally
4	10 yr/F	T_2N_0M	Right petrous bone and ear canal	Biopsy only	6,000 rads betatron x-rays; 28 fractions, (1,780 rets)	Actinomycin D, vincristine	Presented with lung metastases; died 8 mo later; local primary controlled
5	13 mo/F	$T_3N_1M_0$	Right posterior auricular region and mastoid	Excision of soft tissue mass only	5,100 rads to temporal bone and neck; cobalt, 28 fractions, (1,530 rets)	Actinomycin D, vincristine, Cytoxan	Alive and well; N.E.D.* 8 yr following irradiation
6	7 yr/M	T_3N_1	R nasopharynx	Biopsy only	5,800 rads, 30 fractions (1,680 rets)	VAC regimen 2 yr	Alive and well; 5 yr N.E.D.
7	11 mo/F	T_2N_0	Right mental area	Wide local excision of mass	Preoperative; Postoperative, 3,500 rads (1,300 rets)	VAC regimen 2 yr	Alive and well; 5 yr N.E.D.
8	14 yr/M	T_1N_1	Left side of neck	Modified L radical neck dissection	Postoperative radiation 5,640 rads (1,600 rets)	VAC regimen 2 yr	Alive and well; 4 yr N.E.D.
9	15 yr/M	T_3N_0	R maxillary antrum	Biopsy only	6,170 rads, 32 fractions (1,700 rets)	VAC regimen 2 yr, maintenance	Alive and well; 2 yr N.E.D.

No evidence of disease.

TABLE 7.5. DATA ON 11 CASES OF RHABDOMYOSARCOMA OF THE LARYNX

Author	Age (yr)	Sex	Site	Treatment	Result
1. Harris[41]	3	F	Posterior larynx	Total laryngectomy	3 yr, alive and well
2. Pearson et al.[42]	54	M	Larynx	Total laryngectomy	Died three weeks postop
3. Ibid	10	M	Ant. commissure below left true cord	Partial laryngectomy	4-yr cure
4. Cady[44]	—	—	—	Total laryngectomy	
5. Masson and Soule[37]	7	M	Subglottis	Radiation therapy	7½ yr, alive and well
6. Batsakis and Fox[45]	3	M	Subglottis	Total laryngectomy and chemotherapy	16 mo, alive and well
7. Rodriguez and Zinskind[46]	57	M	Large mass right cord and commissure	Total laryngectomy	No postop followup data
8. Pochedly[47]	2½	F	Hypopharynx	Radiation therapy	Died 8 mo from metastases
9. Heyn et al.[39]	6	M	Larynx	Surgery, radiation and chemotherapy	Alive 71 mo
10. Ibid	3	M	Larynx	Surgery and chemotherapy	Alive 66 mo
11. Liebner[34]	7	M	Posterior larynx	Laryngectomy with recurrence; radiation and chemotherapy	17 yr, alive and well

of Illinois Hospital, and a regimen of actinomycin D and Oncovin was begun for his persistent neoplasm. He received a further course of palliative 1,500 rads in five fractions prior to his death, which was due to extension of the tumor to the base of the skull. The other child was a 7-year-old boy (Patient 6, Table 7.4), who had a nasopharyngeal rhabdomyosarcoma on the right side with pterygoid erosion and lymph node involvement (T_3N_1). It is now five years since he was treated with irradiation and adjuvant chemotherapy, and he still shows no evidence of disease.

This unfavorable response to management in the first patient was not unusual and has been noted by many other authors (Table 7.6).[48-55] In an earlier report, Masson and Soule[37] had no survivors out of 15 patients with nasopharyngeal rhabdomyosarcoma. Edland[49,50] described two cases of nasopharyngeal rhabdomyosarcoma. One was in a 9-year-old girl who received 4,300 rads in 34 days and died within three months of disseminated disease and an uncontrolled primary. The other was in an 11-year-old boy whose primary was controlled with 6,900 rads in 52 days but in whom lung metastases developed. Lindberg[51] found that the primary

was not controlled in five of his six cases. In three of the five, a dose of 5,000 rads was given in five weeks, along with adjuvant chemotherapy. One child in whom the primary tumor was controlled with 6,000 rads given over a period of seven weeks, died of metastases. Lindberg[51] concluded that children presenting with primary lesions of the nasopharynx have a uniformly poor prognosis, regardless of the treatment modality used. However, he did recommend at least 6,000 rads in six weeks as the best radiation opportunity for local control. Of Nelson's[48] two patients, one had local recurrence five years and two months after initial treatment with surgery and irradiation, and was treated by intracavitary radium to a dose of 5,000 rads, resulting in complete regression. At the time of publication of the report, the regression had persisted for six months. Holton and associates[52] observed complete regression in a 2-year-old child with a stage II-B lesion. The child had had an incomplete resection, followed by irradiation with 4,950 rads. He was still disease-free 17 months after initial therapy. An even more optimistic result was reported by Donaldson and associates.[38] In seven of their eight patients, local control of the primary tumor, rang-

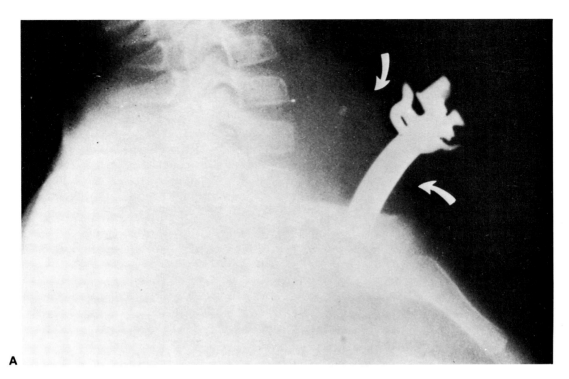

A

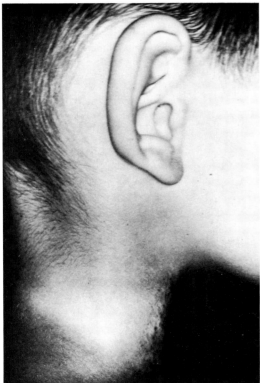

B

Figure 7.8. **(A)** Lateral roentgenogram of lower neck of a 7-year-old boy who had had a laryngectomy for embryonal rhabdomyosarcoma eight months previously. Arrows delineate a large recurrence that is dislodging the tracheotomy tube. The tracheal air column below the tube is narrowed, due to early tumor extension inferiorly. *(Courtesy of Illinois Medical Journal 121:531, 1962.)* **(B)** Four years after successful control of recurrence with electron beam therapy. Patient is still alive and well 20 years after radiation treatment.

ing from 11 to 63 months, was achieved following radiation therapy. The radiation doses were between 5,000 and 6,000 rads. Because of the poor prognosis for patients with these lesions, Donaldson and co-workers[38] advocated adjuvant chemotherapy, consisting of vincristine, actinomycin D, and cyclophosphamide (VAC), for two years.

Ghavimi and associates[55] treated three rhabdomyosarcomas of the nasopharynx (Table 7.6). Two of the patients with stage II lesions were disease-free 26 and 22 months later, respectively. The first, a 3-year-old boy, received 7,000 rads over a period of 94 days, and chemotherapy for 23 months. The total chemotherapy regimen consisted of cycles of sequential administration of actinomycin, adriamycin,

vincristine, and cyclophosphamide, with periods of rest. The second child, a 7-year-old girl, was given 6,500 rads over a period of 74 days and received chemotherapy for 22 months. The third, a 7-year-old boy, had a stage III lesion of the nasopharynx (involvement of the base of the skull and cervical nodes) and received 4,800 rads in 50 days. He died within six months after treatment of the primary. Postmortem examination showed recurrent tumor at the primary site as well as metastases. Das Gupta has treated two children with nasopharyngeal rhabdomyosarcoma with 6,000 rads to the primary and a pulsed VAC regimen. One has been disease-free for five years and the other died of metastatic disease two and one half years later (Table 13.10, Chapter 13). It appears that a dose of at

TABLE 7.6. REVIEW OF PUBLISHED CASES OF RHABDOMYOSARCOMA OF THE NASOPHARYNX

Author and References	Year	Patient Incidence in Series	Treatment	Comments
Masson & Soule[37]	1965	15 of 88	No details given of radiation or surgery	No significant survival rate
Nelson[48]	1968	2 of 24	Surgery and radiation, 5,000 rads	(1) 5 yr, 2 mo; recurrence
Edland[49,50]	1965	2 of 20	Radiation and chemotherapy 6,900 rads/52 days	Local control. Lung metastasis, 5,000 rads/29 days Alive and well 5 yr
Lindberg[51]	1969	6 of 34	Radiation and chemotherapy (3) 5,000 rads in 5 weeks (1) radiation only, 6,000 rads in 8 weeks	5 of 6, local primary failure. In one, primary control, but died of distant metastases; 6,000 rads/7 weeks
Donaldson et al.[38]	1975	8 of 19	Radiation 5,000–6,000 rads in 5–6 weeks. Chemotherapy 2 yr;	7 of 8, local primary control 11 to 63 mo, alive and well
Holton et al.[52]	1975	1 of 19	Incomplete resection	17 mo, alive and well
Jaffe et al.[53]	1973	8 of 28	6,000 rads; mitomycin-C	Age 7 yr, 9 mo; 8-yr survival, hypopituitarism
			6,000 rads; vincristine-actinomycin D	Age 4 yr, 9 mo 2 yr, 9 mo survival
			Wide excision; 4,158 rads; actinomycin D-vincristine	Age 9 yr, 6 mo; 16-yr survivor; osteogenic sarcoma of mandible 10 yr later
			6,650 rads; actinomycin D-vincristine	Age 3 yr, 10 mo 2 yr, 6 mo survival
Smith[54]	1974	1 child (2 adults had other sites)	5040 rads in 6 weeks 8 × 7 cm portals	6 mo, died; primary uncontrolled
Ghavimi et al.[55]	1975	3 of 29	Radiation 7,000 rads/94 days 6,500 rads/74 days 4,800 rads/50 days and chemotherapy, 2-yr plan	26 mo, alive and well 22 mo, alive and well Died, 6 mo

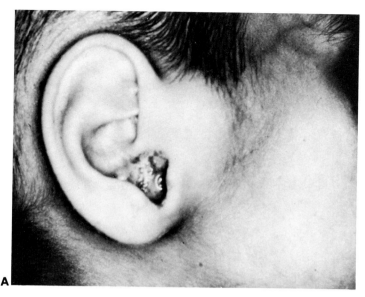

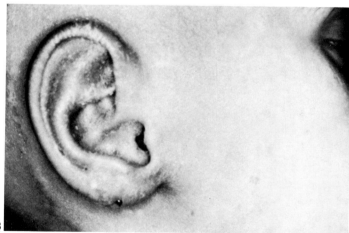

Figure 7.9. (A) Right ear of a 5-year-old boy, showing a polypoid mass protruding through the external canal. Note anterior extension of the tumor. The child had associated otitis media, multiple cranial nerve involvement, and metastasis to the cervical nodes. There was roentgenographic evidence of destruction of the petrous bone (Table 7.4, Patient 3). **(B)** Patient after receiving 5,700 rads (80 percent isodose line) (1,700 rets) electron beam therapy. Note dry desquamation, disappearance of external canal, and preauricular masses. The child died of metastatic disease six months later. Autopsy showed the local tumor was controlled and there was no evidence of residual tumor in the temporal bone.

least 6,000 rads is essential to control primary nasopharyngeal tumors.

Rhabdomyosarcoma of the Maxillary Antrum. The only case of maxillary antrum rhabdomyosarcoma was in a 15-year-old boy (Table 7.4, Patient 9). There was osseous destruction of the antrum (T_3N_0). He has responded well to excision, radiation therapy (6,170 rads), and adjuvant chemotherapy. There was no evidence of disease at two-year followup.

Rhabdomyosarcomas of the Middle Ear and Mastoid. Table 7.4 summarizes our experience with rhabdomyosarcomas of the middle ear and

mastoid. In 1966, Potter[56] reviewed 14 patients from the literature and added a 3-year-old patient. In 1973, Jaffe and associates[53] reported three cases in children: a 3-year-old girl, a 4-year-old boy, and an 8-year-old boy, respectively, and reviewed the natural history of 37 patients from the literature. The longest survival time after diagnosis was found to be 23 months.[50] One of our patients (No. 5, Table 7.4) has survived eight years and continues to do well.

Rhabdomyosarcoma of the middle ear and mastoid occurs predominantly in children. The age range extends from about 1 year to 12 years, the average being 4.4 years. Clinical manifestations are usually those of a chronic suppurative otitis media. A triad of otitis media, polypoid mass (sarcoma botryoid), and bloody discharge is found in most patients. Paralysis or paresis of the facial nerve invariably occurs during the course of the disease. Multiple cranial nerve involvement is not uncommon.[53] Many of these tumors present as a direct extension through the temporal bone. If the tumor in the ear canal, middle ear, or the mastoid erodes inferiorly, then a contiguous parapharyngeal mass is found extending into the nasopharyngeal or oropharyngeal mucosa. In one of our patients (No. 3, Table 7.4) the mass presented anteriorly to the external auditory canal (Fig. 7.9A and 7.9B). This patient also had multiple cranial nerve involvement indicative of intracranial extension (posterior cranial fossa). The destruction of the temporal bone that follows is usually osteolytic. Because of the generally extensive involvement at the time of initial clinical examination, attempts to excise these lesions are usually fruitless.[53] Although radiation therapy has not been adequately tried, this method probably has the best chance of locally controlling the primary tumor. Potter[56] commented that embryonal rhabdomyosarcoma of the middle ear in children is invariably fatal. Jaffe et al.[53] emphasized that there was no mode of therapy that offered a potential for cure. The longest survival reported was that of a 30-month-old boy who received 4,710 rads (4 Mev) in 14 days.[57] A radical mastoidectomy four months later revealed no tumor. He was alive 12 years later with findings of hypopituitarism. We consider this radiation dosage, given in such a short time, to be excessive. Potter[56] reported that 5,000 rads were delivered to the right ear of his patient through opposing 6 × 6 cm portals in 33 days. There was visible local regression, but at operation, six weeks after completion of radiotherapy, the air cells of the mastoid process were filled with tumor, and there was tumor in the region of the lateral sinus and jugular fossa. In contrast, Conte and Sagerman[58] reported that long survival is possible. Their patient, a 4-year-old girl, had an inadequate radical mastoidectomy on the left side, with some residual tumor. A tumor dose of 5,500 rads was given in 23 sessions. These authors utilized a direct field and a wedge pair, 6 × 8 cm, with a hinge angle of 55 degrees. At the time of their report, 42 months after treatment, the child was still well.

Our own patient, who is disease-free after eight years, was treated in a similar fashion and with a comparable dosage for her age. Ragab and associates[59] reported a four-year survival following radical mastoidectomy, radiation therapy (5,200 rads), and chemotherapy. This handful of case reports illustrates the generally bad prognosis for children with rhabdomyosarcoma of the middle ear and mastoid area.

Rhabdomyosarcoma of the Extremities and the Trunk

McNeer and co-workers,[10] in 1968, analyzed the treatment data on their 109 patients with rhabdomyosarcoma of the extremities and trunk seen at Memorial Sloan-Kettering Cancer Center between 1935 and 1959. Only 29 had received some form of radiation therapy. In three, radiation therapy alone was used, and one of the three was a five-year survivor. The results are shown in Table 7.7. Interpretation of these data in present-day context is difficult. Preoperative radiation therapy was probably used only for large infiltrative tumors (stages II-B, III-A, and III-B), which could account for the increased incidence of local recurrence. Suit et al.,[12] in 1975, reviewed the M.D. Anderson Hospital data on rhabdomyosarcoma of the extremities and the trunk and found that, of a total of 12 patients treated primarily by conservative excision and radical radiation, none lived free of disease for as long as 24 months, but only one showed failure of local therapy. In their most recent publication, Lindberg and associates[25] updated M.D. Anderson Hospital's data on rhabdomyosarcoma from all sites. The incidence of local recurrence was 29 percent and none of their 17 patients lived disease-free as long as two years. We have treated only two patients with extremity rhabdomyosarcoma: one was a 3-year-old child and the other a 30-year-old adult. Both had metastatic disease. However, Das Gupta has managed 21 patients with embryonal rhabdomyosarcoma of the trunk and extremities (Chapter 13). None of the patients with extremity tumors was treated by amputation. A 62 percent two-year and 57 percent five-year disease-free survival rate was achieved.

In 1975, Ghavimi and co-workers[55] at Memorial Sloan-Kettering Cancer Center reviewed the influence of multidisciplinary therapy on the end results in 29 children younger than 15

TABLE 7.7. RESULTS OF TREATMENT OF RHABDOMYOSARCOMA OF THE TRUNK AND EXTREMITIES*
MEMORIAL SLOAN-KETTERING CANCER CENTER

Type of Treatment	No. Patients	5 Yr, N.E.D.†	End Results	
			10 Yr, N.E.D.	Local Recurrence
Surgery only	80	41/69 (59%)	24/52 (46%)	19/80 (24%)
Radiation only	3	1/3 (33%)	0/3	2/3 (66%)
Preoperative radiation and surgery	11	7/11 (64%)	3/8 (38%)	4/11 (36%)
Surgery and postoperative radiation	15	9/15 (60%)	3/9 (33%)	4/15 (27%)

*Adapted from McNeer et al., 1968.[10]
†No evidence of disease.

years of age who had rhabdomyosarcoma. These authors showed that use of excision, radiation therapy, and chemotherapy improved the end result, compared with results obtained in 108 children not treated in this fashion between 1960 and 1970 at the same institution.

All 29 children were treated by the appropriate surgical procedure and all received chemotherapy. In addition, nine had node dissection and 19 received radiation therapy (dosages ranged from 5,000 to 7,000 rads). Only two were treated by amputation. At the time of the report, all 29 patients had been disease-free for periods ranging from 4 months to 42 months or longer. Five patients died within 5 to 15 months of diagnosis. All five had either stage III or stage IV disease.

Attempts to salvage the extremities in patients with embryonal rhabdomyosarcoma have also been made by Holton and co-workers.[52] They used 15 to 20 Mev electrons, giving 2,000 to 5,000 rads in four or five weeks. In the four children with tumors of the upper extremities, they included the whole upper extremity, axilla, and lower neck. By varying the separation of the abutting fields they were able to improve the uniformity of the dose. These children have survived for 47, 24, 24, and 22 months, respectively, and only one has evidence of recurrent disease. This method has allowed the children to retain at least a partially functional limb.

Based on the available data[12,15,52,54] as well as the clinical material Das Gupta has reviewed elsewhere in this book, it is possible to reaffirm that a satisfactory end result, that is, disease-free survival and limb salvage, is best accomplished by use of a multimodality therapy consisting of wide excision, radiation therapy, and adjuvant chemotherapy.

Rhabdomyosarcoma of the Genitourinary Tract

The only patient with sarcoma botryoides (embryonal rhabdomyosarcoma) of the urinary bladder treated by the author was a 4-month-old girl who received a preoperative midline tumor dose to the whole pelvis and vagina of 800 rads in four fractions in four days. She was treated by anterior exenteration and maintained on a regimen of chemotherapy for one year. She is still alive and well more than ten years after treatment (Chapter 13). El-Mahdi and associates[60] reported the 25-year survival of a patient with sarcoma botryoides of the vagina treated by radiation therapy alone. The patient was 13 months old when irradiated, and the mid-pelvic soft tissue dose was recalculated to be 2,200 rads. The pelvic bone dose was 4,600 rads (200 Kvp, HVT, 0.9 mm³). As a result of the pelvic irradiation during infancy, this patient has hypoplastic external genitalia, an infantile vagina and uterus, and hypofunction of the ovaries. However, she does have normal urinary and bowel function. The normal functions apparently outweigh any disadvantages of reduced pelvic growth or the presence of an infantile vagina. Schweisguth[61] described two children in whom the use of interstitial implants for localized vaginal rhabdomyosarcoma controlled the primary tumor. Radical surgery was thus avoided in these two children, saving the bladder and rectum. One, a girl who was treated at age 11 years, was three years late in menstruating and the only morbidity was a moderate vaginal stenosis. We agree with Pratt and co-workers[62] that excellent salvage can be accomplished with a combination of conservative excision, adequate radiation therapy, and adjuvant chemotherapy.

The bladder, prostate, and paratesticular

tissues are frequent sites of urogenital embryonal rhabdomyosarcoma in children.[52,55] Ghavimi and associates[55] reviewed the results of multidisciplinary treatment of a series of 27 children who had embryonal rhabdomyosarcoma of the urogenital tract between 1960 and 1971. Eleven of these children had paratesticular sarcomas and six had tumors of the bladder or prostate. Seven of those with paratesticular sarcoma, three with sarcoma of the bladder, and one with sarcoma of the prostate had been free of tumor for periods ranging from 18 months to 10 years from the date of diagnosis. A multidisciplinary approach—surgery, radiation therapy, and multiple drug therapy—offers the best chance for prolonged survival and cure. In Chapter 13, a case of rhabdomyosarcoma of the prostate is described in a 4-year-old boy. This child was seen in consultation (by Das Gupta) and was principally treated by radiation therapy and chemotherapy after establishing the diag-

nosis with a needle biopsy. The local tumor was adequately controlled for a long period of time with radiation therapy alone. However, two years ago an exenterative procedure became necessary because of local recurrence. Although definitive guidelines cannot be drawn, it is reasonable to suggest that radiation therapy will play an increasingly important role in the management of prostatic rhabdomyosarcomas.

Ghavimi and co-workers[55] found that in 3 of 11 paratesticular sarcomas (27 percent), retroperitoneal lymph nodes contained metastatic rhabdomyosarcoma. The Radiation Therapy Department of the University of Illinois has treated three children with paratesticular rhabdomyosarcoma. Lymphangiography was performed in all three, but none had metastatic involvement of the retroperitoneal nodes. In contrast, one of our patients, a 12-year-old girl, had a rhabdomyosarcoma of the perianal region, and lymphography demonstrated in-

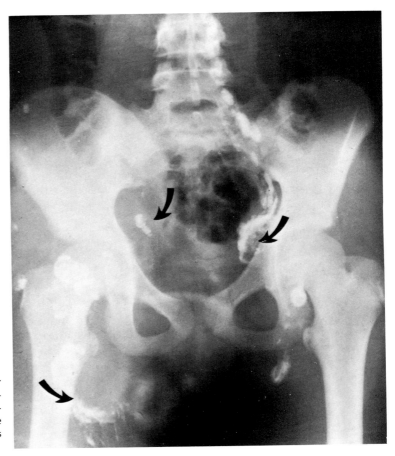

Figure 7.10. Anterior-posterior lymphogram of pelvis of a 12-year-old girl. The right perianal rhabdomyosarcoma has involved the right groin and both iliac regions (arrows).

TABLE 7.8. RESULTS OF DIFFERENT FORMS OF TREAMENT IN NEUROFIBROSARCOMA*

Types of Treatment	No. Patients	5 Yr, N.E.D.†	10 Yr, N.E.D.
Radiation only	4	3/4	2/3
Preoperative radiation and surgery	5	1/5	1/5
Surgery and postoperative radiation	14	11/14 (79%)	7/10
Surgery only	20	10/17 (59%)	7/14

*Adapted from McNeer et al.,[10] 1968.
†No evidence of disease.

volvement of the inguinal, iliac, and periaortic lymph nodes (Fig. 7.10). Suit[63] advocated lymphangiogram studies on patients with rhabdomyosarcoma and high-grade synovial sarcoma. He stated that approximately 15 percent of patients in these groups exhibit metastases to the regional lymph nodes as the first sign of metastatic disease. The role of supplemental use of radioactive lymphangiography has not been adequately investigated.

MALIGNANT PERIPHERAL NERVE TUMORS

McNeer et al.,[10] in 1968, described 23 patients with neurogenic sarcoma who were treated with some form of radiation therapy. Of these, only four were treated by radiation therapy alone; three of the four were long-term survivors (Table 7.8). Two had received 2,000 rads each and the third, 2,500 rads. It is not possible to interpret the results in Table 7.8, since the size of the tumor, anatomic location, and histologic grade of all these tumors are not available. In 1970, Das Gupta and Brasfield[64] reported the end results of radiation therapy in 69 patients with malignant schwannoma treated at Memorial Sloan-Kettering Cancer Center. The radiation dosage varied from 3,000 to 9,000 rads, depending on the location and size of the tumors. Three patients were treated by interstitial radiation therapy. Fifteen of the 69 received preoperative radiation therapy (2,000 rads); 7 of these 15 (46 percent) survived five years and 3 (20 percent) survived 10 years (Table 7.9). Fifty-four patients were initially treated by radiation therapy; of these, 22 (41 percent) lived for five years and 17 (31.4 percent) for 10 years. Of the 54, 31 (57 percent) required wide excision of the primary tumor site, since radiation alone did

not control the primary tumor. Of the 31 so treated, 21 were disease-free at five years and 16 at seven years.

In 1975, Suit and co-workers[12] and Lindberg et al.[32] reported on the effectiveness of local resection and radical dose radiation therapy for neurofibrosarcomas. Suit and co-workers[12] found that four (21 percent) of 19 patients had local recurrence. In nine of the 19 the primary tumor was less than 5 cm in diameter and there was no evidence of local recurrence; 12 of the 19 (63 percent) lived free of disease for two years. In 1975, Lindberg and associates[32] reported a 25 percent local recurrence rate, and in 1981, while updating the original 1975 data,[25] observed that in a series of 60 patients with neurofibrosarcoma the local recurrence rate still was 33 percent and absolute two- and five-year survival rates were 72 percent and 50 percent, respectively. Both Suit[12,30] and Lindberg[25,32] and their co-workers suggested that in a given tumor the stage and microscopic grading are more important than

TABLE 7.9. MALIGNANT SCHWANNOMA—END RESULTS AND TYPE OF TREATMENT (201 PATIENTS)*†

Type of Treatment	No. Patients‡	5 Yr, N.E.D.§	10 Yr, N.E.D.
Surgery alone	132 (124)	62	40
Radiation and surgery combined	15 (12)	7	3
Radiation therapy alone	54 (48)	22	17

*Adapted from Das Gupta and Brasfield.[69]
†In 31 patients treatment was palliative.
‡Numbers in parentheses represent patients eligible for 5-year followup.
§No evidence of disease.

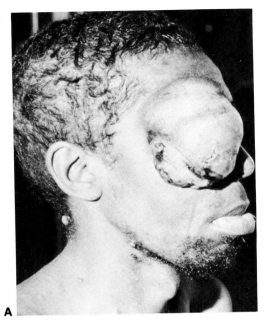
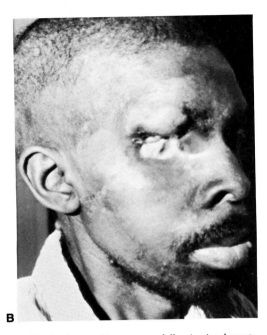

A   **B**

Figure 7.11. **(A)** A 29-year-old man who had massive recurrence of right orbital neurofibrosarcoma following inadequate excision and chemotherapy. **(B)** Right orbit was irradiated using a pair of intersecting wedge fields. A total dose of 6,800 rads was delivered over 55 days. There was some regression of the gross tumor in the right orbit.

the histologic or histogenetic types. We question this concept, since the natural histories of fibrosarcomas and liposarcomas and malignant schwannomas are neither similar nor comparable. However, before embarking on a proposed plan of treatment it is extremely important to histologically grade a tumor after it is correctly classified. In our assessment, malignant tumors of the peripheral nerves in general are not as radioresponsive as malignant mesenchymal tumors (Fig. 7.11A and 7.11B).

NEUROBLASTOMA

Neuroblastoma probably is the most common solid tumor of childhood.[65,66] Its behavior is unique and, in spite of trials of several chemotherapeutic agents with or without radiation therapy, the survival rate has not improved in the past decade.[67-69] The overall survival in most series depends upon the anatomic location of the primary tumors. Children with extra-abdominal neuroblastomas usually have a higher survival rate than those with the abdominal

type.[70-73] The results of treatment of abdominal neuroblastoma are more discouraging than those of Wilms' tumor.[74,75] The prognosis for patients with neuroblastoma depends on the clinical stage of the tumor. The most commonly used staging system is that proposed by Evans and co-workers.[76] Koop and Schnaufer[66] reported a 20 percent overall survival rate for patients with abdominal neuroblastomas. The survival rates according to stage were as follows: stage I, 90 percent; stage II, 33 percent; stage III, 30 percent; stage IV, 2.4 percent. In recent years, however, the Children's Cancer Study Group (CCSG) has shown in prospective studies that the age of the child at the time of diagnosis has a profound influence on the prognosis. The survival rate, when computed according to age, was found to be 90 percent in children in the first and second years of life but fell to 47 percent after that.[77] It has been shown that this improvement is certainly not due to the addition of chemotherapy.[78] Therefore, it appears that more accurate staging, adequate excision, and, finally, radical radiation therapy are probably responsible for the improved survival rate.[77]

Liebner and Rosenthal[79] reported the value of serial determinations of catecholamines in following the response to radiation therapy in the management of childhood neuroblastomas (Fig. 7.12A to 7.12C). We think this marker is a useful guide in planning radiation therapy.

SYNOVIAL SARCOMA

Synovial sarcoma, with all its variants (Chapter 4), has been the subject of a therapeutic controversy over the years.[80-85] Because of the rarity of clinical material it has been difficult to develop a uniformly acceptable therapeutic plan. The section dealing with synovial tissue tumors describes the experience of one of us (Das Gupta) with 26 cases of synovial sarcoma, four cases of clear cell sarcoma of the tendon sheath, and eight cases of epithelioid sarcoma. In most of these cases the patients have been treated with radical excision, regional node dissection, and adjuvant chemotherapy (Chapter 15). Our experience with radiotherapeutic management of both primary and metastatic tumors is therefore not extensive. However, we have an ongoing protocol of limb salvage for synovial sarcoma, in which both preoperative and postoperative radiation therapy is being utilized (Chapter 8). Eight patients have been treated according to this protocol, and the primary tumor has been effectively controlled in all (Table 8.22, Chapter 8).

Synovial sarcomas usually metastasize hematogenously, but anaplastic types have a 15 to 25 percent incidence of lymph node metastases. It is of value to perform lymphangiogram studies on these patients.[63] There is a strong tendency for the sarcoma to recur locally, and radiation is often considered in their management. Pack and Ariel[82] reported that best results were obtained with wide excision and irradiation. Berman[80] advocated adequate local excision followed by a postoperative radiation tumor dose of 4,500 rads in four to five weeks. He also recommended elective irradiation of the regional lymph nodes. He managed 3 of his 12 patients in this manner and all were disease-free at three, seven, and eight years, respectively. McNeer and associates[10] reported that, in five patients, radiation therapy alone resulted in two long-term survivors of ten years. One patient received 7,000 rads and the other 4,500 rads and an interstitial implant of 11.5 miC of radon. They also reported a somewhat higher 10-year survival rate for those receiving postoperative radiation therapy. Some of this enthusiasm for irradiating synovial sarcomas was questioned by Cadman and associates.[81] They found that no cures were achieved by irradiation alone and were not convinced of its palliative value. Nevertheless, their patients who received postoperative radiation therapy had a 50 percent local recurrence rate (16 of 32), compared with 91.5 percent (54 of 59) of those who did not receive it. In 1972, van Andel[84] reviewed the literature on 450 treated cases of synovial sarcoma and added 28 of his own. From this study he recommended the following management: preoperative irradiation with a tumor dose of 400 rads twice, followed by limited excision, and, after histologic confirmation of the diagnosis, completion of the radiation therapy with 5,000 to 6,000 rads in five to six weeks. He suggested that if regional nodes were enlarged they should be included in the field of irradiation. Radical excision of the primary site was advocated three to six weeks after completion of radiation therapy. However, we question the wisdom of irradiation prior to a histologic diagnosis. The author did not elaborate on those patients who, after receiving radiation therapy, were found on biopsy to have either a benign tumor or a different type of sarcoma.[84] The merit of irradiation was also suggested by Raben and coworkers.[83] Their management program consisted of wide local excision and postoperative radiation therapy. MacKenzie[85] studied 58 synovial sarcomas and observed a five-year survival rate of 51 percent. No correlation was found between the histologic picture and the prognosis. Suit and associates[12] described the clinical behavior of 15 synovial sarcomas according to their size and histopathologic grade. A correlation between local recurrence and survival time was evident. A review of the published reports on synovial sarcomas[12,80-85] suggests that this tumor is probably more radiosensitive than was previously thought, and that radiation therapy is probably a useful adjuvant to surgical treatment. Lindberg et al.[25] recently provided data on 24 patients with synovial sarcoma. Following conservative excision and radical radiation therapy, there was a local recurrence rate of 12.5 percent. The absolute two- and five-year disease-free survival rates were 75 percent and 58 percent, respectively.

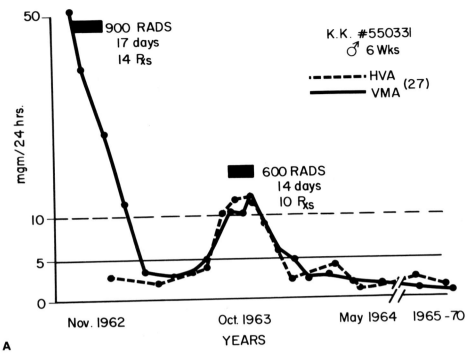

A

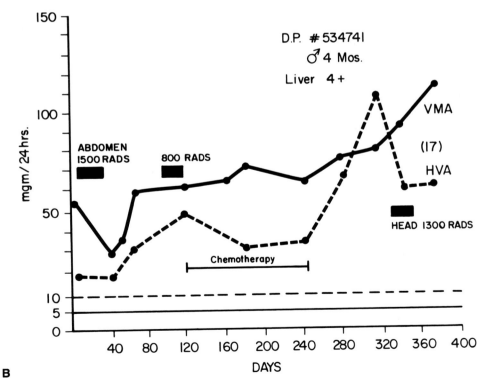

B

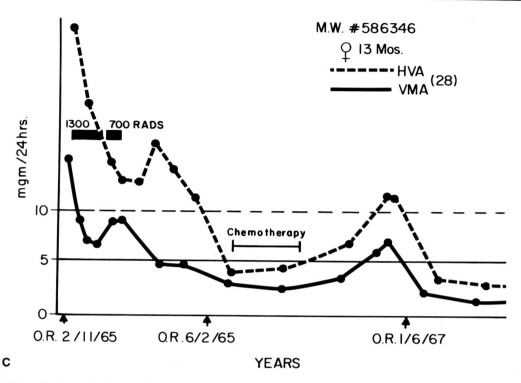

Figure 7.12. (A) Effect of radiation therapy on the urinary VMA and HVA excretion in a 6-week-old male infant with neuroblastoma. The infant also had metastatic involvement of the liver (stage IV-S). Note interval of one year between two courses of radiation therapy; we were able to predict recurrence of the tumor with this marker, however. During the second course of treatment liver was considerably smaller and much smaller volume was radiated. Patient is alive and well 17 years later. **(B)** Effect of irradiation and chemotherapy on the urinary excretion of VMA and HVA in a 4-month-old male infant with liver involvement (stage IV-S). The infant died approximately two years after initial treatment. Note lack of response to treatment when compared with Figure 7.14A. **(C)** Effect of excision, irradiation, and chemotherapy on the urinary excretion of HVA and VMA in a 13-month-old female infant with a stage III abdominal neuroblastoma. She is alive and well, 14 years after her first surgery. *(Courtesy of Cancer 32:623, 1973.)*

TUMORS OF THE ANGIOMATOUS TISSUE

The early radiotherapy literature is replete with instances of the use of radiation therapy to control the growth and progression of benign angiomatous tumors and malformations. However, it has been documented that enlargement can occur during the first six months of life, with ultimate spontaneous regression in 90 percent and complete disappearance in most children.[86] Aggressive treatment, with unnecessary sequelae, should therefore be avoided. In certain unusual circumstances and locations in which the hemangioma fails to regress and interferes with vital functions such as mastication or vision, radiation therapy has been given, often with

gratifying results. It is essential to emphasize that any undue desire to irradiate or operate must be checked, and the main objective of treatment should be masterly inactivity toward the angioma, with support to the child and the parents. For example, in a laryngeal hemangioma a temporary tracheostomy probably will remove the immediate respiratory obstruction, and with time the angioma will regress. In the unlikely event that the lesion fails to regress, and other methods of management have failed, radiation therapy might be considered (Fig. 7.13A and 7.13B). The possibility of a second primary cancer in the irradiated field must be considered before embarking on the use of radiation therapy in the management of these benign lesions.

The hemangioendothelioma of infancy is a

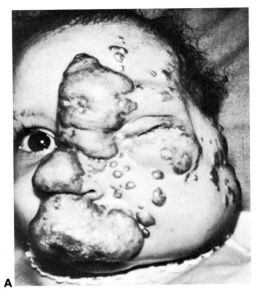
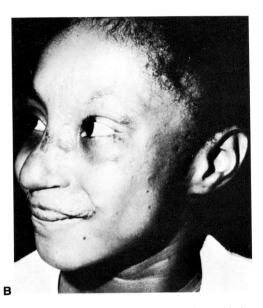

Figure 7.13. **(A)** One-year-old girl with extensive hemangioma of the face and neck. Note large submandibular component. Because of the refractory nature of this hemangioma she was referred for radiation therapy. The involvement was divided into four areas, each of which received 800 rads in 10 fractions over a period of four months. **(B)** Same patient 10 years later. Mild residua remain from previous involvement.

benign tumor, although in some instances the immediate clinical features are suggestive of a highly malignant vascular tumor. The majority of these tumors are self-limiting, however, and do not require any form of radical therapy, be it excision or irradiation. In the past we successfully treated a 4-day-old female infant with a large tumor of the scapular region by radical radiation therapy.[87]

Rarely, malignant hemangioendotheliomas or angiosarcomas are encountered in children.[88–89] When they occur in adults the outcome is frequently fatal, especially if they are primarily located in a viscus. Stout and Lattes[90] observed that malignant hemangioendotheliomas in adults had a 56 percent fatal outcome, whereas in their 14 cases arising in children only four, or 28 percent, were fatal. Although radiation therapy plays an important role both in curative and palliative management of angiosarcoma of the liver and spleen, those of the extremities are better treated by resection.

Hemangiopericytomas are best treated by excision. Primary radiation therapy is indicated only in cases of unresectable tumors or in cases of incomplete excision. Buschke and Parker[91] stated that the variation in biologic behavior

makes short-term studies of control in this tumor type of little value. They could control a small hemangiopericytoma of the tongue and oropharynx with a dose of 5,500 rads in six weeks, but failed to do so in a tumor of the pelvic soft tissue with a dose of 6,000 rads in six and one half weeks. Friedman and Egan[92] studied 10 tumors irradiated in five patients and added three cases from the literature. From these 13 tumor responses they concluded that a lethal radiation dose for hemangiopericytoma probably lies in the range of 7,500 to 9,000 rads given in 30 to 60 days. For palliation, a minimum tumor dose of 3,000 rads in 18 days was recommended. Mira and co-workers[93] studied the response of hemangiopericytoma to radiation therapy in 11 patients treated at Memorial Sloan-Kettering Cancer Center. Response of greater or lesser degree was noted in 26 of 29 radiation therapy courses administered. These included 14 instances of complete tumor regression. Dose and tumor size were the main factors influencing response. The tumors tended to regress slowly and incompletely; yet effective relief of symptoms and long-term local control (average duration 27 months) usually was achieved. These authors found that a dosage above 3,600 rads, or NSD over 1,375 rets, led to eventual complete regression.

KAPOSI'S SARCOMA

The typical clinical presentation is the appearance of multiple vascular, rubbery, bluish-red nodules, with or without pigmented plaques in the skin and subcutaneous tissues of the distal extremities (Fig. 7.14A to 7.14C). These nodules grow, coalesce, and ulcerate. Although the skin is the usual site of involvement, all organs, particularly the gastrointestinal tract, may be affected. Progression is slow and death may occur from systemic disease, but more often death is due to factors related to advanced age.

Since 1962, the University of Illinois Radiation Therapy Division has treated 11 patients with moderately advanced Kaposi's sarcoma. Nine were men with a mean age of 70 years; and two were women 56 and 78 years old, respectively. Among the men, four had advanced disease of the lower extremities. Three of the four retained their extremities even in the face of early osseous involvement. However, the remaining elderly man required amputation of his leg. He had originally been treated elsewhere for Kaposi's sarcoma of the hands and feet.

Cohen[94] studied the dose, time, and volume parameters in radiation therapy for Kaposi's sarcoma. He noted that these nodules are usually highly responsive, and obtained local control in 83 percent of patients treated with the single dose equivalent of 1,000 rads. He recommended a dose of 2,500 rads in three weeks for an entire extremity. Superficial radiation is used for skin nodules, and 200 to 300 kv of radiation for deeper lesions. Vogel and associates[95] showed that Kaposi's sarcoma is also a chemotherapy-responsive tumor, with either actinomycin D alone or in combination with vincristine.

TECHNIQUES

The effects of radiation on tissue are dependent upon the final total dose, the total number of days over which it is delivered, the fraction size (the number of rads given at a treatment), and the volume of tissue irradiated. Attempts have been made to quantitate these concepts with various mathematical formulas (Ellis-NSD).[96–97]

However, all such efforts at quantification have numerous shortcomings and, ultimately, clinical judgement must supervene.

The aim of treatment planning is to deliver tumoricidal doses of radiation to a tumor volume while keeping the doses to the surrounding tissues as low as possible. This may be accomplished by rotating or arcing the gantry to obtain the desired dose distribution, or using multiple fixed fields to avoid critical structures. Occasionally the implantation of radioactive isotopes directly into a soft tissue sarcoma or tumor bed is used in addition to external radiation. This has the advantage of delivering a high local dose to a confined volume.

A simulator should be used to plan the desired treatment portals, since this may provide fluoroscopic aid in defining tumor volumes and ensure reproducibility of the fields and the treatment machine. Weekly verification films should be taken to ensure reproducibility of the treatment set-up. Supervoltage equipment should be used because of its skin-sparing, increased depth dose characteristic and relatively decreased absorption in bone. Electrons or superficial equivalent may be used to boost scar regions or areas of skin thought to be involved with tumor or at high risk for involvement. Each opposing portal, nonopposing pair, any three-field arrangement, or pair wedges would have the daily tumor dose being contributed in part by each of the portals. By this technique the tolerance of normal structures is improved. For further details the reader is referred to a monograph on the subject.[98]

Immobilization of the patient is important, and proper techniques should be used to ensure that the daily treatment is repeated accurately. This aspect of treatment planning becomes extremely important in childhood sarcomas. Various casts and molds have been designed to ensure the immobility of the child and thereby increase accuracy.*

There is continual change in the technical aspects of treatment of soft tissue sarcomas. With increasing knowledge of the natural history of these tumors and the application of multimodality therapy, the end results are improving.

---

*Advances made in our casting techniques are described in detail in Liebner EJ, Haas RE, DeSio, V. Immobilization of pediatric radiotherapy patients. Applied Radiology 9(4):40, July/August 1980.

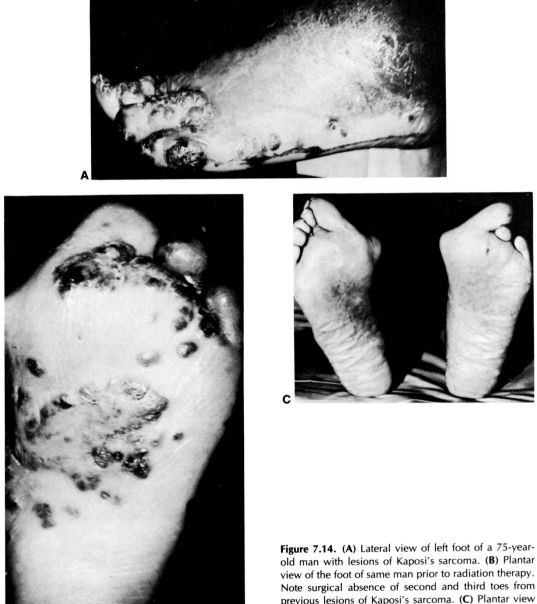

Figure 7.14. **(A)** Lateral view of left foot of a 75-year-old man with lesions of Kaposi's sarcoma. **(B)** Plantar view of the foot of same man prior to radiation therapy. Note surgical absence of second and third toes from previous lesions of Kaposi's sarcoma. **(C)** Plantar view of both feet taken eight years after radiation therapy. The whole left foot received 3,000 rads in five weeks in 25 fractions.

Sophisticated methods of irradiation of the entire extremities have been developed. We have provided here only a brief outline of the general principles of techniques in use today. The interested reader should consult other reports for further details.[10,12,16,25,29,32,98-100] In treatment planning, the use of xeroradiography and computerized axial tomography, especially for deep-seated lesions, is helpful in detecting the presence of satellite nodules or residual tumor. As mentioned earlier in the discussion of rhabdomyosarcoma and synovial sarcoma, because of the higher incidence of lymph node metastases, lymphangiography might be of value. In patients with tumors with a relatively high incidence of node metastases, the regional node-bearing area should be considered in the initial large volume that is to be irradiated. In most patients there will probably be no need to include the nearest joint unless invasion of the joint has occurred. If possible, the patella should not be irradiated. Attempts should be made to keep the radiation dosage to a minimum in surface areas that are subject to constant wear and tear of function, such as the sole of the foot, the anterior tibial skin, and the Achilles tendon.

If there is an incision it should be completely healed. The entire circumference of an extremity should be avoided. Friedman[100] described a method of using a Lucite bent hemicylinder applied to the lateral (remote) aspect of the arm. However, wedge filters, compensator filters, cerrobend molds, and proper field arrangements can also be used to minimize the amount of normal tissue irradiated.[101] Those using electron beam therapy may wish to treat the total volume encompassed in a wax model to produce uniform thickness of the entire part.[52] By these various approaches one tries to avoid

a severe constricting fibrosis with resultant varying degrees of edema below the irradiated fields (Fig. 7.15). The tourniquet method has no advantage in terms of local recurrence rate, and a number of significant complications have been reported.[7]

DOSE CONSIDERATION

In general, the best results for radiotherapy of primary soft tissue sarcomas are after resection of all macroscopic tumors.[102] Generally, margins of resection should be treated with 5,000 rads when possible, with successive "cone down volume" to 6,000 to 7,000 rads. It is best to give 200 rads a day for five days a week. When an anterior-posterior pair of parallel opposed fields are used, each field is treated daily with one-half the dose (100 rads). In the initial part of the treatment a generous margin of 6 to 8 cm about the scar should be used. This large volume is treated to 5,000 rads in five weeks. After that, the volume should be reduced, eg, 3 to 4 cm in all directions about the scar. Following this, the smaller volume can be given additional irradiation up to 6,000 rads. If desired, the final dose at the immediate primary lesion can be in the range of 6,300 to 7,000 rads over a period of six and one half to seven and one half weeks. Lindberg and associates,[25] using these improved techniques and radical-dose radiation therapy, had only 67 of 300 patients (22 percent) with local regrowth of their soft tissue sarcomas during a followup in excess of two years. Eighty-four percent of the patients thus treated retained a useful limb free of pain or edema.

In contrast, Suit and his colleagues[16] proposed the use of preoperative radiation therapy

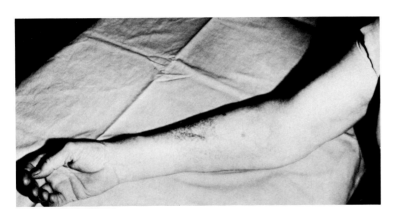

Figure 7.15. Right forearm of a 54-year-old woman, taken 10 years after photon and electron beam radiation treatments. Note absence of edema. There is moderate fibrosis and telangiectasis at the site of maximum dosage. The original tumor, a 5 × 5 cm mass, received 5,000 rads in five weeks to the midplane of the forearm. After a rest period of three weeks a smaller portal, 7 × 10 cm to include the primary, was used to deliver an additional 3,000 rads via electron beam in three weeks.

as an alternative for the management of adult soft tissue sarcomas. In this program, after establishing the histologic diagnosis by an incision biopsy, the primary tumor is irradiated. The dose consists of 5,000 to 6,000 rads over a period of 5 to 6 weeks at a daily dose of 200 rads for 5 days a week. The first 5,000 rads are given over a fairly generous field, including the tumor and the probable boundary, outlining extension into the surrounding tissues. The next 500 to 1,000 rads are delivered to a reduced field, covering the demonstrable tumor by only a small margin. A conservative resection is performed two to three weeks later, followed by a booster dose of 1,000 to 1,500 rads to the tumor bed given intraoperatively by the interstitial implantation technique or electron beam, or postoperatively by small field external photon beam. With very few exceptions, partial regression was found at the time of the operation. The greatest degree of histologic change was observed in high-grade tumors and in lesions that had received more than 4,000 rads.[103] In a series of 52 patients treated by this program, Suit[103] found that 6 (11.5 percent) showed local failure and 20 (38 percent) had distant metastases. Seven of the 52 (13 percent) had wound-healing problems, with one requiring amputation.

COMPLICATIONS OF COMBINED THERAPY

The rate of complications of combined surgery and radiation therapy is dependent on meticulous treatment planning, total radiation dose, and, more importantly, the type and extent of normal tissue within the radiation portal. In a large series of 200 patients with sarcoma of the extremities, the overall rate of complications was 6.5 percent.[25] The most significant complications were soft tissue necrosis (three patients), fibrosis (three patients), and fracture (two patients). The peripheral edema, soft tissue necrosis requiring amputation, and nerve and vascular damage were seen rarely (one patient in each category). In the early years of radiotherapy for soft tissue sarcoma, the full width of the extremity was treated and 6 of 18 patients required an amputation to relieve severe pain and edema secondary to constricting fibrosis.[24] By sparing as much normal tissue as possible, the incidence of complications is diminished. It is also essential to limit the radiation dose to crit-

ical organs such as kidney, stomach, small bowel, and spinal cord to their tolerance limits during the treatment for retroperitoneal sarcomas.

INNOVATIONS IN RADIOTHERAPY

Currently, only locally advanced or recurrent sarcomas that are refractory to surgery are treated with innovative treatments such as neutrons and hyperthermia. Neutrons are high LET particles, with a significant mass and no charge. This results in dense ionization in the tissues traversed by these particles, causing significant damage to the tumor. Advanced tumors with a large proportion of hypoxic tumor cell populations are particularly vulnerable to neutrons. The experience with neutron therapy of soft tissue sarcomas is still in its infancy, but the preliminary results are encouraging. Salinas et al.[104] treated 29 patients with soft tissue sarcoma to a dose of 6,000 to 7,000 rads (gamma equivalent). Of these 29 patients, 20 (69 percent) were locally controlled and in 4 (14 percent) skin necrosis developed. It is worthy of note that of 12 patients who had subsequent histologic evaluation of the tissue, 6 had no residual tumor histologically.

Catterall[105] described 28 sarcoma patients treated with 1,560 neutron rads in 12 fractions over four weeks, achieving 75 percent local control with 32 percent major complications. This increase in complications was attributed to the depth dose characteristics and quality of their 16-MeV$_{d-Be}$ neutron beam. In Japan, Morita et al.[106] treated 12 patients with soft tissue sarcoma and achieved a local control rate of 58 percent (7/12). At the Fermi National Acceleratory Laboratories (Batavia, Illinois), Hendrickson and his colleagues[107] treated 16 patients with advanced soft tissue sarcomas. Nine of the 16 (56 percent) had a complete response and 8 of these 9 patients were disease-free after one year. Although additional confirmatory data are needed, neutron therapy should be seriously considered for all locally advanced and inoperable sarcomas.

Hyperthermia at temperatures from 42–44°C has been shown to be tumoricidal in vitro[108-109] and in man[108,110] with various solid tumors. Heat causes alteration in both DNA and RNA synthesis as well as depression of multiple cellular enzymatic systems required for cell metabolism and division. Its major modes of action may be due to increased cell lysosome membrane permeability, causing selective internal destruction of the cancer cell.

Investigations are under way to evaluate the cytotoxic effects of heat, either alone or in conjunction with irradiation; the proper sequencing of these two treatment modes is not yet available.[111,112]

The use of regional chemotherapy and radiation therapy as a method of preserving the limb in patients with soft tissue sarcoma is being actively investigated in most centers.[113] In Chapter 8, this subject is dealt with in further detail.

The potential advances would greatly enhance the value of radiation in the management of soft tissue sarcomas. More optimum time-dose relations must be achieved for sarcomas at various sites by appropriate manipulation of the time, fraction number, and the dose.[114] If hypoxic cell sensitizers can improve the therapeutic ratio, greater local control will be attained and normal tissue reactions reduced.[115]

In summary, the former pessimism regarding the role of radiation therapy in the primary control of malignant mesenchymal tumors should be replaced with a more positive attitude. Radiation therapy is not a substitute for adequate excision, but it is a valuable adjuvant. The preservation of a functional extremity is the reward with the combined modality approach. However, further improvement in survival should come from effective control of distant micrometastases and early detection.

REFERENCES

1. del Regato JA: Radiotherapy of soft tissue sarcomas. JAMA 185:216, 1963
2. Suit HD, Lindberg RD, Fletcher GH: Prognostic significance of extent of tumor regression at completion of radiation therapy. Radiology 84:1100, 1965
3. Das Gupta TK: Management of soft tissue sarcomas. (Editorial). Surg Gynecol Obstet 137:1011, 1973
4. Bagshaw MS, Doggett RLS: A clinical study of chemical radiosensitization. In Vaeth JA (ed): Frontiers of Radiation Therapy and Oncology, vol 4. Basel/New York, Karger, 1969, p 164
5. Brenner SM, Miller SP, Custodio D: Soft tissue sarcoma: Treatment with methotrexate and radiation. New York J Med 70:855, 1970
6. Byail RD, Hanham IW, Newton K, et al: Combined treatment of soft tissue and osteosarcomas by radiation and ICRF-159. Cancer 34:1040, 1974
7. Suit HD, Lindberg RD: Radiation therapy administered under conditions of tourniquet-induced local tissue hypoxia. Am J Roentgenol 102:17, 1968
8. Van Den Brenk HAS, Kerr RC, Madigan JP, Cass NM, Richter W: Results from tourniquet anoxia and hyperbaric oxygen techniques combined with megavoltage treatment of sarcomas of bone and soft tissue. Am J Roentgenol 96:760, 1966
9. Scanlon PW: Split-dose radiotherapy for radioresistant bone and soft tissue sarcoma: Ten years' experience. Am J Roentgenol 114:544, 1972
10. McNeer GP, Cantin J, Chu F, Nickerson JJ: Effectiveness of radiation therapy in the management of sarcoma of the soft somatic tissues. Cancer 22:391, 1968
11. Sagerman RH, Tretter P, Ellsworth RM: The treatment of orbital rhabdomyosarcoma of children with primary radiation therapy. Am J Roentgenol 114:31, 1972
12. Suit HD, Russell WD, Martin RG: Sarcoma of soft tissue: Clinical and histopathologic parameters and response to treatment. Cancer 35:1478, 1975
13. Windeyer B, Dische S, Mansfield CM: The place of radiotherapy in the management of fibrosarcoma of the soft tissue. Clin Radiol 17:32, 1966
14. Atkinson L, Garvan JM, Newton NC: Behavior and management of soft connective tissue sarcomas. Cancer 16:1152, 1963
15. Morton DL, Eilber FR, Townsend CM, et al: Limb salvage from a multidisciplinary approach for skeletal and soft tissue sarcoma of the extremity. Ann Surg 184:268, 1976
16. Suit HD, Proppe KH, Mankin JH, Woods WC: Preoperative radiation therapy for sarcoma of soft tissues. Cancer 47:2269, 1981
17. Perry H, Chu FC: Radiation therapy in the palliative management of soft tissue sarcoma. Cancer 15:179, 1962
18. Friedman M, Egan JW: Irradiation of liposarcoma. Acta Radiol 54:225, 1960
19. Moss WT, Brand WN, Battifora H (eds): Radiation Oncology, 4th ed. St. Louis, Mosby, 1973, p 602
20. Edland RW: Liposarcoma. A retrospective study of fifteen cases, a review of the literature, and a discussion of radiosensitivity. Am J Roentgenol 103:778, 1968
21. Reszel PA, Soule EH, Coventry MB: Liposarcoma of the extremities and limb girdles. J Bone Joint Surg 48-A:229, 1966
22. Brasfield RD, Das Gupta TK: Liposarcoma. Cancer 20:3, 1970
23. Enterline HT, Culberson JD, Rocklin DB, Broley LW: Liposarcoma: A clinical and pathological study of 53 cases. Cancer 13:992, 1960
24. Suit HD, Russell WO, Martin RG: Management of patients with sarcoma of soft tissue in an extremity. Cancer 31:1247, 1973
25. Lindberg RG, Martin RA, Romsdahl MM, Barkley Jr HT: Conservative surgery and postoperative radiotherapy in 300 adults with soft tissue sarcomas. Cancer 42:2391-2397, 1981
26. Cade S: Soft tissue tumors: Their natural history and treatment. Proc Roy Soc Med 44:19, 1951

27. Pritchard DJ, Soule EH, Taylor WF, Ivins JC: Fibrosarcoma—A clinicopathologic and statistical study of 199 tumors of the soft tissue of the extremities and trunk. Cancer 35:888, 1974

28. Benninghoff D, Robbins R: The nature and treatment of desmoid tumors. Am J Roentgenol 91:132, 1964

29. Hill DR, Newman H, Phillips TL: Radiation therapy of desmoid tumors. Am J Roentgenol 117:84, 1973

30. Suit HD, Russell WO: Radiation therapy of soft tissue sarcoma. Cancer 36:759, 1975

31. Massoud GE, Awwad HK: Nasopharyngeal fibroma: Its malignant potentialities and radiation therapy. Clin Radiol 11:156, 1960

32. Lindberg RD, Martin RG, Romadahl MH: Surgery and postoperative radiotherapy in the treatment of soft tissue sarcoma in adults. Am J Roentgenol 123:123, 1975

33. Sutow WW: Cancer of the head and neck in children. JAMA 190:414, 1964

34. Liebner EJ: Embryonal rhabdomyosarcoma of head and neck in children. Cancer 37:1777, 1976

35. Ellis F: Dose, time, and fractionation: A clinical hypothesis. Clin Radiol 20:1, 1969

36. Cassady RJ, Sagerman RW, Tretter P, Ellsworth RM: Radiation therapy for rhabdomyosarcoma. Radiology 91:116, 1968

37. Masson JK, Soule EH: Embryonal rhabdomyosarcoma of the head and neck: Report of 88 cases. Am J Surg 110:585, 1965

38. Donaldson SS, Castro JR, Wilbur JR, Jesse RH Jr: Rhabdomyosarcoma of the head and neck in children. Cancer 31:26, 1973

39. Heyn RM, Holland R, Newton WA, et al: The role of combined chemotherapy in the treatment of rhabdomyosarcoma in children. Cancer 34:2128, 1974

40. Fernandez CH, Sutow WW, Merino OR, George SL: Childhood rhabdomyosarcoma. Analysis of coordinated therapy and results. Am J Roentgenol 123:588, 1975

41. Harris HH: Rhabdomyosarcoma of the larynx: Report of a case. Arch Otolaryngol 74:205, 1961

42. Pearson RW, Gamme EB, Thayer W: Rhabdomyosarcoma of the hypopharynx. Arch Otolaryngol 64:238, 1956

43. Glick HN: Unusual neoplasm in the larynx of a child. Ann Otolaryngol 53:699, 1944

44. Cady B, Rippey JH, Frazell EL: Non-epidermoid cancer of the larynx. Ann Surg 167:166, 1968

45. Batsakis JG, Fox JE: Rhabdomyosarcoma of the larynx. Arch Otolaryngol 91:136, 1970

46. Rodriguez LA, Zinskind J: Rhabdomyosarcoma of the larynx. Larnygoscope 80:1733, 1970

47. Pochedly C, Suwansirikul L, Piacitelli J: Rhabdomyosarcoma producing respiratory obstruction. JAMA 217:969, 1971

48. Nelson AJ: Embryonal rhabdomyosarcoma: Report of 24 cases and study of the effectiveness of radiation therapy upon the primary tumor. Cancer 22:64, 1968

49. Edland RW: Embryonal rhabdomyosarcoma. Five-year survival of patients treated by radiation and chemotherapy. Am J Roentgenol 99:400, 1967

50. Edland RW: Embryonal rhabdomyosarcoma. Am J Roentgenol 93:671, 1965

51. Lindberg RD: Rhabdomyosarcoma in children: Treatment and results. In Neoplasia in Childhood. Chicago, Year Book Medical Publishers, 1969, p 201

52. Holton CP, Chapman KE, Lackey RW, et al: Extended combination therapy of childhood rhabdomyosarcoma. Cancer 32:1310, 1973

53. Jaffe N, Filler RM, Farber S, et al: Rhabdomyosarcoma in children. Improved outlook with a multidisciplinary approach. Am J Surg 124:426, 1973

54. Smith DM: Rhabdomyosarcoma of the head and neck. Canad J Otolaryngol 3:618, 1974

55. Ghavimi F, Exelby PR, D'Angio GJ, et al: Multidisciplinary treatment of embryonal rhabdomyosarcoma in children. Cancer 35:677, 1975

56. Potter GD: Embryonal rhabdomyosarcoma of the middle ear in children. Cancer 19:221, 1966

57. Barnes PH, Maxwell MJ: Embryonal rhabdomyosarcoma of middle ear: Report of a case of 12 years' survival, with a review of the literature. J Laryngol Otol 86:1145, 1972

58. Conte PJ, Sagerman RH: Embryonal rhabdomyosarcoma of the middle ear with long-term survival. N Engl J Med 284:92, 1971

59. Ragab AH, Vietti TJ, Kassane JM, Sessions DG: Rhabdomyosarcoma of the middle ear. A four-year survival. Cancer 39:648, 1972

60. El-Mahdi AM, Marks R Jr, Thornton WM, Constable WC: Twenty-five year survival of sarcoma botryoides treated by irradiation. Cancer 33:653, 1974

61. Schweisguth O: Panel on rhabdomyosarcoma and neuroblastoma. In Golden JO (ed): Cancer in Childhood. Toronto, Holt, Rinehart and Winston, 1973, p 196

62. Pratt CB, Hustu HO, Fleming ID, Pinkel D: Treatment of childhood rhabdomyosarcoma with surgery, radiotherapy, and combination chemotherapy. Cancer Res 32:606, 1972

63. Suit HD: Soft tissue sarcoma. (Chap 13.) In Fletcher GH (ed): Textbook of Radiotherapy. Philadelphia, Lea and Febiger, 1973, pp 786-789

64. Das Gupta TK, Brasfield RD: Solitary malignant schwannoma. Ann Surg 171:419, 1970

65. Evans AE: Congenital neuroblastoma. J Clin Path 18:54, 1965

66. Koop CE, Schnaufer L: The management of abdominal neuroblastoma. Cancer 35:905, 1975

67. Breslow N, McCann B: Statistical estimation of prognosis for children with neuroblastoma. Cancer Res 31:2098, 1971

68. Koop CE, Kiesewetter WB, Horn RC Jr: Neuroblastoma in childhood—an evaluation of surgical management. Pediatrics 16:652, 1955

69. Sutow WW: Prognosis of neuroblastoma in childhood. Am J Dis Child 96:299, 1958

70. Fortner J, Nicastri A, Murphy ML: Neuroblastoma—Natural history and results of treating 133 cases. Ann Surg 167:132, 1968

71. Koop CE, Hernandez JR: Neuroblastoma—Experience with 100 cases in children. Surgery 56:726, 1964

72. Lingley JF, Sagerman RH, Snatulli TV, Wolff JA: Neuroblastoma—Management and survival. N Engl J Med 277:1227, 1967

73. Perez CA, Vietti TJ, Ackerman LV, Kulapongs P, Powers WE: Treatment of malignant symphathetic tumors in children: Clinicopathological correlation. Pediatrics 41:452, 1968

74. Maurer HM: Current concepts in cancer. N Engl J Med 299:1345, 1975

75. Pinkel D: Curability of childhood cancer. JAMA 235:1049, 1976

76. Evans AE, D'Angio GJ, Randolph J: A proposed staging for children with neuroblastoma. Cancer 27:374, 1971

77. Evans AE, Albo V, D'Angio GJ, Finkelstein JZ, Leiken S, Santulli T, Weiner J, Hammond GD: Factors influencing survival of children with nonmetastatic neuroblastoma. Cancer 38:661, 1976

78. Evans AE, Albo V, D'Angio GH, et al: Cyclophosphamide treatment of patients with localized and regional neuroblastomas. A randomized study. Cancer 38:655, 1976

79. Liebner EJ, Rosenthal IM: Serial catecholamines in the radiation management of children with neuroblastoma. Cancer 32:623, 1973

80. Berman HL: The role of radiation therapy in the management of synovial sarcoma. Radiology 81:997, 1963

81. Cadman NL, Soule EH, Kelly PJ: Synovial sarcoma. An analysis of 134 tumors. Cancer 18:613, 1965

82. Pack GT, Ariel IM: Synovial sarcoma (malignant synovioma): A report of 60 cases. Surgery 28:1047, 1950

83. Raben M, Calabrese A, Higginbothham NL, Phillips R: Malignant synovioma. Am J Roentgenol 93:145, 1965

84. Van Andel JG: Synovial sarcoma: A review and analysis of treated cases. Radiol Clin Biol 41:145, 1972

85. Mackenzie DH: Synovial sarcoma. A review of 58 cases. Cancer 19:169, 1966

86. Lister WA: The natural history of strawberry nevi. Lancet 1:1429, 1938

87. Liebner EJ: Hypertrophic hemangio endothelioma of infancy. Am J Roentgenol Rad Ther Nucl Med 86:5870593, 1961

88. Kauffman SL, Stout AP: Hemangiopericytoma in children. Cancer 13:695, 1960

89. Kauffman SL, Stout AP: Malignant hemangioendothelioma in infants and children. Cancer 14:1186, 1961

90. Stout AP, Lattes R: Tumors of soft tissue. Atlas of Tumor Pathology, Series 2, Fasc 1. Washington DC, AFIP, 1967, p 137

91. Buschke F, Parker RG: Radiation Therapy in Cancer Management. New York. Grune and Stratton, 1972, p 361

92. Friedman M, Egan JW: Irradiation of hemangiopericytoma of Stout. Radiology 74:721, 1960

93. Mira JC, Chu FCH, Fortner JG: Radiotherapy for hemangiopericytoma. Cancer 39:1254, 1977

94. Cohen L: Dose, time and volume parameters in irradiation therapy of Kaposi's sarcoma. Br J Radiol 35:485, 1962

95. Vogel CL, Primack A, Dhru D, et al;: Treatment of Kaposi's sarcoma with a combination of actinomycin-D and vincristine. Cancer 31:1382, 1973

96. Ellis F, Sorensen A: A method of estimating biological effect of combined intracavitary low dose rate radiation with external radiation in carcinoma of the cervix uteri. Radiology 110:681, 1974

97. Orton OG, Ellis F: A simplification in the use of NSD concept in practical radiotherapy. Br J Radiol 46:529, 1973

98. Rubin P, Casarett G: A direction for clinical radiation pathology. Vol 6, Radiation Effect and Tolerance, Normal Tissue. In Vaeth JM (ed): Frontiers of Radiation Therapy and Oncology. Baltimore, University Park Press, 1972, p 1

99. Parker RG: Tolerance of mature bone and cartilage in clinical radiation therapy. In Vaeth JA (ed): Frontiers of Radiation Therapy and Oncology. Radiation Effect and Tolerance, Normal Tissue. vol. 6. University Park Press Baltimore, 1970, p. 312

100. Friedman M: Technic for large-dose irradiation of connective tissue sarcoma of the extremity. Radiology 84:1113, 1965

101. Wang CC, Fleischli DJ: Primary reticulum cell sarcoma of bone with emphasis on radiation therapy. Cancer 22:994, 1968

102. Leibel SA, Tranbaugh RF, Wara WM, Beckstead JH, et al: Soft tissue sarcomas of the extremities: Survival and patterns of failure with conservative surgery and postoperative irradiation compared to surgery alone. Cancer 50:1076, 1982

103. Suit HD: Soft tissue sarcomas: The role of radiation therapy. Hosp Prac 17:114, 1982

104. Salinas R, Hussey DH, Fletcher GH, Lindberg RD et al: Experience with fast neutron therapy for locally advanced sarcomas. Rad Oncol Biol Phys 6:267, 1980

105. Catterall M: Observation on the reaction of normal and malignant tissue to a standard dose of neutron. Proceedings of 3rd meeting on fundamental and practical aspects of fast neutrons and other high LET particles in clinical radiotherapy. The Hague. Sept 1978. Europ J Cancer 1979

106. Morita S, Tsunemoto H, Kurisu A, Umegaki Y, Nakayano N: Results of fast neutron therapy at NIRS. Presented: 4th High LET Radiotherapy Seminar. Sponsored by U.S.-Japan Cooperative Cancer Research Program, Philadelphia, June 19-20, 1978

107. Hendrickson FR: Use of high energy particles for inoperable or recurrent soft tissue tumors. Personal communication

108. Cavaliere R, Ciocatto EC, Giovanella BC, Heidelberger C, et al: Selective heat sensitivity of cancer cells: Biochemical and clinical studies. Cancer 20:1351, 1967

109. Giovanella BC, Morgan AC, Stehlin JS, Williams LJ: Selective lethal effects of supranormal temperatures on mouse sarcoma cells. Cancer Res 33:2568, 1973

110. Storm FK, Harrison WH, Elliott RS: Hyperthermia in cancer treatment: Normal tissue and solid

tumor effects in animal models and clinical trials. Cancer 39:2245, 1979

111. Stewart FA, Denekamp J: Fractionation studies with combined x-rays and hyperthermia in vivo. Br J Radiol 53:346, 1980

112. Stewart FA, Denekamp J: The therapeutic advantage of combined heat and x-rays on a mouse fibrosarcoma. Br J Radiol 51:307, 1978

113. Eilber FR, Mirra JJ, Grant TT, Weisenburger T, Morton DL: Is amputation necessary for sarcomas: A seven-year experience with limb salvage. Ann Surg 192:431, 1981

114. Peschel RE, Fisher JJ: Optimization of the Time-Dose relationship. Sem Oncol 8:38, 1981

115. Phillips TL: Sensitizers and protectors in clinical oncology. Sem Oncol 8:65, 1981

8

Chemotherapy

Tapas K. Das Gupta

In the past, chemotherapy of soft tissue sarcomas was associated with occasional success, but in general the literature was replete with less than glowing reports. The efficacy of any form of chemotherapy as the sole treatment in soft tissue sarcomas is still considered doubtful. As recently as 1977, Krakoff[1] classified soft tissue sarcomas in the category of borderline responders to chemotherapy. Although there is enough reason for such pessimism in adult soft tissue sarcomas, recent reports of excellent end results[2-15] with chemotherapy for childhood sarcomas, notably embryonal rhabdomyosarcoma,[2,16-21] justify reappraisal of its value in the treatment of soft tissue sarcomas in general.

Over the years most clinical oncologists have considered soft tissue sarcomas as a single entity, all with the same natural history and all responding in the same manner to the same type of therapy, be it surgery, chemotherapy, or irradiation. This erroneous concept has resulted in error in planning the management of this disease, especially the metastatic type. Histologists have long argued that the term soft tissue sarcoma represents a myriad of clinicopathologic entities, each with a distinct biologic behavior, and that the management should be tailored to the histogenetic origin. If this premise is accepted and applied to the management of these tumors, then the role of chemotherapy becomes increasingly clear.

An analysis of reported responses of specific histologic types of metastatic malignant mesenchymal tumors in adults to various chemotherapeutic agents is shown in Tables 8.1 through 8.5.[3-5,17,18,22-39] Some of the data in these tables are confusing because of the small numbers of patients and the use of drug combinations without defining the activity of a given drug. Additionally, the response rate was not computed in measurable lesions in all instances. Therefore, it is not possible to discern the actual efficacy of the drugs used in liposarcomas, fibrosarcomas, and leiomyosarcomas. It is apparent, though, that most agents, or combinations of agents, showed promise in the management of rhabdomyosarcomas. Gottlieb and associates[22] also reported that five of nine patients with synovial sarcoma responded to chemotherapy. The response in angiosarcomas was not convincing (Table 8.5).

Wasserman and co-workers[40] tabulated the relative efficacy of a number of drugs used for treating various sarcomas and compiled a roster that is of great help in developing chemotherapy regimens (Table 8.6). It is evident from this table that only a few agents are of proven value, and the majority of drug regimens used in this country are a combination of some of these agents. More recently, other agents and different combinations have been tried in the management of soft tissue sarcomas, but so far no

TABLE 8.1. CHEMOTHERAPEUTIC REGIMENS FOR LIPOSARCOMA

Drug(s)	Dosage	Time Increments	Comments	Response	Duration (mo)
Actinomycin D[31]	15 mcg/kg (0.015 mg/kg) IV	Per day	Given for 5 days. Cycle is repeated every 4 to 6 weeks	2/5	3 to 4
Adriamycin* and DTIC[22]	60 mg/m² IV 250 mg/m²	Day 1 Days 1 to 5	Drugs are administered every 21 days	7/8	17 + (median)
Adriamycin,* DTIC, vincristine[24,25]	60 mg/m² IV 250 mg/m² IV 1.5 mg/m² IV (maximum single dose, 2 mg)	Day 1 Days 1 to 5 Days 1 and 5	Drugs are given in a 28-day cycle	2/4	Not specified

*Given to 500 mg/m² total dose.

TABLE 8.2. CHEMOTHERAPEUTIC REGIMENS FOR FIBROSARCOMAS

Drug(s)	Dosage	Time Increments	Comments	Response	Duration (mo)
Actinomycin[31]	0.5 mg/day IV	Days 1 to 5	Drugs are administered every 6 weeks	2/7	3 to 4
Adriamycin,* DTIC[22] methotrexate[30]	60 mg/m² IV 250 mg/m² 2.5 mg-10 mg	Day 1 Days 1 to 5 Per day	Drugs are administered orally for 2 to 15 days	11/25 5/7	13 + (median) No effect seen on survival
Adriamycin,* DTIC, vincristine[25,26]	60 mg/m² IV 250 mg/m² IV 1.5 mg/m² IV (maximum single dose is 2 mg)	Day 1 Days 1 to 5 Days 1 and 5	Drugs are administered every 21 days	3/6	1 to 23 +

*Given to a total dose of 500 mg/m².

TABLE 8.3. CHEMOTHERAPEUTIC REGIMENS FOR LEIOMYOSARCOMA

Drug(s)	Dosage	Time Increments	Comments	Response	Duration (mo)
Adriamycin* Actinomycin D[31]	75 mg/m² IV 0.5 mg IV	Day 1 Daily for 5 to 12 days	Drug given every 21 days	2/6 12/27	7.5 + (median) 2 +
Methotrexate[30] Adriamycin* and DTIC[22]	0.3 to 1.4 mg/kg 60 mg/m² IV 250 mg/m² IV	Twice weekly Day 1 Days 1 to 5	Intravenously Drugs administered every 21 days	4/11 19/38	3 + 17 + (median)
Adriamycin,* DTIC, vincristine[23,25]	60 mg/m² IV 250 mg/m² IV 1.5 mg/m² IV (maximum 2.0 mg/dose)	Day 1 Days 1 to 5 Days 1 and 5	Drugs are administered every 21 days	5/10	5 + (median)

*Given to a total dose of 500 mg/m².

TABLE 8.4. CHEMOTHERAPEUTIC REGIMENS FOR RHABDOMYOSARCOMA

Drug(s)	Dosage	Time Increments	Comments	Response	Duration (mo)
Actinomycin D[17,18,31,33]	0.015 mg/kg IV	Days 1 to 5	Given every 6 weeks	23/24	Not defined. No response seen until after 2 cycles
Vincristine[3]	1.5 mg/m^2	Per week	Single dose not to exceed 2 mg	17/21	1 to 18 months
Mitomycin[34]	0.4–1.0 mg/kg	Daily	2 to 10 days	4/11	3
Cytoxan[27,35]	30 mg/kg I.V.	Weekly	Given over 28 days as one cycle	10/12	2 to 6
Adriamycin,* DTIC[22]	60 mg/m^2 I.V. 250 mg/m^2 I.V.	Day 1 Day 1 to 5	Drugs are administered in a 21-day cycle	7/18	13+ (median)
Adriamycin,* DTIC, Vincristine[23]	60 mg/m^2 I.V. 250 mg/m^2 I.V. 1.0 mg/m^2 I.V.	Day 1 Days 1 to 5 Days 1 and 5	Drugs are administered in a 21-day cycle.		
Vincristine,	2 mg/m^2 I.V. (maximum single dose 1.5 mg)	Weekly	For 12 doses	13/19	18 to 62
Actinomycin D,	0.075 mg/kg I.V. over 5 days (max. single dose 0.5 mg/day)	Days 1 to 5	Every 3 months for 5 cycles		
Cytoxan[7,18]	10 mg/kg/day	Days 1 to 7 I.V. or p.o.	Every 6 weeks for 2 years		

*Given to a total dose of 500 mg/m^2.

TABLE 8.5. CHEMOTHERAPEUTIC REGIMENS FOR ANGIOSARCOMA

Drug(s)	Dosage	Time Increments	Comments	Response	Duration (mo)
Vincristine[5,38]	2.0 mg IV	1 to 2 × weekly		3/7	No effect on survival
Cytoxan[27,35,37]	200 mg	Daily		1/4	6
Adriamycin,* DTIC[24]	60 mg/m^2 IV 250 mg/m^2 IV	Day 1 Days 1 to 5	Drugs administered every 21 days	3/9	18+ (median)
Cytoxan, vincristine[5,38]	300 mg/m^2 IV 1.5 mg/m^2 IV		Maximum dose 2 mg	1/2	10+

*Given to a total dose of 500 mg/m^2.

TABLE 8.6. CHEMOTHERAPY RESPONSE IN SOFT TISSUE SARCOMA*

Drugs	Activity	No. Responses/ No. Evaluable Patients	Response Rates (%)	Comments
Actinomycin D	+ +	20/83	24	Commonly used for treatment of sarcomas
Adriamycin	+ +	88/351	25	Same as above
Cyclophosphamide	+ +	48/93	52	Same as above
Vincristine	+ +	25/53	47	Commonly used
CHL	+	7/28	25	
DTIC	+	15/127	12	Commonly used
DBD	+	7/44	16	
Methotrexate	—	2/39	5	Role being reappraised
M CCNU	—	4/72	6	
HXM	—	1/43	2	
BCNU	Not evaluated	1/17	24	
CCNU	Not evaluated	1/22	5	
STZ	Not evaluated	1/7	—	
L-ASP	Not evaluated	0/1	—	
S-AZC	Not evaluated	0/4	—	

*Adapted from Wasserman et al., 1975.[40]
+ + Adequate evaluation – drug very active.
+ Adequate evaluation – some drug activity present.
– Adequate evaluation – drug inactive.

new agent has been isolated that can be considered notably superior to the agents described in Table 8.6. However, the efficacy of Cis-platinum in the overall management of sarcomas is presently being investigated, and this agent may prove to be of value.

Prior to 1970, the most commonly used chemotherapeutic agents in soft tissue sarcomas were cyclophosphamide, actinomycin D, and vincristine, given alone or in combination. In 1970, Jacobs[41] reviewed several individual series and found that 56 of 238 patients (23.5 percent) had shown an objective response to these drugs. However, when the childhood cases of rhabdomyosarcoma were eliminated, the response rate was found to be only 18 percent (32 of 179 cases), and only a small number of long-term remissions was reported.

In 1969, Di Marco, Gaetani, and Scarpinato[42] reported encouraging results in initial trials with adriamycin in the treatment of soft tissue sarcomas. Definite activity was also noted during the initial investigations with 5-(3,3-dimethyl–triazeno) imidazole-4-carboxamide (DTIC), a synthetic congener of the naturally occurring purine precursor 5-(or 4)-aminoimidazole 4-(or 5)-carboxamide.[26,43,44] During initial single-agent trials with adriamycin and DTIC,

response rates of 29 percent and 15 percent, respectively, were achieved by most centers.[22,24,26,36,43-49] When the bony sarcomas were excluded from this analysis, adriamycin was shown to produce a response rate of 22 percent and DTIC, 15 percent (Table 8.7). Since neither of these drugs was thought to be cross-resistant, and in view of their relatively different side effects, a study of their combined use in advanced sarcomas was carried out by Gottlieb and co-workers[24] (Table 8.8). Of 78 patients with all types of soft tissue sarcomas, only 5 (6.4 percent) showed complete remission; there was partial remission in 28 (36 percent). There was no instance of complete remission in synovial cell sarcoma, fibrosarcoma, mesothelioma, neurofibrosarcoma, or the miscellaneous types. Table 8.9 shows the responses to this regimen according to the site of metastasis. In contradistinction to metastatic tumors from other sites (eg, breast), there appeared to be no difference in response based on the dominant site of metastases. Gottlieb[23] reviewed the results of the M.D. Anderson Hospital and Southwest Cancer Chemotherapy Study Group (SWCCSG) in 1974 and concluded that out of 200 evaluable patients with all types of soft tissue and bone sarcomas, 22 showed complete response and 63

TABLE 8.7. SUMMARY OF RESPONSE IN SARCOMAS TO ADRIAMYCIN OR DTIC*

Diagnosis	No. Patients	Adriamycin CR/PR[†]	References	No. Patients	DTIC CR/PR*	References
Sarcoma, unspecified and misc.	37	−/5	24,42,47	7	−/−	43,48
Rhabdomyosarcoma	16	−/2	36,42,47	13	−/2	24,49
Fibrosarcoma	5	−/3	36,43	11	−/1	24
Liposarcoma	4	−/2	36,43	2	−/−	24
Leiomyosarcoma	3	−/−	36,43	24	1/5	24
Synovial cell sarcoma	3	1/2	36,43	1	−/−	24
Total	68	1/14 (22)%		58	1/8 (15.5%)	

*Adapted from Gottlieb et al., 1972.[24]

†CR = Complete remission; PR = Partial remission.

partial response, the overall rate being 42.5 percent. The M.D. Anderson Hospital and SWCCSG modified their two-drug regimen with the addition of a third drug, vincristine, and compared the response rates to the two-drug and three-drug schedules. Analysis of both partial and complete responses in advanced soft tissue sarcomas showed that, of the 149 patients treated with the adriamycin-DTIC combination, 67 (45 percent) showed some degree of response. Of the 32 patients treated with vincristine-adriamycin-DTIC, 18 (56 percent) responded (Table 8.10). Although these two protocols (Nos. 445 and 7210) did not show any significant differences in response rate, these investigators recommended the three-drug combination for the majority of patients.

In 1973, Benjamin and co-workers[46] reported a 41 percent response rate in several types of soft tissue sarcomas with the use of adriamycin alone. Gottlieb et al.,[26] in 1976, reviewed the role of DTIC as a single agent in the treatment of soft tissue sarcomas and concluded that, at best, it showed modest activity only in Kaposi's sarcoma and leiomyosarcoma. However, in combination with adriamycin it showed some increase over the response rate with adriamycin alone. They found also that DTIC lengthened the duration of remission. Although the role of vincristine in combination with actinomycin D and cyclophosphamide is well established in the treatment of childhood sarcomas,[3-7,9-13,16-19,27,33,35,50-56] its proper place as an agent in the management of adult soft tissue sarcomas remains un-

TABLE 8.8. RESPONSE, BY DIAGNOSIS, OF TREATMENT WITH COMBINATION OF ADRIAMYCIN AND DTIC*

Diagnosis	No. Evaluable	Complete Response	Partial Response	Overall Response Rate (%)
Synovial cell sarcoma	2		2	100
Rhabdomyosarcoma	5	1	2	60
Undifferentiated sarcoma	13	1	5	46
Fibrosarcoma	11		5	46
Liposarcoma	7	1	2	43
Mesothelioma	7		3	43
Neurofibrosarcoma	10		4	40
Leiomyosarcoma	16	1	5	38
Angiosarcoma	5	1		20
Miscellaneous	2			0
Total	78	5 (6.4%)	28 (36%)	

*Adapted from Gottlieb et al., 1972.[24]

TABLE 8.9. RESPONSE BY SITE OF METASTASES*

Site of Major Metastases	No. Cases	Response (%)
Lung	58	43
Liver	17	41
Nodes	14	36
Soft tissue	17	41
Bone	14	36

*Adapted from Gottlieb et al., 1972.[24]

clear. Additionally, when vincristine and DTIC are added to adriamycin, there are some undesirable side effects, namely, increased gastrointestinal toxicity and marrow suppression.

A review of the published data on chemotherapy of adult soft tissue sarcomas suggests, although the conclusions are sometimes too optimistic, that adriamycin constitutes the most effective single agent, and the addition of DTIC probably improves the response rate, duration of response, or both, in a reasonable number of patients. In 1977, Pinedo and Kenis[25] reviewed the literature on chemotherapy of advanced soft tissue sarcomas in adults and, in summary, expressed the generally held view that the most effective regimen is a combination of cyclophosphamide, vincristine, adriamycin, and DTIC.[25,28,57] However, this four-drug combination has not been directly compared with any combination of two or three agents or against adriamycin alone. Furthermore, a comparative study of the relative risk/benefit ratios of single and combined agents has not yet been published.

A correct histogenetic classification of a given soft tissue sarcoma should be the fundamental basis for planning the method of management. The present chapter is the result of our experience at the University of Illinois in treating more than 300 primary and metastatic soft tissue sarcomas and tumors of peripheral nerve origin. On the basis of this experience we have developed certain guidelines, and these will be the main theme of this chapter. We do not propose to deal with the clinical pharmacology or cell kinetics of the various agents used in the treatment of soft tissue sarcomas, nor do we attempt a comprehensive review of all the published case reports purporting complete or partial remission of a tumor following use of a myriad of combinations of chemotherapeutic agents.

From our observations on the effectiveness of chemotherapeutic agents such as actinomycin D, adriamycin, cyclophosphamide, vincristine, DTIC, methotrexate, and CCNU, used either singly or in combination, as well as our review of other studies,[1,7,19,20,22-28,30,31,34-36,41,48,58-61] the responsiveness of various metastatic adult soft tissue sarcomas to chemotherapy was graded as follows: excellent—complete response of a measurable metastatic lesion for a minimum of 12 weeks in at least 40 percent of the tumors evaluated; good or fair—partial response lasting for 12 weeks or more in 40 percent and 30 percent, respectively; poor—inconsistent partial response, not possible to quantitate. The results of our analysis are summarized in Table 8.11.

Chemotherapeutic agents in general had little effect on most adipose tissue sarcomas, nor

TABLE 8.10. COMPLETE AND PARTIAL RESPONSE RATES IN SOFT TISSUE SARCOMA PATIENTS (M.D. ANDERSON HOSPITAL AND SWCCSG DATA)*

Histologic Type	Adriamycin and DTIC (Protocol 445)†	Adriamycin, DTIC, Vincristine (Protocol 7210)†	Combined Response	
Angiosarcoma	3/8*	0/1	3/9	(33%)
Fibrosarcoma	11/23	3/6	14/29	(48%)
Liposarcoma	5/16	2/4	7/20	(48%)
Leiomyosarcoma	17/36	5/10	22/46	(48%)
Neurofibrosarcoma	10/22	—	10/22	(45%)
Rhabdomyosarcoma	7/17	2/3	9/20	(45%)
Synovial cell sarcoma	5/8	6/8	11/16	(68%)
Undifferentiated sarcoma	9/19	6/8	15/27	(56%)
Total	67/149 (45%)	18/32 (56%)	85/181	(46.9%)

*Complete and partial response shown in numerator and number of evaluable patients in denominator—Adapted from Gottlieb, 1974.[23]
†The difference in response rates with protocols 445 and 7210 between different histologic types is not significant at $p = 0.05$.

TABLE 8.11. METASTATIC SOFT TISSUE SARCOMAS—RESPONSE TO CHEMOTHERAPEUTIC AGENTS (BASED ON UNIVERSITY OF ILLINOIS SERIES OF 232 PATIENTS AND COMPARISON WITH OTHER PUBLISHED REPORTS)*

Type of Tumor	No. Patients	Response†					Comments
		Excellent	Good	Fair	Poor	None	
ADIPOSE TISSUE							
Liposarcoma	39			+			Pleomorphic variety (grades 3 and 4) showed partial response. Other types and grades responded poorly
FIBROUS TISSUE							
Fibrosarcoma	41			+			High-grade fibrosarcomas responded, but erratically. Low grade showed poor response
MALIGNANT FIBROUS HISTIOCYTOMA	31		+				Malignant fibrous histiocytoma was responsive
Malignant histiocytoma	3		+				Responded well
MUSCLE TISSUE							
Leiomyosarcoma	22		+				Muscle tumors, both smooth and voluntary varieties, responded to chemotherapy
Rhabdomyosarcoma							Response rate in adults was not so spectacular as in children
Embryonal	21	+					
Pleomorphic	11	+					
Alveolar	3		+				
PERIPHERAL NERVE TISSUE							
Malignant schwannoma	28				+		In general, did not respond to chemotherapy
SYNOVIAL TISSUE							
Synovial sarcoma	9		+				Synovial cell sarcoma and its variants showed some responsiveness
Epithelioid sarcoma	2		+				
Clear cell sarcoma of tendon sheath	2					+	
ANGIOMATOUS TISSUE							
Angiosarcoma and hemangioendothelioma	8			+			Tumors of the blood vessels responded but response varied and accurate assessment was not possible. None of the lymphangiosarcomas was responsive
Hemangiopericytoma	7			+			
Lymphangiosarcoma	2					+	
HETEROTOPIC BONE OR CARTILAGE	3						
Extraosseous osteosarcoma and chondrosarcoma					+		Poor
Total	232						

*For reference see text.

†Excellent response: Complete resolution of any measurable metastatic lesion for 12 weeks or more in 40 percent or more of the cases evaluated.

Good: Partial response of any measurable metastatic lesion for 12 weeks in 40 percent of the cases.

Fair: Partial response of any measurable metastatic lesion for 12 weeks in 30 percent of the cases.

Poor: Response erratic and could not be quantitated.

on grades 1 and 2 fibrosarcomas; however, grades 3 and 4 fibrosarcomas did respond. Malignant fibrous histiocytomas showed a moderate response, and the majority of malignant tumors of muscle tissue were responsive. Peripheral nerve tissue tumors were generally resistant to chemotherapy (Table 8.11).

In some instances the malignant tumors of synovial cell origin showed a good-to-fair response, whereas the few clear cell sarcomas of the tendon sheath were nonresponders. Of the tumors arising from angiomatous tissue, lymphangiosarcomas were the least sensitive to chemotherapy. Of the remaining sarcomas, none appeared to be overtly sensitive to the conventional chemotherapeutic agents.

From this analysis it appears that there is a definite place for chemotherapy in the management of certain adult soft tissue sarcomas. Remarkable palliation can be achieved in some patients with advanced disease, although in others there is little if any beneficial effect.

On the basis of published data[1,7,20,22-28,41,48,57,59,60] and our own material, the role of chemotherapy in the management of adult soft tissue sarcomas can be divided into two distinct categories: (1) in the palliation of some patients with advanced disease, with occasional long-term control; (2) as a systemic adjuvant to primary surgical and/or radiation therapy, or in the form of adjuvant regional therapy—for example, isolated limb perfusion or intra-arterial infusion.

TREATMENT OF METASTATIC SOFT TISSUE SARCOMAS

The effectiveness of chemotherapy in soft tissue sarcomas is interpreted as either a complete response, meaning total disappearance of all measurable lesions and subjective improvement for a period of one month or more, or a partial response, in which case there is at least a 50 percent reduction in the sum of the products of the two largest perpendicular diameters of all measurable lesions. Although both single and combination drug therapy has been applied, the effectiveness demonstrated in childhood sarcomas has not yet been duplicated in adult types. The difference between childhood and adult sarcomas is most evident in the treatment results of rhabdomyosarcoma.[58] For example, with vincristine, cyclophosphamide, and actinomycin D, the response rate in children

varies between 27 and 62 percent,[4-6,27,35,53] whereas in adults it is less than 20 percent.[4-6,27,53] The significant improvement in the treatment of adult soft tissue sarcomas has in all probability been effected solely by the use of adriamycin. The major factor in its effectiveness is its steep dose response curve. In a Southwest Oncology Group study, patients were initially randomized to receive three courses of chemotherapy with adriamycin at either 45 mg/m^2 (28 patients) or 75 mg/m^2 (41 patients). At the low dose, a response rate of less than 20 percent was observed, compared to 37 percent observed with the higher dose. Subsequently, an intermediate dose of 60 mg/m^2 (10 patients) showed a response rate only slightly higher than the low dose (45 mg/m^2). The difference in rate of response between the high and low doses was significant with a p-value of 0.05. For the 3-dose comparison, the p-value was 0.07.[62]

It is argued that single-agent chemotherapy is not adequate for advanced soft tissue sarcomas,[35,37] and combinations with varying cycles and regimens have been, or are being, tried. A brief review of these combination schedules shows that vincristine plus actinomycin D[25,52] is unsatisfactory. A combination of vincristine, actinomycin D, and cyclophosphamide, so effective in childhood sarcomas,[4-6,25] is far less successful in adults.[4-6,27]

The combination of adriamycin and DTIC (ADIC) has resulted in a significant improvement in the treatment of metastatic soft tissue sarcomas. Benjamin and associates[62] updated the original data reported by Gottlieb and associates[24] on the efficacy of the adriamycin and DTIC combination, and found that in 218 evaluable patients a complete response rate of about 11 percent and overall response rate of 42 percent could be achieved. The overall tolerance of this regimen is good. Nausea and vomiting are often severe on the first day, but less than five percent of patients require withdrawal of treatment because of these side effects. Mild stomatitis occurs in the second week in about 15 percent of patients. Occasionally, fever is observed on day 1. The white blood cell count nadir occurs at the end of the second week, with rapid recovery and often a rebound by the end of the third week.

Vincristine has been added to the ADIC regimen because of its known activity as a single agent in soft tissue sarcomas, especially in children. Gottlieb and co-workers[22,24,28] evaluated 86

TABLE 8.12. RESPONSE TO *VADIC* ACCORDING TO HISTOLOGIC TYPE*

Histologic Type	No. Patients	Response Rate Complete (%)	Partial (%)
Liposarcoma	15	15	47
Fibrosarcoma	10	10	60
Leiomyosarcoma	22	22	36
Rhabdomyosarcoma	9	22	67
Neurofibrosarcoma	3	33	33
Synovial cell sarcoma	2	0	50
Angiosarcoma	7	0	57
Mesothelioma	6	0	0
Undifferentiated sarcoma	12	33	59
Total	86	9	47

*Bone sarcomas excluded from the report (adapted from Gottlieb et al.,[22] 1975).

patients treated with this combination and found a complete remission rate of 9 percent (Table 8.12). The addition of vincristine had little influence on the response rate except in fibrosarcomas and in undifferentiated sarcomas.

Supposedly, the most effective combined chemotherapeutic regimen for soft tissue sarcoma consists of cyclophosphamide, vincristine, adriamycin, and DTIC (the CYVADIC regimen). Cyclophosphamide was added because it has some activity as a single drug. Its addition to the VADIC regimen required reduction of the adriamycin dose to 50 mg/m². The cyclophosphamide dose and schedule initially used by the Southwestern Oncology Group was 500 mg/m² on day 1, the dose of DTIC and vincristine being kept unchanged. This four-drug regimen (SWOG-7302) is indicated here as CYVADIC I to distinguish it from a protocol (SWOG-7402)

with a modified schedule (CYVADIC II). In the first 12-month period the SWOG-7302 (CYVADIC I) protocol was applied, 118 patients with soft tissue sarcoma were evaluable; 18 of these (15 percent) showed complete remission and 52 (44 percent), partial remission, the overall response rate being 59 percent (Table 8.13). From the data presented it is impossible to calculate the exact percentage of patients whose disease remained stable or improved slightly, but in a group of 136 patients, including those with sarcoma of the bones, only 22 percent showed progression of disease with the CYVADIC I regimen. The remission rate obtained with the CYVADIC II regimen was lower than that obtained with CYVADIC I (52 percent and 59 percent, respectively). It should be emphasized once again that, for both combination regimens and single-agent treatment, there are in-

TABLE 8.13. RESPONSE TO *CYVADIC I* (SWOG-7302) ACCORDING TO HISTOLOGIC TYPE OF TUMOR*

Histologic Type	No. Evaluable Patients	Response Rate Complete (%)	Partial (%)
Liposarcoma	10	10	60
Fibrosarcoma	23	17	57
Leiomyosarcoma	28	7	68
Rhabdomyosarcoma	15	40	67
Neurofibrosarcoma	13	23	62
Synovial cell sarcoma	3	0	67
Angiosarcoma	5	0	80
Mesothelioma	6	0	33
Undifferentiated sarcoma	15	13	40
Total	118	15	59

*Adapted from Gottlieb et al.[22]

dications that the dose of adriamycin should not be lower than 50 mg/m² and the treatment intervals should not be prolonged for more than three or four weeks. Adriamycin and its metabolites are eliminated over a period of several days, and therefore the high tissue levels of the drug persist for several days. Although addition of vincristine might improve the overall result, the most effective schedule still remains to be determined. The addition of cyclophosphamide to the VADIC regimen, although it slightly improves the response rate, does result in significantly greater myelosuppression, with about 25 percent of the patients having an absolute granulocyte count of less than 500 cell/mm³ for a short period at some time during the course of chemotherapy. Only a few infections with lethal complications are recorded.

A combination of adriamycin, actinomycin D, vincristine, and cyclophosphamide (CYVADACT) has also been tried.

The Southwest Oncology Group compared the efficacy of CYVADIC with CYVADACT in a randomized study.[62] The CYVADIC regimen (193 patients) produced a 14 percent complete and 52 percent overall response, whereas in the group treated by the CYVDACT regimen (199 patients) the complete and overall response rates were 12 percent and 40 percent, respectively. But although the CYVADIC protocol appeared to be effective, the results were only slightly superior to those obtained by the two-drug regimen of adriamycin and DTIC. The ADIC combination was also found to provide better survival rates than did the CYVADACT regimen.

Pinedo and Kenis[25] reported the preliminary results of a protocol of adriamycin-DTIC-cyclophosphamide-actinomycin D, which was being used by the European Soft Tissue Working Party of the Organization on Research and Treatment of Cancer (EORTC). Vincristine was eliminated because of the unacceptable 18 percent incidence of neurotoxicity and the limited beneficial results. The regimen was a dismal failure.

A multitude of combinations and protocols both with and without adriamycin have been tried. Pinedo and Kenis[25] reviewed all these protocols and their effectiveness and concluded that all combinations without adriamycin are inferior to any combination with adriamycin. The effectiveness of adriamycin improves with the addition of DTIC.

An update on the original CYVADIC pilot

study was recently reported by Yap and colleagues.[63] A 50 percent response rate was observed in 125 evaluable patients, and the complete remission rate was 17 percent.

From all available data[22-26,28,57] and from our own experience, the CYVADIC I combination probably is the most useful. However, this conclusion is only temporary and further investigation is in order. For example, in a recent review of 357 patients taken from the literature, Pinedo and van Oosterom[64] found a mean response rate of only 27 percent. It appears that with use of the popular CYVADIC regimen the complete response rate in most centers remains around 10 percent to 14 percent. Furthermore, analysis of end result data published by Gottlieb[23] between an adriamycin and DTIC combination (Protocol 445) and adriamycin, DTIC, and vincristine (Protocol 7210) showed no significant difference in response rate (Table 8.10). Therefore, the optimum method of managing metastatic soft tissue sarcomas remains an unanswered question. Because of these controversies and uncertainties, multiple chemotherapy protocols with various modifications in dose, route of administration, and schedule are being tested. For instance, at the M. D. Anderson Hospital the current schedule consists of Cytoxan 600 mg/m² and adriamycin 60 mg/m², on day 1, and DTIC 1 gm/m² by continuous 96-hour infusion via a central venous catheter. Doses are repeated every 3 to 4 weeks, at recovery of 1500 granulocytes and 100,000 platelets, with a 25 percent increase in adriamycin and Cytoxan if no morbidity occurs, regardless of low counts. Using this aggressive chemotherapy regimen, the investigators at the M. D. Anderson Hospital have observed decreased cardiac toxicity, a 14 percent complete response, and 53 percent overall response.

At Memorial Sloan–Kettering Cancer Center other protocols, eg, adriamycin, methyl–CCNU, and vincristine, or a disease-oriented combination consisting of high-dose methotrexate with vincristine (VIM), adriamycin, and dactinomycin in a sequential fashion have been used with further additions and alterations in the drugs and schedule of administration, with the response rates varying from 27 percent to 44 percent. Recently, these investigators[65] reported on their experience with a combination of adriamycin, DTIC, Cytoxan, methotrexate, and vincristine. Of 36 evaluable patients treated with this program, 4 had complete and 5 had partial response.[65] From these data the authors concluded that CYOMAD offered no therapeutic advantage over the previous protocols. For nonresponsive sarcomas, we believe that a different form of chemotherapy and the addition of hormone therapy or immunotherapy is indicated.

ADJUVANT CHEMOTHERAPY FOR PRIMARY SOFT TISSUE SARCOMAS IN ADULTS

A program of adjuvant systemic chemotherapy has been in progress for the past seven years in the Division of Surgical Oncology at the University of Illinois, based on our overall experience with the responsiveness of advanced sarcomas to various types of chemotherapy (Table 8.11) as well as the experience of other authors[2,5-9,16-20,22-39,60] (Tables 8.1 through 8.10). The data reported herein are based on the results of this study. Table 8.14 shows the types of sarcoma that we have treated with adjuvant chemotherapy.

Our analysis of overall efficacy versus systemic toxicity of the CYVADIC regimen compared with either adriamycin alone or the ADIC combination in the treatment of metastatic sarcomas led us to conclude that, at least for the present, the risk/benefit ratio between the use

of a four-drug combination and a one- or two-agent program has not been clearly defined. Therefore, as an adjuvant in an ambulatory setting, we elected to use a combination of adriamycin and DTIC. The drug regimen essentially was the same as that reported by Gottlieb and co-workers.[22-24] It consists of adriamycin, 60 mg/m^2, on day 1 and DTIC, 250 mg/m^2, given intravenously on days 1 through 5. The entire regimen was repeated every 21 days. Adriamycin was given up to a total dose of 500 mg/m^2 and DTIC was continued for one year or 17 cycles. In the following pages we report the results obtained from this study.

The results of this treatment program were compared with the results in a group of patients with similar types of primary malignant mesenchymal tumors that we treated with resection alone. All tumors were histologically confirmed as grade 3 or grade 4 and all were staged as T_1 (5 centimeters or less) or T_2 (larger than 5 centimeters).

Adjuvant Chemotherapy Group
One hundred thirteen adult patients with primary mesenchymal sarcomas constituted this group. Table 8.15 shows the anatomic location and histologic distribution of the tumors. In 53 patients (47 percent) the primary tumor was T_1 and in 60 (53 percent), T_2. Sixty-seven tumors (59 percent) were grade 3, and 46 (41 percent), grade 4. The initial treatment of all tumors was entirely surgical: 100 patients (88 percent) had wide soft tissue (muscle group) resection, 8 (7 percent) had major amputation, and 5 (4 percent), local wide excision. The adjuvant chemotherapy was delivered either in our own clinic or by the referring physician elsewhere under our guidance. Regular followup was maintained on all patients and all living patients are still under followup. The entire program of adjuvant chemotherapy was carried out on an ambulatory basis.

Surgically Treated Group
One hundred forty-four patients constituted the group treated by surgery alone (Table 8.16). Sixty-one were operated upon prior to initiation of this program, and the remaining 83 have been treated during the same time period as the patients who received adjuvant chemotherapy. The anatomic sites of the primary tumors were comparable to those of the adjuvant chemotherapy group. Sixty-five patients (45 percent) had a T_1

TABLE 8.14. ADULT SOFT TISSUE SARCOMAS TREATED WITH ADJUVANT CHEMOTHERAPY

Tissue of Origin	Histologic Type	Grades
Adipose	Liposarcoma, pleomorphic or round cell types	3 and 4
Fibrous	Fibrosarcoma	3 and 4
	Malignant fibrous histiocytoma	All grades
Muscle	Leiomyosarcoma	All grades
	Leiomyoblastoma	All grades
	Rhabdomyosarcoma (all cell types)	All grades
Synovial	Synovial sarcoma	All grades
	Epithelioid sarcoma	All grades
Angiomatous	Angiosarcoma	All grades
	Malignant hemangioendothelioma	All grades

TABLE 8.15. HISTOLOGIC TYPE AND ANATOMIC SITE OF 113 PRIMARY SOFT TISSUE SARCOMAS TREATED BY ADJUVANT CHEMOTHERAPY AT THE UNIVERSITY OF ILLINOIS HOSPITAL

Histologic Type	Head and Neck	Upper Extremities	Trunk and Retroperitoneum	Lower Extremities	Misc. Sites	Total
Liposarcoma	1	1	2	4		8
Fibrosarcoma	1	2	2	4		9
Malignant fibrous histiocytoma	1	4	2	9		16
Leiomyosarcoma	—	2	4	3	11*	20
Leiomyoblastoma	—	—	1	—	7†	8
Rhabdomyosarcoma	7	4	6	9	—	26
Synovial sarcoma	1	3	1	8	—	13
Epithelioid sarcoma	—	3	1	1	—	5
Angiosarcoma	—	1	—	2	5‡	8
Total	11	20	19	40	23	113

*10 in gastrointestinal tract, one in vagina.
†Gastrointestinal tract.
‡3 in liver, 2 in breast.
Courtesy of Journal of Surgical Oncology, 19:139, 1982.

tumor and 79 (55 percent), a T_2. Eighty-two (57 percent) of the tumors were grade 3; 62 (43 percent) were grade 4.

In this group, 101 (70 percent) were treated by wide soft tissue (muscle group) resection, 29 (20 percent) by major amputation, and 12 (8.3 percent) by wide excision. Two patients with leiomyoblastoma of the stomach had radical subtotal gastrectomy. All patients in this group were treated in our center and had regular followup.

Toxicity. The adjuvant program, in which adriamycin and DTIC were used was, in general, without serious toxicity. The white blood cell count nadir was between days 10 and 14, with recovery by day 21. Dose escalation was not used, except in eight patients in whom the white blood cell count nadir was less than 3.0×10^{-3} mm^3. No septic complications were noted in any patient. Thrombocytopenia was not a problem.

Gastrointestinal toxicity was universal but

TABLE 8.16. HISTOLOGIC TYPE AND ANATOMIC SITE OF 144 SOFT TISSUE SARCOMAS TREATED ONLY BY SURGERY AT THE UNIVERSITY OF ILLINOIS HOSPITAL

Histologic Type	Head and Neck	Upper Extremities	Trunk and Retroperitoneum	Lower Extremities	Misc. Sites	Total
Liposarcoma	1	8	5	7		21
Fibrosarcoma	4	8	3	11		26
Malignant fibrous histiocytoma	6	8	4	8		26*
Leiomyosarcoma	—	2	4	2	10†	18
Leiomyoblastoma	—	—	—	—	2	2
Rhabdomyosarcoma	5	9	10	8	—	32
Synovial sarcoma	1	3	—	9	—	13
Angiosarcoma	—	1	—	2	3‡	6
Total	17	39	26	47	15	144

*5 more cases have since been added, making a total of 31.
†Gastrointestinal tract.
‡3 Liver.
Courtesy of Journal of Surgical Oncology, 19:139, 1982.

TABLE 8.17. DISEASE-FREE SURVIVAL OF 113 PATIENTS WITH SOFT TISSUE SARCOMAS FOLLOWING SURGICAL TREATMENT PLUS ADJUVANT CHEMOTHERAPY (UNIVERSITY OF ILLINOIS SERIES)

Histologic Type	No. Patients	2-Yr N.E.D.*	No. Eligible for 5-Yr Analysis	5-Yr N.E.D.
Liposarcoma†	8	4	8	3
Fibrosarcoma†	9	5	5	3
Malignant fibrous histiocytoma	16	14	12	10
Leiomyosarcoma	20	15	15	11
Leiomyoblastoma	8	8	6	5
Rhabdomyosarcoma	26	20	16	14
Synovial cell sarcoma	13	11	8	7
Epithelioid sarcoma	5	5	4	3
Angiosarcoma	8	5	4	2
Total	113	87 (77%)	78 (61%)	58 (74%)

*No evidence of disease.
†Only grades 3 and 4 liposarcomas and fibrosarcomas included in this study.
Courtesy of Journal of Surgical Oncology, 19:139, 1982.

manageable with standard antiemetics. In only one patient was nausea and vomiting manifest to such a degree that therapy was stopped after 10 cycles. Stomatitis was noted in 16 (14 percent) of the patients, but was never severe enough to require a dose de-escalation.

With the dosage of adriamycin used, the incidence of cardiac toxicity should be rare. In this series, two patients had abnormal electrocardiograms three months following completion of the adjuvant therapy. In neither patient

has clinical congestive heart failure developed, and both continue disease-free.

The overall tolerance of this adjuvant program was excellent, and in only three patients was the adjuvant program abandoned because of the patient's decision not to continue with treatment. However, the three patients are included in the end result data reported.

Results. Tables 8.17 and 8.18 summarize the two- and five-year disease-free survival rates in the two groups of patients. Applying Fisher's

TABLE 8.18. DISEASE-FREE SURVIVAL OF 144 PATIENTS WITH SOFT TISSUE SARCOMAS FOLLOWING SURGICAL TREATMENT (UNIVERSITY OF ILLINOIS SERIES)

Histologic Type	No. Patients	2-Yr N.E.D.†	No. Eligible for 5-Yr Analysis	5-Yr N.E.D.
Liposarcoma*	21	16	21	12
Fibrosarcoma*	26	18	26	16
Malignant fibrous histiocytoma	26	14	14	6
Leiomyosarcoma	18	6	18	6
Leiomyoblastoma	2	2	2	2
Rhabdomyosarcoma	32	15	25	10
Synovial cell sarcoma	13	11	13	9
Angiosarcoma and hemangioendotheliomas	6	3	4	1
Total	144	85 (59%)	122	62 (50%)

*Only grades 3 and 4 liposarcomas and fibrosarcomas are included in this table.
†No evidence of disease.
Courtesy of Journal of Surgical Oncology, 19:139, 1982.

exact test, it is apparent that overall short-term and long-term disease-free survival rates in the adjuvant chemotherapy group are significantly better than in the group treated by resection alone ($p = 0.05$).

LOCAL RECURRENCE. Eight (7 percent) of the 113 patients in the chemotherapy group had recurrence at the site of the primary tumor, seven within two years and the other at 4.5 years. In the surgically treated group, 12 (8 percent) had local recurrence, 8 within two years of excision of the primary tumor and 4 after two years, the longest interval being five and one half years. Analysis of these two groups of patients showed no significant difference in the incidence of local recurrence when adjuvant chemotherapy was added to wide soft tissue resection.

METASTASIS. Twenty-six (33 percent) of the 113 patients who received adjuvant chemotherapy showed evidence of metastatic disease within two years of treatment of the primary tumor. Out of the 78 patients suitable for five-year analysis, 25.6 percent succumbed to metastatic disease. The highest incidence of metastasis occurred in patients with liposarcoma and fibrosarcoma. In contrast, in the surgically treated group, 41 percent showed evidence of metastatic disease within two years and 50 percent within five years (Tables 8.17 and 8.18). Once metastasis occurred, further chemotherapy with various combinations of agents did not effectively prolong control of the disease in either group.

Although this is not a true prospective randomized clinical trial of adjuvant chemotherapy in soft tissue sarcomas, since all the tumors were classified, staged, graded, treated, and followed by us, some general guidelines and conclusions regarding different histologic types probably can be derived from this study.

Liposarcoma

Advanced liposarcoma in general does not respond well to chemotherapy (Tables 8.1, 8.7, 8.8, 8.10 and 8.11). Analysis by Fisher's exact test of both short-term and long-term end results in our two groups shows that there was no significant difference ($p = 0.36$ for two years and 0.59 for five years). When these results with adjuvant chemotherapy are compared with historical controls reported by Enterline et al.[66] and Enzinger and Winslow,[67] in which similar high-grade liposarcomas were treated by resection alone, it appears that the addition of a double-

agent adjuvant program was not effective in improving the disease-free survival rate. In our experience, when the adriamycin-DTIC regimen failed, the addition of vincristine or a change to other regimens did not materially alter the overall prognosis. It appears, therefore, that a search for a more effective combination is in order.

Fibrosarcoma

Nine patients with T_1 and T_2, grades 3 or 4, fibrosarcomas were entered into this adjuvant therapy protocol. In three, the adjuvant program failed during the period of administration, and in another patient metastasis became obvious immediately after completion of the protocol. Of the five now eligible for five-year end result analysis, three (60 percent) show no evidence of disease (Table 8.17). Of the 26 patients who had only radical resection, 16 (62 percent) survived five years without any evidence of recurrence or metastasis (Table 8.18). Analysis of the results obtained from these two groups of patients suggest that the overall end result was not influenced by the addition of the adjuvant chemotherapy program used here ($p = 0.72$ and 0.28 for two and five years, respectively).

Malignant Fibrous Histiocytoma

Sixteen patients with malignant fibrous histiocytoma participated in this adjuvant protocol. Fourteen of the 16 (87.5 percent) were disease-free at two years, and 12 of the 16 (75 percent) are now eligible for five-year analysis. Of these, 10 (83 percent) are still disease-free. Although survival for two years with no evidence of disease is generally viewed with optimism, 3 of the 16 patients in this study died of metastatic disease between the second and third years after treatment of the primary tumor. In a similar group of 26 patients treated by resection alone, 53 percent survived disease-free for two years, and of the 14 patients eligible for five-year analysis, 6 (43 percent) are still disease-free (Table 8.18). Analysis of the end results by applying Fisher's exact test shows the differences to be significant ($p = 0.05$). In the collective series of 200 patients reported by Weiss and Enzinger,[68] only 51 (26 percent) were disease-free at the end of five years. Our end results with adjuvant treatment (Table 8.17), compared with our own data without adjuvant treatment (Table 8.18) and with the data reported by Weiss and Enzinger,[68] indicate that the proportionate increase in disease-free survival with the addition of adjuvant therapy is significant at both the two-year and five-year levels. Unless definite evidence to the contrary is obtained from randomized national clinical trials, patients with malignant fibrous histiocytoma should receive some form of adjuvant chemotherapy. Possibly, a three- or four-drug adjuvant regimen may even further improve the disease-free survival in this histogenetic subtype of soft tissue sarcoma. Final conclusions, however, must await a randomized clinical trial.

Leiomyosarcoma

Twenty patients with leiomyosarcoma were treated with adjuvant chemotherapy (Table 8.17). Eleven (73 percent) of the 15 eligible for five-year analysis are disease-free. In a similar series of 18 patients treated by resection alone, 6 (33 percent) are disease-free at five years (Table 8.18). The difference in disease-free survival both for two and five years, when subjected to Fisher's exact test, was found to be significant at $p = 0.02$ and 0.05, respectively. Although Suit and coworkers[69,70] found that none of their three patients with leiomyosarcoma survived free of disease for two years, 15 (75 percent) of our 20 patients showed no evidence of recurrence or metastases at the end of the two-year period (Table 8.17). Leiomyosarcomas are infrequent in the extremities, and we have treated only five such cases, one of which could not be salvaged. It appears that leiomyosarcomas in the trunk and extremities can be well controlled with adjuvant chemotherapy. Discouraging results with adjuvant chemotherapy for leiomyosarcomas of the gastrointestinal tract and retroperitoneum[71] probably are related to delayed diagnosis and the size of the primary tumors.

Leiomyoblastoma

In general, the criteria used to designate malignancy in leiomyoblastomas are vague. Therefore, an extremely careful evaluation must be made before the patient is placed on a chemotherapy regimen. On the basis of the criteria described previously, eight of our patients were classified as having malignant leiomyoblastoma and were treated with adjuvant chemotherapy. Six of the eight were eligible for five-year analysis at the time of this writing. Five of the six (83 percent) still show no evidence of recurrence or metastasis (Table 8.17). It is not possible from our own material to provide any comparative

TABLE 8.19. ADJUVANT CHEMOTHERAPY FOR RHABDOMYOSARCOMA (UNIVERSITY OF ILLINOIS SERIES OF 26 PATIENTS*)

Histologic Type	No. Patients	2-Yr N.E.D.†	5-Yr N.E.D.
Embryonal	9	7	5/6
Pleomorphic	12	8	5/6
Alveolar	5	5	4/4
Total	26	20	14/16

*Number in numerator represents actual disease-free survivors, and in denominator, those eligible for 5-year analysis.
†No evidence of disease.

data from a group treated by resection alone, since we have only two such patients in our files, both of whom had leiomyoblastoma of the stomach. Both patients are still disease-free after five years. Because of the basic difficulty in establishing strict criteria to assess the true malignancy of the lesions, it is suggested, at least for the present, that adjuvant chemotherapy be individualized until more data on the biology of these tumors are acquired.

Rhabdomyosarcoma

Rhabdomyosarcoma in adult patients is known to respond to systemic chemotherapy,[2,18,21-25,28-29,33,35] although not so well as in children.[2-4,7,16-19] For the sake of analysis, the three types of rhabdomyosarcoma (embryonal, pleomorphic, and alveolar) were studied separately (Table 8.19).

Embryonal Rhabdomyosarcoma. Nine such patients were treated with adjuvant chemotherapy (Table 8.19). Seven (77 percent) were still disease-free two years later. Of six who became eligible for five-year analysis, five (83 percent) showed no evidence of disease. During chemotherapy local recurrence developed in one patient, and the disease progressed in one out of the seven patients who were free of disease at two years.

Pleomorphic Rhabdomyosarcoma. Twelve patients with this type of rhabdomyosarcoma were treated with adjuvant chemotherapy. Eight of the 12 (67 percent) survived disease-free for two years, and five of six eligible for five-year analysis were still disease-free. One had local recurrence and was salvaged by a second local excision; in another, local recurrence appeared concomitantly with systemic metastases.

Alveolar Rhabdomyosarcoma. Only five patients with alveolar rhabdomyosarcoma were treated with adjuvant chemotherapy in this series (Table 8.19). All were free of disease at two years. Of the four eligible for five-year survival analysis, none had either recurrence or metastasis.

When all three subtypes are combined into one single category of adult rhabdomyosarcoma in the adjuvant chemotherapy group of 26, it is found that 20 (77 percent) were disease-free at the end of two years and 14 of 16 (87 percent), at the end of five years. In contrast, in the group of 32 patients treated only surgically, disease-free survival for two and five years was 47 and 40 percent, respectively. These differences are highly significant (p = 0.04 and 0.01, respectively, for two and five years). Suit and co-workers[69,70] had no five-year disease-free survivors out of a group of 12 patients. McNeer et al.[72] had a 41 percent five-year disease-free survival rate in a total of 69 patients. From our own material, with and without the use of adjuvant chemotherapy in adult rhabdomyosarcoma of all types, and from comparison with other retrospective analyses, it appears that there is sufficient justification for use of adjuvant chemotherapy for all rhabdomyosarcomas.

Synovial Sarcoma

Thirteen patients with synovial sarcoma received adjuvant chemotherapy. At two years, 11 (85 percent) were still disease-free. Of 8 eligible for five-year analysis, 7 (87 percent) showed no evidence of recurrence or metastasis. Of the 13 patients, 2 (15.3 percent) had local recurrence within two years and showed progression of disease during chemotherapy (Table 8.17). In our group of patients who were treated without adjuvant chemotherapy (Table 8.18), 11 of 13 (85 percent) were disease-free at the end of two years, and 9 of 13 (69 percent) at the end of five years (Table 8.18). The difference in end results in these two groups was not significant (p = 0.60 and 0.61, for two and five years, respectively). Suit and co-workers[69,70] treated 15 patients with conservative excision and radical radiation therapy and achieved a 67 percent two-year survival rate. McNeer et al.,[72] in their retrospective analysis of 56 patients, found that radical surgery provided a five-year disease-free rate of 46 per-

cent. In the series reported by Mackenzie[73] and by Gerner and Moore,[74] five-year disease-free survival rates of 51 percent and 24 percent, respectively, were reported.

Analysis of our data with surgical treatment alone suggests that a well-planned resection of the primary tumor produces a good salvage rate. No apparent improvement in the end result was noted with adjuvant chemotherapy. However, a large number of patients with synovial sarcoma should be investigated before a definitive statement can be made.

Epithelioid Sarcoma

Epithelioid sarcoma is a relatively rare entity that has been recognized only recently. We have treated only eight patients. Five of these received adjuvant chemotherapy (Table 8.17). The remaining three received chemotherapy for advanced disease; they survived for four years, three years, and nine months, respectively (Table 15.6, Chapter 15). The data from these three patients and the data published by Pratt and co-workers[75] can be used as historical controls. These investigators[75] reported that 6 of 12 patients survived disease-free for two years, and 4, for five years. In our present adjuvant chemotherapy series, all five patients were disease-free for two years, and four were free of disease at five years or longer. The fifth is not yet eligible for five-year analysis. The use of adjuvant chemotherapy for epithelioid sarcoma clearly merits further investigation.

Angiosarcoma and Malignant Hemangioendotheliomas

It is difficult to establish a role for adjuvant chemotherapy in these entities. Eight of our patients were treated with an adjuvant chemotherapy program. Five of the eight (62 percent) were disease-free for two years, and two of the four who were eligible for five-year analysis showed no evidence of disease. In three of the eight, the tumor was located in the liver and none survived. Of six patients with angiosarcoma in various anatomic sites (including one in the liver) who were treated by resection alone, three lived apparently disease-free for two years (Table 8.18); one of the four (25 percent) eligible for five-year analysis is still free of disease (Table 8.18). When subjected to Fisher's exact test, the disease-free survival rates in the two groups were not significantly different. Of interest, however, is the fact that all five patients in whom

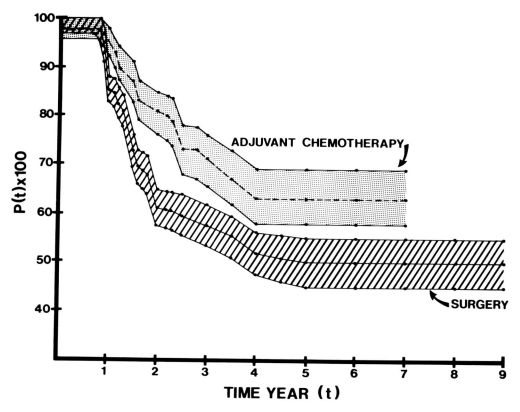

Figure 8.1. Overall corrected disease-free survival rate in adult soft tissue sarcomas in adjuvant chemotherapy and surgical resection group. *(Courtesy of Journal of Surgical Oncology 19:139, 1982.)*

the primary tumor was in superficial soft tissues appeared to have benefited from the use of this adjuvant chemotherapy program.

End Results. The end results of adjuvant chemotherapy with an adriamycin-DTIC combination in a series of 113 malignant mesenchymal tumors located in various anatomic sites show that 87 (77 percent) of the patients lived free of disease for two years. Of 78 patients suitable for five-year end result analysis, 58 (74 percent) are alive and free of disease. In contrast, of the 144 patients treated by resection alone, 85 (59 percent) were disease-free for two years, and of the 122 suitable for five-year end result analysis, 60 (50 percent) were disease-free. The two- and five-year disease-free survival rates in both groups were analyzed by the method of Kaplan and Meier.[76] Figure 8.1 shows the overall corrected disease-free survival in the two groups. It is apparent that the interval of disease-free survival in the adjuvant chemotherapy group is

significantly higher than in the group treated by resection alone ($p < 0.05$).

Comparative analysis of the local recurrence rate and disease-free survival between the adjuvant chemotherapy group and the surgical treatment group provides some guidelines in the management of soft tissue sarcomas. A combination of adriamycin and DTIC is of little use in liposarcoma and fibrosarcoma and is of questionable value in angiosarcoma and leiomyoblastoma; however, this drug combination appears to exert a beneficial effect on malignant fibrous histiocytoma, rhabdomyosarcoma, and leiomyosarcoma. The role of adjuvant chemotherapy in synovial and epithelioid sarcomas is still unclear and is being further investigated.

In the 58 adjuvant chemotherapy patients living disease-free for five years or more (Table 8.17), we have not encountered any long-term side effects due to administration of adriamycin and DTIC. Neither of our two patients who showed cardiotoxicity has become symptomatic; however, neither is as yet a long-term survivor. We have not so far encountered any second primary cancer in any of these 58 patients.

In our experience, this combination of adriamycin and DTIC can be used with safety on an ambulatory basis in adults. The role of multiple agent chemotherapy in those tumors in which adriamycin and DTIC did not influence the outcome requires careful scrutiny before these drugs are used indiscriminately.

The optimism for adjuvant treatment of soft tissue sarcomas generated in recent years has resulted in a number of ongoing protocols.[77,78] At the M. D. Anderson Hospital, the value of nonradical surgery and radiation therapy plus adjuvant combination chemotherapy is under study. Rosenberg and co-workers[79] are investigating the effects of combined modality therapy. Soft tissue sarcomas of the extremities and those of the head, neck, and trunk are being studied separately in two randomized trials, with use of the same protocols for combined-modality therapy. In each of these protocols the role of adjuvant chemotherapy or immunotherapy, or both, is also being evaluated. The initial results on 86 evaluable patients show that adjuvant chemotherapy improved both disease-free survival and overall survival in patients with sarcomas of the extremities. However, no benefit was found for patients with sarcomas of the head and neck and the trunk.[80]

Our own experience has encouraged us to continue with a randomized trial using adriamycin and DTIC. The present schedule consists of adriamycin 60 mg/m² intravenously on day 1 and DTIC, 250 mg/m² intravenously days 1–5. The total dose of adriamycin used is 500 mg/m² and DTIC of 11,250 mg/m² in 6–7 months. Our data are too premature to draw any conclusions.

REGIONAL CHEMOTHERAPY FOR SOFT TISSUE SARCOMA

A major form of regional adjunctive chemotherapy in the treatment of soft tissue sarcomas is isolated limb perfusion.[32,81] This technique, of limb salvage with or without the use of hyperthermia, has been well described by Stehlin and associates,[82-84] as well as Creech et al.,[81] Ryan et al.,[85] Krementz and co-workers,[86,87] and McBride.[88] Most centers in the United States, including ours, follow the technique and methods

developed by the groups in New Orleans or Houston.

The chemotherapeutic agents currently used for perfusion by most groups are melphalan (1-phenyl-alanine mustard), actinomycin D, and nitrogen mustard, either singly or in combination. Krementz and co-workers[86,87] and Ryan et al.,[85] have used melphalan alone in doses of 0.6–1.0 mg/kg in the upper extremities and 1.0–1.4 mg/kg in the lower extremities. A combination of melphalan and actinomycin D was used by these same authors. In the lower extremities the dose of melphalan was 0.8–1.4 mg/kg and of actinomycin D, 0.006–0.015 mg/kg. In the upper extremities the dose of melphalan and actinomycin D consisted of 0.6–1.0 mg/kg and 0.003–0.007 mg/kg, respectively. Melphalan is added to the circuit in aliquots not exceeding 20 mg at intervals of three minutes until the total dose is reached. Actinomycin D is a rapid-acting drug and is added in small doses (0.1 mg) at two-minute intervals. When nitrogen mustard is used, 25 minutes after the first drug begins to circulate a small dose of nitrogen mustard (10–15 mg) is added in 2-mg aliquots every two minutes and the perfusion is carried on for a further 20 minutes.[85-87] McBride,[88] at the M.D. Anderson Tumor Institute, has used both melphalan and actinomycin D extensively in a median dose of melphalan, 1.3 mg/kg, and actinomycin D, 0.03 mg/kg in the lower extremities; and 0.7 mg/kg of melphalan and 0.02 mg/kg of actinomycin D in the upper extremities. Adriamycin has also been used recently in isolated limb perfusion, but no group has yet developed enough experience to define the median dose required. At the University of Illinois the dosage is calculated on the basis of the surface area of the extremity. For example, 20 percent of the total systemic dose of 60 mg/m² is used in the perfusion circuit for a lower extremity sarcoma. However, further experience is required for calculation of the optimum dose of adriamycin in isolated limb perfusion.

The results of isolated limb perfusion have been variously interpreted by different authors in reporting their experience. Krementz and co-workers[86,87] treated 113 cases of sarcoma with isolated limb perfusion, of which 12 were osseous sarcomas and 5 were lymphomas. It is difficult to accurately assess their data in terms of correlation with histologic classification, a difficulty which the authors themselves expressed. Their end results from the standpoint of cure were considerably better when regional isolated limb perfusion was used as an adjuvant to excision. In stage II tumors, with perfusion alone the disease-free five-year survival rate was 47 percent compared with 59 percent in patients who were treated by perfusion and wide excision of the primary tumor. It appears that they indeed obtained good results with synovial sarcomas; however, the inclusion of desmoids and lymphomas in this group makes it difficult to assess the data. McBride[88] reviewed the results of perfusion in 76 patients treated at the M.D. Anderson Hospital from 1960 through 1972. He argued that histologic classification of soft tissue tumors is not required, since the diagnosis frequently changes when the material is reviewed, a position which does not seem tenable in these days of routine use of electron microscopy and other sophisticated techniques. Admittedly, there are still a number of tumors in which the histogenesis is in doubt, but in the overwhelming majority of patients an accurate diagnosis can be established and the proper treatment program initiated. McBride's[88] data suggested that approximately 74 percent two-year and 57 percent five-year salvage was obtained at the M.D. Anderson Hospital. However, according to that hospital's staging system, patients with stage I-A had a 75 percent two-year survival rate, and with stage III-B there were no two-year survivors. Stehlin and co-workers[84] reviewed their experience with 37 soft tissue sarcomas in which hyperthermic perfusion was used. There were nine liposarcomas, seven synovial sarcomas, six rhabdomyosarcomas, four fibrosarcomas, three alveolar soft part sarcomas, two each of leiomyosarcoma, Kaposi's sarcoma, and unclassified sarcomas, and one each of malignant schwannoma and lymphangiosarcoma. Seventeen of these patients were treated by perfusion, irradiation, and delayed radical excision of either the primary tumor or the site of its origin. Nine patients had previously had excisional biopsy of either the primary tumor or local recurrence elsewhere. Seven of the 37 patients were treated by hyperthermic perfusion followed by radiation therapy. Although the results of isolated limb perfusion, alone or as a surgical adjuvant, cannot be adequately evaluated from these data, the five-year salvage rate was 61.9 percent in these patients, some of whom had locally advanced disease. After definitive treatment, 6 of

the 37 (16 percent) had local recurrence, and in another 5 (14 percent) failure of treatment was manifested by systemic disease.

Our own results at the University of Illinois with isolated limb perfusion are not yet extensive enough to draw any definitive conclusions. However, we are assessing various types of limb salvage procedures in sarcomas that we have for the present operationally defined as chemotherapy-sensitive (Table 8.14). Isolated limb perfusion of both the upper and lower extremities is one of the methods being assessed. The usual practice is to establish the diagnosis, perform the isolated limb perfusion, then follow immediately with a wide soft tissue (muscle group) excision.

In an attempt to salvage an extremity, the role of preoperative intra-arterial infusion with a chemotherapeutic agent as an adjuvant to excision and radiation therapy has also been investigated by several groups.[89-92] Morton and co-workers[93] tried intra-arterial adriamycin and radiation therapy prior to radical excision as the treatment of primary sarcomas of the extremities. This treatment was then supplemented with postoperative adjuvant chemotherapy or chemo-immunotherapy.[93] These authors, using a Harvard pump, gave 30 mg of adriamycin over a period of 24 hours for three consecutive days to a total dose of 90 mg. The dosage was reduced to 20 mg/day for lesions distal to the elbow and knee. Following the intra-arterial infusion, the site was irradiated with 350 rads/day for 10 days and the operation was performed on day 21. Two weeks postoperatively the patients were placed on a regimen of methotrexate, 100 mg/kg of body weight, given intravenously over a period of 24 hours, with citrovorum rescue four hours later, 12 mg intravenously every six hours for three days. Vincristine, 1.5 mg/m², was given intravenously one hour prior to methotrexate infusion. Two weeks after the moderate dose of methotrexate, adriamycin, 45 mg/m², was given intravenously for two consecutive days, for a total dose of 90 mg/m². This cycle was repeated every two weeks until the maximum 500 mg/m² total dose was achieved. Methotrexate was given monthly for one year. This extensive treatment program was used in 14 patients, 8 of whom had various types of soft tissue sarcoma. Analysis of their data[93] points up the superior end results in patients treated with intra-arterial adriamycin, preoperative ra-

TABLE 8.20. SOFT TISSUE SARCOMA: RESULTS OF TREATMENT WITH COMBINED INTRA-ARTERIAL ADRIAMYCIN, RADIATION THERAPY, AND SURGERY

Classification	No. Patients	N.E.D.* Median 18 mo†	(%)‡
Stage I			
Grade 1	6	6/6	100
Grade 3	36	27/35	75
Stage II	6	5/6	83
Stage III	3	0/3	0
Total	51		
Total grade 3	45	32/45	71

*No evidence of disease.
†Followup (2–57 months, median = 18.0 months).
‡Percentage of patients continuously free of disease; all recurrences were distant metastases.
Adapted from Morton DL, et al.[94]

diation therapy, and local excision, over those patients treated by excision alone. Immunotherapy with BCG and allogeneic sarcoma cell vaccine was administered in approximately half of these patients during the postoperative period. Morton and co-workers[94] recently updated the end result data from their ongoing study (Table 8.20). One cannot say whether they would have obtained similar results with wide excision and adjuvant chemotherapy. They used a vigorous adjuvant program and the complications consisted of lymphedema of the extremity in 12 percent (6 of 51 patients), spontaneous fracture of normal bone in 8 percent, and wound necrosis in 20 percent. Five patients (10 percent) required amputation.

Additional data have been generated on the use of intra-arterial infusion of adriamycin in soft tissue sarcomas.[89-92] Haskell and co-workers[90] used a dose of 45–107 mg/m² as a continuous infusion over a period of 1.5 to 3 days, followed by surgery or radiation therapy. Di Pietro and associates[91,92] tried a dose of 0.3 mg/kg/day for 10 consecutive days and 14 mg/kg on alternate days for 10 days for a single cycle in each patient. Shah and co-workers[89] used a variety of adriamycin dose schedules in eight sarcoma patients; in six there was partial response and in two, none. Although these small numbers of patients cannot be used to determine the role of intra-arterial infusion with adriamycin as a preoperative surgical adjuvant for the treatment

TABLE 8.21. DOSE SCHEDULE OF INTRA-ARTERIAL ADRIAMYCIN AND TOXIC EFFECTS*

Schedule No.	Dose Schedule	No. Courses	Local Toxicity	Arterial Thrombosis	Mucositis	Gastrointestinal Symptoms (nausea/vomiting)	Neutropenia (<4000 cells/mm³)	Thrombocytopenia (<100,000 cells/mm³)	Alopecia
1	20–30 mg/m²/day × 3 days, q 3 wk†	13	0	0	1	3	4	2	13
2	75–140 mg/m²/wk†	15	1	1	0	0	0	0	15
3	10.7 mg/m², continuous daily infusion × 5 wk	1	0	0	0	0	0	0	1
4	14 mg/m², continuous infusion × 5 wk	1	0	0	1	1	1	1	1
5	75 mg/m², 3 wk†	6	0	1	1	1	0	0	6
6	75 mg/m²/day × 7 days†	1	0	0	0	0	0	0	1
7	40 mg/m²/day × 4 days†	1	0	0	0	0	0	0	1
8	15–20 mg/m²/day × 5 days, q 3 wk	2	2	0	2	1	2	0	2
9	25–45 mg/m²/wk†	3	0	0	0	0	0	0	2

*Shah et al., 1977.[89]
†Daily dose was a 6–8 hr infusion.

of any form of soft tissue sarcomas, the authors have documented the dose schedules and the toxic effects quite thoroughly (Table 8.21).

Currently, we have an ongoing program of preoperative intra-arterial infusion and radiation therapy for chemoresponsive locally advanced extremity sarcomas. The protocol is as follows: After adequate histologic diagnosis, the tumor is staged and a percutaneous intraarterial catheter is appropriately placed. Adriamycin, 15 mg/day for 10 days (total 150 mg) is administered by continuous infusion. Concomitantly, radiation therapy of 3,000 rads is given to the site of the primary tumor and the length of the entire bone. Following completion of this preoperative regimen, usually within two weeks, a muscle group excision is performed. Two weeks after wound-healing, a further course of 2,000 rads is given to the extremity. Four to six weeks later the adjuvant program with adriamycin and DTIC is begun and is continued for six months. In this program, the total adriamycin dosage is thus divided as a preoperative intra-arterial infusion and postoperative intravenous adjuvant.

So far, we have treated 27 patients in this manner, but the regimen is too recent to draw any conclusions. The raw data are tabulated in Table 8.22. This multimodality program has failed in 6 (22 percent) of the 27 patients, but there has been no instance of local recurrence. This would suggest that local control probably can be achieved in most cases. Although wound-healing is delayed after this treatment regimen, we have not yet encountered any problems serious enough to cast doubt on the value of this limb salvage program. The systemic toxicity that results from the adjuvant program is similar to that already described.

Only one patient has refused to continue with the postoperative adjuvant program. On the basis of our preliminary data, it appears that this multimodality approach is justified; however, several questions still remain to be answered. For example: (1) Are the results of regional perfusion better than those with continuous arterial infusion? If they are equally effective, then comparative cost requires consideration. (2) Are radical excision and adjuvant chemotherapy (page 321) less effective, or are the results similar? A systematic, well-controlled program to answer these questions should be initiated before assessing the efficacy of these various combinations.

TABLE 8.22. INTRA-ARTERIAL ADRIAMYCIN INFUSION, RADIATION THERAPY, AND OPERATION FOR SOFT TISSUE SARCOMAS OF THE EXTREMITIES (UNIVERSITY OF ILLINOIS SERIES OF 27 PATIENTS)

Histologic Type	No. Patients	Location	Size	Grade (s)	N.E.D.† (yr)	Comments
Upper Extremity						
Malignant fibrous histiocytoma	2	Arm	5 cm	3 and 4	3 and 5	Alive and well
Rhabdomyosarcoma	1	Arm	5 cm	3	2½*	Living with metastatic disease
Leiomyosarcoma	1	Arm	5 cm	3	1½	Alive and well
Synovial sarcoma	3	Arm and forearm	3–5 cm	3 and 4	2½, 1½*, and 2	One now dead
Lower extremity						
Malignant fibrous histiocytoma	3	Thigh	5 cm	3 and 4	1,* 3, and 4½	One patient now dead
Rhabdomyosarcoma	6	Thigh and leg	4–5 cm	3 and 4	5, 4, 3½, 3½, 2,* and 1.2*	One patient dead and one other living with metastatic disease
Leiomyosarcoma	3	Thigh and leg	2–5 cm	3	4, 5, 2½*	One now dead
Synovial sarcoma	8	Leg	3–5 cm	3	5, 2½, 2, 1½, 1½, 1, 1, and 9 mo	All alive and well

*Patient dead of, or living with, metastatic disease. For 6 of 27 (22%) the program failed.
†No evidence of disease.

REFERENCES

1. Krakoff IH: Cancer chemotherapeutic agents. CA 27:130, 1977
2. Donaldson SS, Castro JR, Wilbur JR, Jesse RH: Rhabdomyosarcoma of head and neck in children. Combined treatment by surgery, irradiation, and chemotherapy. Cancer 31:26, 1973
3. Pratt CB, James DH Jr, Holton CP, Pinkel D: Combination therapy including vincristine (NSC-67574) for malignant solid tumors in children. Cancer Chemother Rep 52:489, 1968
4. Sutow WW: Cyclophosphamide (NSC-26271) in Wilms' tumor and rhabdomyosarcoma. Cancer Chemother Rep 51:407, 1967
5. Sutow WW, Berry DH, Haddy TB, et al: Vincristine sulfate therapy in children with metastatic soft tissue sarcoma. J Pediat 38:465, 1968
6. Sutow WW, Vietti TJ, Donaldson MD, et al: Evaluation of chemotherapy in children with metastatic Ewing's sarcoma and osteogenic sarcoma. Cancer Chemother Rep 56:67, 1971
7. Wilbur JR, Sutow WW, Sullivan MP, Gottlieb JF: Chemotherapy of sarcoma. Cancer 36:765, 1975
8. Rosen G, Suwansirikul S, Kwon C, et al: High-dose methotrexate with citrovorum factor rescue and adriamycin in childhood osteogenic sarcoma. Cancer 33:1151, 1974
9. Benjamin JT, Johnson WD, McMillan CW: The management of Wilms' tumor: A comparison of two regimens. Cancer 34:2122, 1974
10. Harrison J, Myers M, Rowe M, Vermund H: Results of combination chemotherapy, surgery, and radiotherapy in children with neuroblastoma. Cancer 34:485, 1974
11. Sutow WW: Chemotherapy in neuroblastoma. J Pediat Surg 3:182, 1968
12. Burgert EO Jr, Mills SD: Chemotherapy of malignant lesions unique in children. Mayo Clin Proc 41:361, 1966
13. Lawhorn TI, Sonte HH, Martin JD Jr: Chemotherapy in solid tumors of childhood. Oncology 26:250, 1972
14. Jaffe N, Paed D: Recent advances in the chemotherapy of metastatic osteogenic sarcoma. Cancer 30:1627, 1972
15. Tan C, Wollner N, King O, Ilano D: Adriamycin, a new antibiotic in treatment of childhood leukemia and other malignant neoplasms. Proc Am Assoc Cancer Res 11:79, 1970 (abstr)
16. Pratt CB: Response of childhood rhabdomyosarcoma to combination chemotherapy. J Pediat 74:791, 1969
17. Grosfeld JL, Clatworthy W Jr, Newton WA Jr: Combined therapy in childhood rhabdomyosarcoma: An analysis of 42 cases. J Pediat Surg 4:637, 1969
18. Heyn RM, Holland R, Newton WA Jr, Tefft M, et al: The role of combined chemotherapy in the treatment of rhabdomyosarcoma in children. Cancer 34:2128, 1974
19. Wilbur JR: Combination chemotherapy for embryonal rhabdomyosarcoma. Cancer Chemother Rep 58:281, 1974
20. Wilbur JR, Sutow WW, Sullivan MP: The changing treatment of rhabdomyosarcoma in children, particularly in the treatment of inoperable rhabdomyosarcoma of the nasopharynx and oropharynx. In: Neoplasia of Head and Neck. Proc 17th Annual Clinical Conference, 1972, Houston, Texas. Chicago, Year Book Medical Publishers, 1974
21. Hays DM: The management of rhabdomyosarcoma in children and young adults. World J Surg 4:15, 1980
22. Gottlieb JA, Baker LH, O'Bryan RM, et al: Adriamycin (NSC 123121) used alone and in combination for soft-tissue and bony sarcoma. Cancer Chemother Rep (part 3) 6:271, 1975
23. Gottlieb JA: Combination chemotherapy for metastatic sarcoma. Cancer Chemother Rep 58:265, 1974
24. Gottlieb JA, Baker LH, Quagliana JM, et al: Chemotherapy of sarcomas with a combination of adriamycin and dimethyl triazeno imidazole carboxamide. Cancer 30:1632, 1972
25. Pinedo HM, Kenis Y: Chemotherapy of advanced soft-tissue sarcomas in adults. Cancer Treat Rev 4:67, 1977
26. Gottlieb JA, Benjamin RS, Baker LH, et al: Role of DTIC (NSC-45388) in the chemotherapy of sarcomas. Cancer Treat Rep 60:199, 1976
27. Hill DL: A Review of Cyclophosphamide. Springfield (Ill), Thomas, 1975
28. Gottlieb JA, Bodey GP, Sinkovics JG, et al: An effective new 4-drug combination regimen (CY-VA-DIC) for metastatic sarcomas. Proc Am Assoc Cancer Res 15:162, 1974
29. Kucuksu N, Thomas W, Ezdinli EZ: Chemotherapy of malignant diffuse mesothelioma. Cancer 37:1265, 1976
30. Andrews NC, Wilson WT: Phase II Study of methotrexate in solid tumors. Cancer Chemother Rep 51:471, 1967
31. Cupps RE, Ahman DL, Soule EH: Treatment of pulmonary metastastic disease with radiation therapy and adjuvant actinomycin D. Cancer 24:719, 1969
32. Rochlin DB: The therapy of sarcomas by isolation perfusion. Acta Unio Internat Contra Cancrum 20:487, 1964
33. Watne AL, Badillo J, Koike A, et al: Clinical studies of actinomycin D. Ann NY Acad Sci 89:445, 1960
34. Carter DK: Mitomycin C. Cancer Chemother Rep 53:99, 1968
35. Haddy TB, Nora AH, Sutow WW, Vietti TJ: Cyclophosphamide treatment for metastatic soft-tissue sarcoma. Intermittent large doses in the treatment of children. Am J Dis Child 114:301, 1967
36. Middleman E, Luce J, Frei E III: Clinical trials with adriamycin. Cancer 28:844, 1971
37. Bergsagel DE, Levin WC: A prelusive trial of cyclophosphamide. Cancer Chemother Rep 8:120, 1960
38. Burgoon CF Jr., Soderberg M: Angiosarcoma. Arch Derm 99:773, 1969
39. Wharam MD, Phillips TL, Jacobs EM: Combination chemotherapy and whole lung irradiation for pulmonary metastases from sarcomas and germinal cell tumors of the testis. Cancer 34:136, 1974

40. Wasserman TH, Comis RL, Goldsmith M, et al: Tabular analysis of the chemotherapy of solid tumors. Cancer Chemother Rep 6:399, 1975

41. Jacobs EM: Combination chemotherapy of metastatic testicular germinal cell tumors and soft part sarcomas. Cancer 25:324, 1970

42. Di Marco A, Gaetani M, Scarpinato B: Adriamycin (NSC-123-127): a new antibiotic with antitumor activity. Cancer Chemother Rep 53:33, 1969

43. Kingra GS, Comis R, Olson KB, et al: 5-(3,3-dimethyl–triazeno) imidazole-4-carboxamide (SNC-45388) in the treatment of malignant tumors other than melanoma. Cancer Chemother Rep 55:281, 1971

44. Skibba JL, Ramirez G, Beal DD, et al: Preliminary clinical trial and the physiologic disposition of 4(5)-(3,3-dimethyl–triazeno)-imidazole-5-(4)-carboxamide in man. Cancer Res 29:1944, 1969

45. Benjamin RS, Wiernik PH, Bachur NR: Adriamycin: A new effective agent in the therapy of disseminated sarcomas. Med Pediat Oncol 1:63, 1975

46. Benjamin RS, Riggs CE Jr, Bachur NR: Pharmacokinetics and metabolism of adriamycin in man. Clin Pharmacol Ther 14:592, 1973

47. Bonadonna G, Monfardini S, DeLena M, Fossati-Bellani F, Beretta G: Phase I and preliminary Phase II evaluation of adriamycin (NSC 123127). Cancer Res 30:2572, 1970

48. Gottlieb JA, Serpick AA: Clinical evaluation of 5-3,3-dimethyl–triazeno) imidazole-4-carboxamide in malignant melanoma and other neoplasms. Comparison of twice-weekly and daily administration schedules. Oncology 25:225, 1971

49. Luce JK, Thurman WG, Isaacs L, Talley RW: Clinical trials with the antitumor agent 5-(3,3-dimethyl–triazeno) imidazole-4-carboxamide (NSC 45388). Cancer Chemother Rep 54:119, 1970

50. Chanes RE, Condit PT, Bottomley RH, Nisimblat W: Combined actinomycin D and vincristine in the treatment of patients with cancer. Cancer 27:613, 1971

51. Finklestein JZ, Hittle RE, Hammond GD: Evaluation of a high-dose cyclophosphamide regimen in childhood tumors. Cancer 23:1239, 1969

52. Korbitz BC, Davis HL Jr, Ramirez G, Ansfield FJ: Low doses of vincristine (NSC-67574) for malignant disease. Cancer Chemother Rep 53:249, 1969

53. Livingston RB, Carter SK: Single Agents in Cancer Chemotherapy. New York, IFI/Plenum, 1970

54. Moore GE, DiPaolo JA, Kondo T: The chemotherapeutic effects and complications of actinomycin D in patients with advanced cancer. Cancer 11:1240, 1958

55. Evans AE, Heyn RM, Newton WA, Leikin SL: Vincristine sulfate and cyclophosphamide for children with metastatic neuroblastoma. JAMA 207:1325, 1969

56. Tefft M, Fernandez CH, Moon TE: Rhabdomyosarcoma: Response with chemotherapy prior to radiation in patients with gross residual disease. Cancer 39:665, 1977

57. Benjamin RS, Gottlieb JA, Baker LH, Sinkovics JG: CYVADIC vs CYVADACT—A randomized trial of cyclophosphamide (CY), vincristine (V), and adriamycin (A), plus dicarbazine (DIC) or acti-

nomycin-D (DACT) in metastatic sarcomas. Proc Am Assoc Cancer Res 17:256, 1976

58. Sutherland C, Morgan LR, Carter D, Krementz E: Combination chemotherapy of metastatic bone and soft tissue sarcomas. Proc Am Assoc Cancer Res 17:137, 1976

59. Beretta G, Bonadonna G, Bajetta E, et al: Combination chemotherapy with DTIC (NSC-45388) in advanced malignant melanoma, soft tissue sarcomas, and Hodgkin's disease. Cancer Treat Rep 60:205, 1976

60. Goldman RL, Zones SE, Heusinkveld RS: Combination chemotherapy of metastatic malignant schwannoma with vincristine, adriamycin, cyclophosphamide, and imidazole carboxamide: A case report. Cancer 39:1955, 1977

61. Wang J, Cortes E, Sinks L, Holland JF: Therapeutic effect and toxicity of adriamycin in patients with neoplastic disease. Cancer 28:837, 1971

62. Benjamin RS, Baker LH, Rodriquez V, Moon TE, et al: The chemotherapy of soft tissue sarcomas in adults. In Management of Primary Bone and Soft Tissue Tumors. The 21st Annual Clinical Conference on Cancer. Year Book Medical Publishers, Chicago, 1977, p 309

63. Yap B, Baker LH, Sinkovics JG, Rivkin SE, et al: Cyclophosphamide, vincristine, adriamycin, and DTIC (CYVADIC) combination chemotherapy for the treatment of advanced sarcomas. Cancer Treat Rep 64:93, 1980

64. Pinedo HM, van Oosterom AT: Treatment of advanced soft tissue sarcomas in adults: past, present and future. In Therapeutic Progress in Ovarian Cancer, Testicular Cancer and the Sarcomas, van Oosterom AT et al (eds). (Boerhaave Series, vol 16), Leiden University Press 1980, p 425

65. Lynch G, Magill GB, Sordillo P, Golbey RB: Combination chamotherapy of advanced sarcomas in adults with "CYOMAD" (S7). Cancer 50:1724, 1982

66. Enterline ET, Culberson JD, Rochlin DB, Brady LW: Liposarcoma: A clinical and pathological study of 53 cases. Cancer 13:932, 1960

67. Enzinger FM, Winslow DJ: Liposarcoma: Study of 103 cases. Virchows Arch Path Anat 335(40):367, 1962

68. Weiss SW, Enzinger FM: Malignant fibrous histiocytoma. An analysis of 200 cases. Cancer 41:2250, 1978

69. Suit HD, Russell WO: Radiation therapy of soft tissue sarcomas. Cancer 36:759, 1975

70. Suit HD, Russell WO, Martin RG: Sarcoma of soft tissue: Clinical and histopathological parameters and response to treatment. Cancer 35:1478, 1975

71. Bedickian AY, Valdivieso M, Khankhanian N, Benjamin RS, Bodey GP: Chemotherapy for sarcoma of the stomach. Cancer Treat Rep 63:411, 1979

72. McNeer GP, Cantin J, Chu F, Nickson J: Effectiveness of radiation therapy in the management of sarcoma of the somatic tissues. Cancer 22:391, 1968

73. Mackenzie DH: Synovial sarcoma: A review of 58 cases. Cancer 19:169, 1966

74. Gerner RE, Moore GE: Synovial sarcoma. Ann Surg 181:22, 1975

75. Pratt J, Woodruff JM, Marcove RC: Epithelioid sarcoma: An analysis of 22 cases indicating the prognostic significance of vascular invasion and regional lymph node metastasis. Cancer 41:1472, 1978

76. Kaplan EL, Meier P: Nonparametric estimation from incomplete observations. J Am Statist Assoc 53:457, 1958.

77. Yap BS, Baker L, Sinkovics JG, et al: Cyclophosphamide, vincristine, adriamycin, and DTIC: Combination chemotherapy for the treatment of advanced sarcomas. Chemo Treat Rep 64(1):93, 1980

78. Bramwell VHC, Voute PA, Rosenberg SA, Pinedo HM: Adjuvant treatment of soft tissue sarcoma in children and adults. Recent Results Cancer Res 68:431, 1979.

79. Rosenberg SA, Kent H, Costa J, et al: Prospective randomized evaluation of the role of limb-sparing surgery, radiation therapy, and adjuvant chemoimmunotherapy in the treatment of adult soft tissue sarcomas. Surgery 84:62, 1978

80. Rosenberg SA, Tepper J, Glatstein E, et al: Adjuvant chemotherapy for patients with soft tissue sarcomas. Surg Clin North Am 61:1415, 1981

81. Creech O Jr, Krementz ET, Ryan RF, Winblad JN: Chemotherapy of cancer: Regional perfusion utilizing an extracorporeal circuit. Ann Surg 148:616, 1958

82. Stehlin JS Jr: Hyperthermic perfusion with chemotherapy for cancers of the extremities. Surg Gynecol Obstet 129:305, 1969

83. Stehlin JS Jr, Clark RL Jr, White EC, et al: Regional chemotherapy for cancer: Experiences of 116 perfusions. Ann Surg 151:605, 1960

84. Stehlin JS Jr, de Ipolyl PD, Giovanella BC, et al: Soft tissue sarcomas of the extremity: Multidisciplinary therapy employing hyperthermic perfusion. Ann J Surg 130:643, 1975

85. Ryan RF, Krementz ET, Creech O Jr, et al: Selected perfusion of isolated viscera with chemotherapeutic agents. Surg Forum 8:158, 1958

86. Krementz ET, Carter RD, Sutherland CM, Hutton I: Chemotherapy of sarcomas of the limbs by regional perfusion. Ann Surg 185:555, 1977

87. Krementz ET, Carter RD, Sutherland CM, Ryan RF: Malignant melanoma of the limbs: An evaluation of chemotherapy by regional perfusion. In: Neoplasms of the Skin and Malignant Melanoma. Chicago, Year Book Medical Publishers, 1976, pp 375–400

88. McBride CM: Sarcomas of the limbs: Results of adjuvant chemotherapy using isolation perfusion. Arch Surg 109:304, 1974

89. Shah P, Baker LH, Vaitkevicius VK: Preliminary experiences with intra-arterial adriamycin. Cancer Chemo Rep 61:1565, 1977

90. Haskell CM, Silverstein MJ, Rangel DM, et al: Multimodality cancer therapy in man: A pilot study of adriamycin by arterial infusion. Cancer 33:1485, 1974

91. Di Pietro S, De Palo GM, Molinari R, et al: Clinical trial with adriamycin by prolonged arterial infusion. Tumori 56:233, 1970

92. Di Pietro S, De Palo GM, Gennari L, et al: Cancer chemotherapy by intra-arterial infusion with adriamycin. J Surg Oncol 5:421, 1973

93. Morton DL, Eilber FR, Townsend CM Jr, et al: Limb salvage from a multidisciplinary treatment approach for skeletal and soft tissue sarcomas of the extremity. Ann Surg 184:268, 1976

94. Morton DL, Eilber FR, Grant T, Weisenberger TH: Multimodality therapy of malignant melanoma, skeletal and soft tissue sarcomas using immunotherapy, chemotherapy, and radiation therapy. In Jones SE, Salmon SE (eds): Adjuvant Therapy of Cancer, II. New York, Grune and Stratton, 1979, p 497

9

Immunology and Immunotherapy

Robert Epstein

The evolution of humoral and cellular immunity provided vertebrates with potent host defense mechanisms. Initial medical exploitation of immunologic principles was largely centered on the identification, prophylaxis, and therapy of bacterial and viral disease, but as early as 1908 Ehrlich[1] could postulate the potential for immunologic intervention in cancer. Grounds for optimism regarding immune defenses against tumors could be found at the turn of the century in reports of resistance to tumor challenge following regression of canine venereal sarcomas, in reports of treatment of this tumor by immunologic techniques, and in reports of encouraging attempts in man to produce tumor regression by immunization, serotherapy, and the injection of bacterial toxins.[2-5] More than half a century later, an expanded and scientifically sophisticated field of tumor immunology reawakened general enthusiasm for potential immunologic approaches to human neoplasms.[6,7] Although enthusiasm persists, immunotherapeutic goals have proved elusive and serious gaps of fundamental information exist.[8] Because of the voluminous recent literature available in the field of tumor immunology, it is the purpose of this chapter to briefly provide the reader with an orientation to the evolution, existing concepts, and open questions underlying the immunology of soft tissue sarcomas.

The years between periods of activity regarding immunologic approaches to human neoplasms were marked by steady growth in understanding basic mechanisms and in defining antigenic characteristics of malignant tissues in animal systems and in man.[9,10] By 1929, it had become clear that in many experimental systems the production of immunologic tumor regression was based on later-to-be-defined histocompatibility differences that existed when tumors were transplanted into randomly bred hosts. Such results could not be directly extrapolated to autochthonous tumor growth.[11] The subsequent increased experimental use of inbred rodent strains provided a means by which tumor antigenicity could be evaluated under controlled genetic conditions, and tumor lines could be studied in animals syngeneic to the original host. Most current information indicating unique antigens present on malignant cells is based on the use of these inbred rodent strains.

Parallel progress occurred with the discovery that some malignancies occurring in chickens, rabbits, frogs, mice, and cats were caused by viruses.[12,13] In addition, the isolation of polynuclear aromatic hydrocarbons and azo dyes as chemical carcinogens gave investigators techniques for regularly inducing tumors of a variety of histologic types for immunologic study.[14,15] Subsequently, tumor-specific transplantation antigens (TSTA), of known chemical or viral origin, were clearly demonstrated in animal systems.[16-19] Successful prophylactic immunization against some animal tumors was accomplished and intensive efforts to intervene immunologically in the course of progressively growing neoplasms were begun.[6,20] In man, evidence for tumor-associated antigens (TAA) has been described for many tumors, including soft tissue sarcomas.[10,21] However, precise chemical definition of these antigens, their analogy to rodent model TSTA, and even their uniqueness for malignant cells remain an area of debate.[8]

NATURE OF THE IMMUNE RESPONSE TO CELL SURFACE ANTIGENS

The events leading to an immune response involve (1) antigenic challenge, (2) recognition of antigen by immunocompetent cells of the host, (3) activation and proliferation of these cells, and (4) effector mechanisms of antibody production, delayed hypersensitivity, and memory. The response is governed by still incompletely understood cellular interactions dependent on the structure, quantity, and mode of presentation of the antigen.[22] Underlying genetic factors appear to provide for the heterogenicity of responses observed in randomly bred species to a given challenge.[23] Figure 9.1 represents a simplified version of stimulation of the immune response by putative tumor antigens. Cell surface or soluble (shed) antigens may activate either or both of two populations of lymphocytes.[24] B-lymphocytes (derived from the bursa of Fabricius in birds and the bone marrow in mammals) carry immunoglobulin receptors and are responsible for the production of specific antibodies. T-(thymus-dependent) lymphocytes are intimately involved in cell-mediated immunity (delayed hypersensitivity). Interactions between antigens and accessory cells (macrophages and helper T-lymphocytes) are required to initiate most B-cell responses. Evidence indicates that a T-cell subpopulation also suppresses B-cell immune responses under certain conditions.[25-27] Antigenic activation of T- and B-cells is followed by DNA, RNA, and protein synthesis (blastic transformation), leading to cell division. The end results of antibody production or cell-mediated destruction of target tissue then occurs. Having once gone through this

process, the organism reacts more promptly and intensely to rechallenge by the same antigen.

Cell-mediated immunity (CMI) is defined as a special form of inflammatory response that is independent of antibody and can be transferred by infusion of viable sensitized lymphocytes.[28] The tuberculin reaction and primary rejection of allogeneic tissue grafts are the prototypes for this form of immunity. Therefore, CMI has been the focus of immunotherapeutic considerations in cancer. T-lymphocytes and macrophages appear to be the primary cell types involved and have been shown to function by direct contact killing.[29] In addition, activated lymphocytes produce a number of soluble factors (lymphokines), which appear important to the reaction.[30] These include (1) lymphotoxins, which produce direct toxic effects on target cells, (2) macrophage migration inhibition factor (MIF), which immobilizes macrophages in the area of inflammation, (3) blastogenic factor, which stimulates activation of additional lymphocytes to blastic transformation, and (4) transfer factor, which is immunologically specific for recruiting new lymphocytes to the sensitized state. The initial activation of the lymphocytes depends on immunologically specific events. Subsequent effector amplification of the response involving lymphokines and macrophages (with the exception of transfer factor) appears to be of a more nonspecific nature. More recently, an additional subpopulation of lymphocytes naturally toxic to tumor cells has been defined in rodents.[31] These natural killer (NK) cells lack the usual B- and T-cell surface markers and vary in number with the age and major histocompatibility genotype of the host. Their significance in resistance to evolving malignant proliferation is an area of growing interest.

Although delayed hypersensitivity reactions are not directly mediated by antibodies, increasing importance has been placed on the role of humoral immunity in potentiating or inhibiting reactions to cell surface antigens. Depending on the experimental conditions and the tumor system studied, antibodies can be shown to (1) directly lyse cells in the presence of complement (complement-dependent cytotoxicity), (2) potentiate cell growth (enhancement), (3) inhibit cell-mediated immunity (blocking), and (4) act synergistically with lymphocytes or macrophages to destroy target cells (arming).[32-36] The interaction of antibody and effector cells is illustrated by the killer cell activity of a popula-

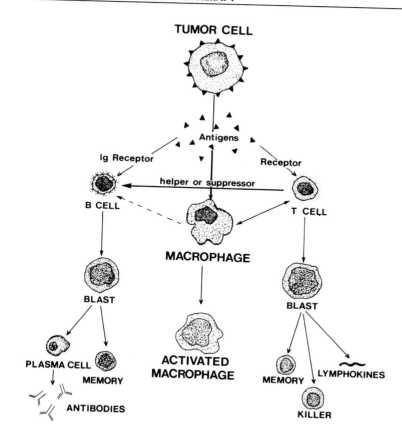

TUMOR CELL

Antigens

Ig Receptor

Receptor

helper or suppressor

B CELL

T CELL

MACROPHAGE

BLAST

BLAST

PLASMA CELL

MEMORY

ACTIVATED MACROPHAGE

MEMORY

LYMPHOKINES

ANTIBODIES

KILLER

Figure 9.1. General scheme of immune response to tumor-associated antigens. Although B- and T-lymphocyte populations provide a framework for consideration of effector mechanisms of humoral and cellular immune responses, interactions between subpopulations of cells governing recognition of antigen processing and helper and suppressor effects are essential to the system.

tion of lymphocytes, which is dependent on the presence of antibody directed at the tumor target tissue.[37] Again, the significance of this observation of antibody-dependent cellular cytotoxicity (ADCC) remains to be put in perspective with other host mechanisms of tumor control.

Both cellular and humoral factors have also been advanced as modulating inhibition of effective host defenses against tumors. Current information suggests that serum factors in the form of circulating immune complexes, free antigen, or enhancing antibodies may block cell-mediated immunity.[38-40] In addition, the role of suppressor T-lymphocytes in preventing or turning off humoral or cellular immune responses has become a serious consideration.[27]

Our present understanding of host-tumor relationships reveals a number of cellular and humoral activities and interactions that can be interpreted as leading to inhibition or potentiation of malignant cell growth (Figs. 9.2 and 9.3). However, production of lytic and protective ef-

fects on tumor cells in vitro is of uncertain significance in the intact host.

EVIDENCE THAT TUMORS ARE IMMUNOGENIC

Table 9.1 summarizes some of the principal techniques used to demonstrate tumor-associated antigens in experimental animal systems and in man. In vitro methods continue to undergo intensive reassessment and technical development. However, even with current methods, host reactivity has been reported in most well-studied tumor systems.

In vivo, the major criterion for immunologic responsiveness has been resistance to rechallenge following tumor removal or immunization.[16-19] Basic studies carried out in the 1950s in animal sarcoma systems defined some of the principles governing such resistance. First, resistance to chemically induced soft tissue sar-

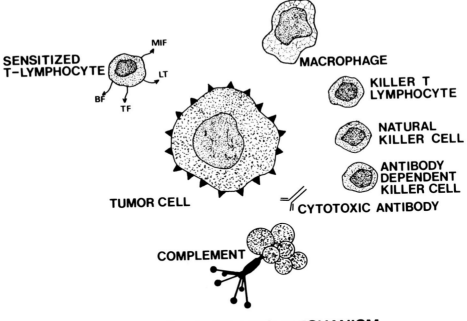

Figure 9.2. Effector components that may be important for immunologic destruction of tumor cells.

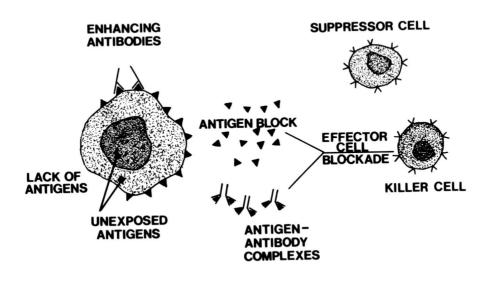

Figure 9.3. Possible mechanisms that permit tumor cells to escape immunologic destruction.

TABLE 9.1. GENERAL METHODS USED TO DEMONSTRATE TUMOR-ASSOCIATED ANTIGENS IN SOFT TISSUE SARCOMAS

A. In vivo
  1. Tumor rechallenge following immunization
  2. Skin-testing with tumor cells or extracts
B. In vitro
  1. Assays correlating with CMI
     a. Tumor cell killing by lymphocytes in tissue culture systems
     b. Lymphocyte blastogenic response to tumor cells or extracts
     c. Leukocyte migration or adhesion inhibition
  2. Assays of humoral immunity
     a. Immunofluorescence
     b. Complement-fixation
     c. Complement-dependent cytotoxicity

comas was generally specific to the individual tumors, ie, an animal resistant to one methylcholanthrene (MC)-induced fibrosarcoma was not resistant to other tumors similarly produced.[17] In contrast, cross-resistance was shown between sarcomas produced by a given viral agent. Tumors produced in mice by the Moloney sarcoma virus (MSV) have antigenic specificity that will effectively immunize against other MSV tumor challenges.[41] Secondly, when chemical carcinogens are used, variations in the extent of immunogenicity occur in sarcomas induced by different agents and even among tumors produced by the same chemical.[17,42] Third, when resistance occurred, it was relative and could be overcome by increasing and sometimes decreasing the tumor cell challenge.[43,44] Fourth, in vivo demonstration of resistance could not be shown for a spontaneously arising fibrosarcoma in C3Hf/He mice.[17] The implications of these early studies for human neoplasms remain significant. Thus, prophylactic immunization might be feasible if human sarcomas were of viral origin, but would not be practical, for example, in chemical carcinogenesis. The inability to demonstrate transplantation resistance in a variety of rodent tumors (particularly of spontaneous origin) and the circumvention of it in others also suggested problems for immunotherapy. However, despite limitations, the fact that tumor resistance often was demonstrated has established tumor transplantation antigens as a feature of a wide variety of experimentally induced sarcomas. Specificity and potency of the antigens described were related to defined etiologic agents. In addition to arising spontaneously, experimental sarcomas can be produced by all classes of known carcinogens, including viral agents, chemicals, and irradiation.[13,15,45] Therefore, a unifying etiology for human soft tissue malignancies cannot be surmised from rodent systems. Moreover, transplantation immunity has been particularly difficult to demonstrate in spontaneous tumors of rodents and lacks definitive proof in man.[8,46,47]

Because transplantation experiments of the kind performed in rodents cannot be carried out in man, in vivo studies of tumor antigenicity have involved a number of attempts to assay delayed hypersensitivity to autochthonous tumors by skin-testing. Skin-testing with extracts of chemically induced sarcomas in guinea pigs regularly produces delayed hypersensitivity reactions which correlate with transplantation resistance that is tumor-specific.[48] Although standardization of testing procedures in man presents many problems, evidence for specific reactivity exists for a number of human neoplasms.[49-53] Among the soft tissue sarcomas, skin reactivity to KC1 extracts of autologous tumor cells has been observed in most histologic types.[52]

Skin-testing has also been used to measure the capacity of tumor-bearing patients to respond to recall antigens (eg, tuberculin, Candida, mumps, etc.), as well as to be sensitized by synthetic antigens, eg, dinitrochlorobenzene (DNCB). The majority of published studies support the thesis that general depression of cell-mediated immunity, as assessed by skin tests, may be associated with the presence of a neoplasm, particularly when lesions are nonoperable or recur early following surgery.[54,55] In studies by Eilber et al.,[56] patients with advanced sarcomas had a significantly reduced response to DNCB. Depression of DNCB preoperatively in sarcoma patients has also been reported by Twomey.[57] Other studies have tended to confirm findings of depressed ability to sensitize patients with large tumor burdens to DNCB, although such findings are not universal.[58,59] Anergy to recall antigens has been a less consistent finding, and correlation between individual skin tests for delayed hypersensitivity is difficult to assess. At best, no firm evidence exists that nonspecific skin test abnormalities are detectable at the inception of tumor growth.

In vitro assay systems have provided the major methods for identifying tumor-associated antigens in man. The demonstration that tumor cells were destroyed when incubated with sensitized lymphocytes in vitro was followed by quantitative assays. These included the inhibition of tumor colony growth in culture by test lymphocytes, and cytotoxicity assays of tumor cell death.[60,61] In addition to direct tumor cell effects, evidence for immune responsiveness can be obtained by measurements of DNA synthesis in lymphocytes stimulated by putative tumor antigens,[52] and by the inhibition of leukocyte migration or adhesion.[62,63]

Studies in animal sarcoma systems and in man defining cell-mediated responses to tumor-associated antigens have used in vitro growth inhibition or cytotoxicity techniques.[34,58,64] In MC or plastic-induced sarcomas in mice, inhibition of tumor colony formation by sensitized lymphocytes was found to be specific for individual tumors, whereas virally induced sarcomas revealed typical cross-reactivity.[34,64] In man, a series of studies by Hellstrom et al.[65] showed tumor colony growth inhibition by autologous lymphocytes in patients bearing a wide range of cancers, including sarcomas. An important finding was that lymphocytes of patients with similar histologic categories of tumors showed cross-reactivity in inhibiting allogeneic tumor cells. Activity of lymphocytes from sarcoma patients to tumor lines was confirmed in the cytotoxicity assay.[58,66] Again, cross-reactivity appeared to be the rule. More recent evidence, however, has raised the question of the specificity of lymphocyte cytotoxicity toward tumor cells of a given histologic type.[67-70] Active lymphocytes that were not tumor-type specific were found in a high proportion of cancer patients and normal subjects. In general, cells from cancer patients were found to be less reactive than those from normal persons. Considerable additional clarification is necessary before firm conclusions can be drawn regarding the significance of these assays to the tumor-host relationship. Given the growing number of mechanisms that may lead to cytotoxic reactions, and the possible multiple antigenic targets for such reaction, it is not surprising that slight variations in techniques may lead to differing results.

The stimulation of lymphocyte blastic transformation by autologous tumor cells in culture has also been used as an in vitro measure of cell-mediated immunity to tumor antigens. In studies by Vanky and co-workers[52] of 95 patients with sarcomas of various types, lymphocyte stimulation was seen in 35 percent of cases.

Correlation with tumor skin-testing results was noted. Evidence of cross-reactivity in mixed lymphocyte-tumor cultures was suggested for patients with fibrosarcoma. In these and other studies of blastogenic responses to suspected tumor antigens, stimulation is often marginally increased and does not compare with that seen with tests for major transplantation antigens.

Leukocyte migration or adhesion inhibition techniques appear to have a high degree of sensitivity for detection of tumor antigens in rodent tumors and in man.[71,72] Recent studies comparing skin-testing and adherence inhibition (AI) in patients with melanoma and epidermoid carcinoma revealed a correlation between the two tests, with greater sensitivity of the in vitro assay.[72] Systematic studies of patients with soft tissue sarcomas are not yet available.

The tests for detection of CMI remain difficult to perform and to critically evaluate. An excellent detailed review of these techniques and their limitations has been published.[73]

The antigenicity of soft tissue sarcomas has largely been studied by serologic methods. Sera from patients bearing soft tissue sarcomas were most frequently examined for the presence of antibodies by immunofluorescence, complement fixation, or cytotoxic assays.[74-76]

Early studies with cultured cell lines of osteogenic sarcoma, liposarcoma, and fibrosarcoma indicated that sera from almost 100 percent of patients with sarcomas gave positive reactions. Cross-reactivity between sera suggested that a common sarcoma antigen was recognized, and the observation of C-type particles in a subculture of liposarcoma cells seemed to support a viral etiology.[75,77,78] In addition, cell-free suspensions of cultured sarcomas were capable of producing foci of transformed cells in fibroblast monolayers.[79] Other findings included an almost equally high rate of reaction when sera from close associates or relatives were tested, whereas controls were positive in about 25 percent of tests. Additional studies confirmed the presence of positive serologic reactions of patients with sarcoma, particularly when cultured rather than fresh tumor tissue was used.[74,80] Considerable confusion exists as to the specificity of these reactions, their frequency in control populations, the extent of cross-reactivity between tumor types, and the relationship of antibody activity to etiologic and prognostic factors of the disease.[76,80-82] For example, although almost universal positive immunofluorescence has been reported against cultured sarcoma cells with sera from normal subjects, Laprevotte and associates[82] described only negative results in a careful study of 19 sera samples tested against a panel of 14 human sarcoma lines.

Additional problems in the interpretation of early results have become evident as the difficulties inherent in the techniques have been clarified. These include the recognition that naturally occurring antibodies in heterologous serum incorporated in cell culture media may provide for positive reactions, as may blood group antigens and the presence of mycoplasma contamination.[83-85] With these reservations regarding the need for continued efforts at adequate control and careful conformation, evidence for several antigenic specificities on sarcoma cells have been advanced.[86-88] These include (1) specificities thought to represent a Forssman-type antigen present on sarcoma cells and recognized by most homologous and heterologous sera; (2) antigens that may be carcinoembryonic in origin, recognized by the sera of most patients with sarcomas, less than half of those with other tumors, and about 10 percent of normals; (3) antigens detected by complement fixation, occurring with approximately the same frequency as the above but showing a different reaction pattern. Similar to the findings originally reported by Eilber and Morton,[55] rising titers of complement-fixing antibodies may be seen after surgical tumor removal.

At present, major issues posed by early studies of the immunology of soft tissue sarcomas remain unresolved. It is of interest that mice with chemically induced sarcomas showing tumor-specific transplantation resistance can produce sera with cross-reacting cytotoxic activity.[89] In man, confirmatory evidence for a viral antigen common to sarcomas is lacking. Reactivity of sarcoma cells with a large number of sera from normal controls and from patients with epithelial neoplasms has again raised questions of sarcoma-specific antigens, and the technical considerations require further exploration. Nevertheless, the information to date at least suggests that these neoplasms regularly have qualitative or quantitative changes that are detectable by assays for cell-mediated and humoral immunity. Reactivity has a high frequency and, as indicated, may reveal a variety of differing antigenic systems. Whether these include tumor-specific transplantation antigens induced by viral or chemical agents is currently

unknown. A feasible method of producing high-titered antisera for specific cell surface antigens on sarcoma cells would be a major advance. The introduction of techniques for cloning rodent myeloma cells hybridized with spleen cells (hybridomas) sensitized to relevant tumors represents an exciting possible way to unravel the complexities of the serologic factors in sarcomas. This elegant technique, originally described by Kohler and Milstein,[90] is being increasingly applied to the human neoplasms.[91] To date, monoclonal antibodies have been produced to antigens associated with melanoma,[92-104] colorectal carcinoma,[94,96,105-110] neuroblastoma,[111-113] glioma,[114] mammary carcinoma,[115,116] leukemia,[117-119] sarcoma,[120] carcinoembryonic antigen;[121] and alpha-feto protein.[122] Monoclonal antibodies will become an increasingly important factor, not only in the characterization of tumor-associated antigens, but also in the study of the relationships of such tumor antigens to normal cellular components.[123]

Monoclonal antibodies may bring a new level of accuracy to the immunologic diagnosis of cancer and are presently providing a new approach to localization of primary and metastatic tumors. Radioimaging of tumors in mice by use of an iodine-labeled monoclonal antibody has been done by several investigators.[124-127] Similarly, gamma ray scintigraphy has been used to localize metastases in patients receiving radiolabeled monoclonal antibody to tumor-associated antigens.[43,44]

IMPORTANCE OF THE IMMUNE RESPONSE TO HOST DEFENSES AGAINST TUMORS

Although the association of specific antigens with soft tissue sarcomas and other malignancies appears to be demonstrated by the in vivo and in vitro tests outlined above, a major question remains as to what part, if any, immunologic mechanisms play in mediating the induction and clinical course of naturally occurring neoplasms.

During the 1950s the concept of immunosurveillance as a host defense mechanism was initially formulated and subsequently elaborated upon in detail.[128,129] In essence, the concept holds that cell-mediated immunity subserves an important function through the detection and elimination of neoplastic cells as they arise.

Clinical disease occurs when immunologic surveillance mechanisms are impaired. This concept has received wide acceptance, with considerable supportive evidence.

Consistent with the immunosurveillance hypothesis is the increased incidence of neoplasms reported to occur with primary or induced immunosuppression. A compilation of 118 cases of malignancy occurring in primary immunodeficiency diseases revealed an incidence of lymphoreticular or leukemic neoplasms in over 75 percent. Mesenchymal tumors were reported in four, including one case each of liposarcoma, leiomyosarcoma, undifferentiated sarcoma, and sarcoma of bone.[130] Long-term followup of patients receiving immunosuppressive drugs after tissue transplantation revealed an increased rate of de novo development of malignancy. Six cases of soft tissue sarcomas occurred in a total of 529 tumors.[131]

In experimental animal systems, immunosuppression with antilymphocyte sera or neonatal thymectomy has been shown to promote tumor induction following viral challenge.[132,133] Further experimental support for immunodepression associated with oncogenesis has been the demonstration that both chemical and viral carcinogenic agents have known immunosuppressive properties.[134] The strong association of Kaposi's sarcoma with cytomegalovirus illustrates a possible relationship between immunosuppression and viral interaction in the development of sarcoma in man.[135]

These observations, suggesting the importance of immunosurveillance at the inception of neoplastic growth, have been supplemented by clinical and pathologic findings in human neoplasms suggesting persistent immunologic activity. Among these is the rare occurrence of spontaneous remissions in soft tissue sarcomas and other tumors that may be explained by immunologic mechanisms. Everson and Cole[136] described 17 cases of such spontaneous regression of soft tissue sarcomas and Boyd[137] added another four. In addition to spontaneous regressions, local lymphocytic and histiocytic responses to human tumors have been reported to be a favorable pathologic and prognostic finding.[138,139]

Despite the stimulation for basic research that the immunosurveillance concept has provided, significant reservations exist as to its relevance for common human neoplasms.[140,141]

Immunodeficiency disease and immunosuppression in transplant patients are associated with a predominant increase in less common lymphoreticular neoplasms rather than usual tumor types. The mechanism for tumor production may well be unique under these circumstances. In addition, immunodeficiency in some animal models has not yielded the predicted increase in tumor incidence, and may show a decrease.[142] Decreases of immune reactivity demonstrated by skin-testing and in vitro techniques are seen only in some cancer patients. Rare spontaneous regression and chronic inflammatory histologic findings in tumors are subject to a variety of interpretations other than specific immunologic events. Prehn[143] presented arguments suggesting that immunologic mechanisms paradoxically may stimulate tumor growth. The relevance of immunosurveillance and immunostimulatory theories remains to be clarified but continues to provide a framework in which critical studies can be designed.

The relationship of measurements of general immunocompetency and specific antitumor immunity to the clinical course of growing tumors is currently under intensive investigation. Although statistical associations between various immunologic assays and the clinical stage of disease may have prognostic implications, they do not imply a cause and effect relationship, nor does tumor control necessarily follow from maneuvers to increase immune responsiveness.

In the area of general nonspecific immune findings in sarcoma patients, abnormalities in the number of lymphocytes and proportion of T- and B-cells could not be demonstrated in a prospective study of 134 patients. Eighty-four patients remained free of disease following therapy (ie, surgical, immunologic, and drug) and 50 had tumor progression.[144] Twomey and associates[57] studied DNCB sensitization and PHA lymphocyte stimulation in 100 patients cured of tumors, including three osteogenic sarcomas, four liposarcomas, five fibrosarcomas, and two myosarcomas. DNCB responses were normal and PHA stimulation was somewhat increased in the cured sarcoma patients. Depression of DNCB and PHA responses was noted in a significant percentage of preoperative patients. Eilber and co-workers[55] described 40 patients with bone or soft tissue sarcomas tested with DNCB at initial presentation, following surgery, and during immunotherapy. An excellent correlation was shown between the extent of disease and DNCB responsiveness. Stage I patients demonstrated 85 percent positive reactions, but this fell to 37 percent in stage II patients. Recurrent disease was noted within six months in patients with persistently negative reactions or in those in whom initial positive reactions became negative. On the other hand, more than 75 percent of patients with increasing DNCB reactivity following surgery, or converting from negative to positive reactions, remained free of disease. General correlations between short-term prognosis and nonspecific skin-testing have been reported by others, but this relationship, including DNCB responsiveness, has also been disputed.[58,59] At the moment, precise prognostic implications derived from skin-testing need further documentation.

When one turns to tumor-specific events occurring with soft tissue sarcomas, evidence supports a crude association between assays of host immune response and the evolution of the tumor. Assessment of antisarcoma antibody reactivity by the complement fixation technique was carried out by Eilber and Morton,[145] and by Morton et al.[145] In 10 patients free of disease the antibody titers remained elevated. Those patients undergoing definitive surgery and remaining free of disease demonstrated a fourfold rise in titer, whereas patients with persistent low levels of antibody or those failing to have a significant rise following surgery regularly developed progressive disease. Declining levels of antibody indicated a poor prognosis. Similar findings have been reported by others.[88] Humoral and lymphocyte-mediated tests for cytotoxicity have also shown correlation with short-term prognosis.[58,59,147] In evaluating blastogenic responses to autochthonous sarcoma cells, reactivity noted in about a third of the cases did not correlate with the extent of disease.[52] However, a more recent study by Rella and co-workers,[147] including seven patients with soft tissue sarcoma, indicated that high responders tended to do better. Hellstrom et al.,[65] using the colony inhibition test, have regularly shown active cell-mediated immunity in many human tumors, including soft tissue sarcomas, irrespective of the extent of disease.[65] As noted earlier, the significance of lymphocyte cytotoxic assays against tumor cells remains controversial.[67,68]

At this point, considerable experimental data in animals exist to support the thesis that immune responses to TSTA are of basic impor-

tance to tumor control and can be monitored. The assumption that this is true in man may be reasonable but is unproved.

In attempting to explain the failure of the demonstrated capability for immunologic tumor control thought to be present in most tumor patients, considerable emphasis has been placed on the role of serum factors acting to block cell-mediated immunity.[148] Such serum activity has been demonstrated in animal models in which the presence and progression of tumors is associated with clear evidence of cell-mediated immunity when in vitro testing is carried out in normal sera, but is blocked when sera is used from tumor-bearing animals.[149,150] The blocking phenomenon bears the same specificities and cross-reactive characteristics that apply to chemical and viral experimental oncogenic mechanisms.

Hellstrom et al.[151] demonstrated such serum activity in human sarcomas. Stjernsward and associates[152] showed that blastogenic responses to tumor cells were inhibited when the tests were carried out in autologous serum or serum from other patients with sarcoma. Using a culture of human rhabdomyosarcoma, Sinkovics and co-workers[66,153] were able to show tumor inhibition by lymphocytes of a cured patient and one with progressive disease. Serum from the cured patient potentiated the tumoricidal effect, but serum from the patient with metastatic disease blocked this response. Further studies have implicated the association of serum blocking factors with progressive tumor growth in other patients examined.

The question of identifying the nature of serum blocking factors remains to be solved. Evidence supporting a role for antigen-antibody complexes has been presented in animal sarcoma systems and in man.[38,154,155] Successful tumor ablation is associated with the decline in blocking activity and the appearance of serum factors that can counteract blocking (unblocking factors).[154,156]

The data at the present time on immunologic events occurring during the natural history of human sarcomas permit some tentative conclusions: (1) the progression of malignancy is associated with increasing defects in immunologic competence, primarily of the cell-mediated type, and, conversely, intact responsiveness has more favorable prognostic implications; (2) by a variety of techniques, most patients can be demonstrated to react immunologically to tumor-associated antigens; and (3) serum factors appear to play an important role in the regulation of such responses and may be useful for in vitro assessment of extent of disease. The modulation of responsiveness by suppressor T-cell populations in soft tissue sarcomas has not yet been explored.

IMMUNOTHERAPY

The demonstration of tumor immunogenicity has provided the rationale for historical and current efforts to treat cancer by immunologic techniques.[4,157] Prophylactic and therapeutic possibilities should be distinguished, since measures to prevent the development of specific neoplasms may be totally ineffective in the therapy of established tumors. Immunoprophylaxis can be achieved in some defined viral and chemically induced sarcomas in animal models.[17,19] Immunization against common human neoplasms, however, must await further etiologic and immunologic information. In contrast, immunotherapy of established tumors, even in animal models, has rarely met with success, and then only under specialized circumstances.[158] The many attempts to treat widespread malignancy in man by immunologic techniques cannot be considered successful. Much of the failure in the past can be explained by the limitations of immunotherapy evidenced in experimental systems. Particularly noteworthy in this regard is the ineffectiveness of immunotherapeutic maneuvers when tumor burdens are large.[159,160]

Classification of immunotherapeutic attempts includes those efforts that depend on the stimulation of the host's own immune system against tumor rejection antigens (active immunotherapy) and those that involve the introduction of exogenous cells or substances that are immunologically active against the neoplasm (passive immunotherapy). Active immunotherapy has been attempted by immunization with living or killed tumor cells, by homogenates, and by cells treated in vitro with agents aimed at increasing their antigenicity.[4,161] The cells may be autologous or obtained from different individuals with histologically similar tumors. Additional efforts directed at activating or enhancing immune capabilities of the host to autochthonous tumors include nonspecific immune stimulation by bacteria and their products and the administration of informational molecules such as transfer factor, thymosin, or RNA.[162-165] Restoration of cell-mediated immune responses has been found to be a property of some synthetic molecules. The antihelminthic drug Levamisole is an example of such an agent currently being evaluated in cancer patients.[166] The action of leukocyte-derived interferon as a cell modulator in cancer patients is also under study.[167]

Passive immunotherapy has included the infusion of homologous or heterologous antisera toxic to tumor cells in vitro. As cellular mechanisms of tumor rejection became clear, the infusion of large numbers of immunocompetent cells (usually lymphocytes) was used.[4,168,169] The demonstration of serum blocking effects has led to interest in the administration of serum factors that may be capable of neutralizing (unblocking) this tumor protective mechanism or of plasmapheresis techniques directed at removal of blocking factors.[156,170]

The above array of potential immunotherapeutic modalities and their use in preliminary studies has been extensively reviewed,[6,157,171] but conclusions regarding their usefulness in soft tissue sarcoma therapy are not possible at this time. General considerations are cited below.

The administration of cytotoxic antisera has been almost universally unsuccessful in producing regression of solid tumors in animal models. This might have been predicted from evidence in tissue transplantation, defining cell-mediated immunity as the effector mechanism for graft destruction. Paradoxically, enhanced tumor growth may occur following antibody administration in a variety of rodent sarcoma systems. For example, sarcoma I tumors in C57 BL/K mice can be readily enhanced by either hetero- or isoantisera. Similar effects have been shown for other solid tumor systems.[33] Fefer,[172] however, was able to show in the strongly antigenic Moloney sarcoma system that regression of tumors could sometimes be produced by serotherapy. The conditions resulting in enhancement or occasional therapeutic effects following antibody administration are not precisely defined and appear to be variable for different tumors and rodent strains. In man, serotherapy was one of the earliest modalities tried for treatment of advanced cancer. Heteroantisera were produced by immunization of animals with human tumors. Although a considerable number of patients were treated by the administration of such antisera, it became apparent that beneficial effects occurred rarely, if at all.[4] Recently, the recognition that following tumor ablation certain sera can neutralize the blocking of cell-mediated anti-tumor effects in vitro, and that under some circumstances antisera can enhance mononuclear tumoricidal functions, has renewed interest in antibody manipulation for immunotherapeutic purposes.[36,154,156] Bansal and Sjogren[156] reported sucessful anti-tumor effects in rats bearing polyoma tumor or carrying primary kidney sarcomas treated by "unblocking antibody." Extensive plasmapheresis of patients with disseminated cancer has recently been used for removal of serum blocking factors. Two evaluable patients with fibrosarcoma failed to respond.[168] Because partial responses were observed in some patients with epithelial tumors, studies of plasmapheresis and related techniques of manipulation of "serum factors" can be expected to continue.

The potential of passive immunotherapy with monoclonal antibodies has been shown in mice.[92,107,124] Such therapy in human neoplasia has often been unsuccessful due to undesirable side effects and only transient tumor response.[173] Recently, monoclonal antibodies have been administered to lymphoma[174] and leukemia[175] patients with dramatic, though often temporary, reduction in circulating tumor load.

Delivery of chemotherapeutic agents, isotopes, and hormones to tumor sites via monoclonal antibodies appears to have promise.[176-179] Such an approach should provide a more efficient means of delivery of agents to tumor-bearing sites with minimal side effects. The actual effectiveness of this therapy remains to be proven. There are several theoretical obstacles to successful implementation of this therapy, for example, shedding of antigen by the host tumor to effectively block the antibody, and the attempt by the host to eliminate the foreign protein within the administered monoclonal antibody. Some of these difficulties might be avoided if human monoclonal antibodies are utilized. Recently, the establishment of a human myeloma line capable of producing antibodysecreting hybridomas has been reported.[180]

Numerous attempts have been made in animals and man to induce tumor regression by the administration of lymphocytes. Successful therapy in virally or spontaneously occurring sarcomas in rodents has depended upon the use of lymphocytes (usually from specifically sensitized donors), small tumor loads, and the persistence of transfused lymphocytes in host animals.[158] In man, the prototype of lymphocyte transfusion immunotherapy has been the cross-immunization of tumor-bearing patients by exchange of tumor grafts.[168] Such grafts are rejected by virtue of normal histocompatibility responses. Following rejection, lymphocytes that may be immune to tumor antigens are transfused. Various modifications of this basic protocol have been carried out and summarized.[168,181,182] Patients treated are representative of most tumor types, with osteogenic sarcoma and melanoma receiving particular attention. In general, the patients treated have had advanced disease. In the series of patients summarized by Nadler and Moore,[168] 23 of 118 were said to have responded, including 1 of 9 with soft tissue sarcoma. Other series are less encouraging.[183] The overall experience with this form of therapy presents little evidence of consistent effects. The rapid rejection of allogeneic lymphocytes, the comparatively small numbers of lymphocytes that can be obtained from donors, and the large tumor load that most patients carry militate against success.

In the realm of active immunotherapy, immunization with cells or extracts of autologous or homologous tumors began in the nineteenth century.[4] Although resistance to new tumor implantation may occur concomitantly with the presence of an established neoplasm (concomitant immunity), regression of established tumors has not been regularly produced by classic immunization techniques.[184] Enhancement of the antigenicity of tumor cells by chemical means has, however, been demonstrated in vitro and in vivo.[185] Vibrio cholera neuraminidase (VCN) is an enzyme that removes the sialic acid coat from cell surfaces. Such treatment apparently exposes active antigenic sites normally protected by mucopolysaccharides on tumor cells. Injection of VCN-treated cells in rodent sarcoma systems has induced regression of small established tumors.[160,186] In man, intermittent therapeutic attempts at active immunization during the course of established malignancies have been carried out with marginal, if any, success.[4] However, inoculation of inactivated tumor cells has been reintroduced as part of adjuvant immunotherapy in situations of low tumor burden. Most data have been derived from studies of patients following remission induction for acute leukemia.[187] Prolongation of remission was reported by several groups.[187,188]

Nonspecific stimulators of the immune system have received attention in recent years. Such stimulation can be achieved by the injection of adjuvants, including a number of bacteria and bacterial products.[162] For example, the modified strain of *Bacillus Calmette-Guerin* (BCG), in addition to specifically immunizing to human *M. tuberculosis*, increases cell-mediated and humoral responses to primary antigenic challenge.[189] *C. parvum* and *B. pertussis* vaccines are other bacterial products being evaluated because of similar immunopotentiating effects.[190,191]

For prophylaxis, BCG is effective when administered both prior to, and mixed with, tumor cell challenges in rodent sarcomas and epithelial cancers. Under certain conditions, however, tumor enhancement rather than prevention is noted.[192-195] In man, attempts to assess the prophylactic value of BCG have largely dealt with epidemiologic retrospective studies of population groups immunized to prevent tuberculosis. Initial reports suggesting that BCG immunization was associated with a reduced incidence of childhood leukemia have not been confirmed.[196,197] More encouraging has been the regression of established sarcomas and carcinomas in mice treated with BCG.[159,198] Such chemically induced tumors are lethal to 100 percent of untreated animals. Surgical removal of the primary tumor fails to cure, since metastatic disease occurs early. Following intralesional BCG administration both primary and nodal micrometastases disappear. Cure, however, is highly dependent on the size of the lesion. Primary tumors beyond 1 cm^3 were not curable.[159]

In humans, BCG has been used by intralesional injection of viable organisms and by intradermal techniques. A high percentage of regression of injected lesions occurs, with occasional regression of uninjected lesions as well. BCG therapy has been summarized in melanoma patients with the following results: approximately 80 percent of injected superficial lesions go on to complete regression. In 20 percent of cases, uninjected lesions may also show a decrease in size that is sometimes dramatic.[199] Delayed hypersensitivity reaction to PPD and other microbial agents injected intralesionally has also resulted in regression of local lesions in several cases of Kaposi's sarcoma and fibrosarcoma.[200] Unfortunately, a response to life-threatening visceral disease is not documented for any human tumor type.

BCG given as adjuvant therapy following primary remission induction in either solid or hematologic malignancies has yielded conflicting results.[187,188,201,202] Often such therapy is combined with inoculation of inactivated autologous or homologous tumor cells. Studies of sarcoma patients have usually been compared with nonrandomized or historical controls. Sinkovics and co-workers[203] indicated a decreased rate of progression of soft tissue sarcomas following treatment with BCG or BCG + viral oncolysates of sarcoma cells. Tumor progression was noted in 36 of 49 patients treated by chemotherapy; 16 of 38 patients treated with the additional immunotherapy regime had progressive disease or died. In the series of patients reported by Townsend et al.,[204] a 21 percent three-year survival rate in historical controls was compared with the 59 percent three-year survival rate in patients treated with combined BCG and sarcoma cell immunization. Confirmation of these beneficial effects clearly requires randomized control studies.

In general, BCG therapy has been associated with mild to moderate local and systemic toxicity when administered intralesionally, or by scarification. Pain and inflammation sometimes leading to ulceration are common after local injection. Fever, myalgia, and malaise occurring from several hours to several days later are also common. Life-threatening reactions and generalized BCG infection may occur in patients who have been immunosuppressed by drugs or disease.[204-206]

Other bacteria, such as *C. parvum* and *B. pertussis*, shown to be effective immunostimulants in rodent models, are also under investigation.[125] Preliminary studies in patients with nonlymphocytic sarcomas suggested that *C. parvum* in addition to chemotherapy offered some advantage over chemotherapy alone.[190]

Experimental human immunotherapeutic protocols continue to grow more complex as new modalities are introduced and combined forms of treatment become more common. It is exceedingly difficult to evaluate the preliminary reports because of the numerous variables involved.

A registry of clinical immunotherapy studies and periodic published conferences of active investigative groups have been helpful in keeping information current while guarding against premature conclusions.[157,169,208,209] The reader is referred to these sources for detailed information. A standard immunotherapy recommendation for treating patients with soft tissue sarcomas cannot be given at this time.

CONCLUSIONS

Although important concepts and supporting data have been introduced in the present era of tumor immunology, a critical period of reassessment is under way. Immunity in vivo has been difficult to demonstrate in many spontaneous tumors in animals or in humans. Where such evidence exists, proof of associated humoral and cellular responses to identified tumor specific antigens is incomplete. At best, immunologic reaction to clinically established tumors appears to be a weak defense mechanism that does not seem to be significantly influenced by current immunostimulatory efforts. The response of some local tumors to intralesional therapy involves an inflammatory process difficult to define as a specific immunologic event.

Particular problems exist when considering immunologic and therapeutic aspects of soft tissue sarcomas. Although rare among human neoplasms, morphologic and clinical heterogenicity is evident. Etiologic heterogenicity to known carcinogenic agents is also well documented in animals. In most clinical studies, patients with soft tissue sarcomas are few and represent various tissue types. Small numbers, along with a proposed common etiology, have reinforced the tendency to group all patients with soft tissue sarcomas as uniform subjects for investigation, a practice with obvious limitations.

The above reservations need to be viewed in the light of existing information, which at least suggests immunologic changes associated with soft tissue sarcomas and their therapy. That animal and human sarcoma cells can be targets for immunologic reactions is quite clear from a variety of in vitro testing procedures. The challenge is to clarify the antigens detected in terms of their biologic classification and implications. The immunogenetic systems necessary for the expression of specific surface markers on tumor cells and their relevance to exogenous or endogenous etiologic factors provide an exciting area for future development.

Immunotherapeutic considerations are being focused in new directions, taking into account the accomplishments in rodent models. Of major importance is that, with current immuno-

therapy, low tumor burdens are essential to demonstrate effects. Thus the clinically tumor-free patient with a high probability of recurrence is the subject of an increasing number of studies. Such investigations call for a rare degree of excellence in experimental design if definitive data are to be obtained.

It is hoped that attempts to potentiate host responses to specific tumor antigens by modification of the tumor cell surface will replace most current efforts based on nonspecific immune stimulation. Similarly, manipulation of humoral and cellular elements favorable to tumor control needs to be considered in the context of a deletion or addition of defined plasma components or cell populations specific for tumor interactions.

At the moment, immunologic examination and immunotherapeutic protocols remain in the realm of experimental medicine. One can only anticipate that useful clinical applications will be forthcoming.

REFERENCES

1. Ehrlich P: Uber den jetzigen Stand der Karzinomforschung. In Himmelweit R (ed): The Collected Papers of Paul Ehrlich, vol. 2. London, Pergamon Press, 1957, pp 550–562
2. Smith GB, Washbourn JW: Infective sarcomata in dogs. Br Med J 2:1807, 1898
3. Crile GW, Beebe SP: Transfusion of blood in the transplantable lymphosarcoma of dogs. J Med Res 18:385, 1908
4. Currie GA: Eighty years of immunotherapy: A review of immunological methods used for the treatment of human cancer. Br J Cancer 26:141, 1972
5. Nauts HC, Swift WE, Coley BC: The treatment of malignant tumors by bacterial toxins as developed by the late William B. Coley, reviewed in the light of modern research. Cancer Res 6:205, 1948
6. Southam CM, Friedman H (eds): International Conference on Immunotherapy of Cancer. Ann NY Acad Sci 277, 1976
7. Hersh EM, Gutterman JU, Mavligit G (eds): Immunotherapy of Cancer in Man. Springfield (Ill), Thomas, 1973
8. Weiss DW: The questionable immunogenicity of certain neoplasms: What then the prospects for immunological intervention in malignant disease? Cancer Immunol Immunother 2:11, 1977
9. Friedman H, Southam C (eds): International Conference on Immunobiology of Cancer. Ann NY Acad Sci 276, 1976
10. Hellstrom KE, Brown JP: Tumor antigens. In Sela M (ed): The Antigens, vol. 5. New York, Academic Press, 1979 pp 1-82

11. Woglom WH: Immunity to transplantable tumors. Cancer Rev 4:129, 1929

12. Gross L: Oncogenic Viruses, 2nd ed. Oxford and New York, Pergamon Press, 1970

13. Gross L: Viral etiology of cancer and leukemia: A look into the past, present, and future. G.H.A. Clowes Memorial Lecture. Cancer Res 38:485, 1978

14. Kennaway EL: The identification of a carcinogenic compound in coal-tar. Br Med J 2:749, 1955

15. Miller JA: Carcinogenesis by chemicals: An overview. G.H.A. Clowes Memorial Lecture. Cancer Res 30:539, 1970

16. Foley EJ: Antigenic properties of methylcholanthrene-induced tumors in mice of the strain of origin. Cancer Res 13:835, 1953

17. Prehn RT, Main JM: Immunity to methylcholanthrene-induced sarcomas. J Nat Cancer Inst 18:769, 1957

18. Baldwin RW: Immunity to methylcholanthrene-induced tumors in inbred rats following atrophy and regression of the implanted tumors. Br J Cancer 9:652, 1955

19. Habel K: Resistance of polyoma virus immune animals to transplanted polyoma tumors. Proc Soc Exp Biol Med 106:722, 1961

20. Churchill AE, Payne LN, Chubb RC: Immunization against Marek's disease using live attenuated virus. Nature 221:744, 1969

21. Morton DL, Malmgren RA, Hall WT, Schidlovsky G: Immunologic and virus studies with human sarcomas. Surgery 66:152, 1969

22. Gershon RK: Immune regulation. Symposium on Immune Regulation. Fed Proc 38:2051, 1979

23. Hildemann WH: Genetics of immune responsiveness. Ann Rev Genet 7:19, 1973

24. Miller JF, Mitchell GF, Davies AJS, Claman HN, Chaperon EA, Taylor RB: Antigen-sensitive cells: Their source and differentiation. Transplant Rev 1:3, 1969

25. Ross GD: Identification of human lymphocyte subpopulations by surface marker analysis. Blood 54:799, 1979

26. Waldmann H: Interactions between T and B cells: A review. J Roy Soc Med 72:198, 1979

27. Waldmann TA, Broder S: Suppressor cells in the regulation of the immune response. Prog Clin Immunol 3:155, 1977

28. Dvorak HF: Delayed hypersensitivity. In Zweifach BS, Grant L, McCluskey RT (eds): The Inflammatory Process. New York, Academic Press, 1974, pp 291–345

29. Perlmann R, Holm G: Cytotoxic effects of lymphoid cells in vitro. Adv Immunol 11:117, 1969

30. David JR: Lymphocyte mediators and cellular hypersensitivity. Seminars in Medicine of the Beth Israel Hospital, Boston 288:143, 1973

31. Herberman RB, Djeu JY, Kay HD, Ortaldo JR, Riccardi C, Bonnard GD, Holdne RT, Fagnani R, Santoni A, Puccetti P: Natural killer cells: Characteristics and regulation of activity. Immunol Rev 44:43, 1979

32. Gore PA: Cytotoxicity of antisera. J Path Bact 54:61, 1942

33. Kaliss N: Immunological enhancement of tumor homografts in mice: A review. Cancer Res 18:992, 1958

34. Hellstrom KE, Hellstrom I: Lymphocyte mediated cytotoxicity and blocking serum activity to tumor antigens. Adv Immunol 18:209, 1974

35. Pollack S, Heppner G, Brown RI, Nelson K: Specific killing of tumor cells in vitro in the presence of normal lymphoid cells and sera from hosts immune to tumor antigens. Int J Cancer 9:316, 1972

36. Hellstrom I, Hellstrom KE, Warner GA: Increase of lymphocyte-mediated tumor-cell destruction by certain patient sera. Int J Cancer 12:348, 1973

37. Brier AM, Chess L, Schlossman SF: Human antibody-dependent cellular cytotoxicity: Isolation and identification of a subpopulation of peripheral blood lymphocytes which kill antibody-coated autologuous target cells. J Clin Invest 56:1580, 1975

38. Sjogren HO, Hellstrom I, Bansal SC, Hellstrom KE: Suggestive evidence that the "blocking antibodies" of tumor-bearing individuals may be antigen-antibody complexes. Proc Nat Acad Sci 68:1372, 1971

39. Thomson DMP: Soluble tumor-specific antigen and its relationship to tumor growth. Int J Cancer 15:1016, 1975

40. Beschorner WE, Hess AD, Nerenberg ST, Epstein RB: Isolation and characterization of canine venereal tumor-associated inhibitory and blocking factors. Cancer Res 39:3920, 1979

41. Fefer A, McCoy JL, Perk K, Glynn JP: Immunologic, virologic, and pathologic studies of regression of autochthonous Moloney sarcoma virus-induced tumors in mice. Cancer Res 28:1577, 1968

42. Old LJ, Boyse EA, Clarke DA, Carswell EA: Antigenic properties of chemically induced tumors. Ann NY Acad Sci 101:80, 1962

43. Klein G, Sjogren HO, Klein E, Hellstrom KE: Demonstration of resistance against methylcholanthrene-induced sarcomas in the primary autochthonous host. Cancer Res 20:1561, 1960

44. Old LJ, Boyse EA: Immunology of experimental tumors. Ann Rev Med 15:1967, 1964

45. Upton AC: Radiation carcinogenesis. In Busch H (ed): Methods in Cancer Research, vol. 4. New York, Academic Press, 1968, pp 53–82

46. Hewitt HB, Blake ER, Waker AS: A critique of the evidence for active host defense against cancer, based on personal studies of 27 murine tumors of spontaneous origin. Br J Cancer 33:241, 1976

47. Klein G, Klein E: Immune surveillance against virus-induced tumors and nonrejectability of spontaneous tumors: Contrasting consequences of host versus tumor evolution. Proc Nat Acad Sci 74:2121, 1977

48. Oettgen EF, Old LJ, McLean EP, Carswell EA: Delayed hypersensitivity and transplantation immunity by soluble antigens of chemically induced tumors in inbred guinea pigs. Nature 220:295, 1968

49. Stewart THM: The presence of delayed hypersensitivity reactions in patients toward cellular extracts of their malignant tumors. 2. A corre-

lation between the histologic picture of lympho-cyte infiltration of the tumor stroma, the presence of such a reaction, and a discussion of the significance of this phenomenon. Cancer 23:1380, 1969

50. Fass L, Herberman RB, Ziegler J: Delayed cutaneous hypersensitivity reactions to autologous extracts of Burkitt lymphoma cells. N Engl J Med 282:776, 1970

51. Herberman RB: Delayed hypersensitivity skin reactions to antigens on human tumors. Cancer 34:1469, 1974

52. Vanky F, Klein E, Stjernsward J, Nilsonne U: Cellular immunity against tumor-associated antigens in humans: Lymphocyte stimulation and skin reaction. Int J Cancer 14:277, 1974

53. Reisfeld RA, David GS, Ferrone S, Pellegrino MA, Holmes EC: Approaches for the isolation of biologically functional tumor-associated antigens. Cancer Res 37:2860, 1977

54. Solowey AC, Rapaport FT: Immunologic responses in cancer patients. Surg Gynecol Obstet 14:756, 1965

55. Eilber FR, Morton DL: Impaired immunologic reactivity and recurrence following cancer surgery. Cancer 25:362, 1970

56. Eilber FR, Nizze JA, Morton DL: Sequential evaluation of general immune competence in cancer patients: Correlation with clinical course. Cancer 35:660, 1975

57. Twomey PL, Catalona WJ, Chretien PB: Cellular immunity in cured cancer patients. Cancer 33:435, 1974

58. Kotz R, Rella W, Salzer M: The immune status in patients with bone and soft-tissue sarcomas. Recent Res Cancer Res 54:197, 1976

59. Pritchard DJ, Ivins JC, Ritts RE, Jr.: Immunologic aspects of human sarcomas. Recent Res Cancer Res 54:185, 1976

60. Hellstrom I: A colony inhibition (CI) technique for demonstration of tumor cell destruction by lymphoid cells in vitro. Int J Cancer 2:65, 1967

61. Takasugi M, Mickey MR, Terasaki PI: Quantitation of the microassay for cell-mediated immunity through electronic image analyses. Nat Cancer Inst Monogr 37:77, 1973

62. Block LH, Ruhenstroth-Bauer G: Biological and clinical relevance of human macrophage migration inhibitory factor (MIP). Blut 38:93, 1979

63. Halliday WJ, Maluish AE, Stephenson PM, Davis NC: An evaluation of leukocyte adherence inhibition in the immunodiagnosis of colon-rectal cancer. Cancer Res 37:1962, 1977

64. Hellstrom I, Hellstrom KE, Pierce GE: In vitro studies of immune reactions against autochthonous and syngeneic mouse tumors induced by methylcholanthrene and plastic discs. Int J Cancer 3:467, 1968

65. Hellstrom I, Hellstrom KE, Sjogren HO, Warner GA: Demonstration of cell-mediated immunity to human neoplasms of various histological types. Int J Cancer 7:1, 1971

66. Sinkovics JG, Ahmed N, Hrgovcic MJ, Cabiness JR, Wilbur JR: Cytotoxic lymphocytes. II. Antagonism and synergism between serum factors and lymphocytes of patients with sarcomas as tested against culture tumor cells. Tex Rep Biol Med 30:347, 1972

67. Takasugi M, Mickey MR, Terasaki PI: Studies on specificity of cell-mediated immunity to human tumors. J Nat Cancer Inst 53:1527, 1974

68. Takasugi M, Mickey MR, Terasaki PI: Reactivity of lymphocytes from normal persons on cultured tumor cells. Cancer Res 33:2898, 1973

69. Heppner G, Henry E, Stolbach L, Cummings F, McDonough E, Calabresi P: Problems in the clinical use of the microcytotoxicity assay for measuring cell-mediated immunity to tumor cells. Cancer Res 35:1931, 1976

70. Bukowski RM, Barna B, Deodhar SK, Hewlett JS: Nonspecific lymphocyte cytotoxicity in patients with malignant melanoma, renal cell carcinoma, and sarcomas, and in nontumor patients. Cancer 38:1962, 1976

71. Halliday WJ, Webb M: Delayed hypersensitivity to chemically induced tumors in mice and correlation with an in vitro test. J Nat Cancer Inst 43:141, 1969

72. Burger DR, Vandenbark AA, Finke P, Malley A, Frikke M, Black J, Acott K, Begley D, Vetto RM: Assessment of reactivity to tumor extracts by leukocyte adherence inhibition and dermal testing. J Nat Cancer Inst 59:317, 1977

73. Bloom BR, David JR (eds): In Vitro Methods in Cell-mediated and Tumor Immunity. New York, Academic Press, 1976

74. Moore M, Witherow PJ, Price CHG, Clough SA: Detection by immunofluorescence of intracytoplasmic antigens in cell lines derived from human sarcomas. Int J Cancer 12:428, 1973.

75. Eilber FR, Morton DL: Sarcoma specific antigens: Detection by complement-fixation with serum from sarcoma patients. J Nat Cancer Inst 44:651, 1970

76. Bloom ET: Further definition by cytotoxicity tests of cell surface antigens of human sarcomas in culture. Cancer Res 32:960, 1972

77. Morton DL, Hall WT, Malmgren RA: Human liposarcomas: Tissue cultures containing foci of transformed cells with viral particles. Science 165:813, 1969

78. Eilber FR, Morton DL: Immunologic studies of human sarcomas: Additional evidence suggesting an associated sarcoma virus. Cancer 26:588, 1970

79. Giraldo G, Beth E, Hirshaut Y, Aoki T, Old LJ, Boyse EA, Chopra HC: Human sarcomas in culture. Foci of cultured cells and a common antigen; induction of foci and antigen in human fibroblast cultures by filtrates. J Exp Med 133:454, 1971

80. Moore M, Hughes LA: Circulating antibodies in human connective tissue malignancy. Br J Cancer 18 (suppl 1):175, 1973

81. Oettgen HF, Bean MA, Klein G: Workshop in human tumor immunology. Cancer Res 32:2845, 1972

82. Laprevotte I, Chaut JC, L'Hirondel AM, Bernard C, Peries J, Boiron M: A search for antibodies against human sarcoma cells in patients' sera by indirect immunofluorescence on fixed cells. Eur J Cancer 11:757, 1975

83. Irie RF, Irie K, Morton DL: Natural antibody in human serum to a neoantigen in human cultured cells grown in fetal bovine serum. J Nat Cancer Inst 52:1051, 1974

84. Bloom ET, Fahey JL, Peterson IA, Geering G, Bernhard M, Trempe G: Anti-tumor activity in human serum: Antibodies detecting blood-group-A-like antigen on the surface of tumor cells in culture. Int J Cancer 12:21, 1973

85. Bloom ET: Microcytotoxicity tests on human cells in cultures: Effect of contamination with mycoplasma. Proc Soc Exp Biol Med 143:244, 1973

86. Hirshaut Y, Pei DT, Marcove RC, Mukherji B, Spielvogel AR, Essner E: Seroepidemiology of human sarcoma antigen (S₁). N Engl J Med 291:1103, 1974

87. Mukherji B, Hirshaut Y: Evidence for fetal antigen in human sarcoma. Science 181:440, 1973

88. Sethi J, Hirshaut Y: Complement-fixing antigen of human sarcomas. J Nat Cancer Inst 57:489, 1976

89. Fritze D, Kern DH, Humme JA, Drogemuller CR, Pilch YH: Detection of private and common tumor-associated antigens in murine sarcomas induced by different chemical carcinogens. Int J Cancer 17:136, 1976

90. Kohler G, Milstein C: Continuous cultures of fused cells secreting antibody of predefined specificity. Nature 256:495, 1975

91. Kennett RH, Gilbert F: Hybrid myelomas producing antibodies against a human neuroblastoma antigen present on fetal brain. Science 203:1120, 1979

92. Koprowski H, Steplewski Z, Herlyn DM, et al: Study of antibodies against human melanoma produced by somatic cell hybrids. Proc Nat Acad Sci USA 75:3405, 1978

93. Stelplewski Z, Herlyn MF, Herlyn DM, et al: Reactivity of monoclonal antimelanoma antibodies with melanoma cells freshly isolated from primary and metastatic melanoma. Eur J Immunol 9:94, 1976

94. Herlyn DM, Herlyn MF, Steplewski Z, et al: Monoclonal antibodies in cell-mediated cytotoxicity against human melanoma and colorectal carcinoma. Eur J Immunol 9:657, 1979

95. Herlyn MF, Clark WH, Mastrangelo MJ, et al: Specific immunoreactivity of hybridoma-secreted monoclonal anti-melanoma antibodies to cultured cells and freshly derived human cells. Cancer Res 40:3602, 1980

96. Steplewski Z: Monoclonal antibodies to human tumor antigens. Transplant Proc XII:384, 1980

97. Mitchell KF, Fuhrer JP, Steplewski Z, et al: Biochemical characterization of human melanoma cell surfaces: Dissection with monoclonal antibodies. Proc Nat Acad Sci USA 70:7287, 1980

98. Yeh MY, Hellstrom I, Brown JP, et al: Cell surface antigens of human melanoma identified by monoclonal antibody. Proc Nat Acad Sci USA 76:2927, 1979

99. Brown JP, Wright PW, Hart CE, et al: Protein antigens of normal and malignant human cells identified by immunoprecipitation with monoclonal antibodies. J Biol Chem 255:4980, 1980

100. Loop SM, Nishiyama K, Hellstrom I, et al: Two human tumor-associated antigens, p155 and p210, detected by monoclonal antibodies. Int J Cancer 27:775, 1981

101. Brown JP, Woodbury RG, Hart CE, et al: Quantitative analysis of melanoma associated antigen p97 in normal and neoplastic tissues. Proc Nat Acad Sci USA 78:539, 1981

102. Dippold WG, Lloyd KO, Li LTC, et al: Cell surface antigens of human malignant melanoma: Definition of six antigenic systems with mouse monoclonal antibodies. Proc Natl Acad Sci USA 77:6114, 1980

103. Imai K, Ng AK, Ferrone S: Characterization of monoclonal antibodies to human melanoma-associated antigens. J Nat Cancer Inst 66:489, 1981

104. Imai K, Molinaro GA, Ferrone S: Monoclonal antibodies to human melanoma associated antigens. Transplant Proc XII:380, 1980

105. Herlyn MF, Steplewski Z, Herlyn DM, et al: Colorectal carcinoma-specific antigen: Detection by means of monoclonal antibodies. Proc Nat Acad Sci USA 76:1438, 1979

106. Koprowski H, Steplewski Z, Mitchell K, et al: Colorectal carcinoma antigens detected by hybridoma antibodies. Somatic Cell Genet 5:957, 1979

107. Herlyn DM, Steplewski Z, Herlyn MF, et al: Inhibition of growth of colorectal carcinoma in nude mice by monoclonal antibody. Cancer Res 40:717, 1980

108. Herlyn DM, Koprowski H: Monoclonal anticolon carcinoma antibodies in complement-dependent cytotoxicity. Int J Cancer 27:769, 1981

109. Koprowski H, Herlyn MF, Steplewski Z: Specific antigen in serum of patients with colon carcinoma. Science 212:53, 1981

110. Magnani JL, Brockhaus M, Smith DF, et al: A monosialoganglioside is a monoclonal antibody-defined antigen of colon carcinoma. Science 212:55, 1981

111. Kennett RH, Gilbert F: Hybrid myelomas producing antibodies against a human neuroblastoma antigen present on fetal brain. Science 203:1120, 1979

112. Kennett RH, Jonak ZL, Bechtol KB: Monoclonal antibodies against human tumor associated antigens. In Kennett RH, McKern TJ, Bechtol KB (eds): Monoclonal Antibodies Hybridomas. A New Dimension in Biological Analyses. New York, Plenum Press, 1980, pp 155–168

113. Momoi M, Kennett RH, Glick MC: A membrane glycoprotein from human neuroblastoma cells isolated with the use of a monoclonal antibody. J Biol Chem 255:11914, 1980

114. Schnegg JF, Diserens AC, Carrel S, et al: Human glioma-associated antigens detected by monoclonal antibodies. Cancer Res 41:1209, 1981

115. Colcher D, Hand PH, Nuti M, et al: A spectrum of monoclonal antibodies reactive with human mammary tumor cells. Proc Nat Acad Sci USA 78:3199, 1981

116. Schlom J, Wunderlich D, Teramoto YA: Generation of human monoclonal antibodies reactive with human mammary carcinoma cells. Proc Nat Acad Sci USA 77:6841, 1980

117. Ritz J, Pesando JM, Notis-McConarly J, et al: A monoclonal antibody to human acute lymphoclastic leukaemia antigen. Nature 283:583, 1980

118. Levy R, Dilley J, Fox RI, et al: A human thymus-leukemia antigen defined by hybridoma monoclonal antibodies. Proc Nat Acad Sci USA 76:6552, 1979

119. Kersey JH, LeBien TW, Abramson CS, et al: A human leukemia-associated and lymphohemopoietic progenitor cell surface structure identified with monoclonal antibody. J Exp Med 153:726, 1981

120. Deng C, El-Awar N, Cicciarelli J, et al: Cytotoxic monoclonal antibody to a human leiomyosarcoma. Lancet 21:403, 1981

121. Accolla RS, Carrel S, Mach JP: Monoclonal antibodies specific for carcinoembryonic antigen and produced by two hybrid cell lines. Proc Nat Acad Sci USA 77:563, 1980

122. Tsung YK, Milunsky A, Alpert E: Derivation and characterization of a monoclonal hybridoma antibody specific for human alphafetoprotein. J Immunol Meth 39:363, 1980

123. Allison JP: Contributions of hybridoma technology to cancer immunology. Cancer Bulletin 33(5):226, 1981

124. Bernstein ID, Tam MR: Mouse leukemia: Therapy with monoclonal antibodies against a thymus differentiation antigen. Science 207:68, 1980

125. Moshakis V, McIthinney RJ, Raghavan D, Neville AM: In vivo immunodetection of xenografted human tumors by monoclonal antibodies: Proceedings of an international workshop on monoclonal antibodies to tumor antigens. Br J Cancer 43:559, 1981

126. Goldenberg DM, Deland F, Kim E, et al: Use of radiolabeled antibody to carcino-embryonic antigen for the detection and localization of diverse cancers by external photoscanning. N Engl J Med 298:1384, 1978

127. Belithy T, Ghose T, Agiano J, et al: Radionuclide imaging of primary renal-cell carinomas by ^{131}I-labeled antitumor antibody. J Nucl Med 19: 427, 1978

128. Thomas L: Discussion P.B. Medawar paper, "Reactions to homologous tissue antigens and relation to hypersensitivity." In Lawrence HS (ed): Cellular and Humoral Aspects of the Hypersensitive States. New York, Hoeber, 1959

129. Burnet FM: Immunological Surveillance. Oxford, Pergamon Press, 1970

130. Kersey JH, Spector BD, Good RA: Primary immunodeficiency and malignancy. In Bergama D (ed): Immunodeficiency in Man and Animals. Sunderland (Mass), Sinauer Associates, 1975

131. Penn I: Malignancies associated with immunosuppressive or cytotoxic therapy. Surgery 83:492, 1978

132. Allison AC, Taylor RB: Observations on thymectomy and carcinogenesis. Cancer Res 27:703, 1967

133. Vandeputte M: Antilymphocyte serum and polyoma oncogenesis in rats. Transplant Proc 1:100, 1969

134. Stjernsward J: Immunosuppression by carcinogens. Antibiotic Chemotherapy 15:213, 1969

135. Drew WL, Miner RC, Ziegler JL, Gullet JH, Abrahms DI, Conant MA, et al: Cytomegalovirus and Kaposi's sarcoma in young homosexual men. Lancet 2:125, 1982

136. Everson TC, Cole WH: Spontaneous Regression of Cancer. Philadelphia, Saunders, 1966

137. Boyd W: The Spontaneous Regression of Cancer. Springfield (Ill), Thomas, 1966

138. Tsakraklides V, Olson P, Kersey JH, Good RA: Prognostic significance of the regional lymph node histology in cancer of the breast. Cancer 34:1259, 1974

139. Lane M, Goksel H, Salerno RA, Haagensen CD: Clinicopathologic analysis of the surgical curability of breast cancers: A minimum ten-year study of a personal series. Ann Surg 153:483, 1961

140. Schwartz RS: Medical intelligence. Another look at immunologic surveillance. N Engl J Med 293:181, 1975

141. Prehn RT: Immunological surveillance: Pro and con. In Bach FE, Good RA (eds): Clinical Immunobiology, vol. 2. New York, Academic Press, 1974

142. Rygaard J, Povlsen CO: The mouse mutant nude does not develop spontaneous tumors. An argument against immunological surveillance. Acta Path Microbiol Scand 82:99, 1974

143. Prehn RT: Do tumors grow because of the immune response of the host? Transplant Rev 28:34, 1976

144. Pritchard DJ, Miller GC, Ritts RE, Jr., Ivins JC: Thymus-dependent and nonthymus-dependent lymphocytes in patients with sarcomas. Cancer 40:803, 1977

145. Eilber FR, Morton DL: Immunologic response to human sarcomas: Relation of antitumor antibody to the clinical course. In Amos B (ed): Progress in Immunology. New York, Academic Press, 1971, pp 951–957

146. Morton DL, Holmes EC, Eilber FR, Wood WC: Immunological aspects of neoplasia: A rational basis of immunotherapy. Ann Intern Med 74:587, 1971

147. Rella W, Dotz R, Arbes H, Leber H: Tumor-specific immunity in sarcoma patients. Oncology 34:219, 1977

148. Hellstrom KE, Hellstrom I, Nepom JT: Specific blocking factors—are they important? Biochem Biophys Acta 473:121, 1977

149. Hellstrom I, Hellstrom KE, Evans CA, Heppner GH, Pierce GE, Yang JPS: Serum-mediated protection of neoplastic cells from inhibition by lymphocytes immune to their tumor-specific antigens. Proc Nat Acad Sci 62:362, 1969

150. Baldwin RW, Embleton MJ, Price MR, Robins A: Immunity in the tumor-bearing host and its modification by serum factors. Cancer 34:1452, 1974

151. Hellstrom I, Sjogren HO, Warner GA, Hellstrom KE: Blocking of cell-mediated tumor immunity by sera from patients with growing neoplasms. Int J Cancer 7:226, 1971

152. Stjernsward J, Vanky F, Klein E: Lymphocyte stimulation by autochthonous human solid tumors. Br J Cancer 28 (suppl 1):72, 1972

153. Sinkovics JG, Williams DE, Campos LT, Kay HD, Romero JJ: Intensification of immune reactions of patients to cultured sarcoma cells: Attempts at monitored immunotherapy. Seminar Oncol 1:351, 1974

154. Sjogren HO: Blocking and unblocking of cell-mediated tumor immunity. In Busch H (ed): Methods in Cancer Research, vol. 10. New York, Academic Press, 1973

155. Sjogren HO, Hellstrom I, Bansal SC, Warner GA, Hellstrom KE: Elution of "blocking factors" from human tumors, capable of abrogating tumor cell destruction by specifically immune lymphocytes. Int J Cancer 9:274, 1972

156. Bansal SC, Sjogren HO: Counteraction of the blocking of cell-mediated tumor immunity by inoculation of unblocking sera and splenectomy: Immunotherapeutic effects on primary polyoma tumors in rats. Int J Cancer 9:490, 1972

157. Terry WD, Windhorst D (eds): Progress in Cancer Research and Therapy, vol. 6. Immunotherapy of Cancer: Present Status of Trials in Man. New York, Raven Press, 1978

158. Fefer A: Experimental approaches to immunotherapy of cancer: recent results. Cancer Res 36:182, 1971

159. Zbar B, Bernstein ID, Bartlett GL, Hanna MG, Jr., Rapp EJ: Immunotherapy of cancer: Regression of intradermal tumors and prevention of growth of lymph node metastases after intralesional injection of living *Mycobacterium bovis*. J Nat Cancer Inst 49:119, 1972

160. Rios A, Simmons RL: Active specific immunotherapy of minimal residual tumor: Excision plus neuraminidase-treated tumor cells. Int J Cancer 13:71, 1974

161. Sedlacek HH, Seiler FR: Immunotherapy of neoplastic disease with neuraminidase: Contradictions, new aspects, and revised concepts. Cancer Immunol Immunother 5:153, 1978

162. Bast RC, Jr., Bast BC: Critical review of previously reported animal studies of tumor immunotherapy with nonspecific immunostimulants. Ann NY Acad Sci 227:60 1976

163. Spitler LE, Levin AS, Fudenberg HH: Human lymphocyte transfer factor. In Busch H (ed): Methods in Cancer Research, vol. 8. New York, Academic Press, 1973

164. Goldstein AL, Low TLK, Rossio JL, Ulrich JT, Naylor PH, Thurman GB: Recent developments in the chemistry and biology of thymosin. In Chirigos MA (ed): Progress in Cancer Research and Therapy. Immune Modulation and Control of Neoplasia by Adjuvant Therapy, vol. 7. New York, Raven Press, 1978

165. Pilch YH, deKernion JB, Skinner DG, Ramming KP, Schick PM, Fritze D, Brower P, Kern DH: Immunotherapy of cancer with "immune" RNA. Am J Surg 132:631, 1976

166. Persico FJ, Potter WA: Effect of Levamisole on an in vitro model of cellular immunity. In Chirigos MA (ed): Progress in Cancer Reserach and Therapy. Immune Modulation and Control of Neoplasia by Adjuvant Therapy, vol. 7. New York, Raven Press, 1978

167. Merigan TC: Human interferon as a therapeutic agent. N Engl J Med 300:42, 1979

168. Nadler SH, Moore GE: Immunotherapy of malignant disease. Arch Surg 99:376, 1969

169. Yonemoto RH: Adoptive immunotherapy utilizing thoracic duct lymphocytes. Ann NY Acad Sci 227:7, 1976.

170. Israel L, Edelstein R, Mannoni P, Radot E, Greenspan EM: Plasmapheresis in patients with disseminated cancer: Clinical results and correlation with changes in serum protein. The concept of "nonspecific blocking factors." Plasma Ther 1:57, 1979

171. Chirigos MA (ed): Progress in Cancer Research and Therapy, vol. 7. Immune Modulation and Control of Neoplasia by Adjuvant Therapy. New York, Raven Press, 1978

172. Fefer A: Immunotherapy and chemotherapy of Maloney sarcoma virus-induced tumors in mice. Cancer Res 29:2177, 1969

173. Rosenberg SA, Terry WD: Passive immunotherapy of cancer in animals and man. Adv Cancer Res 25:280, 1977

174. Nadler LM, Stashenko P, Hardy R, et al: Serotherapy of a patient with a monoclonal antibody directed against a human lymphoma-associated antigen. Cancer Res 40:3147, 1980

175. Miller RA, Levy R: Response of cutaneous T-cell lymphoma to therapy with hybridoma monoclonal antibody. Lancet, in press

176. Ghose T, Blair AH: Antibody-linked cytotoxic agents in the treatment of cancer: Current status and future prospects. J Nat Cancer Inst 61:657, 1978

177. Ettinger DS, Order SE, Whoram MK, et al: Phase I-II study of isotopic immunoglobulin therapy for primary liver cancer. Cancer Treat Rep 66(2):289, 1982

178. Krolick KA, Yuan D, Vitella ES: Specific killing of a human breast carcinoma cell line by a monoclonal antibody coupled to the A-chain of ricin. Cancer Immunol Immunother 12:39, 1981

179. Order SE, Klein JL, Alderson P, et al: Use of isotopic immunoglobulin in therapy. Cancer Res 30:3001, 1980

180. Olsson L, Kaplan HS: Human-human hybridomas producing monoclonal antibodies of predefined antigenic specificity. Proc Nat Acad Sci USA 77:5429, 1980

181. Jewell WR, Thomas JH, Morse P, Humphrey LJ: Comparison of allogeneic tumor vaccine with leukocyte transfer and transfer factor treatment of human cancer. Ann NY Acad Sci 227:516, 1976

182. Krementz ET, Mansell PWA, Hornung MO, Samuels MS, Sutherland CA, Benes EN: Immunotherapy of malignant disease: The use of viable sensitized lymphocytes or transfer factor prepared from sensitized lymphocytes. Cancer 33:394, 1974

183. Neff Jr. Enneking WF: Adoptive immunotherapy in primary osteosarcoma. J Bone Joint Surg 57-A:145, 1975

184. Gershon RK: Regulation of concomitant immunity: Activation of suppressor cells by tumor excision. Isr J Med Sci 10:1012, 1974

185. Simmons RL, Rios A, Toledo-Pereyra LH, Stinmuller D: Modifying the immunogenicity of cell membrane antigens. Tumors and transplants. Am J Clin Pathol 63:714, 1975

186. Simmons RL, Rios A, Lundgren G, et al: Immunospecific regression of methycholanthrene fibrosarcoma using neuroaminidase. Surgery 70:38, 1971

187. Fowles RL, Selby PJ, Jones DR, Russell JA, Prentice HG, McElwain TJ, Alexander P: Maintenance of remission in acute myelogenous leukemia by a mixture of B.C.G. and irradiated leukemia cells. Lancet 2:1107, 1977

188. Hersh EM, Gutterman JU, Mavligit GM: Immunotherapy of leukemia. Med Clin N Am 60:1019, 1976

189. Laucius JF, Bodurtha AJ, Mastrangelo MJ, Creech RH: Bacillus Calmette-Guerin in the treatment of neoplastic disease. J Reticuloendothel Soc 16:347, 1974

190. Israel L, Edelstein R: Nonspecific immunostimulation with Corynebacterium parvum in human cancer. In: Immunological Aspects of Neoplasia. Baltimore, Williams & Wilkins, 1975

191. Likhite VV: The delayed and lasting rejection of mammary adenocarcinoma cell tumors in DBA/2 mice with use of killed Bordetella pertussis. Cancer Res 34:1027, 1974

192. Lavrin DE, Rosenberg SA, Connor RJ, Terry WD: Immunoprophylaxis of methylcholanthrene-induced tumors in mice with Bacillus Calmette-Guerin and methanol-extracted residue. Cancer Res 33:472, 1972

193. Wepsic HT, Harris S, Sander J, Alaimo J, Morris H: Enhancement of tumor growth following immunization with Bacillus Calmette-Guerin cell walls. Cancer Res 36:1950, 1976

194. Old LJ, Benacerraf B, Clarke DA, Carswell EA, Stockert E: The role of the reticuloendothelial system in the host reaction to neoplasia. Cancer Res 21:1281, 1961

195. Bast RC, Jr., Zbar B, Borsos T, Rapp HJ: BCG and cancer (Part 1). N Engl J Med 290:1413, 1974

196. Rosenthal SR, Crispen RG, Thorne MG, Piekarski N, Raisys N, Rettig PG: BCG vaccination and leukemia mortality. JAMA 22:1543, 1072

197. Hoover RN: Bacillus Calmette-Guerin vaccination and cancer prevention: A critical review of the human experience. Cancer Res 36:652, 1976

198. Baldwin RW, Pimm MV: BCG immunotherapy of a rat sarcoma. Br J Cancer 28:20, 1973

199. Morton DL, et al: BCG immunotherapy of malignant melanoma; Summary of a seven-year experience. Ann Surg 180:635, 1974

200. Klein E, Holtermann CA, Helm F, Rosner D, Milgram E, Adler S, Stoll HL, Jr., Case RW, Prior RL, Murphy GP: Immunologic approaches to the management of primary and secondary tumors involving the skin and soft tissues: Review of a ten-year program. Transplant Proc 7:297, 1975

201. Eilber FR, Morton DL, Holmes EC, Sparks FC, Ramming KP: Adjuvant immunotherapy with BCG in treatment of regional lymph-node metastases from malignant melanoma. N Engl M Med 294:237, 1976

202. Mastrangelo MJ, Berd D, Bellet RE: Critical review of previously reported clinical trials of cancer immunotherapy with nonspecific immunostimulants. Ann NY Acad Sci 277:94, 1976

203. Sinkovics JG, Plager C, Romero J: Immunology and immunotherapy of patients with sarcomas. In Crispen RG (ed): Neoplasm Immunity: Solid Tumor Therapy. Chicago, Franklin Institute Press, 1977

204. Townsend CM, Eilber FR, Morton DL: Skeletal and soft tissue sarcomas. Treatment with adjuvant immunotherapy. JAMA 236:2187, 1976

205. Bast RC, Jr., Abar B, Borsos T, Rapp HJ: BCG and cancer (Part 2). N Engl J Med 290:1458, 1974

206. Sparks FC, Silverstein MJ, Hunt JS, Haskell CM, Pilch YH, Morton DL: Complications of BCG immunotherapy in patients with cancer. N Engl J Med 289:827, 1973

207. Windhorst D: The international registry of tumor immunotherapy. Med Clin N Am 60:641, 1976

208. Principal Investigators and Titles from Compendium of Tumor Immunotherapy Protocols, no. 7. International Registry of Tumor Immunotherapy. DHEW, NIH, National Cancer Institute. Bethesda, Informatics, 1979

10
Rehabilitation
Tapas K. Das Gupta

The principles of rehabilitation of patients with soft tissue sarcomas and other malignant tumors of the peripheral nervous tissue are similar to those for cancer patients in general. However, because of the histogenetic origin and anatomic location of these tumors, certain specific forms of physical and psychological rehabilitation are required, and only these will be discussed in this chapter.

The majority of these tumors are located in the extremities; consequently, the rehabilitation plan must be based on the methods of management used for each individual type of tumor, as well as on the location within the specific extremity. Although many mesenchymal tumors are now being treated with limb-salvaging procedures (Chapter 8), a large number of patients still require some form of amputation as the primary form of curative therapy (Chapter 6).

Prospective amputees should be seen by the rehabilitation team prior to operation. The patient should be counseled regarding the program that will be followed, the estimated time for recovery from the operation to the prosthetic fitting, and the adaptation made necessary by the amputation. For adults there should be an open and informative discussion regarding the degree of disability, the change of body image, and, if indicated, occupational readjustment.

Once an *informed consent* is obtained from the patient and the family (when indicated), then the actual amputation at the designated level is carried out.

From the physical standpoint, all amputations have two major considerations: first, the association of phantom limb pain; and second, the acquisition of an appropriately fitting prosthesis.

The phantom limb is a phenomenon that has long aroused curiosity. How is it that one feels a limb that is not there? Yet, once one thinks about the anatomy and physiology of the situation, one realizes that the phantom limb phenomenon is to be expected. All the nerves coming from the limb are still there, they still make connections at various levels of the central nervous system, and, finally, these connections connect to that part of the brain where afferent nerve impulses evoke sensation. The phantom limb sensation occurs in 95 percent or more of all people who have had a limb or part of a limb amputated. In that other five percent or less, the limb may still be conjured up by concentrating on it, or by trying to move it.

In most limb amputations, the cut nerves end up in neuromas.[1] One assumes that these nerve fibers are capable of working and that they frequently fire off impulses to the central nervous system. Not only is this a likely assumption, but it is reinforced by the effect of blocking the cut nerves of the neuroma with a local anesthetic. When these nerve fibers are blocked in this way, there is a great reduction, or even a total loss, of the sensation of the phantom limb.

A few people who have had parts of their bodies amputated experience constant pain in the stump or in the phantom, or both. In such patients, blocking the neuromas with local anesthetics almost always stops the pain temporarily. Many suggestions have been proffered as to why some patients have pain and others do not. It could be caused by a difference in the makeup of the neuromas, but this is an unsatisfactory suggestion because no differences in the histologic appearances of pain-producing and painless neuromas have been found.[2]

Wall and Gutnick[2] induced neuromas in the cut sciatic nerves of rats and recorded a compound potential from the posterior rootlets entering the spinal cord. As expected, they found that the nerve fibers of these neuromas were continually active. Their discharge of impulses could be increased by pressure or tapping on the neuromas, and it could be stopped by anesthetizing the neuromas with local anesthetic solution—all similar to the situation in man.

A more interesting finding was the effect of electrical stimulation of the chronically divided nerve. The nerve on which the neuroma had been induced was divided so that it no longer reached the spinal cord. Electrodes were then placed on the nerve and it was stimulated rapidly for a few seconds. The electrical excitation caused a marked reduction in the nerve's spontaneous activity for as long as an hour. This finding may suggest that if the nerve fibers can be induced to fire off maximally, they may stop firing spontaneously for a prolonged period.

During the past few years the transcutaneous electrical stimulation of nerves has been introduced for many painful conditions, including painful amputation stumps and painful phantom limbs. This treatment is based on the gate control theory of pain of Melzack and Wall.[3] The theory states that whether an input to the spinal cord finally causes pain depends on the amount of input in large myelinated efferent fibers on the one hand and small myelinated and nonmyelinated efferent fibers on the other. Both groups of fibers are said to affect the small neurons of the *substantia gelatinosa* of the posterior horn. The large fibers excite these neu-

rons and the small fibers inhibit them. These *substantia gelatinosa* neurons are inhibitory. Thus, when these neurons are inhibited, their inhibitory action on the efferent fibers is not excited and a massive afferent input enters the spinal cord, resulting in pain. In contrast, when these neurons are excited, they exert presynaptic inhibition on afferent fibers, and the input to the spinal cord is moderate and pain does not occur. Excitation of the large afferent fibers thus reduces the input to the spinal cord and closes the gate.

Wall and Gutnick[2] suggested an alternative way in which electrical stimulation might act. It could do so by preventing nerve impulses from being fired off spontaneously, and since it is this firing that causes both the pain and the phantom sensation, both would be stopped by electrical stimulation. The mechanism by which antidromic stimulation stops impulse generation after stimulation has stopped is unknown.[2,4-8] Wall and Gutnick[2] suggested that the excitability of small nerve fibers within the neuron is altered by electrical stimulation because these endings are abnormal and do not behave in the same way as normal nerve fibers.

This appears to be the first logical explanation for the phantom limb pain syndrome, as well as a practical therapeutic recommendation for control of this syndrome. We routinely infiltrate the cut end of the nerve trunks with local anesthesia. Although this is not a panacea, it appears to lower the incidence and the intensity of the phantom limb pain syndrome. We have not yet found a need for transcutaneous electrical stimulation[8-10]; however, in patients with intractable pain its use might be of considerable help.

Pain in the phantom limb probably can be reduced considerably if the patient is psychologically prepared for the operation and if the proper emotional support is given afterwards. The incidence and intensity of this pain are very real to the patient, and neglect by the clinician might be injurious to his or her well-being.

Patients should be fitted with a prosthesis as soon after amputation as feasible. The majority of amputations are done in the lower extremities, and, excluding hemipelvectomy or hip joint disarticulation, the prosthesis can be fitted within eight weeks. Early physical therapy following a temporary prosthesis is of exceptional value in rehabilitating the patient. In the upper extremities, the problem is the lack of available functionally useful prostheses. Be that as it may, if and when an upper extremity amputation is performed, a rigid cast and some form of prosthesis must be used as early as possible after the operation.

With the increasing use of multimodality therapy in recent years, muscle group excision has, in many cases, replaced amputations. In such instances, immediate physiotherapy to re-educate the patients in the use of limbs in the absence of one or a group of muscles is ex-tremely important.

For tumors arising in the somatic tissue of the trunk, excision of the chest wall or the ab-dominal wall, along with other forms of treat-ment, is frequently indicated. In these in-stances, sometimes due to irradiation, scoliosis or kyphoscoliosis occurs. Unless this is recog-nized early and appropriate braces or supports are provided, varying degrees of pulmonary in-sufficiency may develop.

Patients with mesenchymal sarcomas are frequently treated with adjuvant systemic che-motherapy. Usually there is a telltale mark in such therapeutic regimens, and all too fre-quently a pretherapy discussion regarding the drugs is not carried out with the patient. Most patients are afraid of chemotherapy and require psychological support. This type of rehabilita-tive support should be planned prior to initia-tion of any therapy.

The psychological rehabilitation of these patients is indeed difficult and time-consuming, but if it is not provided, the entire treatment program may fail. Therefore, a comprehensive rehabilitation plan must be initiated as soon as the patient is initially seen with a sarcoma.

REFERENCES

1. Ramon y Cajal S: Degeneration and Regeneration in the Nervous System. London, Oxford University Press, 1928
2. Wall PD, Gutnick M: Properties of afferent nerve impulses originating from a neuroma. Nature 248:740, 1974.
3. Melzack R, Wall PD: Pain mechanisms: A new theory. Science 150:971, 1965.
4. Diamond J: The effects of injecting acetylcholine into normal and regenerating nerves. J Physiol (London) 145:611, 1959.
5. Waxman SG, Wall PD: Neurology 23:295, 1973.
6. Basbaum AI: Effects of central lesions on disorders produced by multiple dorsal rhizotomy in rats. Exp Neurol 42:490, 1974.
7. Catton WT: Some properties of frog skin mechanoreceptors. J Physiol (London) 141:305, 1958
8. Wall PD, Johnson AJ: Changes associated with post-tetanic potentiation of a monosynaptic reflex. J Neurophysiol 21:148, 1958
9. Wall PD, Wickelgren B: Afferent hyperpolarization and post-tetanic potentiation of a monosynaptic reflex. J Physiol (London) 196:135, 1968
10. Wall PD, Sweet WH: Temporary ablation of pain in man. Science 155:108, 1967
11. Campbell JN, Taub A: Local analgesia from percutaneous electrical stimulation. Arch Neurol 28:347, 1973
12. Wall PD: Handbook of Sensory Physiology. Berlin, Springer-Verlag, 1973, p 253

11

Tumors of the Adipose Tissue

Tapas K. Das Gupta

PHYSIOLOGY

The concept of adipose tissue as a dynamic organ capable of participating in a number of metabolic processes is now generally accepted. Body fat may be considered a reservoir of stored calories in the form of *triglycerides,* with high calorie density. However, it is apparent that this reservoir is composed of living cells with different functions.

The number of calories converted to fat derives from two variables: energy intake and energy expenditure. The body of a normal young adult man in caloric balance may contain an average of 14 percent pure fat. In normal persons, the relative amount of fat increases with age, and at age 55 is approximately 25 percent of body weight.[1] In obese persons the amount of body fat may reach more than 40 percent of the body weight. The lipids extracted from normal human adipose tissue comprise more than 98 percent triglycerides, 1.3 percent total cholesterol, and 0.1 percent phospholipids.[2]

Twenty-two different fatty acids have been identified in the adipose tissue triglycerides. Six of these—the palmitic, myristic, palmitoleic, steric, oleic, and linoleic—account for 95 percent of the fatty acid composition in man. Dietary effects on the fatty acid composition occur slowly. There exist two separate metabolic compartments in the white adipose tissue. The larger compartment may serve as a relatively inert storage site, exchanging only slowly with dietary fat. The smaller pool, turning over more rapidly, is in equilibrium with dietary, serum, and liver lipids, and may also be the major site of active synthesis from carbohydrates. Lipomas apparently constitute a relatively inert storage site and exchange slowly with dietary fat. This has probably given rise to the erroneous conclusion that adipose tissue metabolism has no influence on subcutaneous lipomas.

Adipose tissues contain the whole series of mammalian enzymes for carbohydrate and lipid metabolism.[3] A review of the dynamic aspects of adipose tissue metabolism suggests that there is a recognizable and reproducible pattern of metabolic regulation of this tissue.

Lipid deposition in the body is a result of two processes: incorporation of preformed lipid from the circulation, and de novo synthesis of lipid from carbohydrate directly in the adipose cell itself. Preformed lipid may be derived from the diet or from lipid synthesized in the liver. After absorption by the intestine, dietary lipids (as long-chain fatty acids and monoglycerides) enter the circulation via the thoracic duct as protein-lipid aggregates. The particles may be removed directly by adipose tissue, or they may be removed by the liver and returned to the circulation with modification of the lipid or protein content. They may be hydrolyzed to free fatty acid and reesterified to triglyceride in the liver and then returned to the circulation for eventual incorporation into adipose tissue.

The triglyceride-protein aggregate, no matter what route it has taken, is hydrolyzed on or within the wall of the adipose tissue, and the glycerol and protein are returned to the circulation. The enzyme catalyzing this hydrolysis, lipoprotein lipase, is located at or near the capillary endothelium, and its activity is increased by carbohydrate feeding and probably by insulin or heparin. This type of hydrolysis provides one control over the adipose pool by regulating the inflow of fatty acids from circulating triglycerides. The fatty acids, once released from circulating triglycerides by lipoprotein lipase, are reesterified into triglyceride inside the adipose cell and then incorporated into the central droplet. Glycerol in its free form cannot be used for triglyceride synthesis, since adipose tissue lacks the enzyme necessary to activate the glycerol to glycerol phosphate. Glycerol phosphate must therefore be derived from glucose metabolism. Thus, there is a second controlling mechanism, since the entry of glucose into the adipose tissue is regulated by insulin.[4] Insulin activity controls another extremely important mechanism in the regulation of the body's lipid content, namely, lipogenesis from glucose. Adipose tissue stores little glycogen, and most of the glucose is converted into fatty acids and stored as such. Under the influence of insulin, these fatty acids are esterified with glycerol phosphate and end up in the central droplet of triglyceride. It is known that zinc insulin injected subcutaneously over a long period produces fatty tumors.

Mobilization of adipose tissue triglyceride may be in a steady-state with the concentration of free fatty acids inside the cell if there is adequate glycerol phosphate. If the supply of glycerol phosphate is inadequate, free fatty acids are released because of inadequate reesterification. Likewise, if lipolysis is accelerated, free fatty acids may accumulate more rapidly than they can be reesterified and, as a result, are released into the circulation. In other words, the release of free fatty acids depends on the relative rates of lipolysis and reesterification.

Adipose tissue may perform functions other than simply serving as an energy storage site. It provides mechanical protection (interarticular pads, buccal cheek pouch), and its role as an insulating agent in subcutaneous sites is well known. The continuous synthesis and breakdown of triglyceride, a heat-producing process, may play a role in thermogenesis. There is evidence that this is indeed true for brown adipose tissue, and a similar role has been suggested for white adipose tissue.

DISEASES OF ADIPOSE TISSUE

Tumors or tumorlike conditions arising in fat present with protean clinical findings because of the universal distribution of fat. Certain endocrinopathies, idiopathic lipopathies, and true neoplasms are clinically similar and often histologically indistinguishable, posing a difficult problem in the management of affected patients. The main diseases of white adipose tissue can be classified as follows: (1) lipopathies, (2) lypodystrophies, (3) primary hyperlipidemia or hypolipidemia producing a tumorlike condition, (4) endocrinopathic disorders, and (5) benign and malignant neoplasms. Only hibernomas (neoplasms) are found to arise in brown adipose tissue.

A detailed discussion of all these disease entities is beyond the scope of this book. They are briefly alluded to and discussed when germane to a presentation on tumors or tumorlike conditions of the adipose tissue.

DISEASES OF WHITE ADIPOSE TISSUE

Lipopathies

The term lipopathies refers to a group of unrelated diseases of fatty tissue, particularly subcutaneous fat. Lipomas have often been included in this category, but in this presentation lipomas will be classified and described in the section on tumors. It is recognized, however, that lipomas may histologically resemble any of the other lipopathies. The following clinical conditions are considered in the group of lipopathies: (1) adiposis dolorosa, (2) relapsing febrile nodular nonsuppurative panniculitis, (3) foreign body granuloma, (4) fat necrosis, (5) systemic multicentric lipoblastosis, and (6) steatopygia.

Adiposis Dolorosa (Dercum's Disease). Dercum,[5] in 1892, described a rare disease charac-

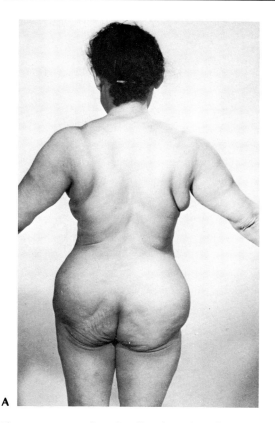
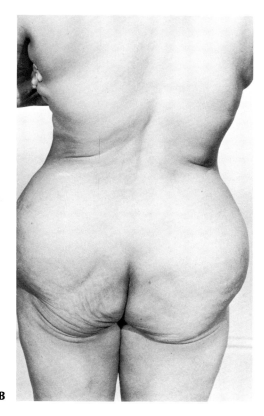

A

B

Figure 11.1. (A) Bilateral axillary fat pad swelling in a 55-year-old woman who complained of incapacitating pain. Relief of symptoms was achieved after excision. **(B)** Same patient, showing accumulation of gluteal fat. This was less tender than the axillary swellings and was not touched.

terized by adiposity, asthenia, pain, and psychic disturbances. The existence of this clinical entity is still denied by many. Adiposis dolorosa occurs largely in women during the menopause. It manifests itself either as nodules or, commonly, as a more or less extensive accumulation of subcutaneous fat. Usually, lumpy encapsulated masses are found on the thighs, abdomen, or in the axillary region (Fig. 11.1A and 11.1B). On the abdomen, these masses hang like an apron, and in other sites they look like hanging sacs. Pack and Ariel[6] found approximately 300 such cases in the literature. Subjective symptoms vary from patient to patient, ranging from mere tenderness to spontaneous severe attacks of pain. The cause of this pain is unknown, but even superficial pressure against fatty masses may elicit it.

A remarkable factor is the severe asthenia brought about by any exertion or attempt to diet. The tenderness and pain cannot be explained on a histologic basis, since histologically the fatty lesions resemble ordinary lipomas and there is no evidence of an increased number of nerve fibers. Various theories have been proposed to explain the nature of this entity, the most popular being related endocrine disturbance, particularly of the pituitary. A hereditary relationship has also been proposed.[7] Although the exact etiologic factor is unknown, the concept of a combined endocrine deficiency seems logical.[8] Pain is the only distinguishing feature by which Dercum's disease can be differentiated from multiple lipomatosis. Because of its extreme rarity, there is no accepted definitive therapy. In some extremely tender areas the excess fat resembling lipomas can be excised, resulting in symptomatic relief for a period of time.

Relapsing Febrile Nodular Nonsuppurative Panniculitis (Weber-Christian Disease). Pfeifer,[9] in 1892, was the first to describe this entity. In 1916, Gilchrist and Ketron[10] reported the second case. However, Weber[11] actually coined the term "relapsing nodular nonsuppurative panniculitis" and Christian,[12] in 1928, added the adjective "febrile." Since then the entity has been called Weber-Christian disease. Lever[13] reviewed the literature and found occasional fatalities. Usually it is self-limited and is characterized by the intermittent appearance of subcutaneous nodules and plaques caused by degeneration of fatty tissue, with subsequent inflammation.

Recurrent subcutaneous nodules located in the extremities, particularly the lower, constitute the characteristic clinical feature of this entity. The overlying skin is usually erythematous (Fig. 11.2). Lever[14] stated that occasionally the skin breaks down and liquid fat drains through the open wound. Clinically, the asymptomatic lesions resemble lipomas. Malaise and slight to moderate pyrexia often accompany the appearance of new nodules. Infrequently, this entity develops in the mesentery of obese persons, and they may have acute abdominal symptoms. Clinical distinction from acute appendicitis is often impossible, since in both diseases the patients have fever, leukocytosis, and tenderness in the abdomen. An exploratory celiotomy shows mesenteric panniculitis in Weber-Christian disease (Fig. 11.3).

The histologic changes can be divided into three stages. In the first stage, there is focal degeneration of adipose cells, accompanied by an acute inflammatory infiltrate. In the second stage, a number of macrophages with foamy cytoplasm and a varying number of lymphocytes, plasma cells, and histiocytes are seen. In the third stage, fibrosis supervenes. In a rare instance in which a patient died as a consequence of this disease, necropsy revealed involvement of perivisceral, mesenteric, and omental fat, as well as involvement of the bone marrow.[14] Usually, however, the disease is self-limited and not severe.

No effective treatment exists for Weber-Christian disease. Steroids will curtail the period of acute manifestation in fulminating cases. In most patients, however, the disease is diagnosed after excision of a tumor.

Foreign Body Granulomas. Many foreign substances, when injected or accidentally im-

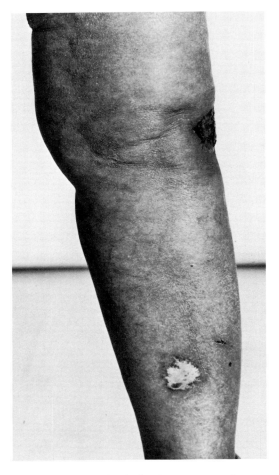

Figure 11.2. Example of relapsing nonsuppurative panniculitis of the left lateral aspect of the knee joint. The overlying skin has broken down, with resultant ulcerating lesions. Liquid fat drained for eight weeks before the wound spontaneously healed. Lower tibial area shows healing.

planted in the subcutaneous tissue, produce a foreign body reaction, and often a localized mass develops. These masses can be misdiagnosed as lipomas, especially in the region of the buttocks, unless history of an injection is elicited. Granulomas that follow injection of an oily substance (called lipid granulomas) occur as irregular, hard, nodular subcutaneous swellings. Although clinically they can be mistaken for adipose tissue tumors, the histologic feature is so characteristic that an error in tissue diagnosis is not likely.

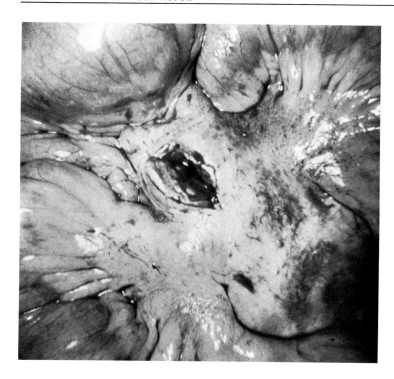

Figure 11.3. Mesentery in a case of Weber-Christian disease. Patient was a 39-year-old woman with a 48-hour history of pain in the abdomen similar to acute appendicitis. On exploration, inflamed mesentery was found. Histologic examination of a wedge of tissue showed inflammatory reaction, with a number of macrophages characteristic of this disease *(Reproduced with permission from Das Gupta, T.K.: Tumors and Tumor-Like Conditions of the Adipose Tissue. In Ravitch, M.M., et al. (eds): Current Problems in Surgery, March 1970. Year Book Medical Publishers, Inc., Chicago.)*

Fat Necrosis. In 1882, Balzer[15] first described fat necrosis as an entity, and ascribed it to acute hemorrhagic pancreatitis. The mechanism of subcutaneous fat necrosis is not clearly understood. An increase in lipase is thought to be the initiating factor, but the cause of the increased tissue lipase content in a specific area of the human body is unknown. Subcutaneous fat necrosis is seen in both adults and children.

Idiopathic fat necrosis sometimes occurs in women with pendulous breasts, presenting as a breast tumor. Adair and Munzer[16] reported its incidence to be 2.76 percent in patients considered to have primary operable carcinoma of the breast. Early fat necrosis is confined to several well-defined fat droplets. Clinically, the firm lesions of fat necrosis resemble carcinoma more than any of the other benign lesions of the breast. Fat necrosis in the subcutaneous tissue of the buttock or abdomen of obese persons is also well recognized. These lesions closely resemble fatty tumors, and diagnosis usually is made following excision.

Subcutaneous fat necrosis is commonly seen in the newborn and should be differentiated from scleroderma neonatorum, edema neonatorum, and scleroderma occurring in infancy. Lesions of fat necrosis usually appear near the end of the first week after birth, although the time of onset may range from 1 to 42 days.[17] The lesions are deep-seated, indurated masses that may vary in size from several centimeters to large plaques. The distribution often is symmetrical, and the sites of predilection are the back, cheeks, arms, thighs, and buttocks. The smaller lesions are freely movable over the underlying structures, and the borders of the lesions ordinarily are sharply defined. In the newborn, the usual form of subcutaneous fat necrosis is self-limited, and no active therapy is required, since most lesions resolve in three to four months.

In some unusual instances, subcutaneous fat necrosis in the newborn is associated with hypercalcemia and serious systemic symptoms. Treatment always poses a problem, and fortunately these patients are rare. The exact mechanism of fat necrosis in the newborn is not understood.[17]

Systemic Multicentric Lipoblastosis. In rare instances, multiple fatty tissue growths are present in subcutaneous as well as visceral fat. These lesions tend to recur after excision. They differ from lipomas in that mesenchymal cells and primitive fat cells are frequently found in microscopic sections. Although these lesions present a primitive appearance, no case of malignant degeneration or metastasis has been recorded.

Steatopygia. This condition (excessive fatness of the buttocks) is normal in women of some cultures. Pack and Ariel[6] commented on a female Bushman who was exhibited as an example of callipygia at the Paris exhibition in 1815, and whom Cuvier[6] described as a "Hottentot Venus." There is no need for therapy, and this condition is mentioned for its ethnic and cultural interest.

Lipodystrophy

This rare disease is mentioned only for the sake of completeness. It is characterized by localized or progressive loss of subcutaneous fat, without subjective symptoms. The cause of progressive lipodystrophy is thought to be a disturbance of autonomic trophic regulation. No therapy exists.

Primary Hyperlipidemia or Hypolipidemia

These entities constitute one of the most fascinating problems in the realm of metabolic disorders, but a detailed classification or discussion is beyond the scope of this book. Suffice it to mention that, in occasional cases of essential hypercholesterolemia, xanthomatous tumors develop in the extremities. These tumors have the clinical features of soft tissue tumors and should be distinguished from common lipomas. Usually they are intradermal, whereas lipomas are subcutaneous.

Endocrinopathic Disorders

Certain fatty accumulations, the result of metabolic derangements such as Frohlich's syndrome (which is caused by pituitary or adrenal disturbances), exophthalmos, abnormal accumulation of fat within the orbit secondary to thyroid disturbances, etc., are not dealt with in this book, since none of these conditions can be confused with tumors of the adipose tissue.

Neoplasms of White Adipose Tissue

A neoplasm of the white adipose tissue can be benign (lipoma) or malignant (liposarcoma).

Lipomas. The etiologic factors of lipomas are unknown, but Ewing[18] suggested that the following are contributory:

1. Heredity (as evidenced by multiple symmetrical lipomas, which are discussed later).
2. Lipogenesis of tissues, as discussed earlier. To what extent the mechanism of normal lipogenesis of tissues is affected so as to result in a lipoma is not known. However, lipoma formation in atrophic organs such as kidneys and breast, or in lymph nodes, has been observed.
3. Formation of multiple lipomas that may occur in cases of, or following, diseases of the thyroid or other endocrine glands. Ewing[18] believed the regional overgrowth of fat in these situations to be related to lipomas in the same manner that diffuse fibromatosis is related to fibromas. This viewpoint, however, cannot be substantiated.
4. Congenital predisposition toward disturbances in the development of fat, including lipomatous overgrowth within such epithelial tissue as the brain. This viewpoint, again, is not universally accepted.
5. Association with systemic disease. This suggestion has appeared in the literature through the years, but no specific abnormality has been defined. Endocrine disturbances as the cause of either solitary or multiple lipomas have always caught the imagination of clinicians, but there is no definite evidence to support this hypothesis insofar as solitary lipomas are concerned.

Ewing,[18] extending his hypothesis concerning etiologic factors, classified adipose tissue tumors as follows: obesity; localized growth of fat tissue; replacement lipomatosis, as noted in atrophic organs such as kidney, bone marrow, etc.; homologous lipomatosis (solitary lipomas, etc.); heterologous lipomas arising from misplaced embryonal cells; overgrowth of fat components in certain mixed tumors, such as teratomas. In contrast, Gellhorn and Marks[19] concluded that disturbance of lipid synthesis is a major factor in fat accumulation in lipomas.

Clinically, lipomas can be classified as (1) solitary, (2) multiple, or (3) congenital diffuse lipomatosis.

Solitary Lipomas. This is the most common type of fatty tumor. Pack and Ariel[6] reported the ratio of lipomas to liposarcomas as 120:1, and Stout[20] saw only 21 (1.4 percent) cases of liposarcoma in a series of 1,454 fatty tumors. Solitary lipomas can arise in any part of the human body. They are subclassified according to the site of origin as (1) subcutaneous (most frequent site), (2) intermuscular and intramuscular, (3) intrathoracic, (4) intraperitoneal and retroperitoneal, (5) intraoral, (6) arising in various organs, (7) arising in the central or peripheral nervous systems, and (8) synovial and bone lipomas.

SUBCUTANEOUS SOLITARY LIPOMAS. In a personal series of 459 lipomas in 320 patients, it was found that lipomas occurred in all parts of

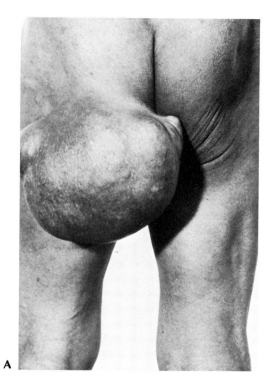

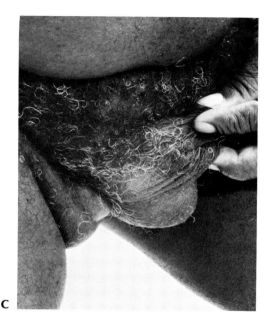

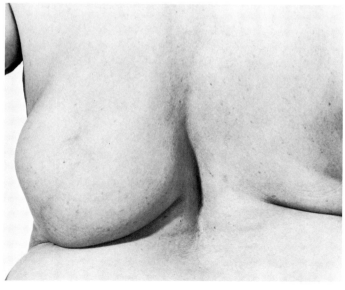

Figure 11.4. (A) Lipoma of the left buttock, which was neglected for a long period of time, resulting in sac-like appearance. **(B)** Lipoma of the dorsilumbar region molding to the location. **(C)** Lipoma of the perineum molding to the fold.

the human body. Pack and Pierson[21] studied the distribution of 352 lipomas in 134 patients and observed no predilection for any particular site.

Generally lipomas can be diagnosed clinically by a long history of a subcutaneous tumor. The tumors are palpable and can be of any size. In smaller lipomas the margins of the tumor can be easily palpated. The shape and size of subcutaneous lipomas are frequently molded according to the location (Fig. 11.4A and 11.4B). Those that arise from the subcutaneous tissue of the perineum, the vulva, or the neck become sacculated and hang like fat bags (Fig. 11.4C). Subcutaneous lipomas that arise in the axilla are often attached to the skin and are difficult to diagnose. Occasionally, lipomas of the breast are confused with carcinoma of the breast or fibrocystic disease. Since breast lipomas are rare, the diagnosis should always be made on the basis of histologic examination. Occasionally, a large lipoma of the breast is seen (Fig. 11.5A and 11.5B); however, care should be taken to exclude the possibility of a liposarcoma.

Booher[22] discussed the clinical manifestation of lipomas of the hands and feet, stressing their relative rarity in these sites. He reviewed the literature up to 1965 and found only 65 cases of palmar lipomas, 19 being in his own patients. In our series of 170 lipomas of the upper extremities, 15 were in the hand (Fig. 11.6). Booher[22] described 32 lipomas of the dorsum and wrist, including five cases of his own. We have encountered only four such cases. Table 11.1 shows the incidence of lipomas in the hand in four large series.[22-24] Lipomas of the feet are rarer still. Booher[22] had only three such cases and we have had only two. Clinical diagnosis of lipomas in these areas is difficult. The lipomas that arise in the head and neck region require special consideration for management. We have had several patients with lipoma of the parotid region. These tumors should be excised by superficial parotidectomy. Lipomas of the forehead, scalp, and neck require care in excision; otherwise, the cosmetic deformity following excision could be far worse than the innocuous small tumor.

Angiolipoma (Fig. 11.7) is a variant of subcutaneous lipoma. The borderline between common solitary lipomas and angiolipomas is still not defined. Clinically, angiolipomas are somewhat tender to the touch and occasionally there is a history of trauma. Howard and Helwig,[25] in a review of the files of the Armed Forces Institute of Pathology, described the distribu-

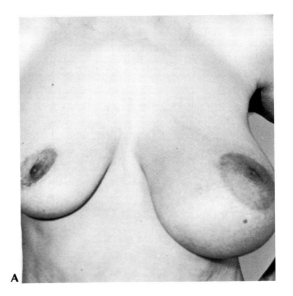

A

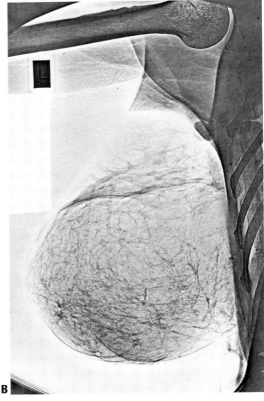

B

Figure 11.5. (A) A 39-year-old woman with a large lipoma of the left breast. **(B)** Xerogram of the same breast.

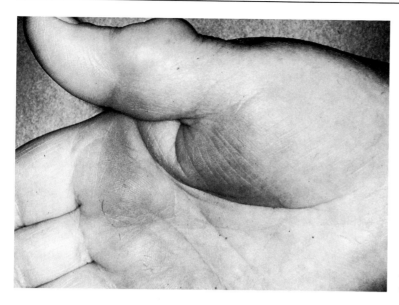

Figure 11.6. Lipoma in the thenar eminence of a 55-year-old man. Of interest, he sought medical opinion because of the ganglion in this thumb. Both lesions were excised without difficulty.

tion of 262 angiolipomas and noted that the tumors arose predominantly in the extremities and trunk, including the retroperitoneum. The management of these tumors is similar to that of common lipomas. However, there is a distinct group of angiolipomas that infiltrate the surrounding tissue (infiltrating angiolipoma). A curative excision of this variety may at times be extremely difficult. Since these are benign tumors, radical excision, amputation, or radiation therapy in which vital tissues are sacrificed is not in order (Fig. 4.5A and 4.5B, Chapter 4.)

Infiltrating angiolipomas are rare. We have treated only four such cases. It appears that, including our four, only 27 cases have ever been reported.[26-32] Table 11.2 summarizes the site, natural history, and different methods of management used in the 27 cases. These are essentially benign tumors. Occasionally, retroperi-

toneal angiolipomas may bleed, leading to an abdominal emergency. In rare instances one or more abdominal viscera require excision. In case 23 (Table 11.2), bleeding at the time of operation necessitated nephrectomy. In case 26, the kidney was already ruptured and nephrectomy was performed for hemostasis. After excision, local recurrence is rare.

INTERMUSCULAR AND INTRAMUSCULAR LIPOMAS. The exact location of a lipoma arising in the depths of the soft tissue is always confusing. These tumors can be either intermuscular, submuscular, or intramuscular. Greenberg[33] classified these deep-seated lipomas into two types, intramuscular and intermuscular. Often it is difficult to establish the exact site of origin, as some may develop within the muscle but extend into the intermuscular spaces (Fig. 11.8). Therefore, Pack and Ariel's[6] suggestion that all these tu-

TABLE 11.1. LIPOMAS OF THE HAND: FOUR SERIES

Authors	Date of Publication	No. Cases	Accompanying Symptoms	Comments
Booher[22]	1965	31	Mass and occasional pain	Excised, one recurrence, no nerve pain
Phalen et al.[23]	1971	15	Mass and pain	Six caused nerve compression; all excised
Paarlberg et al.[24]	1972	59	Mass and occasional pain	Excised
Das Gupta	1981	15	Mass and occasional pain	No nerve deficit, all excised; no local recurrence

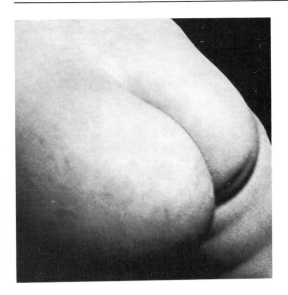

Figure 11.7. Angiolipoma of the left buttock in a child. Note spiderweb distribution of subcutaneous venous plexus. *(Courtesy of Current Problems in Surgery, March 1970.)*

mors be considered intermuscular lipomas is quite satisfactory from both a practical and clinical standpoint.

Intermuscular lipomas have been recognized for many years. In 1913, Kuttner and

Landors[34] reviewed 27 cases from the literature, and since then several other series have been reported.[33,35,36] Congenital intermuscular lipomas have also been described. These tumors have been reported to arise within the inner surface of the cheek, just inside the masseter muscle. Probably most of these represent normal sucking pads of infants.[37]

Greenberg[33] suggested that the intermuscular type grows between the large muscle bundles, probably arising from the intramuscular fascial septa. These lesions form a large central tumor that secondarily infiltrates adjacent muscles. The intramuscular type, on the other hand, originates between the muscle fibers and infiltrates the adjacent muscles by passing through intermuscular septa.

We have treated 34 cases of intermuscular and intramuscular lipomas: 9 in the upper extremities, 17 in the lower extremities, and 8 in the trunk. Kindbloom and co-workers[35] found a similar anatomic distribution in their 43 patients.

The intermuscular lipomas usually are deeply situated but can often be identified by soft tissue roentgenography (Fig. 11.9). They appear as translucent encapsulated masses. Radiolucency is usually characteristic of these tumors, and they are seldom mistaken for cysts

TABLE 11.2. SUMMARY OF 27 INFILTRATING ANGIOLIPOMAS

Case No.	Authors	Year of Publication	Age	Sex	Site of Lesion	Comments
1	Regan, Bickel, Broders[26]	1946	42	F	Right leg	22 × 18 × 11 cm, 2160-gm mass infiltrating skeletal muscles. Resection of tumor with redundant overlying skin. Slight fullness of the operated area at 1-year followup.
2	Ibid.	1946	8	M	Right lower leg	Two huge tumors, 22 × 11 × 6 cm, and 8 × 8 × 4.5 cm. Infiltration of surrounding muscles. Local excision, two recurrences. Wound healed after last wider excision.
3	Greenberg, Isensee et al.[33]	1963	50	F	Right thigh	Firm, nontender, nonencapsulated tumor, 13.5 cm × 10 × 5.5 cm, infiltrating the surrounding muscles. Wide excision. No recurrence.
4	Ibid.	1963	67	F	Left thigh	Yellow, soft nonencapsulated tumor, 7 × 4 × 3 cm, infiltrating skeletal muscles. Wide excision.

Continued

TABLE 11.2. Continued

Case No.	Authors	Year of Publication	Age	Sex	Site of Lesion	Comments
5	Bradley, Klein[28]	1964	30	M	L. scapular region	Ovoid, fatty tumor, 11 × 8 × 8 cm, causing erosion of scapula and pain. No recurrence in 6-year followup.
6	Gonzalez-Crussi, Enneking et al.[29]	1966	27	M	Left heel	A yellow-gray, soft to firm 22 × 14 × 4 cm mass (750 gm) infiltrating vastus lateralis muscle. Wide excision. No recurrence in 4 years.
7	Ibid.	1966	6½	F	Left knee	Soft to firm, pink to red-yellow 7 × 4 × 1.5 cm mass infiltrating quadriceps, joint capsule, and medial collateral ligament, causing tenderness and limitation of movement. Wide excision. No recurrence in 3 years.
8	Ibid.	1966	27	F	Calf muscle	Gray-yellow-pink, 7.5 × 5.5 × 5.5 cm mass (225 gm), infiltrating tibia, gastrocnemius, and causing neurologic deficits in the distal portion of limb. Incomplete excision with two recurrences. Finally treated with wide resection.
9	Ibid.	1966	3	M	Right knee	5 × 3 × 2 cm mass (18.5 gm) infiltrating muscles. Wide excision with recurrence. No recurrence after second resection.
10	Ibid.	1966	26	F	Left heel	Soft, doughy, spongy, white tumor, 5 × 1.5 × 1.5 cm, with 0.2 cm red center, infiltrating the surrounding structure, causing tenderness. Multiple recurrences after local excisions followed by resection of calcaneus and surrounding skeletal muscles. No further recurrence in 13 months.
11	Ibid.	1966	20	F	Lumbar region (L–2 to L–4)	Irregular soft mass, 20 cm in greatest diameter. Extensive bony destruction of the spine. Partial resection followed by radiation therapy (3018 rads in 20 days). No recurrence in 37 months' followup.
12	Pearson, Stellar, Feigin[30]	1970	17	F	Extradural region at T–3	Hard, grayish-purple tumor 1.5- to 2-cm thick. Infiltration of pedicles of T–4 shown by x-ray and histologic examination, causing neurologic deficits. Piecemeal removal of tumor. No recurrence in 9.5 years, with residual neurologic deficits.

Continued

TABLE 11.2. Continued

Case No.	Authors	Year of Publication	Age	Sex	Site of Lesion	Comments
13	Ibid.	1970	22	M	T–3 to T–9 of spine (extradural)	Large extradural mass from T–3 to T–9, 1- to 1.5-cm thick. Minimal bone infiltration histologically, x-ray showed increased density of 5th thoracic body; three operations with profuse bleeding during excision. No recurrence in 9.5 years; minimal neurologic deficits.
14	Ibid.	1970	44	F	T–7 to T–10 of spine (extradural)	Fatty, stringy, easily mobilized nonencapsulated tumor dorsal to the dura, but not attached to it. No bony infiltration. Excision. No recurrence in 14 months; no neurologic deficits.
15	Stimpson[31]	1971	2	F	Pectoralis major muscle	2.5 × 2.5 × 1.5 cm soft tumor with rich vasculature, infiltrating the surrounding muscle. Enucleation with recurrence, followed by wide excision. No second recurrence in 9 months' followup.
16	Ibid.	1971	51	M	Lateral side of thigh	2.5 × 1.5 × 1.0 cm tender tumor infiltrating the surrounding muscle, causing shooting pains. Wide excision. No recurrence in 18 months.
17	Ibid.	1971	53	M	Shoulder	6 × 6 × 3 cm growing lesion infiltrating trapezius muscle. Excision. No recurrence in 18 months.
18	Ibid.	1971	56	F	Triangle of neck	4.0 × 3.5 × 1.5 cm mass simulating left thyroid adenoma clinically. Invaded the strap muscles overlying the normal thyroid. Excision followed by radiation therapy. No recurrence in 12 months.
19	Ibid.	1971	56	M	Right hip	Tender huge mass in right groin extending deep to psoas major and neck of femur, infiltrating skeletal muscles and causing necrosis of muscles. No recurrence in three years; functional deficits.
20	Ibid.	1971	63	F	Right upper arm	Painful mass, 20 × 8 × cm, in right deltoid muscle, infiltrating the surrounding muscles. Excision with recurrence followed by wide excision and radiation therapy (4400 rads). No recurrence in 15 months; neuritic.

Continued

TABLE 11.2. Continued

Case No.	Authors	Year of Publication	Age	Sex	Site of Lesion	Comments
21	Ibid.	1971	63	M	Abdominal wall	Painful mass, 11 × 6 × 2 cm, in left flank, infiltrating the adjacent muscles. Sharp dissection of tumor with recurrence, followed by wider excision. Second recurrence, radiation therapy refused.
22	Lin, Lin[32]	1973	25	M	Left supraclavicular regional	14 × 9 × 7 cm hard to rubbery tan, nonencapsulated tumor infiltrating left brachial plexus, causing neurologic deficits. Excision of tumor and infiltrated muscles. No recurrence in one year; neurologic deficits.
23	Ibid.	1973	37	F	Right lower retroperitoneum	22 × 18 × 6.5 cm, rubbery, pinkish-yellow, partially encapsulated tumor infiltrating the capsule of the right kidney, causing profuse hemorrhage during operation. Right nephrectomy with removal of tumor. No recurrence in three years.
24	Das Gupta	1981	22	M	Right calf	Tumor of right calf, infiltrating the medial head of the gastrocnemius muscle. Gross tumor excised, leaving tumor behind. No recurrence in 3 years.
25	Ibid.	1981	69	F	Retroperitoneum	Left retroperitoneal area, 15 × 10 × 12 cm mass infiltrating the paravertebral muscles and surrounding structures. Excised, with no recurrence in two years.
26	Ibid.	1981	34	F	Retroperitoneum	Diagnosed during pregnancy, created major abdominal catastrophe due to retroperitoneal hemorrhage. Required left nephrectomy and caesarian hysterotomy. Both mother and child doing well one year later. Patient was treated elsewhere and was seen by the author on consultation.
27	Ibid.	1981	59	M	Thigh	Large infiltrating mass in right medial thigh infiltrating adductor muscles. Excision of tumor with margin of the muscles has resulted in apparent cure for 2.5 years.

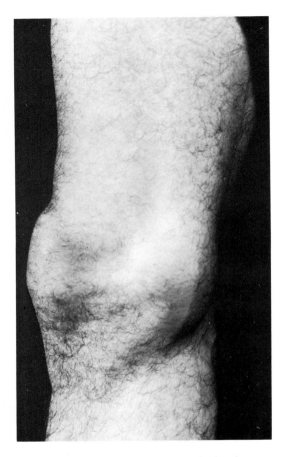

Figure 11.8. Intermuscular lipoma attached to the semitendinosus muscle in a 53-year-old man—an uncommon location. *(Courtesy of Current Problems in Surgery, March 1970.)*

or other types of tumors. In the extremities, the deep lipomas may feel soft and flat when the muscles are relaxed, and hard and spherical when the muscles are contracted. The diagnosis must be made after histologic examination of the tissue.

These tumors tend to recur if inadequately excised. Usually they grow expansively and are not well encapsulated, and frequently fatty offshoots are left behind that lead to recurrence. Recurrence is invariably due to technical error, and every effort should be made to avoid this. They are best excised with a margin of normal muscle.

INTRATHORACIC LIPOMAS. In 1781, Fothergill[38] reported the first case of intrathoracic lipoma. Krause and Ross[39] reviewed the literature in 1962 and, including their own three patients, compiled a series of 80 patients with intrathoracic lipomas. Although solitary lipomas can occur in any site within the thorax, the most common site is the mediastinum,[40] where they can grow to enormous size. The literature is replete with case reports of excision of massive mediastinal lipomas.

Intrathoracic lipoma can be entirely within the thorax or have an hourglass shape, with extension to the neck or through the chest wall into an interspace. The presenting feature of an intrathoracic lipoma depends on the size and location of the tumor. In general, the diagnosis is made by a chest roentgenogram that shows a mediastinal mass. Staub et al.[41] found that approximately 50 percent of patients with mediastinal lipomas are symptomatic, the common symptoms being a nonproductive cough, dyspnea, and a feeling of pressure in the chest. Correct diagnosis usually is achieved after an exploratory thoracotomy and excision of the tumor. Complete excision is almost always possible.

INTRAPERITONEAL OR RETROPERITONEAL LIPOMAS. Benign fatty tumors are occasionally encountered in the peritoneal cavity or in the retroperitoneum. Within the peritoneal cavity, the most likely place would seem to be the omentum, because of the presence there of a large quantity of fatty tissue. In truth, however, omental lipomas are extremely rare. Elfving and Hastbacka[42] found only one tumor that could remotely be considered a lipoma of the omentum. The author has never encountered such a case.

Lipomatous tumors occur more frequently in the retroperitoneal space than in the intraperitoneal region. The retroperitoneal tumors are more often malignant than benign, whereas in other locations the reverse is true. Pack and Ariel[6] reported that out of a series of 19 retroperitoneal fatty tumors, only 2 were benign. Brasfield and Das Gupta[43] found that 35 of a series of 39 retroperitoneal fatty tumors were malignant.

The fatty tumors in this location are clinically quiescent during their early period of development, and because of the nature of the anatomic site, they grow unhampered and attain huge size. Delameter,[44] in 1859, reported a classic case of a 179-pound retroperitoneal tumor in a 36-year-old woman whose original weight was 90 pounds. Symptoms usually are ill defined.

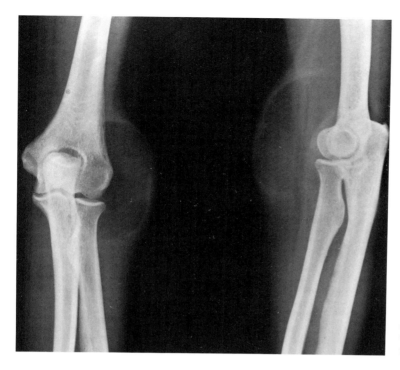

Figure 11.9. Roentgenogram of an intermuscular lipoma located in the antecubital fossa. The tumor was within the muscle bundles and was firm on palpation.

DeWeerd and Dockerty[45] reported the female-to-male ratio in retroperitoneal fatty tumors to be 1.3:1.0; however, in Pack and Ariel's[6] series, the female-to-male ratio was 3:1. The age range commonly was 40 to 50 years. The ideal method of treatment is excision, but both operative mortality and morbidity are associated with operations for large retroperitoneal tumors.

INTRAORAL LIPOMAS. Submucous lipomas in these areas are extremely rare. Seldin and co-workers[46] reported 26 cases, the lesions being distributed as follows: cheek, 11; buccal fold in the region of mental foramen, 2; lower buccal fold, 2; lip, 3; palate, 2; floor of the mouth, 2; and gingiva, 4. Hatziotis[47] reviewed the published material and described 145 cases over a 22-year period ending in 1967. Seven new cases were added by Burzynski et al. in 1971.[48] Greer and Richardson[49] analyzed 16 cases seen at the Boston University School of Dentistry and outlined the criteria for accepting intraoral tumors as lipomas. The management of these lesions is excision.

LIPOMAS ARISING IN THE ORGANS.

1. LIPOMAS OF THE GASTROINTESTINAL TRACT. Lipomas of the gastrointestinal tract, though be-nign and relatively uncommon, require consideration because they mimic several other diseases and tumors of the alimentary tract. In 1963, Mayo and associates[50] collected all the lipomas of the alimentary tract in the Mayo Clinic file and found only 186 cases over a period of 27 years (Table 11.3). They further studied the relationship of gastrointestinal lipomas to other gastrointestinal neoplasms, both benign and malignant. The incidence and type were as follows: gastric carcinoma, 1; colon carcinoma, 47; adenomatous polyps, 35; multiple polyposis, 8; cavernous hemangioma (sigmoid), 2; and villous adenoma (rectum), 1. They also found various other gastrointestinal diseases in this series, for example, duodenal ulcer, ulcerative colitis, and anal fissures.

Feldman[51] studied the relationship of associated conditions in autopsied patients with lipoma of the gastrointestinal tract. Of the 78 cases in his series, 20 were multiple (25.6 percent), growing in widely separated segments of the digestive tract. Frequently, these lipomas were associated with other benign tumors of the gastrointestinal tract: 18 percent with leiomyomas and 23 percent with polyps. A study of the relationship of lipomas to pancreatic disease showed that in 20.5 percent of cases there was

TABLE 11.3. LIPOMAS OF THE GASTROINTESTINAL TRACT (MAYO CLINIC):
DISTRIBUTION BY SITE, SEX OF PATIENT, AND PATHOLOGIC NATURE OF LESION

Site	Sex		Pathologic Diagnosis				Total
	Male	Female	Lipomas	Fibrolipomas	Lipomatosis	Lipoid Granulomas	
Esophagus	2	1	1	2	—	—	3
Stomach	4	2	6	—	—	—	6
Small intestine	21	37	—	—	—	—	58
Duodenum	5	2	6	1	—	—	(7)
Jejunum	2	—	2	—	—	—	(2)
Ileum	7	8	14	1	—	—	(15)
Ileocecal valve	7	27	16	—	18	—	(34)
Large intestine	57	62	—	—	—	—	119
Cecum	7	24	27	—	—	4	(31)
Ascending colon	6	11	16	1	—	—	(17)
Transverse colon	12	12	21	3	—	—	(24)
Descending colon	12	6	18	—	—	—	(18)
Sigmoid colon	10	5	14	1	—	—	(15)
Rectosigmoid	2	1	3	—	—	—	(3)
Rectum	8	3	8	1	—	2	(11)
Total	84	102	152	10	18	6	186

Courtesy of Surgery 53:598, 1963.

evidence of fat necrosis of the pancreas, whereas in the autopsied patients, fat necrosis occurred in only 5.9 percent. Pancreatic cysts occurred in 7.7 percent of the lipoma cases, but in only 3.63 percent of the autopsied patients. Of the 78 cases of gastrointestinal tract lipoma, 18 percent were associated with diabetes, whereas the incidence of diabetes among the autopsied patients was 10.4 percent.

2. ESOPHAGEAL LIPOMAS. Esophageal lipomas are extremely rare. In the series of cases reported by Mayo et al.[50] only three of the 186 were located in the esophagus. Diagnosis was based on histologic examination of the material.

3. LIPOMAS OF THE STOMACH. In 1925, Eliason and Wright[52] compiled a list from the literature of 610 benign stomach tumors and found that lipomas comprised 4.8 percent. These same authors found only one gastric lipoma in 8,000 autopsies. A review of the literature from 1835 to 1940 by Rumold[53] produced 33 cases of submucous gastric lipoma, 17 of which were found at necropsy and 16 at operation. In 1946, Scott and Brunschwig[54] collected five additional cases from the literature that occurred after 1941 and added one case of their own. In 1948, Alvarez, Lastra, and Leon[55] collected four more cases from

the literature following the report of Scott and Brunschwig[54] and described a case of their own, bringing the total to 44. In 1958, Pack and Ariel[6] commented on 58 cases of gastric lipomas. Since then, occasional case reports have appeared in the literature. Thompson and Oyster[56] calculated the incidence of gastric lipomas to be 1.1 percent of all benign gastric tumors. Suffice it to point out that no single clinician has a large personal experience to draw from. In our files there are only two cases.

The tumors usually are seen in older persons and are about equally distributed between the sexes. Structurally, lipomas of the stomach are no different from subcutaneous lipomas. They may range in size from a few millimeters to nine or ten centimeters in diameter. They can be sessile or pedunculated, single or multiple. When they are submucous, they protrude into the lumen of the stomach and may cause erosions and ulcerations of the mucosa, with bleeding.[57] Submucosal and pendunculated lipomas can produce pyloric obstruction or intussusception.[58]

The gastric lipomas are juxtaposed to the pylorus or antrum in about 60 percent of cases. Although they can arise anywhere in the stomach wall, about 96 percent are submucosal. Pain

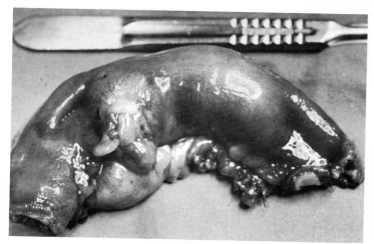

Figure 11.10. (A) Segment of ileum; the intramural tumor is obvious. Overlying serosa smooth and not infiltrated. **(B)** The lumen opened along the antemesenteric border, showing the lipoma in situ. *(Courtesy of H. Abcarian, M.D. Cook County Hospital, Chicago.)*

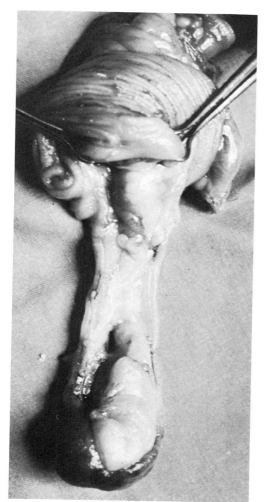

is the usual symptom; occasionally, ulceration of a polypoid tumor may produce hematemesis and melena. Roentgenologic examination of a symptomatic patient might point to the presence of a benign tumor. Although the diagnosis can frequently be made by endoscopy and biopsy, assessment of a gastric lipoma can be made only at the operating table. Removal by polypectomy, enucleation, or partial gastrectomy is curative.

4. LIPOMAS OF THE SMALL INTESTINE (FIG. 11.10A AND 11.10). Lipomas of the small intestine are rare and are seldom solitary. Furste and co-workers[57] described a series of 19 cases of gastrointestinal lipomas, of which 11 were in the small intestine. Mayo et al.[50] had 21 such cases in their series of 186. The two most common symptoms in lipomas of the small intestine as in all other small intestinal tumors, are bleeding and intussusception. Symptomatic patients should be treated by exploratory laparotomy and appropriate resection. Ling and co-workers[59] reported one case of intestinal lipomatosis diagnosed preoperatively. In this case, the patient had resection of the segment containing the ileocecal intussusception, with part of the distal ileum. The specimen was 195 cm long and contained 107 submucosal lipomas.

5. LIPOMAS OF THE ILEOCECAL REGION AND COLON. Although a lipoma of the colon is relatively rare, it is generally agreed that this tumor is one of the most common forms of benign mesenchymal tumors of the colon.[50,60] D'Jarid[60] reviewed the cases published between 1844 and 1958 and found 278. Analysis showed that these

tumors occurred about equally in both sexes and the age at onset was usually in the sixth decade. A high proportion of lipomas involved the ileocecal junction and the colon. In the series reported by Mayo and his colleagues,[50] 110 of 186 were in the large intestine. These tumors are commonly single (Fig. 11.11A and 11.11B). Intermittent intussusception is the characteristic symptom of colonic lipomas, almost all of which are submucosal in location.

A correct preoperative diagnosis of intestinal lipoma is rarely to be expected. In cases of obscure intermittent abdominal pain with periods of complete freedom, a diagnosis of intussusception due to a benign tumor should be considered. The possibility of these tumors being adenomas is greater than the likelihood of their being lipomas. Radiographic studies usually show either a polypoid tumor or the characteristic filling defect of a colonic intussusception.

6. LIPOMAS OF THE GENITOURINARY TRACT. Lipomas of the kidney, ureter, and bladder have all been described. In the kidney, angiolipomas are the most common type.[61] It has been suggested that lipomas develop in atrophic kidneys.[6]

A. RENAL ANGIOLIPOMA. Angiolipomas constitute the most controversial of the benign tumors of the kidney. They are often encountered in the kidneys of patients with the tuberous sclerosis complex, and are usually asymptomatic. In patients in whom the renal neoplasm is not associated with tuberous sclerosis, the tumors can become quite large and symptomatic, necessitating resection. Price and Mostofi[61] found 30 cases in the files of the Kidney Tumor Registry of the Armed Forces Institute of Pathology. This lesion occurs more frequently in women than in men. We have only three cases of renal angiolipoma in our files.

The clinical picture ranges from an acute abdominal emergency to that of renal colic. In one of our patients the abdominal symptoms were misconstrued as tubal pregnancy. Roentgenographic examination of the urinary tract may be of considerable help in diagnosis. These tumors are usually large and the characteristic feature is the associated hemorrhage within the renal parenchyma. Adequate treatment usually entails a nephrectomy. No instance of recurrence after nephrectomy has been reported.

Lipomas of the female genital tract are a well-accepted clinical entity and may occur anywhere in the tract.[62] The rarity of lipoma in the fallopian tube is obvious, inasmuch as only 13 such cases have been reported.[63] Lipomas of the female external genitalia are more common than those of the genitourinary tract, and a number of such cases have been reported.[64] Lipomas of male genitalia are uncommon. Although lipomas of the spermatic cord are encountered not infrequently, lipomas of the scrotum and testes are indeed rare. There is some controversy concerning the classification of scrotal lipomas because of uncertainty in the determination of the exact primary site. Thus the term paratesticular (covering all structures) has been advocated[65] and is used herein.

7. LIPOMAS OF THE RESPIRATORY TRACT. Lipoma of the upper respiratory tract is rare. In the past, a number of cases have been mistakenly classified as lipomas. Zakrewski,[66] in 1965, found 68 reported cases of lipomas of the larynx, of which 54 were in the extrinsic and 14 in the intrinsic larynx. He also reported one case of a subglottic lipoma. These tumors behave like all other submucosal lipomas and the symptoms of obstruction and irritation are relieved by excision. Pulmonary or endobronchial lipomas are extremely rare[67] and are seldom diagnosed before death.

8. LIPOMAS OF THE HEART. This rare form of lipoma is usually diagnosed postmortem. Although most commonly these tumors are incidental necropsy findings, Estevez and associates[68] found a total of 37 cases of cardiac lipoma, including two of their own, in which the patients were symptomatic and died as a result of the cardiac lipoma.

9. LIPOMAS OF THE SPLEEN. Easler and Dowlin,[69] reported one case of primary lipoma of the spleen, and found only one other case in the literature. We have no case in our files.

LIPOMAS OF THE CENTRAL AND PERIPHERAL NERVOUS SYSTEM. Rokitansky,[70] in 1856, accidentally found the first case of a lipoma of the corpus callosum. Intracranial lipomas are extremely rare, and about 50 percent occur in the corpus callosum. Ewing[71] collected six patients with intracranial lipoma of the pia. The exact number of reported brain lipomas is hard to establish. Manganiello and co-authors[72] reported a total of 69 lipomas of the corpus callosum. Clinical diagnosis of intracranial lipoma is extremely difficult and all documented cases should be published. It has been stated that corpus callosum lipomas often produce symptoms of obstructive hydrocephalus.

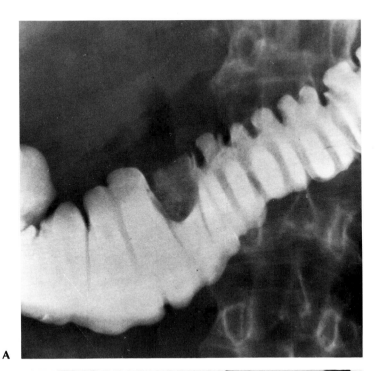

A

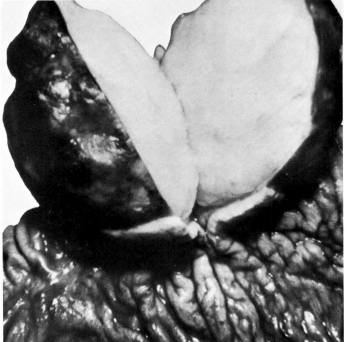

B

Figure 11.11. (A) Roentgenogram of a lipoma of the colon. The smooth contour suggests a benign tumor, but such a preoperative diagnosis should be made with extreme caution. **(B)** A large solitary lipoma of the transverse colon in a 47-year-old man. Patient presented with symptoms of bowel obstruction. An intussusception was found, which could be reduced. The segment containing the lipoma was excised. *(Courtesy of Current Problems in Surgery, March 1970.)*

Intraspinal lipomas, which constitute a small percentage of all primary intraspinal tumors, can be either intradural or extradural. The intradural lipomas are of greater interest because they occur in a region supposedly devoid of fat cells. Ehni and Love[73] collected only 29 cases of intradural lipomas. Usually they are congenital and commonly there is a long history of symptoms. Collins and Henderson[74] stated that symptoms usually appear at one of three age periods: before the third year, in adolescence, and at about the age of 40 years. They often are present for many years before producing serious disability. The extradural lipomas, on the other hand, are not congenital; they occur at all ages and usually have a short history. There is no characteristic segmental distribution, and they often are associated with the multiple lipomas of obesity. In 1973, Thomas and Miller[75] published their experience of 60 intraspinal lipomas from the Mayo Clinic. They suggested that a history of discomfort of long duration, a midline soft tissue mass, roentgenologic evidence of bony anomaly, and myelographic demonstration of a large dural sac and low-lying conus medullaris are all suggestive of an intraspinal lipoma. They recommended excision, and a 10-year followup showed the results to be favorable. However, when excision was not feasible, a decompressing laminectomy was recommended.

Lipomas of the peripheral nerves are extremely rare. Only recently have these tumors been described.[76-80] However, the diagnosis has been confused with fatty infiltration of the nerves by many authors.[77,80-83] Lipofibromatous hamartoma infrequently can give rise to macrodactyly. Stout's[84] admonition that such a diagnosis should be accepted with skepticism still holds true.

SYNOVIAL AND BONE LIPOMAS. Synovial lipomas are not infrequently present within the joint capsule, the popliteal space being one of the common sites.[64] These lipomas can arise within the joint either by penetrating the synovial membrane or as a result of overgrowth of fat within the intra-articular synovial tissue. Extra-articular lipomas are occasionally seen around the hip and knee joints. Intra-articular lipomas are also known as lipoma arborescens. They produce a characteristic treelike growth within the synovial membrane. Pack and Ariel[6] emphasized the necessity for distinguishing this type of lipoma from villous synovitis, an inflammatory overgrowth of the synovia. Lipoma arborescens can simulate pigmented villono-

dular synovitis, rheumatoid arthritis, and synovial hemangioma. Arthrography and arthroscopy have been used to make a preoperative diagnosis of lipoma arborescens.

Lipomas of the bone are seldom encountered. Bartlett[85] reported two patients in whom the lipomas arose from the periosteum and extended into the contiguous soft tissues. Dahlin,[86] in 1978, described five cases of lipomas of bones, including the roentgenographic findings. Association of a translucent mass in intimate contact with the diaphysis of a long bone and a hyperostotic reaction penetrating the tumor are classic findings. After excision the patient's progress is good. Occasionally, lipomas occur in the sacroiliac joint, producing symptoms of low back pain.[87] These tumors probably represent benign variants of periosteal fibrous tissue. Lipomas arising in bone should not be confused with ossifying lipomas. In such cases, areas of bone formation are infrequently encountered in the center of a long-standing subcutaneous lipoma (Fig. 11.12).

Multiple Lipomas. Multiple lipomas are unquestionably inherited and the mode of inheritance is a simple dominant gene.[88] The number varies from two or three to as many as 500 in one person. Although usually small and subcutaneous, they become large and confluent, producing a knobby contour of the extremities of the trunk that may be disfiguring. Pack and Ariel[6] described one patient with about 400 such lipomas. Several patients with hundreds of lipomas have been treated in our center.

In patients with von Recklinghausen's disease, a large number of lipomas are encountered along with cutaneous neurofibromas, and often clinical distinction between the two types is impossible without histologic examination. Adair et al.[89] suggested that multiple lipomas are connected with peripheral nerves and are essentially neurolipomas of neurogenic origin. These authors were impressed by the symmetrical arrangement of multiple lipomas, often corresponding to the course of a peripheral nerve; by their appearance in situations in which fat is usually absent; by their occurrence in young adults; and by a familial tendency to both multiple lipomas and neurofibromatosis, with pigmented cutaneous lesions present in both conditions. However, there is no evidence to support a thesis that multiple lipomas or lipomas in general have any relation to peripheral nerves. Multiple lipomas may be associated with angiomas

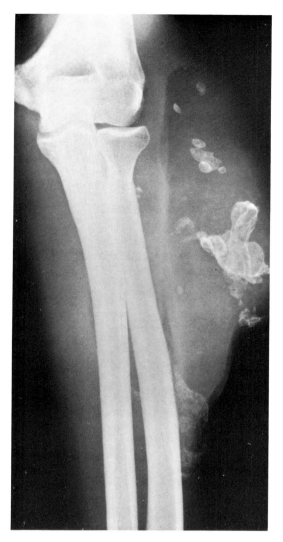

Figure 11.12. Areas of ossification in a long-standing solitary lipoma of the forearm. (See also Fig. 4.6, Chapter 4.)

and, less frequently, with diaphyseal aclasis; or they may be associated with multiple endocrine abnormalities.[90] Pain may suddenly develop in one of the lipomas and gradually extend to involve more and more discrete lipomas. This is not related to adiposis dolorosa.

The treatment of multiple lipomas is a perplexing problem. It is often technically impossible to excise all the hundreds of lipomas, even though total excision might be desirable from a cosmetic viewpoint. The inevitable question is,

do these tumors ultimately become malignant? Fortunately, they rarely do. We have come across only one such instance, a description of which follows:

Case Report.

A 43-year-old man was referred to us in 1973 for consultation regarding the management of two separate primary liposarcomas. He gave a family history of multiple lipomas. He had had his painful lipomas excised at regular intervals over the previous 10 to 15 years. Recently, however, two tumors, one in the neck and the other in the anterior abdominal wall, had rapidly increased in size. His surgeon excised these two lesions and found them to be liposarcomas. A review of the slides confirmed the histologic diagnosis. Examination of the patient showed multiple small lipomas and several large ones. Excision of these tumors was recommended, along with wider excision of the already diagnosed liposarcomas. The patient underwent the suggested therapy and is still doing well seven years later. Examination of all the resected lesions showed that he had nine independent primary liposarcomas.

It is not possible to define guidelines for the management of multiple lipomas. Generally, in view of the rarity of malignant degeneration, the reason for excision should be either pain relief or cosmetic.

Congenital Lipomatosis. This is a malformation of the adipose tissue in which the lipoblasts not only form discrete tumors, but infiltrate the surrounding structures. For clarity of description, the patients are grouped according to the anatomic locations in which lipomatosis is most commonly seen. These are as follows:

1. Congenital diffuse lipomatosis of the extremities
2. Congenital lipomatosis of the trunk
3. Pelvic lipomatosis

CONGENITAL DIFFUSE LIPOMATOSIS OF THE EXTREMITIES. This variety of lipoma is usually confined to one or two limbs and commonly is associated with corresponding gigantism (Fig. 11.13). Frequently, it is found with a cavernous hemangioma. The condition becomes apparent soon after birth and usually there is progressive enlargement. The lipomatous tumors commonly infiltrate the surrounding musculature and have an unusual propensity for recurrence, even after relatively wide excision. We have en-

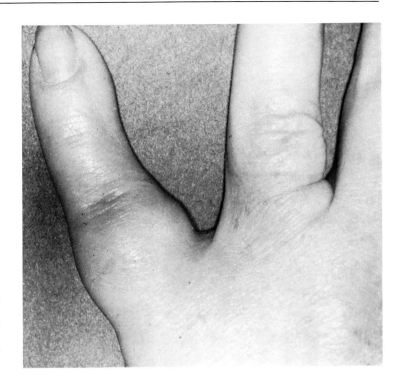

Figure 11.13. Lipoma of the palm and index finger in a patient with multiple lipomatosis. The local gigantism of the index finger is evident and was not altered even after excision of the lipoma at the base of the finger.

countered one patient[64] who required a forequarter amputation (Fig. 11.14).

Lipomatosis of discrete parts of the skeletal muscle has been described in Maffucci's syndrome. Cameron and McMillan[91] described a patient with the symptoms of Maffucci's syndrome who had a tumorlike adipose infiltration of the semitendinous muscle and short head of the biceps femoris.

CONGENITAL LIPOMATOSIS OF THE TRUNK. The underlying pathologic findings are similar to those of lipomatosis of the extremities. In the majority of patients, the tumors are found in the lumbodorsal and scapular regions. Nixon and Scobie[92] reported three cases, all in the lumbodorsal region. Another type of lipomatosis that may occur at any age is Madelung's disease (Fig. 11.15), in which the neck and axillae are symmetrically enlarged. The disease has also been called adenolipomatosis, since it occurs in the neck, axillary, and antecubital regions, although it has no relation to lymph nodes.

PELVIC LIPOMATOSIS (FIG. 11.16A TO 11.16E). Pelvic lipomatosis as a distinct clinical entity has been recognized only since Fogg and Smyth[93] first described it in 1968. However, Engels[94] was

the first to recognize the entity on a radiologic basis. It is essentially a benign condition in which there is an abundance of fatty tissue in the perirectal and perivesical spaces in the pelvis.

The cause of this disorder is unknown. Although four patients in the series reported by Engels underwent laparotomy and had large amounts of fatty tissue in the pelvis, they also had extensive pelvic adhesions, and he concluded that these adhesions were the underlying cause of the distortion of the bladder and sigmoid colon. Rosenberg et al.[95] reported a case of sciatica in a 50-year-old man in whom they had made a diagnosis of Dercum's disease. The patient had painful tender masses on the arms, legs, and right side of the rectum. A barium enema and urographic studies were suggestive of pelvic lipomatosis. Fogg and Smyth[93] suggested that pelvic lipomatosis is comparable to Weber-Christian disease and sclerosing lipogranulomatosis. It is apparent that different authors have applied various fanciful theories regarding the causation of this unusual clinical entity. However, in reality, no known systemic or local factor or factors can be shown to have a cause and effect relationship. Certainly these

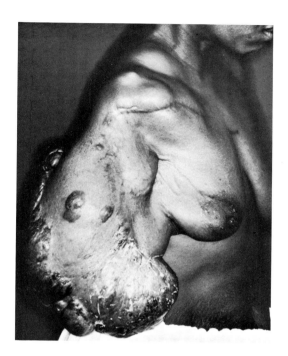

Figure 11.14. A 42-year-old woman who had had gigantism of the right upper extremity since infancy. She had had multiple operations, and lipomatous tissue was sequentially excised. At age 8, she had an above-elbow amputation. She was first seen with this massive lipomatous enlargement 34 years after above-elbow amputation. The remainder of the upper arm was heavy and painful. She complained of pain, tenderness, and loss of balance. Because of the extreme discomfort, a forequarter amputation was resorted to. *(Courtesy of Current Problems in Surgery, March 1970.)*

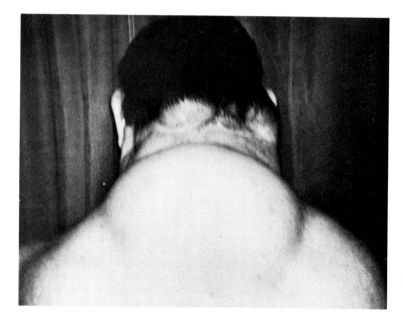

Figure 11.15. Typical case of Madelung's deformity. Note the Buffalo hump on the back. *(Courtesy Current Problems in Surgery, March 1970.)*

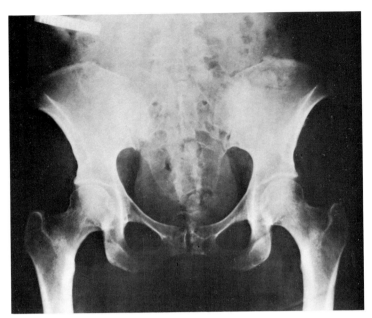

Figure 11.16. (A) Anteroposterior roentgenogram of the pelvis in pelvic lipomatosis. Note the ground glass shadow of the pelvic fatty tissue, the outline of which is smooth.

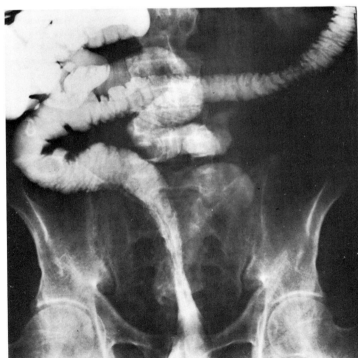

Figure 11.16. (B) Barium enema in a man with pelvic lipomatosis. The vertical straightening and foreshortening of the rectosigmoid is obvious and frequently is diagnostic.

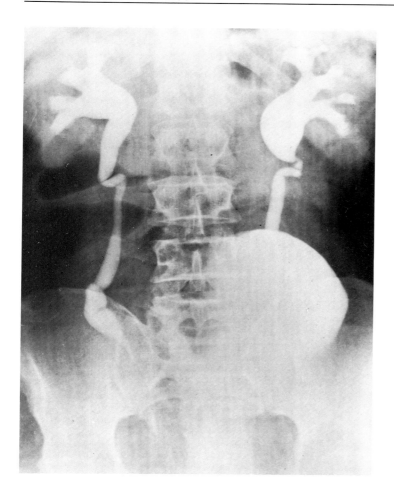

Figure 11.16. **(C)** Displacement of right ureter.

are not pelvic lipomas, although in one of our patients it was tempting to consider this as a variant of infiltrating angiolipoma. It is necessary, however, to keep an open mind regarding pelvic lipomatosis, since none of these patients has as yet had the advantage of a long-term followup.

The term pelvic lipomatosis aptly describes the anatomic and pathologic essence of this entity, which consists of an excessive proliferation of fibroadipose tissue in the pelvis. Cook et al.[96] reviewed 29 published cases, 27 in men and 2 in women. At the University of Illinois, we have seen five cases, all in men. Clinical correlation varies, with symptoms of lower urinary tract obstruction, vague pelvic pain, constipation, and even hypertension. However, in a large number of these patients the diagnosis of pelvic lipoma-

tosis is considered only after roentgenograms are obtained for evaluation of these nonspecific complaints.

Physical findings are not consistent, but an ill-defined mass in the suprapubic region has been found most frequently. Prostatic enlargement has been mentioned by some authors.[95-99] Elongation of the membranous and bulbous portions of the urethra has also been observed.[100]

Several authors have mentioned the difficulty of performing cystoscopy because of the elongated bladder or the distorted trigone, or both.[94,96-99] Cystoscopic findings ranged from normal to marked bullous edema.[96] Most authors report that examination of the colon shows tubular narrowing and vertical straightening, with upper displacement of the rectum and the

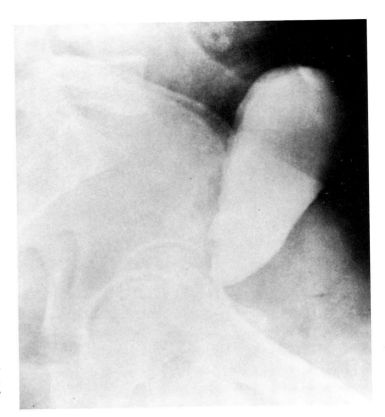

Figure 11.16. **(D)** Dye-filled urinary bladder in pelvic lipomatosis. The bladder appears vertically elongated.

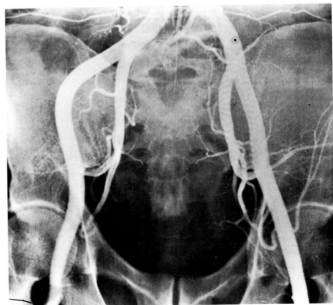

Figure 11.16. **(E)** Aortogram in pelvic lipomatosis, showing the displacement of the iliac vessels. Displacement of the right iliac is most marked.

sigmoid colon. Sigmoidoscopy, when performed, reveals no intrinsic lesion, but merely a straightening of that part of the colon.

Plane films of the abdomen demonstrate increased radiolucency in the pelvis; the lucency indicates increased fatty tissue. The bladder appears vertically elongated as a result of fatty infiltration of the pelvis. Hydronephrosis and hydroureters are found when the fat impinges upon the pelvic structures. In our patients, marked hydronephrosis or hydroureters have not been a major problem.

Cook and co-workers,[96] in their review of the various forms of treatment used for these patients, found that 20 patients were operated upon and showed masses of fat in the pelvis. In one patient we found the pelvis totally occupied by globulated fatty tissue without any specific macroscopic or microscopic characteristics. Although reports are found in which urinary diversion has been necessary because of lower urinary tract obstruction, in only one of our patients was this required.

In our judgment, pelvic lipomatosis is a relatively innocuous entity and aggressive therapy is unnecessary. Possibly most of these cases can be diagnosed by x-rays and an operation can be avoided. There is no place for either radical operation or radical radiation therapy. Furthermore, neither urinary nor fecal diversion should be performed unless the patient is symptomatic in either of these areas.

Treatment of Lipomas. The management of these lesions is operative. The solitary subcutaneous lipomas should be locally excised. Although enucleation via a small incision is usually adequate, care should be taken to avoid leaving fragments of lipomatous tissue behind.

Intermuscular lipomas should be excised, along with a portion of the muscle; however, no major nerve or blood vessel need be sacrificed. Gastrointestinal lipomas should be locally excised via gastrotomy or enterotomy, unless obstruction requires bowel resection.

Multiple lipomas should be excised if they are larger than 5 cm, or if they grow rapidly and produce symptoms. Excision for cosmetic reasons should be an individual decision for each patient. Congenital lipomatosis may require no treatment; however, functional or cosmetic disability may require partial removal, or digital or extremity amputation. Associated orthopedic procedures to stop overgrowth of bone may also be required.

Benign lipoblastomas are usually lobulated and found in the lower extremity. Local excision with a rim of normal fat is the treatment of choice.

Liposarcomas.

Anatomic Distribution. Liposarcomas seem to have a predilection for the deeper soft tissues, unlike benign solitary lipomas, which more commonly arise in the subcutaneous tissues. In Brasfield and Das Gupta's[43] series of 236 patients at Memorial Sloan-Kettering Cancer Center, the distribution of the liposarcomas consisted of 142 (60 percent) in the lower extremities and 39 (17 percent) in the upper extremities (Table 11.4).

In most series[43,64,101–105] the highest incidence of liposarcomas has been found in the lower extremities, the upper extremities, retroperitoneum, and trunk, in that order. The sites of occurrence of the 95 liposarcomas in our series at the University of Illinois are shown in Table 11.4. It is evident that the distribution of these tumors in the various anatomic sites corresponds with the distribution pattern reported in other series.[43,64] In the lower extremities (Table 11.5), the thigh and the buttock are the most common sites. In the upper extremities, there is no apparent predilection for any specific anatomic site. An uncommon site for liposarcoma is the head and neck region. In 1979, Saunders and co-workers[106] reviewed the literature and found 25 such cases, to which they added 4 of their own, making a total of 29. We have treated only two patients with liposarcoma of the head and neck region.

Clinical Features. In the series of 236 patients reported from Memorial Sloan-Kettering Cancer Center,[43] the sex ratio was 62.7 percent male to 37.3 percent female. In the University of Illinois series of 95 patients, 50 were women. In women in their fifth decade, a rapid-growing mass in the thigh is most apt to be a liposarcoma. The age at onset may be as early as six months, with a peak incidence of 55 percent occurring between the ages of 40 and 60 years.[64] The tumor is seen in all races and nationalities, and no predisposing epidemiologic factor is known.

A liposarcoma usually starts as an inconspicuous swelling of the soft tissues and continues to grow steadily (Fig. 11.17A to 11.17E). The patient's usual complaint is the gradual enlargement of a perceptible tumor. Pressure symptoms are felt only when the tumor reaches

TABLE 11.4 ANATOMIC DISTRIBUTION OF LIPOSARCOMA IN TWO SERIES

Site	Memorial Sloan-Kettering Cancer Center,[43] 1970 (236 Patients)	Das Gupta, 1981 (95 Patients)
Head and neck	4 (1.6%)	2 (2.1%)
Trunk	20 (3%)	16 (17%)
Retroperitoneal region	35 (14.5%)	9 (9.4%)
Upper extremities	39 (16%)	21 (22.1%)
Lower extremities	142 (59%)	47 (49.4%)
Total	240*	95

Four patients had multiple primary liposarcomas.

a certain size. It is almost impossible to arrive at a correct diagnosis by physical examination alone. However, liposarcomas are firmer, more deeply situated, and are more widely attached to the surrounding tissues than are common solitary subcutaneous lipomas. The retroperitoneal tumors are always diagnosed after operative intervention, although a preoperative tentative diagnosis of a malignant tumor based on high statistical incidence, CAT scan, and angiography is often made. The principles of diagnosis, staging, and pathologic classifications are discussed in Chapters 3 to 5.

Treatment.

SURGICAL. The fundamental principle in the primary management is radical excision, based on anatomic location, size, and local spread of the tumor. In the extremities, the choice of an appropriate type of operation depends on numerous factors, such as regional location, degree or grade of malignancy, fixity to the surrounding tissue (or mobility), the stage of the

TABLE 11.5 DISTRIBUTION OF LIPOSARCOMAS IN THE LOWER EXTREMITIES

Site	Memorial Sloan-Kettering Series,[43] 1970	Das Gupta, 1981
Thigh	99	28
Buttocks	13	11
Groin	12	3
Leg	16	4
Foot	2	1
Total	142	47

primary tumor, and the presence or absence of regional metastases.

The dissection should be performed with meticulous, gentle care, and retraction should always be away from, rather than toward, the tumor. The soft tissues encompassing the liposarcoma must never be handled roughly. The majority of primary liposarcomas can be well treated by means of wide soft tissue resection. Although amputation of an extremity for a liposarcoma is a mutilating procedure and should be performed only when absolutely indicated, if and when required, the operation should not be denied to the patient. Frequently, an initial inadequate operation results in local recurrence and lowers the overall salvage rate of patients with this type of tumor (Fig. 11.17E).

The technical considerations for wide excision and its variants for major amputations are described elsewhere. Unless all indications and contraindications for each of the types of operations are taken into consideration, the results of treatment will be less than optimal.

RADIATION THERAPY. In general, the most important role of radiation therapy in the management of primary liposarcoma is in an adjuvant setting. Edland[107] considered radiation therapy more useful as an adjunct to surgery than as a primary form of treatment. Pack and Ariel[6] suggested that the radiosensitivity of liposarcoma is greater than the radiocurability. In their series of 12 patients treated entirely by radiation therapy, only two had complete regression of the tumor: one had a cure of ten years or more. Sixteen percent of their patients had complete clinical regression and 60 percent had partial regression of their primary tumor when preoperative radiation therapy was used. However, microscopic examination of the re-

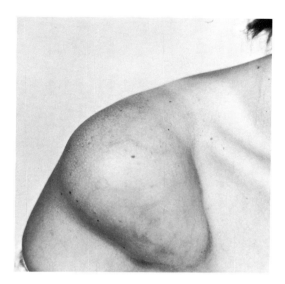

Figure 11.17. (A) The tumor started as an insidious soft subcutaneous swelling. After it attained the present size, it was excised and a well-differentiated liposarcoma was found.

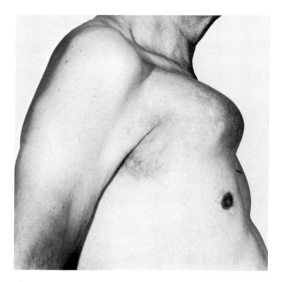

Figure 11.17. (C) Liposarcoma of the chest wall in a 54-year-old man. Medical attention was sought when the mass rubbed against the arm and was a source of irritation.

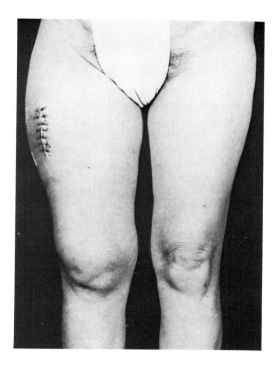

Figure 11.17. (B) Liposarcoma of right thigh in a 48-year-old woman. The primary tumor was 8 cm in maximum diameter before a wedge biopsy was performed.

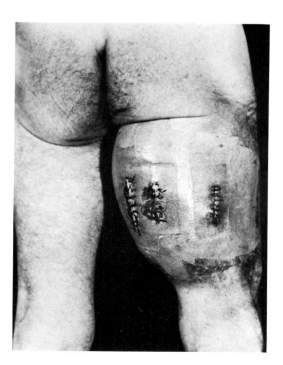

Figure 11.17. (D) Liposarcoma of the right posterior thigh. Patient had multiple biopsies before being referred to us.

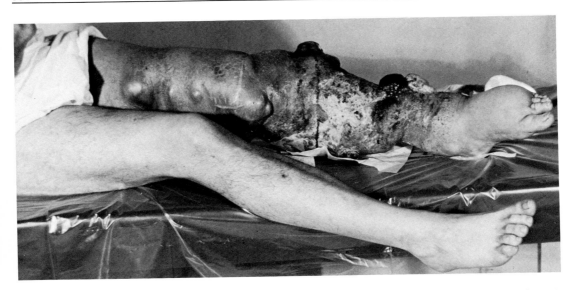

Figure 11.17. (E) A neglected case of liposarcoma in a 52-year-old man. He had 18 local excisions prior to his visit to the University of Illinois Hospital. A palliative hip joint disarticulation was performed. Following amputation he remained symptom-free for nine months and died of metastatic liposarcoma 14 months after amputation.

sected specimens showed residual tumor in a majority of the patients. McNeer and associates[108] concluded that radiation therapy has an adjuvant role in the treatment of liposarcomas. Preoperative irradiation sometimes converts unresectable tumors into resectable ones, as in the case of bulky retroperitoneal tumors (Fig. 11.18).

The role of postoperative radiation therapy has been recently evaluated by Lindberg and associates.[109] There is definite indication for the use of curative radiation therapy following excision of certain histologic types and grades of liposarcomas. The topic is discussed in detail in Chapter 7.

CHEMOTHERAPY. In general, primary liposarcomas do not respond well to any form of conventional systemic chemotherapy. Local infusion or perfusion with any specific agent has not been tried extensively enough to provide dependable data. This subject is discussed in detail in Chapter 8.

End Results. The clinical behavior of liposarcomas can be prognosticated by the type and the grade of the tumors. Histologic classification of liposarcomas, as proposed by several authors,[101-105] has tended to show that the five-year survival rate is the highest in well-differentiated tumors, and the recurrence rate, the lowest. In the accompanying tables, the five-year survival

rate for patients with four different types of tumors and the recurrence rate in these categories is compared in three relatively large series (Tables 11.6 and 11.7).

Enzinger and Winslow[103] reported that in patients with myxoid liposarcomas, the local recurrence rate was 53 percent and the five-year survival was 77 percent. With the round cell type, the local recurrence rate was 85 percent and the five-year survival rate, 18 percent. For the well-differentiated type, the local recurrence rate was 53 percent and the five-year survival rate, 85 percent. In the pleomorphic type the tumor recurred locally in 73 percent of cases, and the five-year salvage rate was only 21 percent. Similarly, the data from the Mayo Clinic shows that the survival rate and rate of local recurrence were dependent on histologic type (Tables 11.6 and 11.7). A 60 percent five-year survival rate and 15 percent local recurrence rate in well-differentiated liposarcoma was considered a good result. In our later group, both the five-year survival rate and the local recurrence rate in all histologic types of liposarcoma have considerably improved (Tables 11.6 and 11.7).

Seventy-seven patients in our series could be staged and graded according to the system proposed by the American Joint Committee for Staging and End Results Reporting.[110] Table 11.8

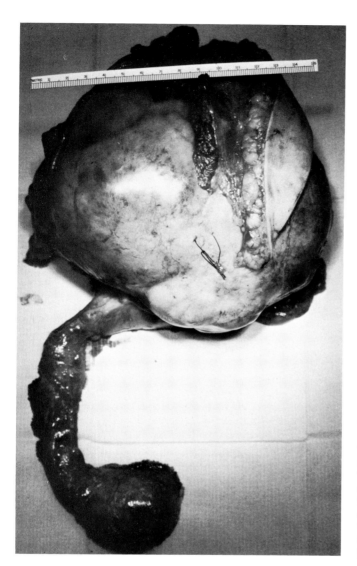

Figure 11.18. A huge retroperitoneal liposarcoma that originated in the right spermatic cord. The patient was 58 years old when first seen with a mass extending from the root of the penis to the right subcostal margin. Clinically, the tumor appeared unresectable. A course of preoperative radiation therapy was given. The tumor shrank considerably and three weeks later was resected. Patient is still well nine years after the operation and is leading an active professional life.

TABLE 11.6 FIVE-YEAR SURVIVAL OF LIPOSARCOMA PATIENTS BY HISTOLOGIC TYPES: DATA FROM THREE INSTITUTIONS

Tumor Type	Enzinger and Winslow[103] AFIP, 1962 (103 Patients)	Reszel et al.,[104] Mayo Clinic, 1966 (221 Patients)	Das Gupta, 1981 (95 Patients)*
Myxoid	77%	47.3%	80%
Round cell	18%	—	25%
Well differentiated	85%	60.0%	83%
Pleomorphic	21%	33.3%	43%

*Eight patients received adjuvant chemotherapy (Chapter 8).

TABLE 11.7 RATE OF LOCAL RECURRENCE OF LIPOSARCOMA BY HISTOLOGIC TYPE

Tumor Type	Enzinger and Winslow[103] AFIP, 1962 (103 Patients)	Reszel et al.[104] Mayo Clinic, 1966 (221 Patients)	Das Gupta, 1981 (95 Patients)*
Myxoid	53%	43%	11%
Round cell	85%	—	10%
Well differentiated	53%	15%	0
Pleomorphic	73%	30%	9%

Eight patients received adjuvant chemotherapy (Chapter 8).

shows that all 15 patients with T_1G_1 tumors lived free of disease for five years, compared with only one of four patients with stage IV disease. Although the biologic behavior of a liposarcoma is dependent on the T and G values of the primary (Chapter 4), it cannot be overemphasized that most poorly differentiated liposarcomas show varying microscopic features, and too much reliance on the prognosis or prediction of biologic behavior on the basis of what is seen in only a few sections is bound to be a source of disappointment unless a properly designed therapeutic approach is undertaken.

Brasfield and Das Gupta[43] found that 92 (50 percent) of their 184 patients eligible for five-year followup were still disease-free. Twelve

TABLE 11.8 FIVE-YEAR RESULT IN 77 PATIENTS WITH LIPOSARCOMA ACCORDING TO STAGE AND GRADE[110] (UNIVERSITY OF ILLINOIS SERIES)

Stage	No. Patients	No. Surviving Free of Disease
$T_1G_1N_0M_0$	15	15 (100%)
$T_2G_1N_0M_0$	20	18 (90%)
$T_1G_2N_0M_0$	13	12 (92%)
$T_2G_2N_0M_0$	8	6 (75%)*
$T_1G_3N_0M_0$	9	6 (66%)†
$T_2G_3N_0M_0$	8	5 (62%)‡
$T_3G_3N_0M_0$	4§	1 (25%)
Total	77	63 (82%)

One patient needed a second excision of the local recurrence before five years.
†*Two patients needed a second excision of local recurrence before five years.*
‡*Two patients needed same as above.*
§*Three of four needed more than one excision of the locally recurrent tumor with which they were originally seen.*

patients (7 percent) lived for five years or more with recurrent tumor. An overall survival rate of 54 percent was obtained. Seventy-six patients (41 percent) died of liposarcoma and four (2 percent) died of unrelated causes.

In the present series of 95 patients, 87 were treated by surgery alone. Of 77 eligible for a five-year end result study, 63 (82 percent) were found to be free of disease. Eight patients (10 percent) were treated for recurrent tumor before five years (Table 11.8). These results are compared with the series reported by Pack and Ariel,[6] Enterline and co-workers,[102] and Brasfield and Das Gupta,[43] in Table 11.9. It is evident that, with the progression of time, the results of surgical treatment for primary liposarcoma have improved.

The accent in the management of primary liposarcoma has been on operative treatment. In all major reported series, the authors[20,43,64,101-105,111] in general agreed with the concept of excisional therapy. Most series, however, have been reported either by surgeons[43,64,104,105] or by pathologists,[20,101-103] and the possibility of bias cannot be ruled out. In any event, the results obtained in the University of Illinois series of an overall five-year cure rate of 82 percent following excision cannot be disregarded.

The operative methods used vary according to the anatomic location of the tumor. However, the end results, based on location of the tumor, do not show great variability. Pack and Ariel[6] suggested that the highest cure rates occur in cases of liposarcoma of the arm and foot and the lowest in those of the buttocks and groin. The most likely explanation for such a finding in Pack and Ariel's series is early recognition and treatment of the liposarcomas of the hands and feet.

The end results based on the method of

TABLE 11.9 FIVE-YEAR END RESULTS IN ELIGIBLE PATIENTS WITH LIPOSARCOMA IN FOUR SERIES

	Pack and Ariel,[6] 1958	Enterline et al.,[102] 1960	Brasfield and Das Gupta,[43] 1970	Das Gupta, 1981
No. patients eligible	64	40	184(of 236)	77(of 95)
No. patients living free of disease at five years	2(3%)	5(12.5%)	92(50%)	63(82%)
No. patients free of disease at five years with treatment for locally recurrent tumors in-between	2(3%)	5(12.5%)	12(6.5%)	8(10%)
Dead with liposarcoma	39(61%)	18(45%)	76(41%)	14(18%)
Dead of unrelated causes	—	5(12.5%)	4(2%)	1(1%)
Overall five-year survival rate	39%	42.5%	56.5%	82%

operative treatment at the University of Illinois series are shown in Table 11.10. The category of wide excisions also includes chest wall and abdominal wall resections. Amputation in this context refers only to limb ablative procedures. Major amputations have decreased in frequency and the most commonly performed operation at the University of Illinois is wide excision or a variant thereof, resulting in limb salvage in most instances. A comparison of the present data with the earlier analysis of Memorial Sloan-Kettering Cancer Center material shows that the results have improved.

Analysis of 54 primary amputations in the Memorial Sloan-Kettering series[43] shows a 41 percent salvage at the end of five years. The majority of these amputations were performed after the initial therapy was found to be inadequate. Fifteen of those patients needed either a forequarter amputation or a hemipelvectomy as secondary operations and, of these, nine (60 percent) survived for five years or longer. In the present series, nine patients required a limb ablative procedure, in each case for a locally recurrent tumor after failure of both local resection and radiation therapy.

Node dissection is seldom necessary. In the present series only 14 patients had node dissection with the wide excision. In most of these patients the primary tumors were either in or adjacent to a node-bearing area, for example, axilla, groin, upper end of the thigh, or the breast.

From a study of the University of Illinois material and a review of other published studies,[43,64,102-105] it appears that if aggressive operative intervention is initially performed, patients with liposarcoma have a good to excellent prognosis. In general, operative intervention entails wide excision, or a variant of it. Infrequently, however, a major amputation becomes necessary, and even in such circumstances, the salvage rate justifies these radical procedures. Reszel and associates,[104] reviewing the Mayo Clinic experience of 55 years, stated as follows:

TABLE 11.10. TYPES OF CURATIVE OPERATION AND END RESULTS IN 259 PATIENTS WITH LIPOSARCOMA

	Memorial Sloan-Kettering Series		University of Illinois Series	
Type of Operation	No. Patients	5-Yr N.E.D.*	No. Patients	5-Yr N.E.D.
Wide excision	74	34 (46%)	23	17 (74%)
Muscle group excision	23	13 (57%)	31	28 (90%)
Wide excision with node dissection	31	13 (42%)	14	11 (78%)
Amputation	54	22 (40%)	9	7 (77%)
Total	182	82 (45%)	77	63 (82%)

*No evidence of disease.

"Based on the data relative to recurrence, metastases, and death, it appears to us that, during the 55 years covered by this study, surgical treatment of liposarcomata has not been aggressive enough either at the Mayo Clinic or at other institutions. We think that greater effort should be made to eradicate the primary growth at the time of initial operation, since inadequate removal invites recurrence and, in all but grade I tumors, very possible metastases." These authors also cautioned against not using primary amputation for the treatment of liposarcomas. Brasfield and Das Gupta[43] reported that 22 of 194 (11.3 percent) determinant patients were treated by curative radiation therapy. Ten of the 22 (45 percent) survived five years free of disease. Sixty-nine other patients received adjunctive radiation therapy along with excision: Eleven patients received preoperative therapy and four (36 percent) survived five years. One of the four developed recurrence and metastases soon after the fifth year and died. Fifty-eight patients were treated by postoperative radiation therapy, 25 (43 percent) of whom lived five years or more. Two developed local recurrence. It is difficult to express an opinion based on this type of retrospective analysis because, in the majority of these patients, radiation therapy was used without a formal plan. The basic aim of both excision and radiation therapy is local control of the primary tumor and long-term cure. In this context, both preoperative and postoperative radiation therapy have been tried by several authors.[109,112,113] In selected cases, this combined modality of local excision and appropriate radiation therapy has been found useful.[109,112,113]

Local Recurrence. Of the 77 liposarcoma patients eligible for appropriate staging and five-year end-result analysis in the University of Illinois series, 8 (10 percent) had local recurrence following initial treatment of the primary (Table 11.8). Local recurrence rates for liposarcoma have been reported as 33.3 percent by Pack and Pierson,[21] 48 percent by Enterline and co-workers,[102] 70 percent by Reszel et al.,[104] and between 53 and 85 percent in the series reported by Enzinger and Winslow.[103] This marked reduction in the incidence of local recurrence in the University of Illinois series is mostly due to an initial aggressive surgical approach.

Histologic prognostic criteria for patients with liposarcoma were developed by Enterline and his associates.[102] Later, Enzinger and Winslow[103] and Reszel and co-workers[104] ana-lyzed their cases and tried to develop some general prognostic guidelines. The American Joint Committee for Cancer Staging and End-result Reporting has developed a comprehensive staging system[110] (Table 11.8). It appears that a small, well-differentiated liposarcoma (T_1G_1 or T_1G_2) has less potential for local recurrence and distant metastases, and the patient thus has a better chance for cure. Therefore, it is logical to propose that an initial curative wide excision should be the therapy of choice. In contrast, less differentiated or pleomorphic forms of the tumor (T_2G_2 or T_2G_3) have a higher potential for local recurrence and metastases, with less chance for cure. Therefore, these tumors require not only aggressive initial resection, but adjuvant radiation therapy as well. The end results obtained in the University of Illinois patients suggest that adequate wide excision should constitute the mainstay in the management of most liposarcomas in all anatomic locations and of varying sizes and grades.

Retroperitoneal Liposarcomas. Of all the lipomatous tumors, retroperitoneal liposarcomas have aroused the most interest, possibly because their location hampers both diagnosis and management.

Lipomatous tumors are one of the most common forms of retroperitoneal tumor. Only 4 of 30 retroperitoneal lipomatous tumors reported by Brasfield and Das Gupta were histologically benign.[43] Ockuly and Douglass[114] estimated that approximately 35 percent of retroperitoneal fatty tumors are of perirenal origin, which is logical since the largest amount of fat accumulates in the perirenal region.

Retroperitoneal fatty tumors occur more frequently in women than in men. Adair, Pack, and Farrow[89] reported the incidence in females to be 73 percent. In our present series of nine patients, six are women. These tumors occur in patients of all ages, but most frequently in those between the ages of 40 and 60 years. The oldest patient in our group is 81 years of age (Table 11.11).

Characteristically, retroperitoneal liposarcomas are "silent" during their early growth, and are capable of attaining tremendous size. Generally their presence becomes known by reason of their increasing growth, which causes progressive swelling of the abdomen, a palpable mass, and later, pain. Thirty of 35 patients in the series reported by Brasfield and Das Gupta[43] were first seen because of swelling of the ab-

TABLE 11.11. END RESULTS IN THE TREATMENT OF NINE PATIENTS WITH RETROPERITONEAL LIPOSARCOMA

Patient	Age/Sex	Anatomic Extent	Surgical Treatment	Radiation Treatment	Metastases or Local Recurrence	End Result	Comments
1	47/F	R. perirenal area, infiltrating kidney and Gerota's fascia	Wide excision with nephrectomy and resection of a segment of liver	—	—	5½ yr N.E.D.*	Extensive resection performed for the primary tumor
2	39/F	L. upper quadrant infiltrating stomach and spleen	Excision with splenectomy and partial gastrectomy	4,000 rads	Lung and local recurrence	18 mo dead	Massive local recurrence, received chemotherapy as well
3	81/M	R. iliac fossa	Excision	—	Local recurrence 18 mo later	N.E.D. 6 yr after second excision	Doing well after second excision
4	64/M	R. iliolumbar region extending from the scrotum	Excision	Preop radiation therapy (R.T.)		9 yr N.E.D.	See case report, Figure 11.18
5	56/F	L. iliac fossa extending to ovarian ligament, etc.	Total excision plus hysterectomy	Preop R.T.	Lung metastases	2 yr dead	Widespread metastases, including brain
6	64/M	L. perirenal area infiltrating splenic flexure	Excision, resection of left kidney and splenic flexure	Postop R.T. 4,000 rads	Recurrence and metastases	2½ yr dead	Patient died in postop period; specimen weighed 55 pounds
7	68/F	Paravertebral, invading inferior vena cava	Excision with inferior vena cava excision (reexcised)	—	Local recurrence 1½ yr	3½ yr N.E.D. after second excision	Patient 5 yr N.E.D. after excision of one local recurrence
8	54/F	Paravertebral, predominantly left side	Excision	—	—	5 yr N.E.D.	Slow-growing tumor
9	72/F	Presacral area	Excision	—	Local recurrence, lung metastases 9 mo	14 mo dead	Original excision inadequate

*No evidence of disease.

389

domen. Enzinger and Winslow[103] found abdominal enlargement as the initial observation in 23 patients. The tumor may compress the adjacent structures, resulting in related symptoms. Larger and more highly malignant tumors cause weight loss, anorexia, and asthenia.

The diagnosis of retroperitoneal liposarcoma is difficult to make and frequently is possible only after an exploratory celiotomy. It has been suggested that a retroperitoneal liposarcoma can be distinguished from other tumors in this location by its translucency in the roentgenogram. Although this suggestion is based on sound theoretical reasoning because of the low specific gravity of fat and water absorption coefficient, in practice, the roentgenogram is rarely diagnostic. However, sonograms, intravenous pyleograms, inferior venacavograms, aortic angiograms, and CAT scans can often define the extent of the tumor, as well as provide sufficient information on its nature.

The treatment of retroperitoneal liposarcoma is excision. Every effort should be made to remove the entire tumor. Preoperative radiation therapy is indicated in large tumors. In patients in whom excision is inadequate and the histologic classification justifies it, postoperative radiation therapy should be used.

The end result of treatment of retroperitoneal liposarcomas is poor. Pack and Ariel[6] had 2 patients out of 17 (12 percent) living free of disease after five years. Table 11.11 shows the clinical features and the end result of nine cases of retroperitoneal liposarcomas treated by the author.

Liposarcomas in Unusual Locations. Although, theoretically, liposarcomas can be found in any part of the body, in certain sites they occur very rarely, if at all. Bone, the periorbital region, and the female breast are examples. A brief review of acceptable cases of liposarcoma in these regions follows:

LIPOSARCOMA OF THE BONE. Pack and Ariel[6] stated that Ewing, in 1928, described a patient with supposed liposarcoma of the bone marrow. Stewart[115] reported three additional cases in 1931. However, Stout,[116] in 1949, was reluctant to accept a diagnosis of primary liposarcoma of bone. This diagnosis has remained in doubt ever since. Goldman[117] reviewed the literature in 1964 and found 11 cases that could be accepted as true liposarcomas of the bone. To these he added one of his own. Catto and

Stevens[118] and Ross and Hadfield[119] added one case each. Ross and Hadfield's[119] case was unusual since it also produced neoplastic bone and was regarded as an osteoliposarcoma. In 1970, Schwartz and co-workers[120] reviewed the literature and reported an additional case of their own. Because of the extreme rarity of this entity, its biologic behavior is not well known.

LIPOSARCOMA OF THE BREAST. Of the 95 patients in the University of Illinois series, only one had liposarcoma of the breast. This patient required not only a mastectomy, but excision of the underlying chest wall. Histologically, this was a well-differentiated liposarcoma. Five years after chest wall excision she is still doing well. In the earlier reported series of 236 patients,[43,64] liposarcoma of the breast was found in two patients. Recently, Rasmusen and Jensen[121] found 34 published cases of primary liposarcoma of the breast and added one of their own. These authors have described the clinical data in these 35 patients. The usual history is of a progressively enlarging tumor of the breast. Excision of the breast usually suffices; infrequently the extent and local infiltration necessitates resection of the pectoral muscles and chest wall, and an axillary dissection.

LIPOSARCOMA OF THE PLEURA. In 1942, Ackerman and Wheeler[101] described a case of liposarcoma of the pleura. Gupta and Paolini[122] reported an additional case. In a review of the literature, they were unable to find any other case of primary liposarcoma of the pleura. We have not treated any such patient.

INTRATHORACIC AND CARDIAC LIPOSARCOMAS. An intrathoracic liposarcoma is extremely rare. Currie,[123] in 1964, collected only 26 cases and added one of his own. In the same year, Cicciarelli and associates[124] reported eight cases from the Mayo Clinic. Razzuk and co-workers,[125] in 1971, reported one case and reviewed the literature. These authors found 44 cases of intrathoracic liposarcoma. The tumor originated in the mediastinum in 43 cases and in the pulmonary hilum in 1 case. All but two cases were in adult patients. The ages ranged from 13 to 63 years, with no significant sex predominance. The majority of patients were symptomatic. The onset and nature of the symptoms were related to the size and location of the tumors. Some patients remained relatively asymptomatic until the terminal stage. Symptoms included cough, chest pain, dyspnea, and, occasionally, symptoms of superior vena cava obstruction. Survival from the time of onset of symptoms in the 21 patients that were followed ranged from two months to 14 years. All but two patients were dead at the time of the original report. Five patients survived longer than five years, one was alive and well 6.5 years after operation, two lived for nine years, and two for 14 years.

The clinical history of intrathoracic liposarcoma is not particularly characteristic. The diagnosis is usually confirmed by means of an exploratory thoracotomy and adequate biopsy.

The results of therapy in 23 evaluable cases show that seven patients were treated by excision and four of the seven lived for an average of 6.75 years.[125] Six patients were treated by both excision and irradiation. The average survival time in these six patients was three years. The remaining ten patients were only palliated because of the extent of their disease. None of these patients lived for more than 18 months, the average survival time being one year. To the best of our knowledge, a documented case of primary liposarcoma of the heart has not been reported.

LIPOSARCOMAS OF THE GASTROINTESTINAL TRACT AND OMENTUM. Liposarcomas of the gastrointestinal tract are exceptionally rare. Only one case of gastric liposarcoma[126] and one arising in the transverse colon[127] have been reported. Omental sarcomas are extremely rare, despite the high fat content of the omentum. Only one such case has been encountered in the University of Illinois series. As with the patient reported by Robb,[128] our patient also had a hemoperitoneum due to rupture of the highly vascular tumor in the omentum. Hassan,[129] in 1970, reported a similar case of omental liposarcoma with a hemoperitoneum. This patient had a subcutaneous liposarcoma excised 5.5 years prior to the omental tumor.
prior to the omental tumor.

LIPOSARCOMA OF THE GENITOURINARY TRACT. Edson and associates[130] reported a case of perivesical liposarcoma. The presenting symptoms were prostatitis and frequent failure to respond to a brief course of antibiotic therapy. The patient was operated on with a presumptive diagnosis of prostatic abscess. The true nature of the tumor was discovered after the operation.

LIPOSARCOMA OF THE SPERMATIC CORD AND SCROTUM. Liposarcomas of the spermatic cord are extremely rare.[131] We have treated only one

case. These tumors appear either as a scrotal or as an inguinal mass. Sometimes the enlarging inguinal mass mimics an incarcerated inguinal hernia. Our patient was first seen with a large inguinal mass extending proximally through the inguinal canal into the retroperitoneal space (Fig. 11.18). Wide excision entailing orchiectomy and high ligation of the cord is usually adequate. The prognosis is about the same as for a liposarcoma in other anatomic locations.

Waller[132] reported a case of liposarcoma of the scrotum, an uncommon tumor. If such a case is truly encountered, wide excision would be the therapy of choice.

DISEASES OF BROWN ADIPOSE TISSUE

In humans, disease of the brown adipose tissue is limited to occasional benign tumors or hibernomas. Although brown fat has a thermogenic property and can store either adrenal steroids or catecholamines, no systemic disease similar to the lipopathies of white adipose tissue has been described. It is indeed curious that tumors of the brown adipose tissue are usually benign, even though this apparently is a primitive type of adipose tissue. Rona[133] described two patients who died in shock following removal of a pheochromocytoma. One of these had a massive accumulation of brown fat 8 × 4.5 × 2 cm, weighing 18 gm. The other had similar masses of brown fat in the epicardium. Histologic examination showed that the transformed fatty tissue contained, in addition to adult fat cells, two other cell types: polygonal cells with central nuclei and pleurivacuolar cytoplasm that contained doubly refractile lipids; and cells with argentaffin and chromaffin properties. Extract prepared from the brown fat in one of the two patients exerted a pressor effect on injection into a cat. Hibernoma masquerading as a pheochromocytoma has also been described.[134]

Hibernomas

Hibernomas are found in the subcutaneous tissue of the neck, shoulder, axilla, interscapular region, and mediastinum. These are the areas in which immature fat or brown fat is found in mammals. Mesara and Batsakis[135] collected a total of 26 cases of hibernoma from the literature and reported one of their own. Twelve were in the interscapular region, four in the mediastinum, three in the axillae, four in the buttocks and thighs, two in the abdominal wall, and two in the neck. In 1973, Merlina and Pike[137] reported a case of hibernoma in the thigh of a 24-year-old man. Hibernomas are slow-growing neoplasms. The subcutaneous variety is recognized only after excision of a tumor that appeared to be a solitary subcutaneous lipoma. On the other hand, hibernomas located in the neck or mediastinum may produce pressure symptoms, because of compression of the regional structures. Patients with mediastinal hibernomas occasionally present with symptoms of tracheal compression and cough. Leiphart and Nudelman[134] reported a case of hibernoma adjacent to both kidneys. This case was of particular interest since, by angiography, it had been diagnosed as a right-sided pheochromocytoma. An exploratory procedure revealed two masses of brown fat in the perirenal region with findings characteristic of hibernoma. Furthermore, at the bifurcation of the aorta a 6 × 7 cm mass was found which was interpreted to be a pheochromocytoma. Lawson and Biller[136] found reports on 37 cases of hibernoma, of which 10 were interscapular, 6 were axillary, and 5 cervical or intrathoracic; the remaining 16 cases were distributed in the thigh, buttock, popliteal region, chest wall, and abdominal wall. Hibernomas of the extremities are extremely rare.[137]

In 1967, Lowry and Halmos[138] published a report of a malignant hibernoma in the scapular region of a 24-year-old woman with Turner's syndrome. This tumor was considered to be malignant because of its infiltration into the surrounding muscles. Infiltration is not adequate evidence of malignancy, since the infiltrative qualities of benign intermuscular lipomas and angiolipomas are well established. A primary malignant hibernoma or malignant transformation of a benign hibernoma is still hard to document.[139]

REFERENCES

1. Keys A, Brozek J: Body fat in adult man. Physiol Rev 33:235, 1953
2. Jeanrenaud B: Dynamic aspects of adipose tissue metabolism: A review. Metabolism 10:535, 1961
3. Hashim SA: Metabolism of body fat. NY J Med 16:1339, 1961
4. Steiner G, Cahill GF, Jr: Adipose tissue physiology. Ann NY Acad Sci 110:749, 1963
5. Dercum FX: Three cases of a hitherto unclassified affliction resembling in its grosser aspects obesity, but associated with special nervous symptoms—adiposis dolorosa. Am J Med Sci 104:521, 1892
6. Pack GT, Ariel IM: Tumors of the Soft Somatic Tissues: A Clinical Treatise. New York, Hoeber-Harper, 1958, p 343
7. Lynch HT, Harlan WL: Hereditary factors in adiposis dolorosa (Dercum's disease). Am J Human Genet 115:184, 1963
8. Wohl MG, Pastor N: Adiposis dolorosa (Dercum's disease). JAMA 110:1261, 1938
9. Pfeifer V: Ueber einen Fall von herdweiser Atrophie des subcutanen Feltgewekes. Deutsch Arch Klin Med 1:438, 1892
10. Gilchrist TG, Ketron LW: A unique case of atrophy of the skin, preceded by large phagocytic cells (macrophages). Bull Johns Hopkins Hosp, Baltimore, XXVII, p. 291, 1916
11. Weber FP: A case of relapsing nonsuppurative nodular panniculitis showing phagocytosis of subcutaneous fat-cells by macrophages. Br J Dermat 37:301, 1925
12. Christian HA: Relapsing febrile nodular non-suppurative panniculites. Arch Int Med 42:338, 1928
13. Lever WF: Nodular nonsuppurative panniculitis (Weber-Christian disease). Arch Dermat Syph 59:31, 1949
14. Lever WF: The lipopathies. In Beeson PB, McDermott W (eds): Cecil-Loeb Textbook of Medicine, 11th ed. Philadelphia, Saunders, 1963, p 1336
15. Balzer F: Recherches sur la degenerescence granulograisseuse des tissues dans les maladies infectieuses; parasetisne du xanthelasma et de l'ictere grave. Rev de Med Par ii:307, 1882
16. Adair FE, Munzer TY: Fat necrosis of the female breast. Am J Surg 74:117, 1947
17. Weary PE, Graham GF, Selden RF: Subcutaneous fat necrosis of the newborn. South Med J 59:960, 1966
18. Ewing J: Fascial sarcoma and intermuscular myxoliposarcoma. Arch Surg 31:507, 1935
19. Gellhorn A, Marks PA: The composition and biosynthesis of lipids in human adipose tissues. J Clin Invest 40:925, 1961
20. Stout AP: Liposarcoma—malignant tumor of lipoblasts. Ann Surg 119:86, 1944
21. Pack GT, Pierson JC: Liposarcoma. A study of 105 cases. Surgery 36:687, 1954
22. Booher RJ: Lipoblastic tumors of the hands and feet. Review of the literature and report of thirty-three cases. J Bone Joint Surg 47-A:727, 1965
23. Phalen GS, Kendrick JI, Rodriguez TM: Lipomas of the upper extremity. A series of fifteen tumors in the hand and wrist and six tumors causing nerve compression. Am J Surg 121:298, 1971
24. Paarlberg D, Linscheid RL, Soule EH: Lipomas of the hand including lipoblastomatosis in a child. Mayo Clin Proc 47:121, 1972

25. Howard WR, Helwig EB: Angiolipoma. Arch Dermat 82:126, 1960
26. Regan JM, Bickel WH, Broders AC: Infiltrating benign lipomas of the extremities. Western J Surg 54:87, 1946
27. Dionne G, Seemayer TA: Infiltrating lipomas and angiolipomas revisited. Cancer 33:732, 1974
28. Bradley RL, Klein MM: Angiolipoma. Am J Surg 108:887, 1964
29. Gonzalez-Crussi F, Enneking WF, Arean VM: Infiltrating angiolipoma. J Bone Joint Surg 48-A:1111, 1966
30. Pearson J, Stellar S, Feigin I: Angiolipoma—Long-term cure following radical approach to malignant-appearing benign intraspinal tumor. J Neurosurg 33:466, 1970
31. Stimpson N: Infiltrating angiolipomata of skeletal muscle. Br J Surg 58:464, 1971
32. Lin JJ, Lin F: Two entities in angiolipoma: A study of 459 cases of lipoma with review of the literature on infiltrating angiolipoma. Cancer 34:720, 1973
33. Greenberg SD, Isensee C, Gonzalez-Angulo A, Wallace SA: Infiltrating lipomas of the thigh. Am J Clin Path 39:66, 1963
34. Kuttner H, Landors F: Die chirugie der Quergestrifleu Muskalatur. Dtsch Chir (A) 25:228, 1913
35. Kindbloom LG, Angervall L, Stener B, Wickbom I: Intermuscular and intramuscular lipomas and hibernomas: A clinical, roentgenologic, histologic and prognostic study of 46 cases. Cancer 33:756, 1974
36. Davis C Jr, Gruhn JG: Giant lipoma of the thigh. Arch Surg 95:151, 1967
37. Calhoun NR: Lipoma of the buccal space. Oral Surg 16:246, 1963
38. Fothergill J: Medical and Philosophical Works. London, John Walker, 1781
39. Krause LB, Ross C: Intrathoracic lipomas. Arch Surg 84:444, 1962
40. Cicciarelli FE, Soule EH, McGoon DC: Lipoma and liposarcoma of the mediastinum: A report of 14 tumors including one lipoma of the thymus. J Thor Cardiovasc Surg 47:411, 1964
41. Staub EW, Barker WL, Langston HT: Intrathoracic fatty tumors. Dis Chest 47:308, 1965
42. Elfving F, Hastbacka J: Primary solid tumors of the greater omentum. Acta Chir Scandinav 130:603, 1965
43. Brasfield RD, Das Gupta TK: Liposcaroma. CA-Cancer J for Clin Vol. 20, Jan–Feb, 1970
44. Delameter J: Mammoth tumor. Cleveland Gaz 1:31, 1859
45. DeWeerd JH, Dockerty MB: Lipomatous retroperitoneal tumors. Am J Surg 84:397, 1952
46. Seldin HM, Seldin SD, Rakower W, Jarrett WJ: Lipomas of the oral cavity: Report of 26 cases. J Oral Surg 25:270, 1967
47. Hatziotis JCH: Lipoma of the oral cavity. Oral Surg 31:511, 1971
48. Burzynski NJ, Sigman MD, Martin TH: Lipoma of the oral cavity: Literature review and case report. J Oral Med 26:37, 1971
49. Greer RO, Richardson JF: The nature of lipomas and their significance in the oral cavity: A review and report of cases. Oral Surg 36:551, 1973
50. Mayo CW, Pagtalunan RJG, Brown DJ: Lipoma of the alimentary tract. Surgery 53:598, 1963
51. Feldman M: An appraisal of associated conditions occurring in autopsied cases of lipoma of the gastrointestinal tracts. Am J Gastroenterol 36:413, 1961
52. Eliason EL, Wright VWM: Benign tumors of the stomach. Surg Gynecol Obstet 41:461, 1925
53. Rumold MJ: Submucous lipomas of the stomach. Surgery 10:242, 1941
54. Scott OB, Brunschwig A: Submucosal lipomas of the stomach. Arch Surg 52:254, 1946
55. Alvarez LF, Lastra JA, Leon P: Ulcerated gastric lipoma. Gastroenterology 11:746, 1948
56. Thompson HL, Oyster JO: Neoplasms of the stomach other than carcinoma. Gastroenterology 15:185, 1950
57. Furste W, Solt R Jr, Briggs W: The gastrointestinal submucosal lipoma: A cause of bleeding and pain. Am J Surg 106:903, 1963
58. Hart RJ: Submucous lipoma of the stomach presenting as pyloric obstruction. Br J Surg 54:157, 1967
59. Ling CS, Leagus C, Chahlgren LH: Intestinal lipomatosis. Surgery 46:1054, 1959
60. D'Jarid IF: Lipomas of the large intestine: Review of the literature and report of a case. J Int Coll Surg 33:639, 1960
61. Price EB Jr, Mostofi FK: Symptomatic angiomyolipoma of the kidney. Cancer 18:761, 1965
62. Kanter AE, Zummo BP: Lipomas of gynecologic interest. Am J Obstet Gynecol 71:376, 1956
63. Dede JA, Janovski NA: Lipoma of the uterine tube—A gynecologic rarity. Obstet Gynecol 22:461, 1963
64. Das Gupta TK: Tumors and tumor-like conditions of the adipose tissue. Current Problems in Surgery. Chicago, Year Book Medical Publishers, Inc., 1970
65. Ashby BS, MacGillivray JB: Paratesticular lipoma. Br J Surg 53:828, 1966
66. Zakrewski A: Subglottic lipoma of the larynx. J Laryngol Otol 79:1039, 1965
67. Jonasson L, Soderlund S: Intrathoracic lipoma. Acta Chir Scand 126:558, 1963
68. Estevez JM, Thompson DS, Levinson JP: Lipoma of the heart: Review of the literature and report of two autopsied cases. Arch Path 77:638, 1964
69. Easler RE, Dowlin WM: Primary lipoma of the spleen. Arch Path 88:557, 1969
70. Rokitansky C: Lehbuch der pathologischen Anatomie, vol 2. Vienna, Braumuller, 1856, p 468
71. Ewing J: Neoplastic Disease, 4th ed. Philadelphia, Saunders. 1942
72. Manganiello LOJ, Daniel EF, Hair LQ: Lipoma of the corpus callosum. J. Neurosurg 24:892, 1966
73. Ehni F, Love JG: Intraspinal lipomas. Report of cases, review of literature, and clinical and pathological study. Arch Neurol Psychiat 53:1, 1945
74. Collins DH, Henderson WR: A case of intradural spinal lipoma. J Path Bact 61:277, 1949

75. Thomas JE, Miller RH: Lipomatous tumors of the spinal cord. A study of their clinical range. Mayo Clin Proc 48:393, June 1973

76. Brooks D: Clinical presentation and treatment of peripheral nerve tumors. In Dyck PJ, Thomas PK, Lamber EH (eds): Peripheral Neuropathy. Philadelphia, Saunders, 1975, p 1354

77. Mikhail LK: Median nerve lipoma in the hand. J Bone Joint Surg 46-B:726, 1964

78. Pulvertaft RG: Unusual tumors of the median nerve: Report of two cases. J Bone Joint Surg 46-B:731, 1964

79. Seddon H: Surgical disorders of the peripheral nerves. Edinburgh and London, Churchill/Livingstone, 1972

80. Yeoman PM: Fatty infiltration of the median nerve. J Bone Joint Surg 46-B:737, 1964

81. Callison JR, Thomas OJ, White WC: Fibrofatty proliferation of the median nerve. Plast Reconstr Surg 42:403, 1968

82. Rowland SA: Lipofibroma of the median nerve in the palm. J Bone Joint Surg 49-A:1309, 1967

83. Watson-Jones R: Encapsulated lipoma of the median nerve of the wrist. J Bone Joint Surg 46-B:736, 1964

84. Stout AP: Atlas of Tumor Pathology, sect. 2, fasc 6, Tumors of Peripheral Nerves. Washington DC, AFIP, 1949

85. Bartlett EI: Periosteal lipoma. Arch Surg 21:1015, 1930

86. Dahlin DC: Bone Tumors, 3rd ed. Springfield (ILL), Thomas, 1978, p 149

87. Singewald ML: Sacroiliac lipomata—An often unrecognized cause of low back pain. Bull Johns Hopkins Hosp 118:492, 1966

88. Osment LS: Cutaneous lipomas and lipomatosis. Surg Gynecol Obstet 127:129, 1968

89. Adair FE, Pack GT, Farrow JH: Lipomas. Am J Cancer 16:1104, 1932

90. Ballard HS, Fame B, Hartsock RJ: Familial multiple endocrine adenoma-peptide ulcer complex. Medicine 43:481, 1964

91. Cameron AH, McMillan DH: Lipomatosis of skeletal muscle in Maffucci's syndrome. J Bone Joint Surg 38-B:692, 1956

92. Nixon HH, Scobie WG: Congenital lipomatosis: A report of four cases. J Pediatric Surg 6:742, 1971

93. Fogg LB, Smyth WJ: Pelvic lipomatosis: Conditions simulating pelvic neoplasm. Radiology 90:558, 1968

94. Engels EP: Sigmoid colon and urinary bladder in high fixation: Roentgen changes simulating pelvic tumors. Radiology 72:419, 1959

95. Rosenberg B, Hurwitz A, Hermann H: Dercum's disease with unusual retroperitoneal and paravesical fatty infiltration. Surgery 54:451, 1963

96. Cook SA, Hayashi K, Lalli AF: Pelvic lipomatosis: Case report. Cleveland Clin Quart 40:36, 1973

97. Morettin LB, Wilson M: Pelvic lipomatosis. Am J Roentgenol Rad Ther Nucl Med 113:181, 1971

98. Grimmett GM, Hall MG Jr, Aird CC, Kurts LH: Pelvic lipomatosis. Am J Surg 125:347, 1973

99. Becker JA, Weiss RM, Schiff M Jr, Lytton B: Pelvic lipomatosis: A consideration in the diagnosis of intrapelvic neoplasms. Arch Surg 100:94, 1970

100. Mahlin MS, Dovite DW: Perivesical lipomatosis. J Urol 100:720, 1968

101. Ackerman LV, Wheeler PW: Liposarcoma. South Med J 35:156, 1942

102. Enterline HT, Culberson JD, Rochlin DB, Brady LW: Liposarcoma: A clinical and pathological study of 53 cases. Cancer 13:932, 1960

103. Enzinger FM, Winslow DJ: Liposarcoma: A study of 103 cases. Virchows Arch Path Anat 335:367, 1962

104. Reszel PA, Soule EH, Coventry MB: Liposarcoma of the extremities and limb girdles. J Bone Joint Surg 48-A:229, 1966

105. Phelan JT, Perez-Mesa C: Liposarcoma of the superficial soft tissues. Surg Gynecol Obstet 115:609, 1962

106. Saunders JR, Jaques DA, Casterline PF, Percarpio B, Goodloe S: Liposarcoma of the head and neck: A review of the literature and addition of four cases. Cancer 43:162, 1979.

107. Edland RW: Liposarcoma: A retrospective study of fifteen cases: A review of the literature and a discussion of radiosensitivity. Am J Roentgenol 103:778, 1968

108. McNeer GP, Cantin J, Chu F, Nickson J: Effectiveness of radiation therapy in the management of sarcoma of the soft somatic tissues. Cancer 22:391, 1968

109. Lindberg RD, Martin RG, Romsdahl MM, Barkley HT: Conservative surgery and postoperative radiotherapy in 300 adults with soft tissue sarcomas. Cancer 47:2391, 1981

110. Manual for Staging of Cancer. Chicago, American Joint Committee for Cancer Staging and End Results Reporting, 1977

111. Bowden L, Booher RJ: Surgical treatment of sarcoma of the buttock. Cancer 6:89, 1953

112. Suit HD, Proppe KH, Mankin HJ, Woods WC: Preoperative radiation therapy for sarcoma of soft tissue. Cancer 47:2269, 1981

113. Suit HD, Russell WO: Radiation therapy of soft tissue sarcomas. Cancer 36:759, 1975

114. Ockuly EA, Douglass FM: Retroperitoneal perirenal lipomata. J Urol 37:619, 1937

115. Stewart FW: Primary liposarcoma of bone. Am J Clin Path 7:87, 1931

116. Stout AP: 1949 Tumor Seminar. J Missouri Med Assoc 46:259, 1949

117. Goldman RL: Primary liposarcoma of bone. Am J Clin Path 42:503, 1964

118. Catto M, Stevens J: Liposarcoma of bone. J Path Bact 86:248. 1963

119. Ross CF, Hadfield G: Primary osteo-liposarcoma of bone (malignant mesenchymoma): Report of a case. J Bone Joint Surg 50-B:639, 1968

120. Schwartz A, Shusters M, Becker SM: Liposarcoma of bone: Report of a case and review of the literature. J Bone Joint Surg 52-A:171, 1970

121. Rasmussen J, Jensen H: Liposarcoma of the breast. Case report and review of the literature. Virchows Arch Path Anat Histol 385A:117, 1979

122. Gupta RK, Paolini FA: Liposarcoma of the pleura: Report of a case, with a review of literature and views on histogenesis. Am Rev Resp Dis 95:298, 1967

123. Currie RA: Mediastinal liposarcoma. Dis Chest 46:489, 1964

124. Cicciarelli FE, Soule EH, McGoon DCJ: Lipoma and liposarcoma of the mediastinum: A report of 14 tumors including one lipoma of the thymus. J Thor Cardiovasc Surg 47:411, 1964

125. Razzuk MA, Urschel HC, Race GH: Liposarcoma of the mediastinum: Case report and review of the literature. J Thor Cardiovasc Surg 61:819, 1971

126. Abrams MJ, Tuberville JS: Liposarcoma of the stomach. Southern Surg 10:891, 1941

127. Neel HB: Liposarcoma of the transverse mesocolon: Report of a case. Minn Med 35:867, 1952

128. Robb WAT: Liposarcoma of the greater omentum. Br J Surg 47:537, 1960

129. Hassan MA: Subcutaneous liposarcoma of forearm followed by liposarcoma of omentum. Br J Surg 57:393, 1970

130. Edson M, Friedman J, Richardson JF: Perivascular liposarcoma: A case report. J Urol 85:767, 1961

131. Datta NS, Singh SM, Bapna BC: Liposarcoma of the spermatic cord: Report of a case and review of the literature. J Urol 106:888, 1971

132. Waller JI: Liposarcoma of the scrotum. J Urol 87:139, 1962

133. Rona G: Changes in adipose tissue accompanying pheochromocytoma. Canad Med Assoc J 91:303, 1964

134. Leiphart CJ, Nudelman EJ: Hibernoma masquerading as a pheochromocytoma. Radiology 95:659, 1970

135. Mesara BW, Batsakis JG: Hibernoma of the neck. Arch Otolaryngol 85:199, 1967

136. Lawson W, Biller HF: Cervical hibernoma. Laryngoscope 86:1258, 1976

137. Merlina AF, Pike RF: Hibernoma of the thigh. J Bone Joint Surg 55-A:406, 1973

138. Lowry, WSB, Halmos PB: Malignant tumors of brown fat in a patient with Turner's syndrome. Br Med J 4:720, 1967

139. Enterline HT, Lowry LD, Richman AVE: Does malignant hibernoma exist? Am J Surg Path 3:265, 1979

12
Tumors of the Fibrous Tissue

Tapas K. Das Gupta

Tumors and tumorlike conditions arising from the fibrous tissue have a protean manifestation. Seldom do these tumors have a clinically uniform pathognomonic presentation. Certain tumorlike conditions, strictly speaking, do not fall in the category of neoplasms, but they require classification and description, since they can mimic both benign and malignant neoplasms to an extent that even the most experienced pathologist may have difficulty with diagnosis. These entities will be discussed under three broad headings: (1) benign tumors or tumorlike lesions, (2) histologically benign but clinically malignant tumors, and (3) malignant fibrous tissue tumors.

BENIGN TUMORS OR TUMORLIKE LESIONS

Fibroma
True fibrous tissue proliferation leading to the formation of a so-called fibroma is indeed rare. This cutaneous tumor occurs as a pedunculated polypoid structure and usually is excised for cosmetic reasons (Fig. 12.1). Fibromas rarely occur beneath the skin, despite the abundance of fibrous tissue. The majority of fibromas in the somatic tissues are of the mixed variety, for example, neurofibroma or fibrolipoma. In con-

trast, the tumor in its pure form can occur in the kidney, liver, or ovary. A fibroma of the ovary is characterized by ascites and pleural effusion (Meig's syndrome).

Fibromatosis
The term fibromatosis describes a number of individual clinical entities. From a clinical standpoint these entities can be classified as follows:

JUVENILE VARIANTS
1. Congenital fibromatosis, both localized and generalized
2. Fibromatosis coli (sternomastoid tumor, congenital torticollis)
3. Juvenile aponeurotic fibroma
4. Juvenile nasopharyngeal angiofibroma
5. Recurring digital fibrous tumor with inclusions
6. Progressive myositis fibrosa
7. Pseudosarcomatous fasciitis

ADULT VARIANTS
1. Keloid
2. Palmar and plantar fibromatosis
3. Penile fibromatosis
4. Idiopathic retroperitoneal fibrosis
5. Pseudosarcomatous fasciitis
6. Progressive ossifying myositis
7. Paradoxical fibrosarcoma of skin
8. Elastofibroma

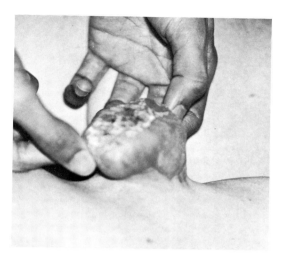

Figure 12.1. A pedunculated fibroma of the skin of the forearm.

Juvenile Variants of Fibromatosis.

Congenital Fibromatosis. In their localized form these tumors usually are confined to an extremity and sometimes are erroneously designated as congenital fibrosarcomas.[1-5] But they definitely are benign and radical therapy must be avoided. In our experience they are totally self-limiting and spontaneously regress. Nevertheless, the generalized form, as opposed to the localized, may have serious consequences. Occasionally an infant is born with multiple tumors all over the body, and this disease can be fatal. Teng and co-workers,[6] however, reported a case of the generalized form in which the tumors spontaneously regressed. Bartlett et al.[7] described a familial tendency to these tumors in one family.

Fibromatosis Coli (Sternomastoid Tumor, Congenital Torticollis). Fibromatosis coli is a congenital fibrous replacement of the sternomastoid muscle. The replacement may represent a localized swelling (sternomastoid tumor), multiple small swellings, or diffuse involvement of the entire sternomastoid muscle.

The etiologic factors are unknown, but the association of the manifestation with difficult and prolonged labor in childbirth and its occasional relationship to forceps delivery has led to the assumption that probably torticollis (wry neck) is the result of some form of birth trauma. The entity is so rare that a definitive cause and effect relationship to trauma has not been proved.

In 1948, Chandler[8] reviewed 101 cases of torticollis and suggested a hereditary relationship.

The mass usually becomes evident within one to two weeks after birth, gradually increases in size, and reaches its maximum growth by the end of the first month, after which regression sets in. It usually regresses slowly, but occasionally it disappears in a few weeks. An infant in whom the entire sternomastoid muscle is involved, may, after a few months, hold its head toward the affected side and torticollis may set in. Unless care is taken to avoid this postural deformity at the onset, concomitant asymmetry of the eyes, clavicle, and shoulder may develop. There may even be pain, requiring some form of therapy for the associated conditions.

The best treatment for fibromatosis coli of any intensity is to prevent the postural deformity that might occur. Therefore, parents must be instructed to observe the child closely and any tendency toward wry neck must be checked by persuading the child not to hold his or her head on the affected side. Although attempts have been made to excise the localized lesions, this is not necessary, since almost all these tumors sooner or later regress.

Juvenile Aponeurotic Fibroma. Keasby,[9] in 1953, first described this entity arising in the hands and feet of children and called attention to its microscopic similarity to fibrosarcoma. Although it has a propensity for recurring after inadequate excision, it is benign and not life-threatening. It usually presents as a slow-growing tumor in the hands and feet of children, especially the palms or soles. Sometimes these tumors are calcified and roentgenograms show calcific nodules within the main tumor body. Keasby,[9] Keasby and Fanselau,[10] Lichtenstein and Goldman,[11] Goldman,[12] and Allen and Enzinger[13] reviewed the clinicopathologic features of a total of 59 such cases. There are four cases in the files of the University of Illinois, three in the upper extremities and one in the lower (Fig. 12.2). About 70 percent of cases occur in the upper extremities. In this collected series of 63 cases, only one was in the head and neck region. Although the histologic features are of great interest and the tumors frequently infiltrate the surrounding subcutaneous tissue, tendons, and muscles, they actually are benign. Therefore, treatment should be conservative and the major accent must be on obtaining a proper histologic diagnosis. A hurried misinterpreta-

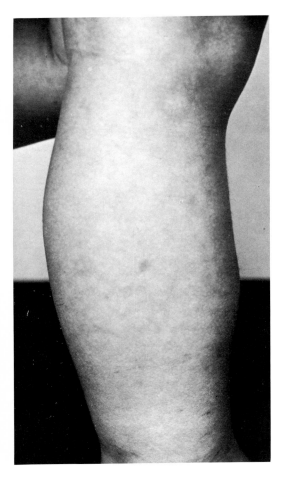

Figure 12.2. A diffuse swelling in the anterior leg of a 12-year-old girl. This was locally excised in 1971 and she is growing normally without any evidence of local recurrence.

tion of the histologic findings, especially when there is local recurrence, may lead to unnecessary amputation in these young patients.

Juvenile Nasopharyngeal Angiofibroma. Nasopharyngeal angiofibroma in the juvenile is an enigmatic tumor characterized by its unusual vascularity and its tendency to bleed (Fig. 4.19, Chapter 4). According to Martin and co-workers,[14] the tumor was first recognized by Chelius in 1847. Subsequently, several case reports appeared in the literature.[15,16] Friedberg,[17] in 1940, reported three cases and first suggested the term angiofibroma. Martin and co-workers,[14] in 1948, reported 29 cases, all in males. The age at onset

ranged from 7 to 10 years. In some cases histologic confirmation was not obtained because of the threat of hemorrhage.

In 1950, Figi and Davis[18] published an additional 51 cases, all in males. About half of these were not diagnosed histologically; the age at onset generally ranged from 9 to 17 years, but in one case was 23 years. Martin[19] described five patients, all of whom were treated with radiation therapy. In 1954, Sternberg[20] reviewed the material from 25 histologically proven cases, all in males. MacComb,[21] in 1963, described an additional nine cases, also all in males. Apostol and Frazell[22] made an exhaustive study of 40 cases and Conley and co-workers,[23] in 1968, described 38 cases.

Today it is generally agreed that nasopharyngeal angiofibroma is preponderantly a tumor of the male adolescent, although rare cases have been reported in older and younger male patients, as well as in young women.[24] To what extent sex hormones play a role, if any, in the growth and development of this tumor is uncertain. A variety of theories have been forwarded,[18–23] none of which has yet been substantiated. The histologic features of this tumor, however, are extremely specific and provide a body of information about its clinical course.

The clinical behavior of the tumor depends largely upon the site of origin and its rate and direction of growth. As long as it remains localized in the nasopharynx, the tumor remains quiescent. Thus many such tumors probably remain unrecognized and their ultimate involution leaves their presence undetected. In contrast, the infiltrative tumors become symptomatic, the main presenting features being nasal obstruction, epistaxis, bulging cheek, bulging palate, exophthalmos, headache, and deafness. In Apostol and Frazell's[22] series, as well as in the series reported by Conley and associates,[23] nasal obstruction and epistaxis were the main presenting symptoms.

The best diagnostic aid is awareness that these tumors occur preponderantly in adolescent boys and produce the above-mentioned symptoms. Examination usually reveals a firm, rubbery, bulging mass in one or both sides of the nasopharynx, extending into the posterior portion of the nasal cavity. Occasionally the surface of the tumor is ulcerated, especially if it has bled recently. Conley and associates[23] found tomography to be the best radiologic aid in defining the extent of the tumor. These authors[23] found 34 different sites of bone destruction in 18 of 38 patients. The pterygoid plate was involved in 11 cases, the maxilla in 9, and the sphenoid, base of the skull, and apex of the orbit in 6, 5, and 3 cases, respectively, thus highlighting the potential local aggressiveness of the tumors.

Microscopic diagnosis by means of preoperative incisional or wedge biopsy is not always required. In a juvenile male patient with all the characteristic clinical findings, the diagnosis can be made by total or subtotal excision of the tumor in the operating room, under the most optimum conditions.

Surgical intervention constitutes the major form of treatment for this tumor. It must be emphasized that these tumors are not supplied by one or more large vessels that can be ligated prior to operative attack. Apostol and Frazell,[22] after reviewing all the operative methods used at Memorial Sloan-Kettering Cancer Center, concluded that the best approach is a modified Weber-Ferguson incision through the anterior wall of the antrum, wide excision of the party wall, and thus into the nasopharynx. The exposure is adequate for visibility and removal of the tumor. Following removal, the nasopharynx and the antrum are packed. The end of the packing is brought out through the nostril for gradual removal.

Radiation therapy for these tumors has been tried in the past but is no longer used. Recent improvement in cryosurgical techniques makes it likely that this method will be used increasingly in selected patients. Estrogens also have been tried; however, it is injudicious to use estrogen in adolescent males over a long period of time.

Recurring Digital Fibromas of Childhood. This is a rare form of juvenile fibromatosis characterized by the appearance of nodular tumors in the fingers and toes of young children. These tumors have a high propensity for recurring, and instances are on record of multiple recurrences after apparently adequate local excision of the initial tumor.

Reye,[25] in 1965, first focused attention on this variant of fibromatosis by reporting six such cases in children. Similar case reports were published by Ahlquist and co-workers[26] and Shapiro.[27] Battifora and Hines[28] reported an additional case in 1971. It is conceivable that other cases have been found and probably have been reported without subclassification into the cat-

egory of recurring digital fibromas. The treatment is local excision and, even in the presence of local recurrence or multicentricity, major excision is not warranted.

Progressive Fibrosing Myositis (Progressive Myositis Fibrosa). Progressive myositis fibrosa is a rare juvenile disorder in which fibrous tissue proliferation infiltrates the surrounding muscles and blood vessels, resulting in degeneration of muscle fibers and leading to various bizarre-shaped tumors. Stewart and MacGregor[29] found only 11 authenticated cases.

The child usually shows progressive and rapid involvement of numerous muscle groups, generally within the first five years of life. Despite the muscle involvement, the patient usually suffers little interference with normal health. There is complete absence of pain, tenderness, or any other systemic manifestation. Although this entity differs from progressive muscular dystrophy, the end result of both disease processes is the same. No known curative treatment exists, but the judicious use of physiotherapy and occupational therapy is indicated.

Pseudosarcomatous Fasciitis. This disease is more prevalent in adults than in juveniles and is described on page 403.

Adult Variants of Fibromatosis.

Keloid. Keloid commonly develops in susceptible persons, usually after trauma. The degree and extent of injury bear no relation to the keloid formation. A relatively minor trauma such as a needle prick can initiate the formation of a keloid. Keloidal diathesis is congenital, but whether it is hereditary is not known. The incidence of keloid is hard to establish, since most cases are not recorded. In certain parts of Africa people are scarified to develop keloids in certain geometric formations.

The clinical appearance of keloids is so characteristic that the diagnosis of this lesion is never in any doubt. Keloids can occur in the skin in any location, but are more prone to occur on the ears and the presternal and intermammary areas (Fig. 12.3). These lesions are relatively fast-growing and have a tendency to spill outside the original site of trauma. Clinically this growth pattern is one of the distinguishing features between a keloid and a hypertrophic scar.

The subjective symptoms are sometimes more annoying than the cosmetic blemish. Pain, itching, paresthesia, and increased epicritic sen-

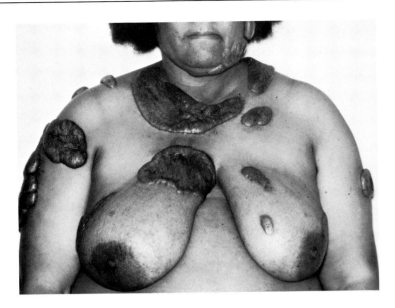

Figure 12.3. Woman with a tendency to develop keloids.

sibility are common. Of interest is the fact that the intensity of symptoms is not related to the size or location of the keloid.

Although Horton and his associates[30] described one case of malignant change in a keloid and cited a second case from the literature, the author has never encountered any such instance.

The treatment of keloids has been an exercise in futility over the years. Excision usually results in another keloid formation. Fibrolytic agents have produced indifferent results, and radiotherapy, although it can sometimes be useful, is fraught with the inherent hazard of treating a benign lesion with radiation therapy. Therefore, before embarking on any treatment regimen the patient should be made aware of the advantages and disadvantages of any therapy planned.

Considerable symptomatic relief is obtained by local injection of triamcinolone acetamide, 10 mg in 1 ml of saline (Kenalog 10 mg). The amount to be injected varies with the size of the lesion, and spraying with ethylchloride prior to injection frequently will prevent the temporary discomfort caused by the injection. In our hands, the best symptomatic results have been obtained when 1 to 1.5 cm segments of the keloid receive 1 to 2 mg of triamcinolone acetamide injected through a No. 25 needle. We repeat the course on a weekly basis for about three or four weeks. If there is no subjective

improvement, we consider this mode of therapy a failure. In larger keloids, excision of the lesion with minimal trauma and the injection of Kenalog in the surrounding tissue, followed by careful skin approximation, appears to provide the best result.

Palmar and Plantar Fibromatoses (Dupuytren's Contracture). Dupuytren,[31] in 1839, described the palmar deformity that bears his name. This is a common deformity in the hand, often leading to flexion contractures of the metacarpophalangeal and interphalangeal joints of the fingers. The etiologic factors are unknown, but apparently trauma is not a cause.[5,32]

NORMAL AND PATHOLOGIC ANATOMY. The palmar fascia, extending from the palmaris longus tendon at the base of the palm into the fingers and thumb to the level of the second phalanx, serves as a protective covering for the palm of the hand. Shortening or contracture of the fascial slips reaching into the fingers results in the characteristic flexion deformity of the metacarpophalangeal and the proximal interphalangeal joints. Palmar skin is firmly attached to the underlying fascia by numerous fasciculi, providing greater stability and accuracy in grasping objects. Subcutaneous fat is scant. The undersurface of the palmar fascia is connected with the deeper structures in the palm by perpendicular fascial septa, the most prominent of which is that to the third metacarpal, which divides the deep palm into the thenar and midpalmar spaces. Other minor septa compartmentalize the vital structures. The flexor digitorum superficialis and profundus tendons and sheaths course in an individual canal or compartment, whereas the neurovascular bundle and lumbrical muscles jointly occupy another.

The circulation of the subcutaneous tissue and skin arises from the superficial vascular arch, with tiny branches perforating the normal palmar fascia. As palmar fibromatosis develops, a skin pucker or dimple may appear, due to involvement of the tiny fasciculi attaching the skin to the palmar fascia. Contraction or shortening pulls the skin down into a dimple or pucker, which later becomes diffusely attached to the overlying skin, replacing the subcutaneous tissue and occluding the tiny perforating vessels. The attenuated circulation of this skin may result in delayed healing of dissected skin flaps, especially if large flaps are developed.

The fibromatous thickening also involves the perpendicular septa deep in the palm. Longitudinal bands or cords of hypertrophied fascia appear over the metacarpal bone and into the base of the finger. In the region of the web space, the main cord may branch out into the base of an adjacent finger, resulting in a flexion deformity of that metacarpophalangeal joint. When the thumb is involved there is an adduction contracture and narrowed thumb cleft along with the flexion deformity of the thumb itself. All the fingers can be affected, but the third and fourth are the most commonly involved.

This disorder occurs in 1 to 2 percent of all people,[33] predominantly in males. Skoog[33] found 85 percent of the patients he studied were middle-aged males, and the age at onset is usually between 40 and 49 years.

The presenting symptom is a nodular subcutaneous enlargement, either in the palm or in one of the fingers. It tends to increase in size and gradually becomes more tender. The development of the flexion deformity may be so insidious that it escapes notice until it has progressed to a moderate degree. A well-developed case of Dupuytren's contracture is so characteristic that diagnosis is obvious.

TREATMENT. The only satisfactory form of therapy is excision of the involved fascia. Although the principle of surgical therapy is simple and apparently uncomplicated, the pendulum of surgical technique has swung back and forth from the early practice of limited excision to the radical excision of the palmar fascia popularized in the 1960s; currently it is back to some form of limited excision. The very number of proponents for each method demonstrates both the complexity of the problem and the fact that each technique has value only for certain selective situations.

The method of making the skin incision has been debated over the years. However, since Conway[34] showed that any horizontal incision, regardless of its relation to the normal palmar crease, will heal well with good functional results if proper surgical care is exerted, the argument over skin incisions has somewhat abated. A horizontal incision near the distal palmar crease, allowing access to the palmar aponeurosis with S-shaped and L-shaped finger incisions, permits exposure for resecting the digital fibrous bands where indicated. Asepsis, hemostasis, and thick skin flaps are the prerequisites for successful surgical therapy. If during the operation the overlying skin is found to be thin and infiltrated by the fibrous tissue, it is better to excise the damaged skin in toto and repair the skin defect. Rhode and Jennings,[32] after reviewing their earlier experience with total excision of the palmar fascia, reverted to local excision. According to these authors, this method did not increase the incidence of recurrence and the functional results were as good as those in patients receiving total excision of the fascia.

Plantar fibromatosis is the fibrous replacement of the plantar aponeurosis and is similar to Dupuytren's contracture of the hand. Compared with palmar fibromatosis, the plantar variety is indeed rare, although the exact incidence is not known, since a large number of these cases are not reported.

The etiologic factors again are obscure, but chronic trauma does not play an important role. The disease usually occurs in adult males after the age of 40 years. A relatively small number of cases are bilateral. Whether these tumors are familial is not clear, although cases have been recorded in multiple members of a family.[33]

A characteristic feature of plantar fibromatosis is subcutaneous nodular thickening, most frequently in the middle portion of the medial half of the sole of the foot (Fig. 12.4). These nodules are usually asymptomatic, but the chronic trauma of continuous standing induces tenderness, which frequently is the presenting symptom. Although the possibility of digital contracture similar to that seen in the

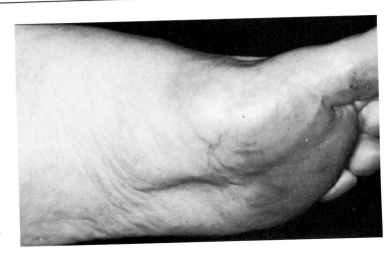

Figure 12.4. Plantar fibromatosis in a 60-year-old man. Note the linear swelling in the medial plantar aspect. He was conservatively treated and during the last eight years no contracture of any of the toes has developed.

hand does exist, the incidence of toe contracture is far less common. Skoog[33] suggested that the anatomic attachment of the plantar fascia is responsible for the low incidence of contracture.

Plantar fibromatosis must be differentiated from fibrosarcoma. Clinically, either lesion can be a slow-growing, diffuse, and nonencapsulated nodular enlargement. Additionally, the age groups are similar. Histologically, the presence of mitoses with plump fibroblasts might lead to an erroneous diagnosis of fibrosarcoma. Pack and Ariel[5] described three cases in which the patients had been subjected to an amputation because of an incorrect diagnosis. However, today such instances are extremely rare.

The only satisfactory treatment of plantar fibromatosis is excision. Fortunately, excision of the plantar fascia is not accompanied by as many rehabilitation problems as for palmar fascia. Adequate wide excision, immobilization, and avoidance of weight-bearing for a short period produces good clinical results. Occasionally, reexcisions are required, but these are not as complicated as in their palmar counterpart.

Penile Fibromatoses (Peyronie's Disease). Peyronie's disease represents a fibromatous infiltration of the sheath of the corpora cavernosa of the penis, frequently extending to Buck's fascia and the tunica albuginea. This form of fibromatosis can infiltrate the skin, producing multiple indurated skin nodules. According to Scott and Scardino,[35] Francois de la Peyronie should be credited with first describing this entity in 1743, although some believe that this disease was described earlier.[33]

The causative factors in the development of Peyronie's disease are unknown. In some instances penile fibromatosis is associated with fibromatosis elsewhere; for example, 3 of 48 patients in the series of Burford et al.[36] had concomitant palmar fibromatosis. A similar association has been reported by other authors.[5,33,35]

Penile fibromatosis usually occurs between the ages of 45 and 60; however, younger and older patients have been encountered. The usual presenting feature is abnormal curvature of the penis, with single or multiple plaquelike nodules on the dorsum of the penis. Due to this penile deformity, erection and intercourse become difficult. Frequently, there is associated pain in the late stage of the disease.

Management of this condition is difficult. Although excision is probably the best treatment, local limited excisions have never provided a permanent control. In the past, various forms of irradiation were tried,[5,33] but none with any tangible good result. Local infiltration with various agents ranging from vitamin E to steroids have all been tried, but not with consistent success. Administration of local steroids, as for keloids, with judicious excision of hard, plaquelike nodules, probably provides maximum relief.

Idiopathic Retroperitoneal Fibrosis (Ormond's Disease). This disease is of uncertain etiology and is characterized by proliferation of the retroperitoneal fibrous tissue. Apparently the disease starts in the pelvic region and progresses cephalad.[37–40] Retroperitoneal fibrosis was first described in 1948 by Ormond.[41] Since then a number of such cases have been reported. Today retroperitoneal fibrosis is accepted as a valid clinical entity of unknown etiology.[42] Usually the fibrous plaque is first seen over the sacral promontory, which then extends upward and laterally, encircling one or both ureters and resulting in obstructive uropathy (Fig. 12.5). Although idiopathic retroperitoneal fibrosis should always be considered in patients with urinary problems, frequently, underlying neoplasia, eg, lymphoma, can be overlooked unless scrupulous attention is given to details, including multiple biopsies of the retroperitoneal fibrous tissue.

The treatment of idiopathic retroperitoneal fibrosis is directed to the urologic problem. The ureters are dissected free of their fibrous plaquelike encasement. This simple surgical maneuver relieves the urinary retention and the urinary problems are usually solved.

A fibrotic process similar to idiopathic retroperitoneal fibrosis has been recognized in the mediastinum,[43,44] and Barrett[45] suggested that Riedel's thyroiditis and pseudotumor of the orbit are further examples of the same disease. Tubbs[46] described a patient with both mediastinal and retroperitoneal fibrosis. Temperley[43] reported a case of multifocal fibrosclerosis that apparently was controlled with the use of steroids. However, steroids have not been useful in established cases of retroperitoneal fibrosis.

Pseudosarcomatous Fasciitis. Pseudosarcomatous fasciitis is usually encountered in adult patients of either sex. Hutter and co-workers,[47] however, had nine patients below the age of 19 out of a total of 64, and we have encountered four patients below the age of 16, one being a 3-month-old infant.

This type of fibromatosis can occur in any anatomic site, but the most common site is the extremities (Table 12.1). The tumors can be present superficially or can be associated with deeper structures, such as the muscles and tendons. In the University of Illinois series of 12 patients with upper extremity pseudotumors, four were in the forearm and all were associated with tendons. Of the eight in the lower extremities, two were in the posterior thigh near the gluteal cleft and were adherent to the gluteal muscles. Hutter and associates[47,48] warned of the possibility of misdiagnosis of sarcoma in these cases of deep-seated fasciitis, and this admonition should be remembered.

Frequently the patients give a history of only a few weeks' duration of the tumor. The tumor enlarges in size rather rapidly, reaching a plateau; subsequent growth is usually slow (Fig. 12.6).

Although the primary mode of therapy is excision, a major ablative procedure is contraindicated since these benign tumors are frequently self-limiting. In a certain proportion of patients, recurrence might result, but even then it is logical to limit the extent of reexcision, since some of these tumors regress spontaneously.

Hutter and associates,[48] in 1962, described

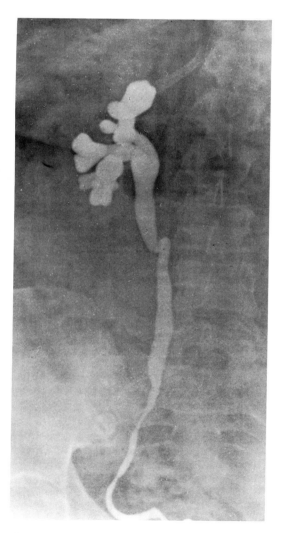

Figure 12.5. Intravenous pyelogram showing the narrowing of the right ureter near the pelvic brim. The diagnosis of retroperitoneal fibrosis was established by an exploratory celiotomy and biopsy.

TABLE 12.1. ANATOMIC DISTRIBUTION OF PSEUDOSARCOMATOUS FASCIITIS IN TWO SERIES

Anatomic Site	Hutter et al.[47]	University of Illinois
Head and neck	4	1
Trunk	9	3
Breast	4	1
Upper extremities	36	12
Lower extremities	13	8
Total	66	25

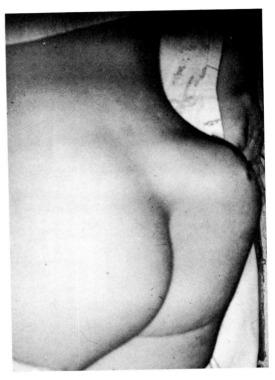

Figure 12.6. This 27-year-old woman first noted a marble-sized mass in the gluteal region in March 1968. In the ensuing two months the tumor grew to the size of a tennis ball. In October 1968, a biopsy elsewhere was interpreted as a sarcoma. She was then referred to the University of Illinois Hospital. Examination showed a 15 × 10 × 6 cm mass. We could not substantiate the outside diagnosis of fibrosarcoma. A second biopsy was suggestive of a histologically benign tumor. The tumor was locally excised and she has remained well for 10 years. Reassessment of the microscopic material confirmed the diagnosis of pseudosarcomatous fasciitis.

four cases in which the pseudosarcomatous fasciitis invaded and infiltrated the periosteum. The term parosteal fasciitis was coined and the entity was well described. These authors concluded that, like its soft tissue counterpart, parosteal fasciitis is also self-limiting and, even though the roentgenographic findings might be ominous, the treatment should be conservative. Toker[49] described another patient with bone infiltration and it is likely that more such cases will be found. Even under such circumstances, the benign interpretation of the tumor does not change.

Progressive Ossifying Myositis. This rare form of disease is similar to the progressive myositis encountered in children. The adult localized variety, however, is characterized by extraskeletal bone formation (Fig. 12.7). As with its counterpart, myositis fibrosa, the etiologic factors are not known. The localized form of myositis ossificans clinically resembles traumatic myositis ossificans, which is more commonly encountered. Active therapy is not indicated in this disorder.

Paradoxical Fibrosarcoma of the Skin (Pseudosarcoma or Atypical Fibrous Histiocytoma of the Skin). The number of synonyms signifies the difficulty experienced in classification. These are benign fibrous tissue tumors commonly seen in the skin of the head and neck of the elderly.[50-52] In spite of their aggressive histologic appearance, they are biologically benign and conservative excision is adequate.

Elastofibroma. Elastofibroma is a rare benign tumor usually encountered in the deltoid region.[53,54] Mirra et al.[55] reviewed the literature up to and including 1974 and found a total of 56 cases, only 2 of which were outside the deltoid region. Older patients usually present with a swelling around the shoulder region of short duration, and histologic examination of the specimen provides the clue to the diagnosis (Fig. 4.22, Chapter 4). Since this is a benign degenerative process, a limited excision, mainly for histologic examination, is adequate therapy.

Fibrous Histiocytic Tumors

Benign fibrous histiocytic tumors are classified as follows: (1) fibrous xanthoma, (2) sclerosing angioma, (3) giant cell tumor, and (4) nevoid histiocytoma.

Fibrous Xanthoma. These tumors are usually seen as small cutaneous or subcutaneous nod-

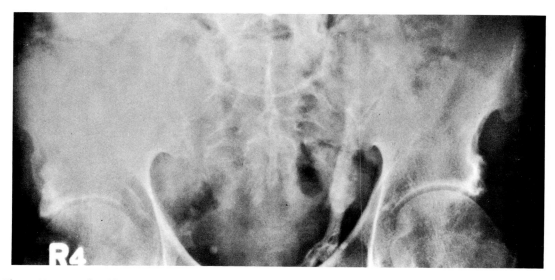

Figure 12.7. Localized bone formation in the soft tissues of the left wall of the pelvis. The patient was asymptomatic. Although skeletal tissue was found in the iliopsoas muscle as well, the exact origin could not be determined.

ules covered by intact skin.[56] They can remain localized over long periods without infiltration of the surrounding subcutaneous tissue. A conservative excision for histologic diagnosis is adequate therapy.

Fibrous histiocytomas or xanthomas have been reported in sites other than subcutaneous tissues, most commonly the lung. Grossman and associates[57] described one case and discussed other case reports in the literature. Although some authors have reported that pulmonary fibrous histiocytomas apparently behave like malignant tumors, unquestionable histologic and clinical proof of malignancy is lacking.

Sclerosing Hemangioma. This is a small subcutaneous vascular tumor usually seen in older age groups; it may arise in any part of the body. Clinically, this tumor is umbilicated and so highly pigmented, due to vascularity or deposition of hemosiderin pigments, that it may resemble a nodular malignant melanoma (Fig. 12.8A). The larger variety of sclerosing angiomas can even mimic a dermatofibrosarcoma protuberans (Fig. 12.8B). Treatment consists of excision of the nodule.

Giant Cell Tumor. These tumors occur most frequently in the digits on both the flexor and extensor surfaces of the tendon sheaths. Although these are fibrous histiocytic tumors, for

the sake of convenience they are discussed in the section on benign tumors or tumorlike conditions of the synovial tissue.

Nevoid Histiocytoma. This is a rare tumor that arises in the torso of young children, and has no special clinical characteristics. It often spontaneously regresses[4] and seldom requires any active therapy.

HISTOLOGICALLY BENIGN BUT CLINICALLY MALIGNANT TUMORS

There are two classes of tumors in this category. One is the fibrous histiocytic variety (dermatofibrosarcoma protuberans) and the other includes the whole gamut of aggressive fibromatoses.

Dermatofibrosarcoma Protuberans (Fibrous Histiocytic Tumors)

Darier and Ferrand[58] first described this relatively rare entity in 1924. However, Hoffman,[59] in 1925, actually named the tumor *dermatofibrosarcoma protuberans*. Since these original descriptions, several case reports and series reports have appeared in the literature.[60–65] Although this is a relatively rare tumor, its clinical features have been adequately documented. McPeak and associates[64] reported that about two new pa-

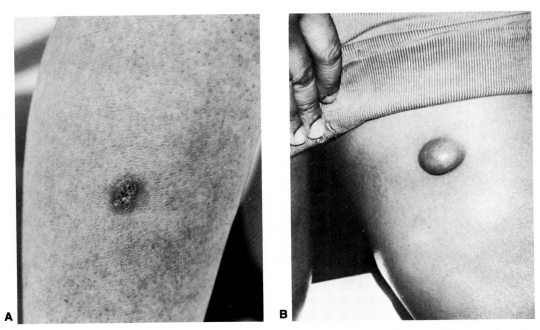

Figure 12.8. (**A**) Sclerosing angioma on the anterior aspect of the leg in a 40-year-old woman. She was referred to us with a presumptive diagnosis of malignant melanoma. (**B**) An umbilicated nodular lesion on the anteromedial aspect of the thigh of a 48-year-old woman. The umbilication and tense overlying skin mimic an early dermatofibrosarcoma protuberans.

tients are seen each year at Memorial Sloan-Kettering Cancer Center in New York. The incidence in our institution is similar.

Sex, Age, and Race. In the author's series of 28 patients, 16 were men and 12 were women. Taylor and Helwig[63] reported a fourfold higher incidence in males, probably because all their patients were from the files of the Armed Forces Institute of Pathology.

The tumor occurs in all age groups, but most frequently between the ages of 20 and 40 years. The youngest patient reported by McPeak et al.[64] was 7 years old. All races appear to be equally affected.

Although the tumor most commonly arises in the trunk (Fig. 12.9A and 12.9D), no anatomic location is spared (Fig. 12.9B, 12.9C and 12.9E). The tumor characteristically appears in early adult life as a small cutaneous nodule. It is rather firm and has a violaceous red color. Pressure on the surface on the nodule causes it to blanch. The periphery of the tumor infiltrates the adjacent

skin and subcutaneous tissue and other circumferentially located nodules may form (Fig. 12.9E). Coalescence of these nodules forms a fibrotic plaque in the dermis (Fig. 12.9D). After a few years the nodular protrusions appear on the surface of the plaque and at this stage their growth frequently accelerates. The overlying skin is stretched and undergoes atrophic changes that lead to heightened susceptibility to trauma, resulting sometimes in superficial ulceration (Fig. 12.9E). In the initial stages, the rate of growth of these tumors is slow; consequently, a lesion on the back may have a history of onset ranging from a few months to several years. A well-developed dermatofibrosarcoma protuberans has such a characteristic appearance that in most instances a correct clinical diagnosis is possible.

Darier and Ferrand's[58] descriptive term *progressive and recurrent dermatofibroma* aptly describes the notorious tendency of these neoplasms to recur after excision. The local recurrence rate of the tumor stems from its infiltrative capability, which is not widely appre-

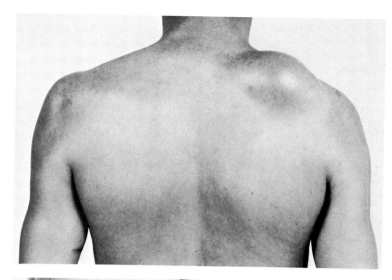

Figure 12.9. (**A**) Primary dermato-fibroma protuberans on the posterior trunk. Patient stated the tumor grew to this size in four years.

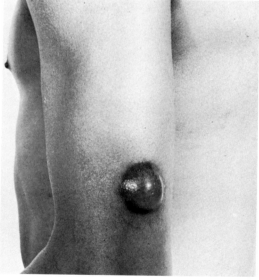

Figure 12.9. (**B**) Early tumor in the arm of a 29-year-old man, clinically thought to be a sclerosing angioma.

ciated. Condensation of connective tissue at the periphery may give a false appearance of encapsulation, but actually the tumor may extend well beyond the apparent margins in fine microscopic projections. Usually this occurs in the adjacent subcutaneous fat, but deep fascia, muscle, and bone are similarly vulnerable. Inability to comprehend the infiltrative potential of this tumor results in local recurrence. McPeak et al.[64] reported that 21 of their patients had a collective total of 75 excisions prior to admission to Memorial Sloan-Kettering Cancer Center. Re-

currences are probably a regrowth of residual disease following incomplete removal. Sometimes patients for whom an apparently total excision of the tumor had been performed have been sent to the University of Illinois, but on further elective excision residual tumors were discovered. Similar experiences have been reported by other authors.[61,62,64]

The ideal treatment for dermatofibrosarcoma protuberans is wide excision. Although it is imprudent to try to define the parameters of excision in mathematical terms, upon review of

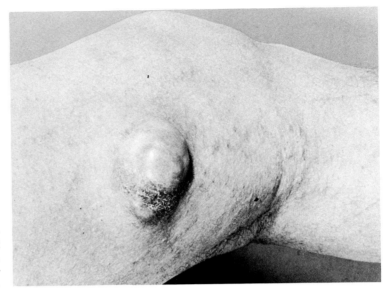

Figure 12.9. (**C**) Dermatofibrosarcoma protuberans in the lower part of thigh in a 38-year-old woman. Note the umbilication of the primary tumor with a satellite nodule.

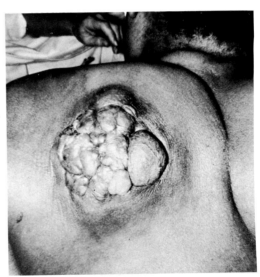

Figure 12.9. (**D**) A long-standing tumor showing the coalescence of a number of nodules, forming a plaque.

the pertinent literature and from our own experience we would recommend a 4-cm margin on all sides, including the deep fascia as well as part of the underlying muscle, if the location of the tumor necessitates such an excision. The skin closure in most cases would therefore require a skin graft. Based on this concept, even after apparent total excision of a primary tumor, if the margins of excision are not according to the guidelines described above, an elective reexcision is advised.

In general, dermatofibrosarcoma protuber-

ans does not metastasize to the regional nodes, and therefore a routine node dissection is not indicated. There are, however, rare instances of a malignant variant with the potential to metastasize, and in such instances node dissection might be required (discussion follows).

Of the 28 patients treated at the University of Illinois, 22 had an intact primary and the remaining six were seen with a locally recurrent tumor. Of the 22 patients treated for the primary tumor, one developed local recurrence (3.5 percent). One of the six patients with locally re-

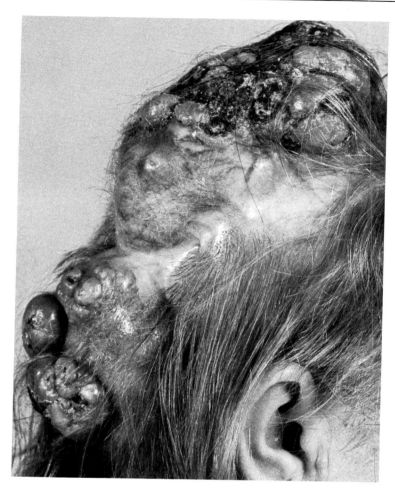

Figure 12.9. (E) A neglected primary tumor with ulceration and necrosis.

current tumor required a massive soft tissue resection for cure. McPeak and co-workers[64] reported three recurrences out of 27 primary tumors (11 percent), and Pack and Taba[61] had eight (20.5 percent) local recurrences out of 39 primary tumors. Although these two groups recognized the need for adequate wide excision, neither performed as wide an excision as is recommended here. In contrast, in Taylor and Helwig's[63] collected series of 98 cases, the local recurrence rate after conservative excision was 49 percent. It appears that conservative excision has no place in the management of these tumors.

Local recurrence usually happens within the first two years after the primary excision, but recurrences have been noted as late as seven or

eight years later. Local recurrence probably constitutes the only major problem in the management of dermatofibrosarcoma protuberans. It is not generally recognized that with every local recurrence the biologic behavior of this tumor changes, and after several recurrences the tumor can become lethal (Fig. 12.10). The primary objective, therefore, is to avoid local recurrence.

The question has often been posed as to whether there is a true malignant variant of a dermatofibrosarcoma protuberans that arises de novo. Although in our opinion the rare malignant variety is the result of multiple inadequate excisions of the primary tumors, we have three instances in our files in which the possibility of primary malignant dermatofibrosarcoma protuberans can probably be assumed. One is a

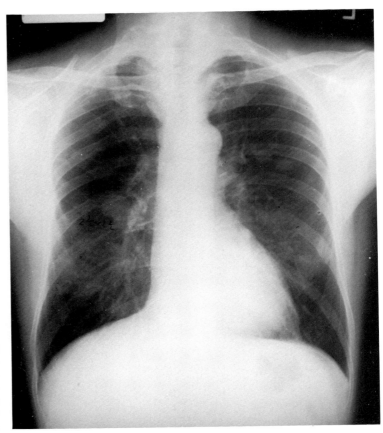

Figure 12.10. This 55-year-old man was inadequately operated upon for a dermatofibrosarcoma of the skin of the forehead. This resulted in a locally recurrent tumor. He was referred to our clinic after three local excisions and a course of radiation therapy when the tumor recurred for the fourth time. Although a review of the original histologic material showed it to be a dermatofiborsarcoma protuberans, by this time the patient had pulmonary metastases. He died six months later.

case in which the patient presented us with a neglected case of dermatofibrosarcoma protuberans of 15 years' duration. The case is briefly illustrated:

CASE REPORT

A 64-year-old man was admitted with complaints of a rapidly growing swelling on the medial side of the right scapula and intermittent bleeding from the mass of several months' duration. The tumor on the back was 8 × 5 × 6 cm, protuberant, nodular, ulcerating, nontender, and firm. It was situated 2.5 cm medial to the inner border of the right scapula. The right axillary lymph nodes were enlarged (5 × 5 cm), hard, matted, and fixed to the chest wall. A chest roentgenogram with tomogram of the lungs revealed a right superior mediastinal mass and various nodular densities in both lung fields suggestive of metastatic disease. Further investigation suggested metastatic disease into the vertebrae and sixth rib and infiltration of the left lobe of the liver. An incisional biopsy

of the main mass and a biopsy of both axillary nodes were performed. The right axillary lymph nodes were totally replaced by metastatic tumor (Fig. 12.11A). The patient was treated with systemic chemotherapy but died within six months of initial diagnosis. An autopsy revealed diffuse involvement of the visceral system (Fig. 12.11B).

Brenner and associates[65] recently described a patient with inguinal node metastases synchronous with a primary intact tumor in the foot. Therefore, an ab initio development of malignant dermatofibrosarcoma protuberans is a possibility, albeit rare. For the present, however, it is more appropriate to consider that, in most cases, multiple local recurrences probably initiate malignant transformation. Table 12.2 summarizes the experience of metastases from dermatofibrosarcoma protuberans in the available cases. The incidence of regional lymphatic metastases is so small that, even in patients with

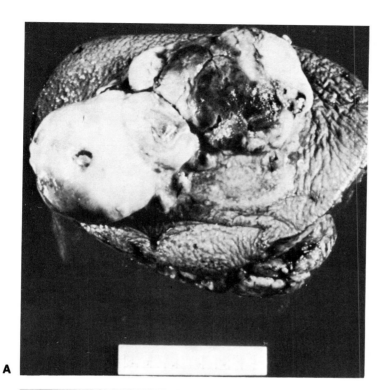

A

Figure 12.11. (**A**) Right axillary lymph node showing metastatic involvement with fungation. (**B**) Involvement of the lung is apparent.

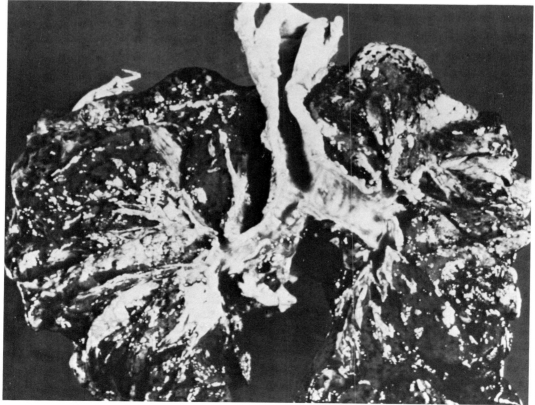

B

TABLE 12.2. WORLD EXPERIENCE WITH DERMATOFIBROSARCOMA PROTUBERANS, INCLUDING HEMATOGENOUS AND LYMPHATIC METASTASES*

Author(s)	Year of Publication	No. Cases	No. Metastases	Metastases	
				Hematogenous	Lymphatic
Darier and Ferrand	1924	3	—	—	—
Hoffman	1925	3	—	—	—
Darier	1926	1	—	—	—
Hertzler	1926	26	—	—	—
Senear et al.	1928	2	—	—	—
Levi	1930	1	1	—	1
Bezecny	1931	3	—	—	—
Michelson	1932	1	—	—	—
Bezecny	1933	1	1	1	—
McMaster	1934	25	—	—	—
Sciacchitano	1935	1	—	—	—
Binkley	1939	6	1	1	—
Costa	1946	1	—	—	—
Gate et al.	1948	1	1	1	—
Mopper and Pinkus	1950	2	—	—	—
Gentele	1951	38	3	2	1
Pack and Tabah	1951	39	—	—	—
Penner	1951	1	1	1	1
Hoffert	1952	3	—	—	—
Woolridge	1957	1	1	—	1
Przybora and Wojnerowicz	1959	13	2	—	2
Taylor and Helwig	1962	115	—	—	—
Adams and Salzsteis	1963	2	2	2	—
Burkhardt et al.	1966	56	2	2	—
Fisher and Hellstrom	1966	2	2	1	1
McPeak et al.	1967	86	5	5	—
Sauter and DeFeo	1971	1	—	—	—
Tamoney	1971	12	—	—	—
Brenner	1975	1	1	—	1
Das Gupta	1981	28	4	3	1
Total		475	27	19	8

*Adapted from Brenner et al.[65]

multiple local recurrences without obvious nodal enlargement, node dissection is not required.

Aggressive Fibromatosis

Desmoid Tumors of the Anterior Abdominal Wall. In 1832, MacFarlane[66] of Glasgow described two tumors occurring between the layers of the abdominal muscles that resembled what we now call desmoid tumors. The term desmoid was first used in the English language in 1847.[67] However, Müller[68] is credited with coining the term in 1838. Paget,[69] in 1856, described a patient with a desmoid tumor of the

abdominal wall and also one of the arm. The phenomenon of local recurrence of these tumors following excision was stressed by both Paget[69] and Bennet.[70] Because of the high incidence of local recurrence, this tumor has occasionally been designated as *recurring fibroid of Paget*. Sanger[71] was the first to point out its predilection for the anterior abdominal wall. Since then the term desmoid has been closely linked with this location.[72,73]

These tumors are rare. Pack and Ehrlich,[73] in 1944, found only 17 desmoid tumors in a series of 50,346 cases of neoplastic disease. Dahn and associates,[74] in 1963, commented on 24 abdominal desmoid tumors encountered during a period of 15 years at an institute of pathology serving approximately one million people. Brasfield and Das Gupta,[75] in 1969, reported 38 cases seen during the years 1931 to 1968 at Memorial Sloan-Kettering Cancer Center. This should provide the reader with an idea of how infrequently this tumor occurs. Despite its rarity, however, there is no doubt that it is a distinct anatomic and clinical entity.

Sex, Age, and Race. Most patients with anterior abdominal wall desmoids are women of child-bearing age.[72-78] Nine patients with abdominal wall desmoids have been treated by the author at the University of Illinois Hospital. Of these, 6 (75 percent) were women of child-bearing age. In our collected series of 38 patients from Memorial Sloan-Kettering Cancer Center, the age distribution ranged from 1 to 81 years, with 26 (68.4 percent) between 20 and 40 years old. The median age was 30 years. In the present series of nine patients (six female and three male), a similar age distribution was observed.

It appears that, in women, multiparity has some influence on the initiation of growth and progression of desmoid tumors of the anterior abdominal wall. In most studies dealing with large numbers of patients, a direct or indirect link with antecedent pregnancy could be demonstrated.[73-75] Our experience at the University of Illinois is similar in this respect.

The majority of patients have a painless tumor in the anterior abdominal wall, such as that seen in Figure 12.12. Two male patients in our series were referred after multiple local recurrences following inadequate excisions. Of the six female patients, two had local recurrence. Brasfield and Das Gupta[75] found 9 of 38 had locally recurrent tumors, 28 had untreated primary tumors, and 1 had had an incisional biopsy. If pain is present, it is usually due to the large volume of the tumor pressing on adjacent structures. Untreated tumors are frequently large. We have seen an unusually large tumor in a 40-year-old man (Fig. 12.13A and 12.13B). As expected, the size is directly proportional to the duration of the tumor.

Localization of these tumors follows a definite pattern. The majority are located in the rectus abdominis muscle (Fig. 12.14) and the anterior layer of the rectus sheath and the linea alba (Table 12.3). The anatomic distribution of desmoid tumors in the anterior abdominal wall suggests that an unhealed injury of the midline musculature (Table 12.3) during repeated preg-

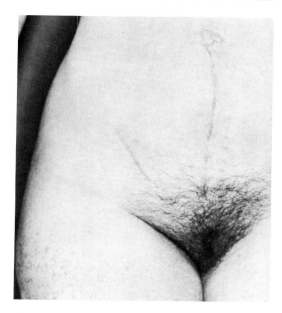

Figure 12.12. Abdominal wall desmoid in a 28-year-old woman. The tumor was predominantly in the right rectus abdominis muscle. After an attempted excision, she was referred to the University of Illinois. An abdominal wall resection was performed.

nancies might play a role in the etiogenesis. This proponderance of tumor occurrence in the rectus abdominis muscle and linea alba can be explained on the basis of the functions of these structures during pregnancy. During pregnancy the fibers of all the abdominal muscles are repeatedly stretched, resulting in injury to the fibers. In the rectus abdominis the fibers are parallel and, as a result, the stretching produces a long-standing injury and less opportunity for healing. Regarding the linea alba, a theoretic explanation could be forwarded that a defect in the process of midline healing within the embryo results in these types of tumors.[79] In the two children in our previous group[75] the desmoid tumors were in the midline. The midline desmoid tumors in adult female patients are most likely associated with diastasis of the recti, an end result of multiple pregnancies.

Diagnosis. In a multigravida patient, a midline anterior abdominal wall tumor with a history of relatively slow growth should be considered a desmoid tumor until proved otherwise by histologic examination of the biopsy specimen.

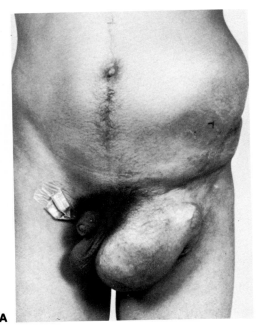
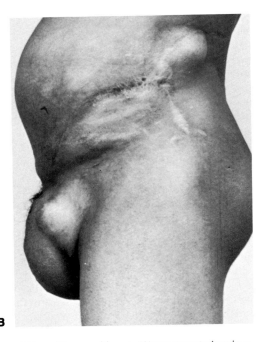

Figure 12.13. An unusual neglected case of abdominal wall desmoid in a 40-year-old man: (**A**) anteroposterior view, (**B**) lateral view. The tumor extended to the inguinal region.

The treatment of an abdominal wall desmoid is radical excision. Adequate surgical management may necessitate resection of a considerable portion of the abdominal musculature, underlying parietal peritoneum, and, under certain conditions, periosteum of the pelvic bones and parts of the small or large intestine. Successful resection of the parietal peritoneum for desmoid tumors was first performed by Sanger[71] in 1884. Although the neoplasm is histologically benign, local recurrences are frequent, so wide excision is mandatory. In case of doubt about the margins of resection in large tumors, histologic examination of the margins is indicated.

The effectiveness of radical excision was evident in the nine patients treated at the University of Illinois. In the four seen with an intact primary there has been no recurrence. The remaining five patients presented with locally recurrent tumors, and in three the recurrence was controlled by an initial abdominal wall resection with wide margins. However, in the other two patients, an additional wide excision was necessary to eradicate all the tumor from the primary site.

Of the patients with intact primaries in Brasfield and Das Gupta's[75] series, only one had a recurrence. In this patient the original tumor was approximately 20 cm in diameter. Three other patients who had recurrences were originally seen with recurrent disease and seeding of the operative site. This remarkably low incidence of recurrence, compared with the 10 to 40 percent reported by Musgrove and McDonald[80] or the 25 percent by Dahn and associates,[74] is justification enough for wide radical excision. Abdominal wall desmoids do not metastasize. Therefore, the only goal in therapy is local control of the primary tumor.

It is suggested that aggressive fibromatosis of the anterior abdominal wall is hormone-dependent and probably can be treated by hormone manipulation. However, only fragmentary data exist to support this concept. Geschickter and Lewis[81] assayed various fibrous tissue tumors for estrogens and gonadotropins. In a desmoid tumor of the anterior wall, they found 13,000 rat units (R.U.) of gonadotropins per kilogram of tumor. Jadrijvic and colleagues[82] induced desmoid tumors experimentally in the abdominal wall by means of estrogens. The tumors apparently disappeared when hormone administration was interrupted. Testosterone,

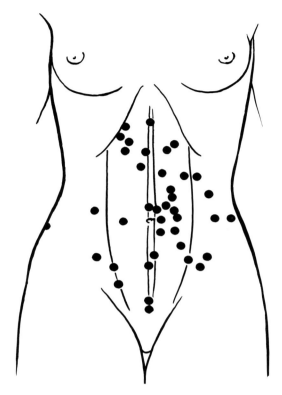

Figure 12.14. Scattergram showing the location of 38 desmoids of the anterior abdominal wall. *(Courtesy of Surgery 65:241, 1969)*

progesterone, and DOCA prevented development of these tumors. Pack and Ehrlich[73] noted regression of a tumor after radiation castration. On the other hand, Strode[76] reported that some desmoid tumors subsided after menarche. Dahn and associates[74] described two patients in whom the tumor apparently subsided with menopause. In the series reported by Brasfield and Das Gupta,[75] there was no evidence that menarche or menopause induced any appreciable regression. In the University of Illinois group of patients, none of the six women was at the menopausal age, so the effect of menopause on these tumors could not be studied. In view of recent data on hormone receptors[83] these isolated experimental findings and clinical observations on the role of hormones in these tumors should be reevaluated.

Extra-Abdominal Wall Desmoids. Nichols,[77] in 1923, was the first author to define the entity of extra-abdominal wall desmoid tumors. He described six patients in whom this tumor occurred in various sites: the thigh, popliteal space, gluteus maximus, adductor longus, pectoralis major, and the serratus anterior muscles, respectively. Musgrove and McDonald,[80] in 1948, analyzed 34 patients with this tumor and categorized the morphologic criteria. Since then, a number of relatively large series of reports have been published[74,84–86] (Table 12.4).

Sex, Age, and Race. Nineteen of the 36 patients (53 percent) treated at the University of Illinois were women and 17 (47 percent) were men. A similar sex incidence was found in our previous study.[86] In that group of 72 patients, 62 percent were women and 38 percent were men.

The age at onset ranges from the neonatal period to old age. We have seen an extra-abdominal wall desmoid tumor in a child of eight months, and our oldest patient was 80 years

TABLE 12.3. RELATION OF DESMOIDS TO ABDOMINAL WALL MUSCULATURE

Muscle	Function	No. Tumors*	
		Brasfield and Das Gupta[75] (1969)	Das Gupta (1981)
External oblique	Compresses abdomen, flexes and laterally rotates spine, depresses ribs	4	2
Internal oblique	Compresses abdomen, flexes and laterally rotates spine, depresses ribs	2†	1
Rectus abdominis	Compresses abdomen, flexes spine	18	4
Transversus abdominis	Compresses abdomen, depresses spine	2†	
Linea alba		8	2

*Six patients had tumor in their surgical scar.
†Both the internal and transverse abdominis muscles involved.

TABLE 12.4. ANATOMIC LOCATION OF EXTRA-ABDOMINAL DESMOID TUMORS IN SEVEN SERIES

Author(s)	Year of Publication	No. Patients	Head and Neck	Upper Extremities	Lower Extremities	Trunk	Miscellaneous	
Nichols[77]	1923	6	—	—	3	3	—	
Musgrove and McDonald[80]	1948	34	5	7	9	13	—	
Ramsey[84]	1955	8	—	3	2	3	—	
Hunt et al.[85]	1960	22	4	9	2	6	1	(tongue)
Dahn et al.[74]	1963	9	5	1	3	—	—	
Das Gupta et al.[86]	1969	72	8	20	16	15	13	
Das Gupta	1981	36	4	14	9	6	3	
Total		187	26	54	44	46	17	

old. However, the peak incidence is between the ages of 20 and 40 years. All races are equally afflicted by aggressive fibromatosis.

Anatomic Distribution. Extra-abdominal wall desmoid tumors may arise in any anatomic location. Table 12.4 shows the pattern of anatomic distribution of these tumors reported in major series since the time of proper recognition in 1923. It is noteworthy that aggressive fibromatosis can be found intra-abdominally and often can be the source of serious management problems. In the combined clinical material in this author's two series (Table 12.4), 11 percent of 108 tumors were in the head and neck region, 31 percent in the upper extremities, 19 percent in the trunk, and 23 percent in the lower extremities. Sixteen (15 percent) were located in miscellaneous sites: three in the retroperitoneal region, one in the broad ligament, three in the breast, two in the omentum, four in the mesentery and small intestine, two in the pelvic floor, and one in the iliac fossa.

The majority of these patients are first seen with a painless tumor, although if in the extremities, the tumor, because of its location, might cause pain. One patient with a desmoid tumor of the arm was first seen with shooting pain because the tumor was located near and infiltrating the median nerve. Extra-abdominal desmoid tumors are slow-growing and the size of the tumor at the time of initial presentation is dependent on duration. Frequently the tumors are quiescent for a long period, thereby escaping recognition, especially if they are located in an unusual site, such as the retroperitoneum.

A history of antecedent trauma is rare. In

only one case in the series of Das Gupta et al.[86] were the authors satisfied that some relationship might have existed. This was in a three-month-old child who was delivered with the help of forceps. Soon after birth, bilateral swelling of the temporal region was detected. The right-sided swelling completely subsided within a week, but the swelling on the left side, after an initial phase of regression, persisted. On examination at three months of age, the infant was

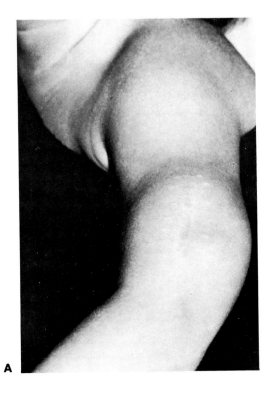

A

found to have a preauricular tumor 2 × 2.5 cm. The lesion was excised and histologic examination revealed the presence of aggressive fibromatosis. Unlike in aggressive fibromatosis of the anterior abdominal wall, which sometimes arises in scars, we have found only one patient in whom an extra-abdominal aggressive fibromatosis probably arose in a scar (Fig. 12.15A and 12.15B).

A correct clinical diagnosis of the primary tumor is almost impossible, but for a recurrent tumor it is not difficult, since most patients give a history of multiple excisions of a slow-growing tumor. The diagnosis of untreated primary tumor is made only after microscopic examination of the biopsy specimen.

Treatment of extra-abdominal wall desmoids consists of a wide, three-dimensional excision. The objective of optimum surgical treatment is to excise the tumor with an adequate margin of surrounding normal soft tissues (Fig. 12.16). Since the histologic structure does not reflect the growth potential of the tumors, once the diagnosis has been established the therapy in all cases must be radical excision. To accomplish this objective, some patients require a muscle group excision or occasionally a major

amputation. Table 12.5 shows the types of surgical treatment used in the author's combined series of 107 patients. The primary tumor of one patient was treated by radiation therapy alone. Seventy of these 107 patients (65 percent) had three-dimensional excision as the primary form of therapy. Twenty-one (20 percent) had muscle group excision, and 15 (14 percent) required a major amputation. However, in the more recent University of Illinois series, amputation was resorted to in only 4 (11 percent) of 36 patients. In most instances a well-planned initial wide soft tissue excision will obviate the need for amputation.

Regional node metastases is not a feature of this tumor, and node dissection is not in order. Infrequently, node involvement is encountered because of local extension of the tumor to an adjacent lymph node.

Fifteen patients were treated by major amputation (Table 12.5), ten by hemipelvectomy, and five by interscapulothoracic amputation; one patient underwent a minor amputation. Of the 15 patients treated by major exarticulation, 11 had locally recurrent tumors and 4 had primary tumors. Four of the patients in the University of Illinois series underwent major amputation

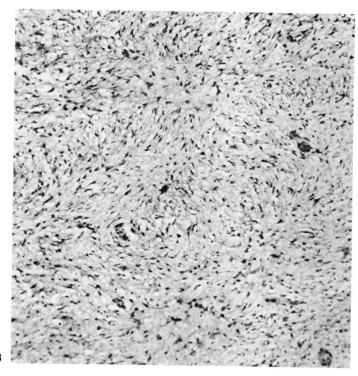

B

Figure 12.15. (A) A mass underneath the scar of a previous excision of an angiolipoma. **(B)** Micrograph of the excised tumor. Patient was treated by wide excision *(Courtesy of Annals of Surgery 170:109, 1969)*

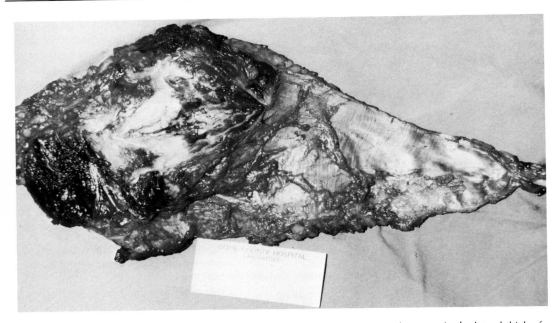

Figure 12.16. A specimen obtained by a wide soft tissue (muscle group) excision of a tumor in the lateral thigh of a 47-year-old man. Note white tumor in the center of the specimen surrounded by normal muscle tissue. *(Courtesy of Dr. P. Szanto, Department of Pathology, Cook County Hospital, Chicago)*

either because of the location of the tumor or because of multiple local recurrences (Fig. 12.17A and 12.17B).

These tumors are only locally invasive, however, and most deaths occur because of local extension. In extremity tumors an initial radical soft tissue excision will control the primary tumor and local recurrence can be obviated in most instances. This will reduce the future need for amputation. In recent years we have taken a relatively conservative attitude toward management of aggressive fibromatosis of the extremities (Fig. 12.18).

In most instances aggressive fibromatosis of the extremities and the trunk can be ade-

quately treated by wide soft tissue resection or muscle group excision. Thirty-two of 36 patients in the University of Illinois series (89 percent) (Table 12.5) were so treated. In the extremities, initial muscle group excision, as defined earlier, will control local disease in most patients. Major amputation becomes necessary usually after initial inadequate resection with locally recurrent tumors.

End Result. Twenty-five of the 36 patients from the University of Illinois Hospital are eligible for five-year followup. Of these, 23 (92 percent) have been free of disease for five years or more (Table 12.6). In our previous study from Memorial Sloan-Kettering Cancer Center,[86] of 52

TABLE 12.5. INITIAL SURGICAL TREATMENT OF 107 DESMOID TUMORS*

Type of Operation	Das Gupta et al.[86] (1969)	Das Gupta (1981)	Total
Wide excision of primary tumor	56	14	70
Muscle group excision	3	18	21
Minor amputation	1	0	1
Major amputation	11	4	15

One patient in this combined series of 108 patients was treated only with radiation therapy.

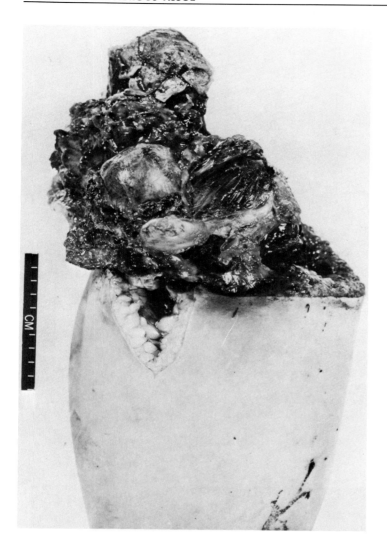

Figure 12.17. (**A**) This 28-year-old woman was found to have a large tumor during pregnancy. The pregnancy was allowed to reach full term and she delivered a normal, healthy child. Following childbirth, she refused to have any operation. Three years later she returned with a large right iliac fossa tumor. A diagnosis of aggressive fibromatosis was made and a hemipelvectomy was performed. Note the large tumor with extensive infiltration of the surrounding tissue, even the ilium.

patients eligible for five-year analysis, 33 (63 percent) had survived for five years or longer without any evidence of local recurrence at the time the paper was published (Table 12.7). Enzinger and Shiraki[87] reported a 43 percent cure in their collected series of 30 patients with only shoulder girdle desmoids.

Four (11 percent) of 36 patients in the University of Illinois series and 18 (25 percent) of 72 in the Memorial Sloan-Kettering series[86] had local recurrence following therapy of the initial tumor. In contrast, in Enzinger and Shiraki's[87] series, the local recurrence rate was 57 percent. A similar high incidence of local recurrence has been reported by other authors.[77,78,81,84,85,88–91] The primary consideration in the treatment of extra-abdominal tumors, as in their abdominal counterpart, is prevention of local recurrence. To avoid recurrence, an adequate excision of the lesion is mandatory. The low incidence in our series justifies an aggressive surgical approach. Frequently the clinician is lulled into a false sense of security because the tumor is reported as microscopically benign. A review of several large series[77,78,84–91] shows that extra-abdominal desmoids can be a direct cause of death, although only rarely. Of the 72 patients in our previous study,[86] two died with recurrent tumor. In Masson and Soule's series,[91] 3 of 34 patients died with aggressive fibromatosis. One of 36 patients in the University of Illinois series died postoperatively. This patient had a large tumor in

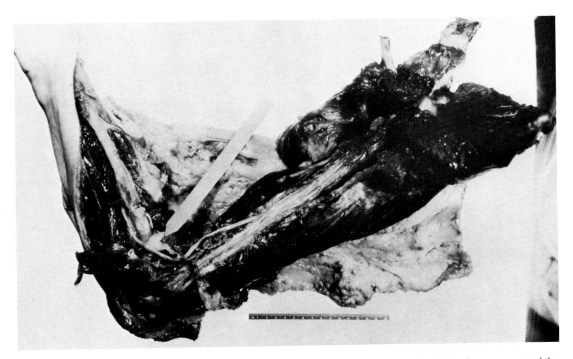

Figure 12.17. (B) This 36-year-old man was seen with a large painful recurrent tumor involving the upper part of the forearm, elbow, and lower third of the arm. An interscapulothoracic amputation was performed. Note extensive infiltration of the surrounding tissues by the tumor. *(Courtesy of Annals of Surgery 170:109, 1969)*

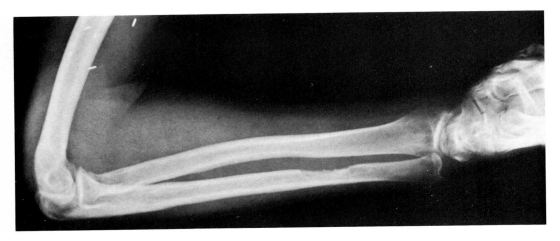

Figure 12.18. A 32-year-old man was referred to us for further therapy following three local recurrences of aggressive fibromatosis of the arm and forearm. The recurrent tumor of the forearm, which is seen infiltrating the ulna, was treated by wide excision of the ulna with a replacement bone graft. The patient has remained free of disease for four years. *(The replacement bone graft was performed by Dr. R. Barmada, Department of Orthopedics, University of Illinois.)*

TABLE 12.6. ANATOMIC LOCATION OF 36 EXTRA-ABDOMINAL AGGRESSIVE FIBROMATOSES, WITH FIVE-YEAR FOLLOWUP

Location	No. Patients*	5 Yr, N.E.D.†
Head and neck region	4 (2)	3
Upper extremities	14 (10)	9
Trunk	6 (5)	4
Lower extremities	9 (6)	5
Miscellaneous sites	3 (2)	2

*Numbers in parentheses represent patients eligible for five-year survival analysis.
†No evidence of disease.

the root of the mesentery, diagnosed during pregnancy. Of the remaining 35, 1 patient with a recurrent desmoid tumor of the neck has advanced local involvement. In this collected group of 142 patients from the two reported series[86,91] and the present group, in 7 (5 percent) death can be attributed to aggressive fibromatosis. It appears that, depending on the anatomic location and the number of recurrences, extra-abdominal wall desmoids can be lethal, and a complacent attitude regarding their management is not justifiable.

Aggressive fibromatosis occurs so rarely in certain specific anatomic sites that it has generated unusual interest among clinicians and pathologists, notably with regard to those tu-

TABLE 12.7. RESULTS IN 72 PATIENTS WITH EXTRA-ABDOMINAL DESMOID TUMORS (MEMORIAL SLOAN-KETTERING SERIES, 1969)

Location	No. Patients*	5 Yr, N.E.D.†
Head and neck region	8 (6)	4
Upper extremity	20 (14)	11
Trunk	15 (12)	8
Lower extremity	16 (13)	7
Miscellaneous sites‡	13 (7)	3

*Numbers in parentheses represent patients eligible for five-year analysis. Eleven patients were lost to followup.
†No evidence of disease.
‡The 13 miscellaneous tumors were distributed as follows: 2 in retroperitoneal region, 1 in broad ligament, 3 in breast, 1 in the omentum, 3 in mesentery and small intestine, 2 in pelvic floor, and 1 in iliac fossa related to iliacus muscle.

Courtesy of Annals of Surgery, 170:109, 1969.

mors that arise in the head and neck region or the intra-abdominal variety. Although the biologic behavior and management principles of these tumors are the same as for aggressive fibromatosis in the extremities and the trunk, it is appropriate to briefly describe the clinical features of those found in rare sites.

Aggressive Fibromatosis of the Head and Neck. Aggressive fibromatosis or an extra-abdominal wall desmoid of the head and neck region is a curious clinical entity. Until recently, this type of neoplasm was documented only rarely in the literature and little emphasis was placed upon its identity and biologic behavior. In recent years a number of large series have been published, providing us with reasonably adequate information concerning the biologic behavior and methods of management of these lesion (Table 12.8).[91-93] Radical excision is probably the only way to treat these patients. However, radical three-dimensional excision of the head and neck region frequently taxes the most innovative surgical mind. There were four deaths in a total of 91 collected cases, and one patient is living with locally advanced disease. This would suggest that the initial treatment planning must consider the high propensity for local recurrence, with resultant morbidity and occasional mortality.

Intra-Abdominal Aggressive Fibromatosis. The intra-abdominal type of aggressive fibromatosis is rarer still, and the diagnosis can be established only after an exploratory celiotomy and open biopsy (Fig. 12.19). Although the majority of patients are initially seen because of a large intra-abdominal tumor without any discomfort, an occasional patient may complain of gastrointestinal symptoms. In one of our female patients, a palpable intra-abdominal mass was preceded by vague abdominal discomfort and chronic loss of weight. An upper gastrointestinal tract series was suggestive of a malabsorption syndrome. She was operated upon and a mesenteric desmoid tumor with extension to the small intestine was found.

The intra-abdominal sites of these tumors vary considerably. In the series reported from Memorial Sloan-Kettering Cancer Center,[86] 10 of 72 cases of aggressive fibromatosis were intra-abdominal. In the present series, three were intra-abdominal. In this combined group of 13

TABLE 12.8. COLLECTED CASES OF AGGRESSIVE FIBROMATOSIS OF THE HEAD AND NECK REGION (FIVE SERIES)

Author(s)	Year of Publication	No. Cases	Type of Treatment	Incidence of Local Recurrence	Death Due to Desmoid	Living with Tumor	N.E.D.[†] at Publication
Masson and Soule[91]	1966	34	22, surgery 8, surgery and irradiation 4, surgery alone	21 of 34 (62%)	3 (9%)	2	29
Conley et al.[92]	1966	40	21, initial local excision 15, initial radical excision 4, type of excision not described	After local excision 11 of 21 (52%) After radical excision, 40%	None	6 (15%)	Not shown
Das Gupta, et al.[86]	1969	8	Wide radical excision	3	1	1	4
Wilkins et al.[93]	1975	5	Excision	0	0	0	1
Das Gupta	1981	4	Wide radical excision	1	0	1*	3

*Locally advanced disease at time of last followup.
†No evidence of disease.

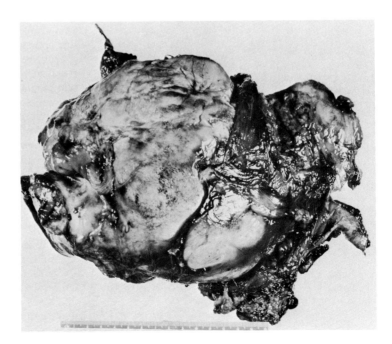

Figure 12.19. Operative specimen of a mesenteric desmoid in a 47-year-old man. A pancreaticoduodenectomy was performed and he is doing well. See also Figure 4.32 in pathology section.

patients with intra-abdominal tumors, 7 had a tumor in the mesentery and omentum, 3 in the retroperitoneum, and 3 in the pelvis. The management principle is similar to that for tumors encountered in other sites, namely, wide excision.

Gardner's Syndrome and Aggressive Fibromatosis. The existence of an autosomal dominant syndrome comprised of colonic polyposis, soft tissue, and bone tumors was recognized by Gardner and Richards[94] in the early 1950s. Since then, a number of case reports have appeared that link the presence of aggressive fibromatosis to Gardner's syndrome.[95–102] When Gardner[97] reviewed his cases in 1962, he added abnormal dentition and postoperative desmoids arising in surgical scars as part of the syndrome. In the interim, Smith,[96] and then Simpson, Harrison, and Mayo,[98] had included mesodermal tumors as part of Gardner's syndrome. They described fibrous tumors seen superficially on the skin, in the mesentery of the small or large intestine, and near or in a surgical scar after colectomy. The tumors usually developed within a year after surgery. Parks and associates,[100] in discussing desmoids in a recent review of the extracolonic abnormalities of familial polyposis, stated, "Surgical trauma is the precipitating factor in their causation."

We have treated six patients with Gardner's syndrome, one of whom was reported in our original study.[86] This patient had polyposis coli and a mesenteric tumor invading the head of the pancreas; a pancreaticoduodenectomy was performed (Fig. 12.19).

Gardner's syndrome appears to be an abnormal proliferation of varying combinations of the three primary *germ* layers. Sebaceous and epidermoid cysts, and tumors of the central nervous system (Turcot's syndrome) are abnormalities of the *ectoderm*. Adenomas of the large bowel and rarely seen duodenal hamartomas and periampullary carcinomas are forms of *entodermal* proliferation.[101] Bone proliferations (in the form of osteomas, odontomas, and supernumerary teeth) and connective tissue proliferation represent disorders of the *mesodermal* element. The connective tissue forms include excessive postoperative intra-abdominal adhesions (approximately 20 percent of patients with Gardner's syndrome are reoperated upon for adhesions), fibromas, and fibrosarcomas in-

volving the mesentery, mesocolon, and retroperitoneum.[100,101,103] Of the approximately 30 reported cases of desmoids of the abdominal cavity associated with polyposis, more than half have been documented as occurring after surgery; in the other cases either this point is not clear or information is not available. Penn and coworkers[104] and Das Gupta et al.[86] found aggressive fibromatosis in patients in whom there was no history of antecedent operation. On reviewing the material at the University of Illinois, we also found several patients with Gardner's syndrome who had intra-abdominal fibrous tissue tumors in the absence of trauma. The polyps in Gardner's syndrome and those in familial polyposis are adenomas, and the roentgenographic picture is identical. The polyps are most prevalent in the rectum and descending colon. Although there are reports of polyps regressing,[95] eventually they regrow. Colonic polyps are usually manifest by the age of 20, and malignant transformation usually occurs about 15 years later.

Aggressive fibromatosis in the breast parenchyma in association with Gardner's syndrome has also been reported.[103] We have encountered three patients with discrete involvement of the breast parenchyma in association with Gardner's syndrome.

Desmoplastic Fibroma and Aggressive Fibromatosis. Jaffe[105] first described this entity in 1958, and several case reports have since appeared in the orthopedic literature.[106] In 1968, Rabhan and Rosai,[106] reviewed this entity in a total of 25 cases, 10 of which were from their own institution. These authors found that the tumor was distributed as follows: mandible, three: clavicle, one; humerus, five; radius, two; scapula, one; vertebra, two; ilium, three; femur, three; tibia, four; and calcaneus, one. Although this is primarily a bone tumor, the anatomic sites of occurrence, as well as the macroscopic features, might easily confuse the examiner, and the tumor might be diagnosed as an aggressive fibromatosis. Microscopic examination can also pose a problem in distinguishing desmoids from desmoplastic fibromas. The biologic behavior of these tumors is similar to that of aggressive fibromatosis. Limited local excision results in recurrence. Wide three-dimensional excision of the tumor with surrounding normal soft and bony tissue usually results in cure.

MALIGNANT FIBROUS TISSUE TUMORS

Fibrosarcoma

Paget,[90] in 1865, designated malignant tumors of fibrous tissue as recurrent fibroids. Cornil and Ranvier,[107] in 1880, considered them as fasciculated sarcomas. Virchow[108] described them as fascial sarcomas (arising from the fascia), usually in a lower extremity, slow-growing, with surgical removal resulting in cure. Birkett[109] and Billroth[110] recorded some of the earlier case histories. From these few case reports describing what apparently were sarcomas of the fibrous tissue, there came an avalanche of case reports all purporting to describe fibrosarcomas. As mentioned in the section on pathology, after all tumors composed of cells capable of acting as facultative fibroblasts are excluded, the true incidence of fibrosarcoma will be found to be much lower than generally thought. The pioneering works of Ewing,[111] Stout,[2,3,112–115] Pack and Ariel,[5,116] and Stout and Lattes[4] provide excellent diagnostic criteria for the diagnosis of fibrosarcomas. Based on the original work of these authors, others[1,117–132] have reviewed their own material in recent years and published their experiences with the incidence and natural history of fibrosarcomas arising in various anatomic sites. It is indeed difficult to calculate the exact incidence of fibrosarcoma. Pack and Ariel[5] found only 39 cases out of a total of 717 sarcomas (5.4 percent); the incidence of dermatofibrosarcoma protuberans in that series was about the same (5.9 percent). Table 12.9 shows the comparative incidence of fibrosarcoma in six collected series.[5,112,133–136]

Fibrosarcomas, like most other soft tissue sarcomas, develop spontaneously, and no apparent etiologic agent has been identified. However, there are a number of documented cases developing in heavily irradiated tissues.

Role of Irradiation in Formation of Fibrosarcomas. Frequently, epidermoid carcinomas develop in irradiated tissues and some areas show spindle cell metaplasia that microscopically can be confused with fibrosarcoma. A review of the literature shows that the true incidence of fibrosarcoma is indeed low. Solway[137] found six cases of post-irradiation fibrosarcoma in the files of the pathology department of the Columbia University College of Physicians and Surgeons. Only 11 such cases were documented up to 1970 (Table 12.10),[137–146] seven of which were the sequelae of treatment of retinoblastoma in children and four of which were in adults. In 1979, Hajdu[147] reported five additional cases of post-irradiation fibrosarcoma in adults.

Congenital Relationship. Congenital and infantile cases of fibrosarcoma have been reported,[1 3,117,125–127] but there is still some controversy as to its true malignant potential. All the cases of congenital fibrosarcoma reported could probably fall within the realm of aggressive fibromatosis. Although Balsaver et al.[125] classified all such cases as grade I fibrosarcomas, an extensive review of the literature shows that even if a generous interpretation for fibrosarcoma is

TABLE 12.9. INCIDENCE OF FIBROSARCOMA IN SEVEN COLLECTED SERIES

Author(s)	Year of Publication	Total No. of Sarcoma Patients	No. of Fibrosarcomas
Stout[112]	1948	218	144(66%)
Pack and Ariel[5]	1958	717	39(5.4%)
Thorbjarnarson[133]	1961	176	82(47%)
Hare and Cerny[134]	1963	200	86(43%)
Coran et al.[135]	1970	30	6(20%)
Ferrell and Frable[136]	1972	117*	23(19.6%)
Das Gupta	1981	681	79(11.6%)
Total		2139	459(21.5%)

These authors included dermatofibrosarcoma protuberans in this category and reported 39 cases, making the incidence 33% of fibrosarcoma in their series.

TABLE 12.10. COLLECTED CASES OF POST-IRRADIATION FIBROSARCOMAS*

Author(s)	Year of Publication	Type of Primary Tumor Requiring Treatment	Age at Time of Radiation Therapy	Dose of Radiation Received	Latent	End Result (mo)
Schoenberg[138]	1927	Retinoblastoma	2 yr	36 mc × 4 mc	27 yr	Died
Pettit et al.[139]	1954	Retinoblastoma	6 mo	Not known	5 yr	9
Forrest[140]	1961	Retinoblastoma	1 yr, 6 mo	6,000 rads × 2	6 yr	18
Ibid.	1961	Retinoblastoma	6 mo	7,800 rads × 2	9 yr	198
Frezzotti and Guerra[141]	1963	Retinoblastoma	4 mo	4,200 rads	4 yr	Not known
Fabrikant et al.[142]	1964	Retinoblastoma	7 mo	2,800 rads	5 yr	30
Regalson et al.[143]	1965	Retinoblastoma	Not known	Not known	16 yr	12
Schwartz and Rothstein[144]	1968	Ca breast	58 yr	Not known	15 yr	11
Oberman and O'Neal[145]	1970	Ca breast	49 yr	2,100 rads ant. and post. intermammary ports; 1,800 rads more, 4 mo later	4 yr	12 (Dead with disease)
Hatfield and Schultz[146]	1970	Ca breast	40 yr	2,400 rads to ant. supraclavicular area, 2,800 rads postsupraclavicular area; 2,600 rads mediastinum and left axillary area	10 yr	24
Ibid.	1970	Goiter	15 yr	4,400 rads to mediastinum	31 yr	31

In 1979, Hajdu[147] reported five additional cases in adults.

allowed, the number recorded is few. Chung and Enzinger[1] found that 20 of 53 cases of infantile fibrosarcomas were present at birth. Including one case from our own experience, only about 41 such cases can be accepted as meeting the histologic guidelines for diagnosing congenital fibrosarcoma.[1,2,5,117,125–127,148–150] These tumors should be treated only by local excision, and any form of mutilating procedure should be avoided.

Age, Sex, and Race. Fibrosarcoma is essentially a disease of adults. In our group of 79 patients, 32 (40.5 percent) were between the ages of 20 and 49 years, 8 percent of the patients were below 9 years of age, and 16 percent between 10 and 19 years. The remaining patients were all over 50 years of age. Fifty-seven percent of our patients were males and 43 percent were females. Pritchard and associates[131] excluded 23 children from their study since, according to

these authors, fibrosarcoma shows a benign behavior in children. However, in our study we found that 5 of the 19 patients below the age of 19 died of metastatic fibrosarcoma. A more detailed description of childhood fibrosarcoma will be found in Chapter 20.

It appears that fibrosarcomas are found in all races in about equal incidence. In our series the distribution was proportional. Crawford and associates[151] reported that fibrous tissue tumors probably have a higher incidence in American blacks than in whites, but this observation has not been substantiated.

Anatomic Distribution. Fibrosarcomas occur predominantly in the lower extremities. Pritchard and co-workers[131] found a 60 percent incidence in the lower extremities, and Werf-Messing and van Unnik,[132] a 32 percent incidence. In the present University of Illinois series the incidence is 39 percent (Table 12.11), the

TABLE 12.11 ANATOMIC DISTRIBUTION OF FIBROSARCOMAS IN FIVE LARGE SERIES

Author(s)	No. of Cases	Head and Neck	Upper Extremities	Lower Extremities	Trunk	Miscellaneous
Pack and Ariel (1958)[5]	39	—	22 (56.4%)	10 (25.6%)	7 (18%)	—
Werf-Messing and van Unnik (1965)[132]	139	20 (14%)	21 (15%)	44 (32%)	32 (23%)	22 (16%)
Bizer (1971)[152]	64	5 (7.8%)	11 (17%)	15 (23%)	15 (23%)	18 (28%)
Pritchard et al. (1974)[131]	199	—	60 (30.2%)	120 (60.3%)	19 (9.5%)	—
Das Gupta (1981)	79	13 (16%)	10 (13%)	31 (39%)	10 (13%)	15 (19%)

thigh being the most common site of occurrence. Pritchard and associates[131] found 73 (37 percent) occurred in the thigh, and in our series, the incidence was 13 of 31 (42 percent). Although fibrosarcomas are found most frequently in the extremities and torso, they can occur in any part of the body where fibrous tissue is present, eg, in the alimentary tract, mesentery, omentum, retroperitoneal region, liver, kidney, urethra, vagina, lung, mediastinum, oral cavity, oropharynx, nasopharynx, orbit, and blood vessels. In our present series, 15 fibrosarcomas were encountered in various uncommon sites (Table 12.12). They are seldom located around major joints, although we did see one patient with fibrosarcoma around the knee joint.

TABLE 12.12. INCIDENCE OF 15 FIBROSARCOMAS IN UNUSUAL SITES (UNIVERSITY OF ILLINOIS SERIES)

Site	No. Patients
Nasopharynx	1
Pharynx	1
Maxillary antrum	1
Buccal mucosa	1
Floor of mouth	1
Retroperitoneum	2
Mesentery	1
Breast	3
Diaphragm	1
Kidney	1
Ovary	1
Dura	1
Total	15

Clinical Features. Fibrosarcomas do not present a characteristic symptom complex that could serve to differentiate this malignant neoplasm from benign tumors or other malignant tumors that involve the somatic tissues. Most commonly, the patient notices a painless mass that starts insidiously, grows slowly, and either reaches a huge size or, more rarely, causes the patient to seek treatment because of pressure against a nerve, producing pain or other disability (Fig. 12.20A to 12.20D). Infrequently, the patient complains of pain for a period before the neoplasm is actually identified. Of our 64 patients in whom the tumors were located in the soft tissues of the head and neck, trunk, or extremities, 50 (78 percent) were initially seen because of a mass. In six patients, pain of a duration ranging from three months to five years preceded the actual discovery of the mass. The remaining eight patients were first seen because of local recurrence after initial therapy elsewhere. In 8 of the 56 patients with intact primary fibrosarcoma, the tumors measured less than 2 cm; in 16, the masses were between 2 and 5 cm; in 14, between 5 and 10 cm; in 10, between 10 and 15 cm; and in 8, more than 15 cm.

Involvement of regional lymph nodes in fibrosarcoma is extremely rare. We have not encountered any in our series of 79 patients. Stout[112] in 1948, reported an 8 percent incidence, but in the earlier series a number of cases were considered as fibrosarcomas when in fact they were not. Pack and Ariel[5] and Pritchard and associates[131] found only one instance each in their respective series of 39 and 199 patients. Bizer[152] also found no evidence of true nodal involvement in his series of 64 patients.

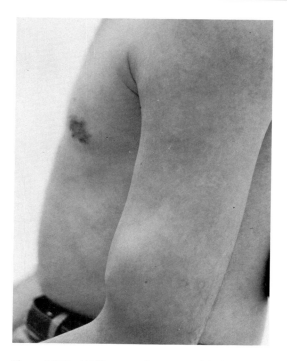

Figure 12.20. (A) Slow-growing tumor of the lower part of left arm in a 34-year-old man. This tumor was noticed about 12 months before attaining its present size. He came to our clinic not because of the tumor but because of associated pain and some muscle weakness. A muscle group excision was performed and he has remained well for six years.

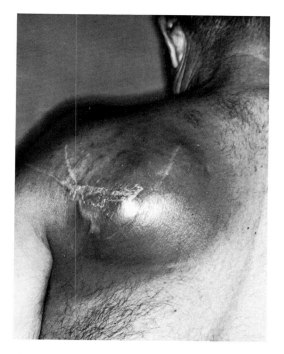

Figure 12.20. (B) A fibrosarcoma of the back of long duration. The exact sequence of events was not known to the patient. After it attained considerable size, an inadequate excision was performed and the tumor recurred. The patient was treated by irradiation before he was sent to us. At the time of this presentation, he already had lung metastases.

Treatment.

SURGICAL. The principle in the management of fibrosarcomas is adequate radical excision of the soft tissues. The extent and type of excision will depend on the anatomic location of the tumor (Fig. 12.21A and 12.21B). Suffice it to emphasize that margins of resection must be free of tumor cells on all sides. Adequacy of margin can be defined as the presence of at least one uninvolved fascial barrier between the tumor and the adjacent normal remaining structures. Determinants of this include the site and size of the tumor, histologic grading, neurovascular involvement, bone or joint involvement, and, finally, multicentricity of origin of some fibrosarcomas. The technical considerations for the specific types of operations are discussed in Chapter 6. Initial surgical treatment at the University of Illinois consisted of 19 wide soft tissue resections, 31 muscle group excisions, and 14 amputations. Eight of the 14 patients subjected to a major amputation were initially seen with locally recurrent tumors.

RADIATION THERAPY FOR FIBROSARCOMA. Radiation therapy alone has a limited role in the management of fibrosarcomas. In our series, 11 patients were treated with radiation therapy (details in Chapter 7). Windeyer et al.[153] reviewed the experience of management by radiation therapy of 58 patients and concluded that adequate excision is still the best treatment. However, they recommended the use of preoperative radiation therapy in patients with large tumors. McNeer and associates[154] did not find irradiation to be of much value in the management of fibrosarcomas, either preoperatively or postoperatively. Suit et al.[155] recently showed that curative radiation therapy has a role in the treatment of primary fibrosarcoma of the extremities.

CHEMOTHERAPY. Although chemotherapy as a primary form of treatment of fibrosarcoma

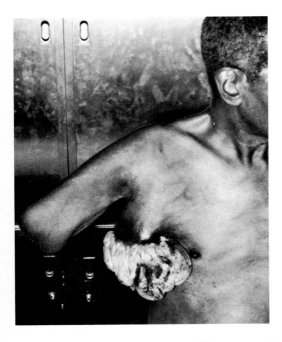

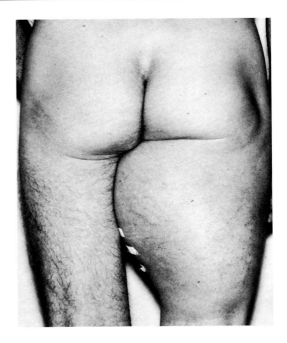

Figure 12.20. (**C**) A neglected case of fibrosarcoma of the chest wall with fungation. There was no evidence of systemic disease at this time and a regional resection was possible. Patient lived for one year, after which time he died of metastases.

Figure 12.20. (**D**) Huge fibrosarcoma of the thigh, which, because of its location and size, was treated with major amputation. Patient lived only three and one-half years free of disease and died of massive lung and liver metastases.

is not effective, it is being used increasingly as an adjuvant to primary surgical treatment. A detailed discussion will be found in Chapter 8.

End Results. In 64 of our 79 patients the fibrosarcoma was in the trunk (10), extremities (41), or head and neck (13). All 64 are now eligible for five-year analysis. Fifty of these (78 percent) have lived five years or longer without recurrence or metastasis. Table 12.13 shows the survival data for each site at two, three, and five years.

An overall end result of 78 percent tumor-free survival for five years without any form of adjuvant therapy speaks well for radical excision. Similar results have been reported by Bizer,[152] Castro and associates,[156] and Pritchard et al.[131] Bizer[152] observed a 78 percent absolute five-year survival for patients treated by radical excision. However, no data as to the number of patients treated by major amputation are available in his study. Castro and associates[156] found that of 75 patients with lower extremity fibrosarcoma treated by muscle group excision, 43 (58 percent) survived free of disease for five years. Pritchard and co-workers[131] similarly ob-

served that radical soft tissue resection provided a good to excellent five-year survival rate. The term "wide excision" in our series includes chest wall resection, abdominal wall resection, and other soft tissue resections. At the University of Illinois, radical soft tissue resection is now being used more frequently than major amputation (Table 12.14).

The natural history of fibrosarcomas can to a large extent be prognosticated by the type and degree of differentiation (histologic grading) of a given tumor (for discussion of grading, see Chapters 4 and 5). In our 64 patients with fibrosarcoma of the soft tissues, 38 had grades 1 and 2 tumors and the remaining 26, grades 3 and 4. Thirty-two of the 38 patients (84 percent) with grades 1 and 2 survived five years free of tumor, compared to 18 of 26 (69 percent) with grades 3 and 4 (Table 12.14). Analysis of 56 patients with untreated primary tumors showed that best results were obtained when the tumors were small and the histologic grades were between 1 and 2 (Table 12.15). Similar results with grading have been reported by Pritchard and associates.[131] These authors showed that, in 161

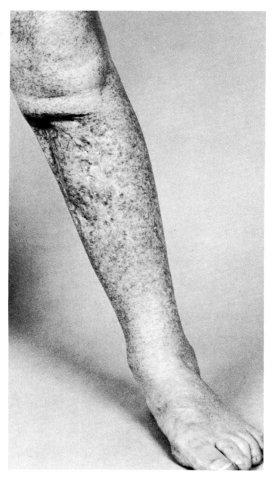

Figure 12.21. (A) Anteromedial aspect of the leg in a 56-year-old woman, showing the site of excision of low-grade fibrosarcoma from this area six years ago. At age 50, she was found to have a 3 × 3 cm grade 2 fibrosarcoma. The operation included resection of the surrounding soft tissue and a part of the tibia. She is still leading an active life six years later.

patients, those with grades 1 and 2 had a significantly better survival rate than those with grades 3 and 4. Recently, Lindberg and co-workers[157] reviewed the M.D. Anderson Hospital experience with conservative surgery and radiation therapy in a series of 300 patients. In their series, the absolute two- and five-year survival rates in patients with fibrosarcoma were 97 and 86 percent, respectively. However, this end result data does not clarify the absolute survival according to stage, histologic grade, and status of the primary tumor.

In our present series, 13 (20 percent) of the 64 patients had local recurrence after excision. Of the 56 patients seen initially with intact primary tumors, only seven had local recurrence. Therefore, the true incidence of local recurrence after treatment of an intact primary in this series was 12.5 percent. The incidence of local recurrence was found to be 56 percent by Pack and Ariel,[5] 50 percent by Bizer,[152] 68 percent by Werf-Messing and Van Unnik,[132] 48 percent by Castro et al.,[156] and 76 percent by Pritchard et al.[131] However, in the Pritchard and co-workers' series,[131] if the 76 patients who were referred originally with recurrent tumors are excluded, then the true incidence of local recurrence is 18 percent. Local recurrence of fibrosarcoma often reflects an inadequate primary excision. The single most significant factor that influences local recurrence is adequacy of excision. Werf-Messing and Van Unnik[132] reported that when the margins were not microscopically checked, the recurrence rate was 70 percent, whereas in cases in which microscopic examination was performed, the recurrence rate was only 10 percent. In some instances local recurrence is synchronous with distant metastases. In our series, 2 (15 percent) of the 13 patients with local recurrence had concomitant pulmonary metastases, and any form of locally directed therapy was useless. However, the remaining 11 patients were treated aggressively, 8 by major amputation and 3 by radical soft tissue excision. Two of the eight in the amputation group and one of the three in the soft tissue resection group died with metastases within one year. In all, 8 of 11 patients (73 percent) who had only local recurrence following original excision could be salvaged for prolonged periods. Castro and associates[156] found a similar salvage rate in recurrent fibrosarcomas of the extremities. Lindberg et al.[157] found that in their series the rate of local failure was 12 percent (almost identical to our own series). It is noteworthy that even after local recurrence a substantial number of these patients can be salvaged.

In the University of Illinois series, eight patients (10 percent) died of fibrosarcoma within two years, and four (5 percent), between three and five years. After five years, two patients (3 percent) had local recurrence and simultaneous pulmonary metastases and another two showed visceral metastases, with the primary site remaining free of tumor. Castro et al.[156] reported that 8 percent of their 74 patients died of sys-

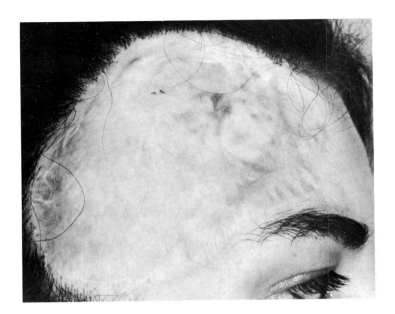

Figure 12.21. **(B)** An area of wide excision of a 4 × 3 cm grade 2 fibrosarcoma in the scalp of a 19-year-old girl. She is doing well seven years later. The outer table was excised. Defect was treated with split-thickness skin graft.

TABLE 12.13. END RESULTS IN 64 PATIENTS WITH FIBROSARCOMA, ACCORDING TO SITE* (UNIVERSITY OF ILLINOIS SERIES)

Site of Primary Tumor	No. Patients	Survival Free of Cancer		
		2 Yr	3 Yr	5 Yr
Head and neck	13	11	9	8 (61.5%)
Upper extremities	10	10	9	9 (90%)
Trunk	10	8	8	7 (70%)
Lower extremities	31	29	28	26 (84%)
Total	64	58	54	50 (78%)

*Fifteen patients with fibrosarcoma in unusual sites are excluded from this group.

TABLE 12.14 ANALYSIS OF TYPES OF TREATMENT VS TUMOR GRADE AND FIVE-YEAR SURVIVAL FREE OF TUMOR OF 64 PATIENTS WITH FIBROSARCOMA OF THE TRUNK, HEAD AND NECK, AND EXTREMITIES (UNIVERSITY OF ILLINOIS SERIES)

Type of Operation	Total No. Patients	No. Patients with Grades 1 and 2	5 Yr, N.E.D.*	No. Patients with Grades 3 and 4	5 Yr, N.E.D.*
Wide excision	19	16	13 (81%)	3	2 (66%)
Muscle group excision	31	20	17 (85%)	11	8 (73%)
Amputation	14	2	2 (100%)	12	8 (67%)
Total	64	38	32 (84%)	26	18 (69%)

*No evidence of disease.

TABLE 12.15 DISEASE-FREE SURVIVAL, ACCORDING TO TUMOR SIZE AND GRADE, OF 56 PATIENTS SEEN INITIALLY WITH *INTACT PRIMARY FIBROSARCOMAS* AND TREATED ONLY BY RADICAL SOFT TISSUE EXCISION (UNIVERSITY OF ILLINOIS SERIES)

Tumor Size	No. Patients	Grades 1 and 2	5 Yr, N.E.D.*	Grades 3 and 4	5 Yr, N.E.D.
< 5 cm	24	16	16	8	6
> 5 cm	26	12	11	13	11
> 5 cm and local infiltration to muscles and bone	6	2	1	5	2
Total	56	30	28 (93%)	26	19 (73%)

*No evidence of disease.

temic metastases after five years. Similar observations have been made by other authors[5,131,132,152] investigating a large number of patients.

Fibrosarcomas of Unusual Locations.

Intra-oral and Pharyngeal Regions. Fibrosarcomas of the oral region are extremely rare, as underlined by the study of O'Day and associates.[158] These authors were able to find only 15 examples in the literature and added six additional cases from the files of the Mayo Clinic. In our files there are five cases: one of the nasopharynx, one of the pharynx, one of the maxilla, one of the buccal mucosa, and one of the floor of the mouth (Fig. 12.22A and 12.22B). Treatment of these lesions entails wide excision with an adequate margin all around the primary tumor. Although it is not possible to elaborate on the prognostic factors on the basis of so few case histories, adequate wide excision should be the primary goal of the initial treatment of fibrosarcomas in these locations.

Fibrosarcoma of the Retroperitoneum and Mesentery. Retroperitoneal fibrosarcomas occur only rarely (Table 12.16).[5,112,132,152,159-162] Analysis of the data in Table 12.16 shows that, in a total of 500 patients with fibrosarcoma in all sites, only 17 (3 percent) were found in the retroperitoneal space. There are no characteristic clinical features of retroperitoneal fibrosarcoma. Usually the patients are first seen with a large retroperitoneal tumor and the diagnosis is established after celiotomy. The accepted form of treatment is exploratory celiotomy followed by total excision of the tumor. It is evident that it is almost impossible to obtain an adequate margin of normal soft tissue at the time of excision of the primary tumor. Consequently, excision

does not yield as good a salvage as in fibrosarcomas of the trunk and extremities. Of the two patients in our series, only one survived more than five years after excision of the tumor. Only 24 percent of eight patients in the series reported by Werf-Messing and Van Unnik[132] lived five years or more.

Fibrosarcoma of the mesentery is extremly rare. Stout[112] found six such cases and we have encountered only one. In our patient, the diagnosis was made at celiotomy and the tumor could not be resected. The patient died with lung metastases within eight months of initial diagnosis.

Fibrosarcoma of Breast. Fibrosarcomas are the most common form of stromal sarcomas of the breast parenchyma. In the University of Illinois series, three patients had fibrosarcoma of the breast. In a combined group of 22 patients (Table 12.17),[119,163,164] 8 (36 percent) survived for five years free of any cancer. These results compare unfavorably with those for fibrosarcomas of other sites.[5,131,132,152] The prime reason for this reported bad end result is inadequate excision of the primary tumor.[163,164] In the three patients we treated, total mastectomy was performed as soon as the diagnosis was established, resulting in one of the three living free of cancer for five years and the other two living and well at three and four years, respectively. If these patients undergo a total mastectomy as the initial form of therapy, the rate of survival free of cancer can be directly correlated with the size and degree of differentiation, as found generally in any of the large series of fibrosarcomas.

Cystosarcoma Phyllodes of the Breast (Fig. 12.23). In 1883, Muller[68] collected several cases of an unusual mammary tumor characterized chiefly by its large bulk, rapid growth following

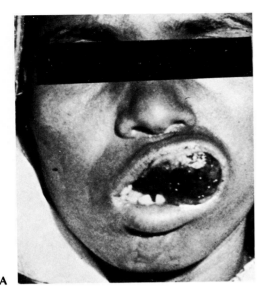

A

Figure 12.22. (**A**) A large fungating intraoral fibrosarcoma probably arising from the floor of the mouth. (**B**) Micrograph of the same tumor. (H&E. Original magnification ×100.)

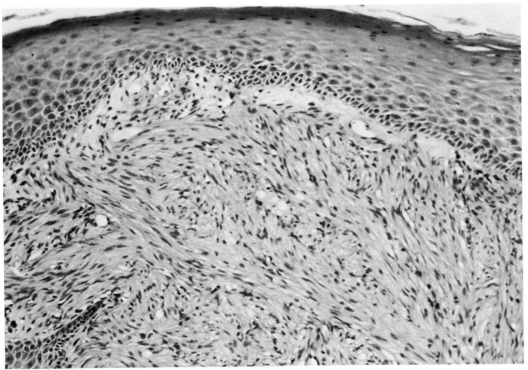

B

TABLE 12.16 INCIDENCE OF RETROPERITONEAL FIBROSARCOMA IN COLLECTED SERIES

Author(s)	Year of Publication	No. Cases	No. Retroperitoneal Fibrosarcomas	Incidence
Andrews[159]	1923	23 retroperitoneal tumors (all types)	5	22%
Frank[160]	1938	107 retroperitoneal tumors (all types)	5	4.7%
McNamara, et al.[161]	1940	8 retroperitoneal tumors (all types)	2	25%
Donnelly[162]	1946	95 retroperitoneal tumors (all types)	19	20%
Stout[112]	1948	218 all sites (fibrosarcomas only)	2	0.9%
Pack and Ariel[5]	1958	103 retroperitoneal tumors (all types)	6	5.8%
Werf-Messing and Van Unnik[132]	1965	139 all sites (fibrosarcomas only)	8	5%
Bizer[152]	1971	64 all sites (fibrosarcomas only)	5	7.8%
Das Gupta	1981	79 all sites (fibrosarcomas only)	2	2.5%

years of quiescence, benign nature, and peculiar gross and microscopic features. He coined the term *cystosarcoma phyllodes* to designate these tumors.

Cystosarcoma phyllodes is an uncommon neoplasm of the breast, composed of a cellular stroma and epithelial-lined duct. Although the tumor can arise de novo, a relationship with fibroadenomas (especially the intracanalicular types) of the breast has been reported by several authors.[163-169] A comprehensive review of the subject of cystosarcoma phyllodes, including our own clinical experience, is not germane to this book. Suffice it to point out that, according to the criteria established by McDivitt and associates,[169] it is appropriate to differentiate between the benign and malignant varieties.[170] The malignant variant of this tumor must not be confused with the stromal fibrosarcoma of the breast described earlier. Malignant cystosarcoma phyllodes metastasizes to the regional nodes, as well as to other viscera. Kessinger et

TABLE 12.17. FIBROSARCOMAS OF THE BREAST (COLLECTED SERIES*)

Author(s)	No. of Cases	Treatment	5 Yr, N.E.D.‡	Comments
Oberman (1965)[163]	5	Excision (some type of mastectomy)	1	1 patient living and well; 3 patients died with metastatic disease
Rissanen and Holsti (1968)[164]†	8	Some form of mastectomy and postoperative radiotherapy	2	5 patients died with metastases; 1 patient died of unrelated causes
da Silva Neto[119] (1970)	6	Some form of excision and mastectomy	4	2 probably died of metastases
Das Gupta (1981)	3	Simple mastectomy	1	2 patients living and well 3 and 4 years postoperative

*Only 3 series are included and compared with University of Illinois material. No attempt is made to make this a comprehensive table of all reported cases of fibrosarcomas of the breast.
†Only 8 cases of their group 1A fit the criteria of fibrosarcoma and are included in this analysis.
‡No evidence of disease.

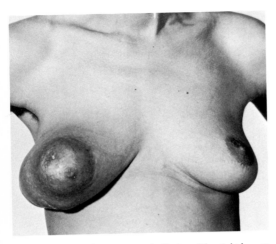

Figure 12.23. Cystosarcoma phyllodes of the right breast in a 38-year-old woman. A wide excision was performed and she has remained well for seven years.

al.[171] reviewed the literature and found 66 cases of metastastic cystosarcoma phyllodes. To this series they added one of their own.

The treatment of malignant cystosarcoma phyllodes is usually total mastectomy if there are no enlarged nodes. If the nodes are enlarged, then a radical mastectomy is indicated.[172] In only five of seven recorded cases was there histologic proof of ipsilateral nodal metastasis.[172]

Fibrosarcoma of the Diaphragm. Fibrosarcoma arising in the diaphragm is also rare. We have only one such instance in our files. This patient, a 51-year-old woman, was referred with a large tumor in the left upper quadrant. An exploratory procedure revealed a localized tumor arising from the inferior leaf of the left diaphragm. The tumor, along with a portion of the diaphragm, was excised. The diaphragmatic defect was closed with Marlex mesh. She remained well for three years, after which retroperitoneal recurrence was noted with pulmonary metastases. The patient died within one year of recognition of the recurrent tumor.

Fibrosarcoma Arising in the Viscera. Fibrosarcomas can arise in any organ with a fibrous stroma. However, only a few documented cases of visceral fibrosarcomas have been reported. Since these cases are rare, a detailed analysis of the symptoms, signs, and natural history is not possible. From a therapeutic standpoint, these tumors should be excised whenever possible.

Probably treatment with adjuvant radiation therapy and systemic chemotherapy might be of some value. In the following sections, fibrosarcomas in some of these viscera are described.

Primary Fibrosarcoma of the Liver. Eleven cases of fibrosarcoma of the liver are recorded (Table 12.18),[173-183] only two of which were treated. One patient responded well to radiation therapy and the second patient underwent resection of the fibrosarcoma. In four other cases fibrosarcoma and carcinoma occurred as two separate tumors. These tumors usually are diagnosed at autopsy (Fig. 12.24A and 12.24B).

Primary Fibrosarcoma of Kidney. Primary fibrosarcoma of the kidney is also rare.[184-186] Unless several different areas of the tumor are microscopically examined a diagnosis of sarcoma should not be made. In our files we have only one instance of primary fibrosarcoma of the kidney. This female patient was sent to us after a recurrence of fibrosarcoma following simple nephrectomy. An angiogram showed massive retroperitoneal recurrence (Fig. 12.25A and 12.25B). She was operated upon, but within six months metastatic involvement of the lungs, pleura, liver, and brain developed and she expired.

Primary Fibrosarcoma of the Ovary. Although fibromas of the ovary with concomitant pleural effusion are not uncommon, a true fibrosarcoma is indeed rare.[186] We have encountered only one such instance and pulmonary metastases developed soon after resection of the primary ovarian tumor.

Primary Fibrosarcoma of the Thyroid. A fibrosarcoma of the thyroid, another rare tumor,[187] is difficult to distinguish from a spindle cell carcinoma. The treatment appears to be removal of the thyroid with an adequate margin of normal neck contents.

Primary Fibrosarcoma of the Spermatic Cord. Arlen and co-workers[188] reviewed the world literature in 1969 and found 21 cases, including one of their own. This tumor presents as a firm, nontender, irregular mass that does not transilluminate and can be separated from the testicle. Orchiectomy with high ligation of the cord is the minimum therapy required. The patient described by Arlen and co-workers[188] was referred four months after orchiectomy with a large inguinal tumor, but died before therapy was instituted.

Fibrosarcomas are extremely rare in male genitalia. Dehner and Smith[189] made an exhaustive study of all soft tissue tumors of the

TABLE 12.18. SUMMARY OF 11 CASES OF HEPATIC FIBROSARCOMA REPORTED IN THE LITERATURE

Author(s)	Year of Publication	Age	Sex	Liver Weight (g)	Cirrhosis	Metastases	Gross Appearance of Tumor	End Results
Shallow and Wagner[173]	1947	60	M	5,200*	—	—	Massive, left lobe solid, firm, central necrosis	Dead
Simpson et al.[174]	1955	66	M	—	—	Lymph nodes, omentum and jejunum	Massive right lobe, cystic, grayish, satellite nodules	Dead
Steiner[175]	1960	45	M	4,100	+	—	—	—
Ojima et al.[176]	1964	62	M	3,190	—	—	Massive, right lobe solid, white	Dead
Snapper et al.[177]	1964	60	M	12,150	—	Lungs	Massive, right lobe solid, pinkish-white, satellite nodule	5 yr, N.E.D.†
Totzke and Hutcheson[178]	1965	56	F	650	—	Lymph nodes	Massive, right lobe, solid, soft pinkish-yellow, satellite nodules	Dead
Belouet and Destombes[179]	1967	38	—	—	—	—	—	—
Cavallo et al.[180]	1968	30	F	2,820	—	—	Two nodules, solid, yellowish-white central necrosis	Dead
Smith and Rele[181]	1972	37	M	7,325	—	—	Massive, right lobe, solid, soft and fleshy	Dead
Walter et al.[182]	1972	66	M	1,780*	—	—	Multinodular lobe, solid, elastic	Living and well 1 yr after lobectomy
Alrenga[183]	1975	51	M	1,200	—	—	Massive, right lobe, solid, firm, grayish-white	Dead

Weight of the operative specimen.
†No evidence of disease.*

penis in the files of the Armed Forces Institute of Pathology and found only 22 cases. Of these, two were fibrosarcomas and one was a dermatofibrosarcoma protuberans. One of the two patients with fibrosarcoma died with pulmonary metastases within one year of therapy and the other patient was lost to followup.

Fibrosarcoma of the Blood Vessels. Primary sarcomas of the blood vessels are rare and fibrosarcomas are rarer still.[190-206] Abell[207] described

one case of fibrosarcoma of the inferior vena cava. Lunning[208] reported one of the femoral vein, and de Vries[209] reported a spindle cell sarcoma, probably a fibrosarcoma, of the small veins of the thigh. Fibrosarcomas of the systemic arteries are also extremely rare.[210-221] Salm,[210] in 1972, reported 13 cases of fibrosarcoma of the aorta, including one of his own. The cases reported by Sladden,[222] Bowles et al.[223] and Blenkinsopp and Hobbs[224] should be excluded from

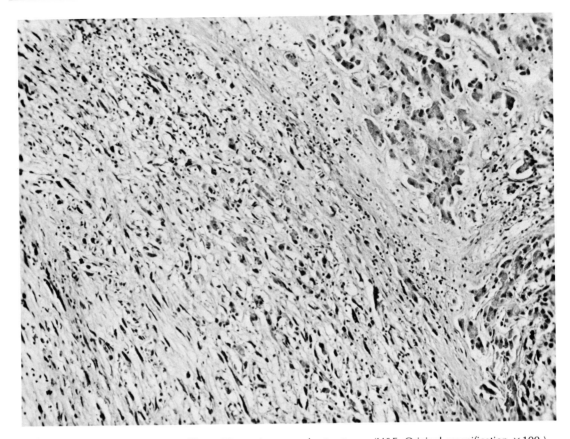

Figure 12.24. (A) Fibrosarcoma of liver. Diagnosis was made at autopsy. (H&E. Original magnification ×100.)

consideration, since they do not satisfy the histologic criteria for fibrosarcoma. Furthermore, in this author's opinion, the cases reported by Auffermann,[213] Detrie,[214] Karhoff,[217] and Kattus et al.[225] do not fulfill the criteria for fibrosarcoma and should also be excluded. There is no denial that these four cases represent sarcomas, but whether they can be considered fibrosarcomas is open to question. Therefore, only eight documented cases of fibrosarcoma of the aorta are recorded in the literature (Table 12.19).

Salm,[210] in a superb analysis of the subject, described three main tumor types, namely, polypoidal and intraluminal, intimal, and adventitial. The intimal and polypoidal types frequently cause clinical vascular occlusions. However, the other types can produce a myriad of symptoms and a clincial diagnosis is almost impossible. In the polypoidal types, if a pre-

operative diagnosis is made, these lesions can be removed. Resection of the segment of the artery containing the tumor, with replacement grafting, is the treatment of choice. Cure following this resection is rare, however.

In 1972, Burns and co-workers[226] reported a case in a 31-year-old man who had repair of a lacerated superficial femoral vessel by a woven Teflon-Dacron graft. Ten years later he was admitted with an 8 × 10 cm mass in the left thigh that was found to be a fibrosarcoma. A wide soft tissue resection was performed and 7 cm of the graft intimately adherent to the tumor was excised. This is probably the only documented case of fibrosarcoma developing after implantation of a vascular graft.

Fibrosarcoma of The Bone. Fibrosarcoma of the bone is a malignant fibroblastic tumor characterized by interlacing bundles of collagen fi-

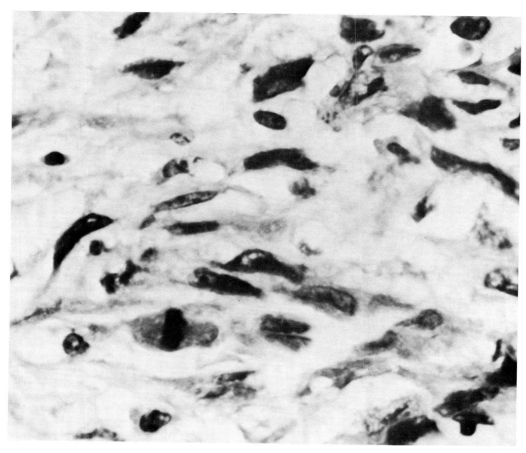

Figure 12.24. (B) Higher magnification of malignant cells with a mitotic figure. (H&E. Original magnification ×500.) *(Courtesy of Dr. D.P. Alrenga, Department of Pathology, Cook County Hospital, and J.B. Lippincott Co.)*

bers, lacking any tendency to form neoplastic bone, osteoid, or cartilage, either in its primary site or in its metastases. Until recently there was some controversy regarding the nature of this tumor.[112,228] Today it is generally agreed that fibrosarcoma of the bone is a distinct entity that can arise as a primary tumor of the skeletal system in either a medullary (central) or periosteal (peripheral) location.[228-230]

Dahlin and Ivins[229] found that fibrosarcomas of the bone constituted 23 percent of the primary bone sarcomas in the files of the Mayo Clinic. Huvos and Higginbotham[231] reported that primary fibrosarcomas of the bone constituted five percent of all bony neoplasms treated at Memorial Sloan-Kettering Cancer Center.

Fibrosarcoma of the bone is found in all age groups and is about equally divided between the sexes. No racial predilection has been found in any of the larger series.[227-231] Any bone can be involved; however, Dahlin and Ivins[229] did not find any tumor in the hands or feet in their series. Usually there is a predilection for long tubular bones; for example, Huvos and Higginbotham[231] found 43 in the femur, 16 in the humerus, and 12 in the tibia in their series of 130 cases. The relative distribution of medullary and periosteal fibrosarcoma is similar. The tumor can be multifocal, and multiple separate areas of involvement can be found in the same bone.[231]

Pain and swelling are the most common

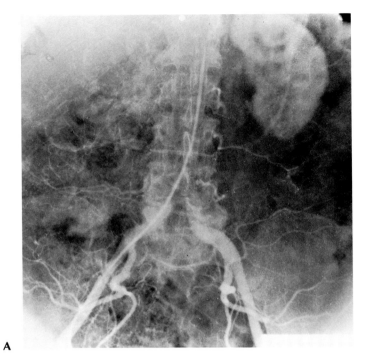

A

Figure 12.25. (A) Aortogram showing the recurrent renal fibrosarcoma of the right. Note the neovascularity in the right lumbar region. **(B)** Micrograph of the original renal fibrosarcoma. (H&E. Original magnification ×100.)

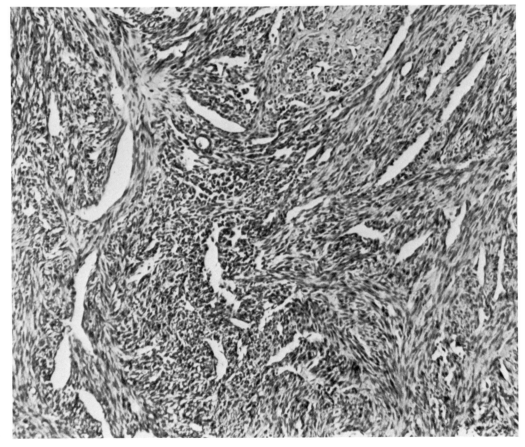

B

symptoms, and associated roentgenologic findings of cystic lesions on the corresponding bone should arouse suspicion of a malignant lesion. The diagnosis can be established only by histologic examination of the biopsy specimen.

The treatment of fibrosarcoma of a long bone has primarily been amputation of the extremity.[228-231] However, when the lesions are located in areas in which an en bloc resection is possible, the tumors are treated accordingly. Huvos and Higginbotham[231] found that, when clinically feasible, an en bloc resection produced survival rates similar to those for major amputation.

Radiation therapy as a primary form of treatment has not been tried extensively. However, from limited trials, the results are not comparable to those achieved with resection. Dahlin and Ivins[229] found that radiation therapy produced definite suppression of tumor growth in several instances. One patient lived for nearly seven years after biopsy and treatment with radium and x-ray before she died of sarcoma of the ilium. Another was lost to followup eight years after subtotal excision and roentgen therapy for a fibrosarcoma of the sacrum. No other long-term survivors were treated by radiation therapy alone.

The end result of treatment of fibrosarcoma of the bone is better than that for osteogenic sarcoma. Cunningham and Arlen[228] reported a 29.6 percent five-year survival. Dahlin and Ivins[229] had an overall survival rate of 28.7 percent. In their series, patients with grade 2 tumors had a 40 percent five-year survival rate; grade 3, 30.8 percent; and grade 4, 13.6 percent. Huvos[231] reported the overall five-year disease-free survival for fibrosarcoma of the bone as 34 percent. The 10-year, 15-year, and 20-year survival rates in their series were 28 percent, 27 percent, and 25 percent, respectively. According to these authors it is more meaningful to use 10- and 15-year survival rates as indicators of cure.

Malignant Fibrous Histiocytoma

Malignant fibrous histiocytoma is now a well-accepted clinicopathologic entity. The other terms commonly used to describe it are *malignant fibrous xanthoma* and *fibroxanthosarcoma*. Weiss and Enzinger[232] suggested that malignant fibrous histiocytoma is the most common soft tissue

sarcoma of late adult life, and that in the past, many of these tumors were erroneously diagnosed as liposarcoma, fibrosarcoma, or rhabdomyosarcoma.

Age, Sex, and Race. These tumors are seen in all age groups, but more commonly in patients between the ages of 50 and 70 years. Both sexes are about equally involved and no racial predilection has been observed in any of the published series[123,232-236] or in our own clinical material.

Location. Malignant fibrous histiocytomas can occur in all parts of the human body (Table 12.20). Occasionally they arise in the subcutaneous tissues above the deep fascia (Fig. 12.26A). The anatomic location plays a role in the size of the initial tumor and has a distinct influence on the prognosis. Superficially located tumors are smaller, whereas the deep-seated ones are larger (Fig. 12.26B). In our series, 26 patients had tumors larger than 5 cm (one was 30 cm: Fig. 12.26C and 12.26D), and in 21, the tumor was smaller than 5 cm. Soule and Enriquez[235] suggested that the size at initial presentation has no prognostic significance. Weiss and Enzinger[232] analyzed the clinical behavior and size of the primary tumor in 151 of the 200 cases from the files of the Armed Forces Institute of Pathology to find a correlation between the size of the tumor and the incidence of local recurrence and metastases. Tumors smaller than 2.5 cm had a 50 percent incidence of local recurrence and 21 percent of metastases. In contrast, for tumors larger than 5 cm, the local recurrence rate was 47 percent and the incidence rate of metastasis 34 percent. From a study of our patients it appears that anatomic location and size play a significant role in the incidence of recurrence and metastases.

The presenting symptom in all our patients was the presence of a tumor of short duration. Weiss and Enzinger[232] also found that in their collected series, the history usually was of less than six months' duration.

Treatment. In all reported series,[123,232-236] including our own, these tumors have been primarily treated by excision. Sixteen of 47 patients in this series have also been treated with adjuvant chemotherapy, and the results have been analyzed in detail (Chapter 8, Table 8.17). We have not treated any patient in this series with curative radiation therapy. Soule and Enriquez[235]

TABLE 12.19. PRIMARY FIBROSARCOMA OF THE AORTA

Author(s)	Year of Publication	Age/Sex	Site	Size	Type
Brodowski[211]	1873	52 M	Thoracic aorta	11 × 8 cm	Adventitial (with intimal spread)
Miura[215]	1891	38 M	Thoracic aorta	9 cm	Intimal (with adventitial spread)
Nencki[216]	1946	46 M	Abdominal aorta	3.5 × 3 × 2 cm	Adventitial
Kovaleva and Press[218]	1959	65 M	Abdominal aorta	From ostia of renal arteries to 2 cm above bifurcation	Intimal
Kaignodova and Berezovskaya[219]	1963	62 F	Thoracic	13 cm	Intimal
Zeitlhofer et al.[220]	1963	3½ mo M	Thoracic and abdominal aorta	6.5 × 2 × 0.5 cm	Intimal
Smeloff et al.[221]	1965	65 F	Thoracic and abdominal aorta	20 cm	Mural and intraluminal
Salm[210]	1972	60 F	Thoracic aorta	3.5 × 2 × 2 cm	Adventitial

had three patients who had preoperative radiation therapy (the tumor regressed in only one) and three who received radiation therapy postoperatively in the tumor bed (two had recurrence). Weiss and Enzinger[232,236] could not ascertain the role of radiation therapy or chemotherapy in their series, since adequate data were not available to them. Lindberg and co-workers[157] recently evaluated the role of postoperative radiotherapy following conservative surgery in patients with malignant fibrous histiocytoma and found the incidence of local recurrence to be 26.6 percent.

In the 47 patients in our series, a wide soft tissue excision was performed, along with regional node dissection when possible. Of 36 cases in the extremities that were treated with some type of muscle group excision and regional node dissection, including one case of a 15-cm lesion in the thigh, eight (22 percent) were found to have microscopic evidence of regional node metastases and were treated with adjuvant chemotherapy. Six of these eight are still free of tumor after five years. A review of the clinical data published by Kempson and Kyriakos,[233] O'Brien and Stout,[123] Soule and Enriquez,[235] and Weiss and Enzinger[232,236] shows a high incidence of local recurrence following local excision, with

Symptoms and Signs	Duration	Metastases	Histologic Type	Significant Necropsy Findings
Thoracic and abdominal pain, paresthesia of hand and feet, cachexia	4 wk	+	Fibrosarcoma	Metastases to peritoneum, liver, kidneys, spleen, pancreas, gastric and intestinal mucosa, and left of ileum
Thoracic and sacral pain, hyperesthesia of left leg, pathologic fracture of right femur, pyrexia emaciation	3 mo	+	Fibrosarcoma	Metastases to kidney, adrenals, mesentery, omentum, 4th lumbar vertebra and right femur
Abdominal pain, spastic constipation, emaciation	3 mo	−	Fibrosarcoma	Simple thrombosis of superior mesenteric artery
Abdominal pain radiating into right leg, hypertension, retinopathy, cachexia	1 yr	+	Fibrosarcoma	Partial occlusion of renal, superior, and inferior mesenteric arteries by intimal tumor; metastases to right acetabulum and right os pubis; renal and hepatic amyloidosis
Pyrexia, anemia	1 yr	+	Fibrosarcoma	Parietal subpleural metastases (with medial and adventitial invasion)
Dyspnea, tachycardia, atony	3½ mo	−	Fibromyxosarcoma	Hypertrophy of left ventricle
Hypertension of right arm, hypotension of legs, enlarged heart	3 mo	−	Fibromyxosarcoma	Patient died during operation
Osseous metastases, pyrexia, and cachexia	2 yr	+	Fibrosarcoma	Widespread osseous metastases of lower half of body; terminal metastases of kidneys, pancreas, and celiac lymph node; malignant thrombosis of celiac artery

TABLE 12.20. ANATOMIC LOCATION OF MALIGNANT FIBROUS HISTIOCYTOMA IN THREE SERIES

Anatomic Site	Soule and Enriquez (1972)[235]	Weiss and Enzinger (1978)[232]	Das Gupta (1981)
Head and neck	1	6	3
Trunk	4	19	7
Upper extremities	8	37	12
Lower extremities	16	98	24
Retroperitoneum	4	31	1
Miscellaneous sites	—	9	—
Total	33	200	47

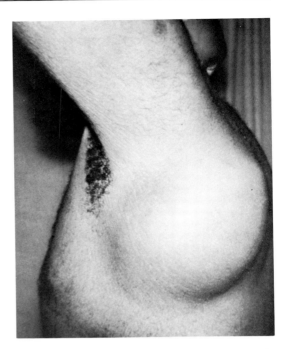

Figure 12.26. (**A**) Malignant fibrous histiocytoma of the left arm and trunk. Note the superficial location of the tumor. A wide excision with a skin graft provided local control.

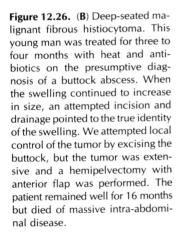

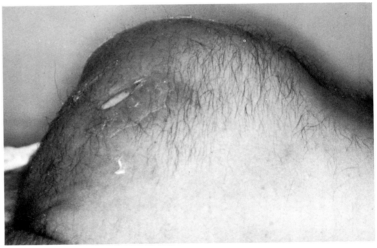

Figure 12.26. (**B**) Deep-seated malignant fibrous histiocytoma. This young man was treated for three to four months with heat and antibiotics on the presumptive diagnosis of a buttock abscess. When the swelling continued to increase in size, an attempted incision and drainage pointed to the true identity of the swelling. We attempted local control of the tumor by excising the buttock, but the tumor was extensive and a hemipelvectomy with anterior flap was performed. The patient remained well for 16 months but died of massive intra-abdominal disease.

resulting amputation. It appears that, if aggressive surgical treatment had been provided initially to these patients, the incidence of local recurrence would probably have been reduced, and a number of amputations could have been avoided. If the primary tumor is located in the hands or feet, sometimes an amputation becomes essential; but in the light of our own studies on the sensitivity of these tumors to radiation therapy and chemotherapy, the need for amputation even in these anatomic settings is becoming less and less.

End Results. Of our 47 patients with malignant fibrous histiocytoma, 34 are eligible for five-year survival analysis. Twenty-six (76 percent) of these 34 are still free of tumor after five years.

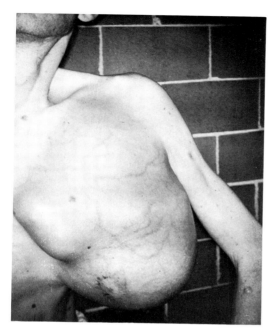

Figure 12.26. (C) A neglected case of malignant fibrous histiocytoma of the chest wall.

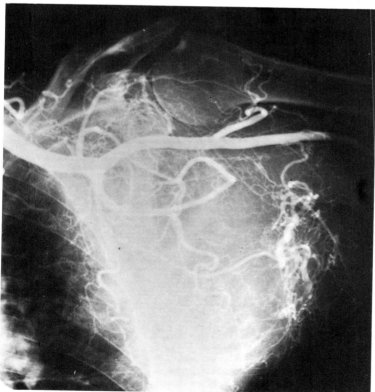

Figure 12.26. (D) Angiogram showing extensive neovascularity. No attempt was made to treat this patient and he died of diffuse metastases three months later.

The end results according to site and size are shown in Table 12.21. The incidence of local recurrence has been reported as ranging between 20 and 44 percent.[123,157,232,234] The recurrence rate of 6 percent (three patients) in our series shows the value of initial aggressive surgical therapy. Most of the reports on this entity have come from pathologists[123,232-236] who did not have the opportunity to plan therapy. Therefore, the term "wide resection," as used by these authors, may not have the same meaning as used in this text. Wide soft tissue resection with preservation of functional limbs (Chapter 6) performed in our patients has consistently led to a lower incidence of local recurrence in all types of sarcoma, including malignant fibrous histiocytoma. Weiss and Enzinger[232] compared local recurrence rates between wide resection and amputation in two groups of 12 and 13 patients, respectively. In the first group, 58 percent had recurrence and the other had none. However, as mentioned above, the validity of this comparison is open to question. Weiss and Enzinger[232] found a two-year survival rate of 60 percent and a local recurrence rate of 42 percent in their collected series of 200 patients. Soule and Enriquez[235] reported a 65 percent five-year survival rate and 38 percent for 10-year survival. It is difficult to calculate the exact survival rate in the series of Kempson and Kyriakos,[233] since their followup data were not complete. Lindberg and associates[157] reported that conservative surgery and postoperative radiation therapy yielded a survival rate of 65 percent and 56 percent for two and five years, respectively. Our clinical data suggest that an initial aggressive therapeutic approach reduces local recurrence as well as improves ultimate survival. Soule and Enriquez[235] emphasized that these tumors can recur or metastasize, or both, even after five years. One of our patients presented with multiple pulmonary nodules 63 months after initial therapy. In this context, the natural history of these tumors is similar to that of fibrosarcoma, in which recurrence and metastases sometimes occur after a prolonged period of quiescence.

Prognostic Factors. Malignant fibrous histiocytoma is an aggressive form of sarcoma and, unless adequately treated initially with wide excision and regional node dissection, the salvage rate from the standpoint of both local recurrence and metastases will be low.

Of the factors controlling the prognosis, the location in relation to the surrounding tissues, the size, and the histologic grading appear to be most significant. If the tumors are located superficially in the subcutaneous tissue or the deep fascia and the size is less than 5 cm, the prognosis for patients with a low-grade tumor, after the therapy outlined above, is better than that for patients with a tumor larger than 5 cm that arises in an underlying muscle or the retroperitoneum, or is of a higher grade (Table 12.22). The role of node involvement still remains unclear. Weiss and Enzinger[232] consider that the incidence is low and therefore elective

TABLE 12.21. END RESULT ACCORDING TO ANATOMIC SITE AND SIZE OF THE PRIMARY TUMORS SEEN IN 47 PATIENTS (UNIVERSITY OF ILLINOIS SERIES)*†

Site	No. Patients	< 5 cm	> 5 cm	2 Yr, N.E.D.§	5 Yr, N.E.D.
Head and neck	3 (1)‡	2 (1)	1 (1)	3	1
Trunk	7 (4)	3 (2)	4 (2)	5	3
Upper extremities	12 (9)	5 (4)	7 (5)	9	8
Lower extremities	24 (19)	11 (9)	13 (9)	19	14
Retroperitoneum	1 (1)	—	1 (1)	1	0
Total	47 (34)	21 (16)	26 (18)	37 (79%)	26 (76%)

Sixteen of these 47 patients received adjuvant chemotherapy (Table 8.18, Chapter 8).
†*All 47 patients were eligible for two-year analysis.*
‡*Numbers in parentheses represent patients eligible for five-year analysis.*
§*No evidence of disease.*

TABLE 12.22. DISEASE-FREE SURVIVAL, ACCORDING TO TUMOR SIZE AND GRADE, OF 34 PATIENTS WITH MALIGNANT FIBROUS HISTIOCYTOMA (UNIVERSITY OF ILLINOIS SERIES)

Tumor Size	No. Patients	Grades 1 and 2	5 Yr, N.E.D.*	Grades 3 and 4	5 Yr, N.E.D.
< 5 cm	16	12	11	4	2
> 5 cm	18	10	8	8	5
Total	34	22	19	12	7

*No evidence of disease.

dissection is not required. In contrast, we found it to be high enough to justify consideration of a node dissection. Our overall five-year salvage rate of 76 percent and the fact that six of eight patients with positive regional nodes have now lived five years free of tumor certainly adds credence to this concept. Furthermore, our data (Chapter 8) suggest that malignant fibrous histiocytoma is a chemotherapy-responsive tumor as well, and use of adjuvant chemotherapy after the initial local treatment will further improve the overall long-range salvage rate.

Miscellaneous Sites. McCarthy and associates[237] recently described 35 primary cases of malignant fibrous histiocytoma of the bone. Spanier and co-workers[238] studied 11 cases and drew some general guidelines for management. In their opinion, a combination of chemotherapy and radiation therapy might be of value. The average survival time was 12 months in six of nine patients who had no secondary treatment of their metastases.

Like fibrosarcomas, malignant fibrous histiocytomas have been found to occur in the oral cavity and the mandible,[239] larynx,[240] genitourinary tract,[241-243] the gastrointestinal tract,[244] and the mediastinum.[245] Since these are rare locations, every case should be recorded in detail for better understanding of its natural history.

Fibrous histiocytoma of the lung[57,246] has also been reported. Grossman and co-workers[57] described such a case and reviewed the pertinent literature. Approximately eight cases have been documented. A review of these case reports suggests that probably the authors were describing either a benign or atypical kind of fibrous histiocytoma. Although microscopic diagnosis of these tumors might be in question,

there is no denying that malignant fibrous histiocytoma of the pulmonary parenchyma is a distinct possibility.[246]

In 1976, Kyriakos and Kempson[234] described seven cases of a tumor which they considered to be a subclassification of malignant fibrous histiocytomas. They termed this entity inflammatory fibrous histiocytoma. All their patients were adult (mean age 52.6 years), only one being younger than 40 years. Four of the seven were women. The tumors were found in the retroperitoneum, anterior chest wall, anterior abdominal wall, femoral area, and oral cavity. The average size was 8.5 cm and, although they appeared encapsulated, they were microscopically infiltrative. The clinical course was protracted, with multiple recurrences and eventual metastases. All seven patients died of the tumor, the average survival time being 53 months.

Malignant Histiocytoma. This rare tumor is a variant of malignant fibrous histiocytoma. Soule and Enriquez[235] reported seven cases. At the University of Illinois there have been only two. The clinical presentation of malignant histiocytoma is similar to that of malignant fibrous histiocytoma. The results of treatment are unsatisfactory. Four of seven patients in the series of Soule and Enriquez[235] died with metastatic disease and three patients were living at the time of their report in 1972. Both our patients died within one year of excision of the primary (Fig. 12.27A and 12.27B). Although one cannot conclude much from such a small number of patients, it appears that these patients should be treated aggressively as soon as the diagnosis is established.

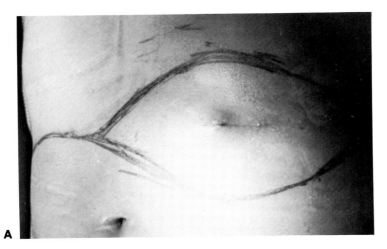

A

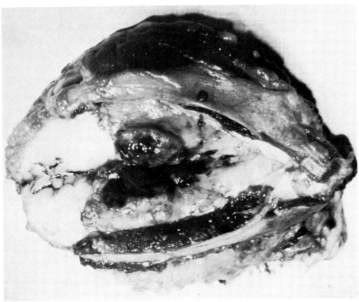

B

Figure 12.27. (**A**) Locally recurrent malignant histiocytoma of the anterior abdominal wall in a 48-year-old woman. Four months previously she had first noticed a small (3 × 2 cm) tumor. An excision of the tumor was performed, but within six weeks the mass recurred. We performed a wide resection of the tumor, including the anterior abdominal wall. (**B**) Gross appearance of the tumor. Within six months of the second excision, she developed massive intra-abdominal disease and pulmonary metastases and died.

REFERENCES

1. Chung EB, Enzinger FM: Infantile fibrosarcoma. Cancer 38:729, 1976
2. Stout AP: Juvenile fibromatoses. Cancer 7:953, 1954
3. Stout AP: Fibrosarcoma in infants and children. Cancer 15:1028, 1962
4. Stout AP, Lattes R: Tumors of the soft tissues. Atlas of Tumor Pathology, series 2, fasc 1. Washington DC, AFIP, 1967
5. Pack GT, Ariel IA: Tumors of the Soft Somatic Tissue: A Clinical Treatise. Hoeber-Harper, New York, 1958
6. Teng P, Warden MN, Cogen WL: Congenital generalized fibromatosis (renal and skeletal) with complete spontaneous regression. J Pediat 62:748, 1963
7. Bartlett RE, Otis RD, Laasko AO: Multiple congenital neoplasms of soft tissues: Report of four cases in one family. Cancer 14:913, 1961
8. Chandler FA: Muscular torticollis. J Bone Joint Surg 30-A:566, 1948
9. Keasby LE: Juvenile aponeurotic fibroma (calcifying fibroma). A distinctive tumor arising in the palms and soles of young children. Cancer 6:338, 1953
10. Keasby LE, Fanselau HA: The aponeurotic fibroma. Clin Orthopaed 19:115, 1961

11. Lichtenstein L, Goldman RL: The cartilaginous analogue of fibromatosis. A reinterpretation of the condition called "juvenile aponeurotic." Cancer 17:810, 1964

12. Goldman RL: The cartilage analogue of fibromatosis (aponeurotic fibroma): Further observations based on seven new cases. Cancer 26:1325, 1970

13. Allen PW, Enzinger FM: Juvenile aponeurotic fibroma. Cancer 26:857, 1970

14. Martin H, Ehrlich HE, Abels JC: Juvenile nasopharyngeal angiofibroma. Ann Surg 127:513, 1948

15. Shaheen HB: Nasopharyngeal fibroma. J Laryngol Otol 45:259, 1930

16. New GB, Figi FA: Treatment of fibromas of the nasopharynx. Report of 32 cases. Am J Roengenol 12:340, 1924

17. Friedberg SA: Vascular fibroma of the nasopharynx (nasopharyngeal fibroma). Arch Otol 31:313, 1940

18. Figi FA, Davis RE: Management of nasopharyngeal fibromas. Laryngoscope 60:794, 1950

19. Martin JS: Nasopharyngeal fibroma and its treatment. J Laryngol Otol 68:39, 1954

20. Sternberg SS: Pathology of juvenile nasopharyngeal angiofibroma. A lesion of adolescent males. Cancer 7:15, 1954

21. MacComb WS: Juvenile nasopharyngeal fibroma. Am J Surg 106:754, 1963

22. Apostol JV, Frazell EL: Juvenile nasopharyngeal angiofibroma. A clinical study. Cancer 15:869, 1965

23. Conley J, Healey WV, Blaugrund SM, Perzin KH: Nasopharyngeal angiofibroma in the juvenile. Surg Gynecol Obstet 126:825, 1968

24. Svoboda DJ, Kirchner F: Ultrastructure of nasopharyngeal angiofibromas. Cancer 19:1949, 1966

25. Reye RDK: Recurring digital fibrous tumors of childhood. Arch Path 80:228, 1965

26. Ahlquist J, Pohjanpelto P, Hjelt L, Hurme K: Recurrent digital fibrous tumor of childhood. Clinical and morphological aspects of a case. Acta Path Microbiol Scand 70:291, 1967

27. Shapiro L: Infantile digital fibromatosis and aponeurotic fibroma. Case reports of two rare pseudosarcomas and review of the literature. Arch Dermat 99:37, 1969

28. Battifora H, Hines JR: Recurrent digital fibromas of childhood: An electron microscope study. Cancer 27:1530, 1971

29. Stewart AM, MacGregor AR: Myositis fibrosa generalisata. Arch Dis Child 26:215, 1951

30. Horton CE, Crawford J, Oakey RS: Malignant change in keloids. Plast Reconstr Surg 112:383, 1953

31. Dupuytren G: Lecons orales de clinique chirurgicale faites a L'Hotel Dieu Paris, Paris, 1832, vol. 1, chap 1. Translated: Permanent retraction of the fingers produced by an affection of the palmar fascia. Lancet 2:222, 1934

32. Rhode CM, Jennings WD Jr: Dupuytren's contracture. Am Surgeon 33:8555, 1967

33. Skoog T: Dupuytren's contraction: With special reference to etiology and improved surgical treatment: Its occurrence in epileptics; note on knuckle pads. Acta Chir Scand Suppl 139, Vol 96, 1948

34. Conway H: Dupuytren's contracture. Am J Surg 87:101, 1954

35. Scott WW, Scardino PL: A new concept in the treatment of Peyronie's disease. South Med J 41:173, 1948

36. Burford EH, Glenn JE, Burford CE: Therapy of Peyronie's disease. Urol Cutan Rev 55:337, 1951

37. Mende S, Volpel M, Rotthauwe I: Idiopathic retroperitoneal fibrosis (Ormond's disease) with unusual extension involving the brain. Beitr Path 153:80, 1974

38. Skeel DA, Shols GW, Sullivan MJ, Witherington R: Retroperitoneal fibrosis with intrinsic ureteral involvement. J Urol 113:166, 1975

39. Cauble WG: Retroperitoneal fibrosis with bowel obstruction: Presentation of one case. Am J Proctol 25:75, 1974

40. Rothman D, Kendall AB: Bilateral ureteral entrapment by perianeurysmal fibrosis: Case reports. Vasc Surg 8:259, 1974

41. Ormond JK: Bilateral ureteral obstruction due to envelopment and compression by inflammatory retroperitoneal process. J Urol 59:1072, 1948

42. Ormond JK: Idiopathic retroperitoneal fibrosis. An established clinical entity. JAMA 174:1561, 1960

43. Temperley JM: Multifocal fibrosclerosis. Br J Clin Pract 28:217, 1974

44. Yacoub MH, Thompson VC: Chronic idiopathic pulmonary hilar fibrosis—A clinical pathologic entity. Thorax 26:365, 1971

45. Barrett NR: Idiopathic mediastinal fibrosis. Br J Surg 46:207, 1958

46. Tubbs OS: Superior vena caval obstruction due to chronic mediastinitis. Thorax 1:247, 1946

47. Hutter RVP, Stewart FW, Foote FW Jr: Fasciitis: A report of 70 cases with follow-up proving the benignity of the lesion. Cancer 15:992, 1962

48. Hutter RVP, Foote FW Jr, Francis KC, Higginbotham NL: Parosteal fasciitis: A self-limited benign process that simulates a malignant neoplasm. Am J Surg 104:800, 1962

49. Toker C: Pseudosarcomatous fasciitis: Further observations indicating the aggressive capabilities of this lesion and justifying the inclusion of this entity within the category of the fibromatoses. Ann Surg 174:996, 1971

50. Finlay-Jones LR, Nicol P, Ten Seldam REJ: Pseudosarcoma of the skin. Pathology 3:215, 1971

51. Woyke S, Domagala W, Olszewski W, Korabiec M: Pseudosarcoma of the skin: An electron microscopic study and comparison with the fine structure of the spindle-cell variant of squamous carcinoma. Cancer 33:970, 1974

52. Bourne, RG: Paradoxical fibrosarcoma of the skin (pseudosarcoma): A review of 13 cases. Med J Australia 50(1):504, 1963

53. Jarvi OH, Saxen AE, Hopsu-Havu VK, Wartiovaara JJ, Vaissalo VT: Elastofibroma—A degenerative pseudotumor. Cancer 23:42, 1969

54. Renshaw TS, Simon MA: Elastofibroma. J Bone Joint Surg 55-A:409, 1973

55. Mirra JM, Straub LR, Jarvi OH: Elastofibroma of the deltoid: A case report. Cancer 33:234, 1974

56. Fretzin DF, Helwig EB: A typical fibroxanthoma of the skin: A clinicopathologic study of 140 cases. Cancer 31:1541, 1973

57. Grossman RE, Bemis EL, Pemberton AH, Narodick BG: Fibrous histiocytoma or xanthoma of the lung with bronchial involvement. J Thor Cardiovasc Surg 65:653, 1973

58. Darier J, Ferrand M: Dermatofibromes progressifs et recidivants, on fibrosarcomes de la peau. Ann de dermat et de syph 5:545, 1924

59. Hoffmann E: Knobby fibrosarcoma of the skin. Dermatology 43:1, 1925

60. Michelson HE: Dermatofibrosarcoma protuberans (Darier, Hoffmann). Arch Dermat Syph 25:1127, 1932

61. Pack GT, Taba EJ: Dermatofibrosarcoma protuberans: Report of 39 cases. Arch Surg 62:391, 1951

62. Woolridge WE: Dermatofibrosarcoma protuberans: A tumor too lightly considered. Arch Dermat 75:132, 1957

63. Taylor HH, Helwig EB: Dermatofibrosarcoma protuberans. Cancer 15:717, 1962

64. McPeak CJ, Cruz T, Nicastri AD: Dermatofibrosarcoma protuberans: An analysis of 86 cases—five with metastasis. Ann Surg 166:805, 1967

65. Brenner W, Schaefler K, Chhabra H, Postel A: Dermatofibrosarcoma protuberans metastatic to a regional lymph node: Report of a case and review. Cancer 36:1897, 1975

66. Macfarlane J: In Robertson D (ed): Clinical Reports of the Surgical Practice of the Glasgow Royal Infirmary, 1832, p 63

67. Onion CT (ed): The Shorter Oxford English Dictionary on Historical Principles, 3rd ed. London, Clarendon Press, Oxford University Press, 1967

68. Müller J: Uber den feinern Bau und die Formen der Krankhaften Greschwulste. Berlin, G Reimer, 1838, p 80

69. Paget J: Fibronucleated tumor of the abdomen of fourteen years' growth; removal. Lancet 1:625, 1856

70. Bennet JH: On cancerous and canceroid growths. Edinburgh, Southerland and Knox, 1849, p 176

71. Sanger M: Uber desmoide Greschwulste der Bauchwand und deren operation mit Resection des peritoneum parietale. Arch Gynak 24:1, 1884

72. Stone HB: Desmoid tumors of the abdominal wall. Ann Surg 48:175, 1908

73. Pack GT, Ehrlich HE: Neoplasms of the anterior abdominal wall with special consideration of desmoid tumors. Internat Abst Surg 79:177, 1944

74. Dahn I, Jonsson N, Lundh G: Desmoid tumors, a series of 33 cases. Acta Chir Scandi 126:305, 1963

75. Brasfield RD, Das Gupta TK: Desmoid tumors of the anterior abdominal wall. Surgery 65:241, 1969

76. Strode JE: Desmoid tumors, particularly as related to their surgical principles. Ann Surg 139:335, 1954

77. Nichols RW: Desmoid tumors: A report of thirty-one cases. Arch Surg 7:227, 1923

78. Mason JB: Desmoid tumors. Ann Surg 92:444, 1930

79. Keith A: Human Embryology and Morphology. London, Edward Arnold Ltd, 1948, p 580

80. Musgrove JE, McDonald JR: Extra-abdominal desmoid tumors. Arch Path 45:513, 1948

81. Geschickter EF, Lewis D: Tumors of connective tissue. Am J Cancer 25:630, 1935

82. Jadrijvic D, Mardones E, Lipschutz A: Antifibromatogenic activity of 19-Nor-α-ethinyltestosterone in the guinea pig. Proc Soc Exp Biol Med 91:38, 1956

83. Chaudhuri PK, Beattie CW, Walker MJ, Das Gupta TK: Presence of steroid receptors in human soft tissue sarcomas of diverse histological origin. Cancer Res 40:861, 1980

84. Ramsey RH: The pathology, diagnosis and treatment of extra-abdominal desmoid tumors. J Bone Joint Surg 37-B:1012, 1955

85. Hunt RTN, Morgan HC, Ackerman LV: Principles in the management of extra-abdominal desmoids. Cancer 13:825, 1960

86. Das Gupta TK, Brasfield RD, O'Hara J: Extra-abdominal desmoids: A clinicopathological study. Ann Surg 170:109, 1969

87. Enzinger FM, Shiraki M: Musculo-aponeurotic fibromatosis of the shoulder girdle (extra-abdominal desmoid): Analysis of thirty cases followed up for ten or more years. Cancer 20:1131, 1967

88. Gonatas NK: Extra-abdominal desmoid tumors. Arch Path 71:217, 1961

89. Bowden L, Booher RJ: The principles and technique of resection of soft parts for sarcoma. Surgery 44:963, 1958

90. Paget J: Lectures on Surgical Pathology, 3rd ed. Philadelphia, Lindsay and Blakiston, 1865

91. Masson JK, Soule EH: Desmoid tumors of the head and neck. Am J Surg 112:615, 1966

92. Conley J, Healey WV, Stout AP: Fibromatosis of the head and neck. Am J Surg 112:609, 1966

93. Wilkins SA Jr, Waldron CA, Mathews WH, Droullas CA: Aggressive fibromatosis of the head and neck. Am J Surg 130:412, 1975

94. Gardner EJ, Richards RC: Multiple cutaneous and subcutaneous lesions occurring simultaneously with hereditary polyposis and osteomatosis. Am J Human Genetics 5:139, 1953

95. Hubbard TB Jr: Familial polyposis of the colon: The fate of the retained rectum after colectomy in children. Ann Surg 23:577, 1957

96. Smith WG: Desmoid tumors in familial multiple polyposis. Proc Staff Meeting Mayo Clin 34:31, 1959

97. Gardner E: Follow-up study of Gardner's syndrome. Am J Hum Genet 14:376, 1962

98. Simpson RD, Harrison EG, Mayo CW: Mesenteric fibromatosis in familial polyposis. Cancer 17:526, 1964

99. Thomas KE, Watne AL, Johnson JG, Roth E, Zimmermann B: Natural history of Gardner's syndrome. Am J Surg 115:218, 1968

100. Parks TG, Bussey HJR, Lockhart-Mummery HE: Familial polyposis coli associated with extracolonic abnormalities. Gut 11:323, 1970

101. Jones TR, Nance FC: Periampullary malignancy in Gardner's syndrome. Ann Surg 185:565, 1977
102. Gold RS, Mucha SJ: Unique case of mesenteric fibrosis in multiple polyposis. Am J Surg 130:366, 1975
103. Haggitt RC, Booth JL: Bilateral fibromatosis of the breast in Gardner's syndrome. Cancer 25:161, 1970
104. Penn D, Federman Q, Finkel M: Fibromatosis in Gardner's syndrome. Am J Gastroenterol 59:174, 1973
105. Jaffe HL: Tumors and Tumorous Conditions of Bones and Joints. Philadelphia, Lea Febiger, 1958, p 298
106. Rabhan WN, Rosai J: Desmoplastic fibroma: Report of ten cases and review of the literature. J Bone Joint Surg 50:487, 1968
107. Cornil V, Ranvier L: A Manual of Pathological History. Philadelphia, Henry C Lea, 1880
108. Virchow R: Die Krankhafter Geschwulste. Berlin, Hirschwald, 1864–65
109. Birkett J: Contributions to the practical surgery of new growths or tumors. II. Fibro-plastic growths. Guy's Hospital Reports. Sec 3, 4:231, 1858
110. Billroth T: Lectures on Surgical Pathology and Therapeutics. London, The New Sydenham Society, 1877–78
111. Ewing J: Neoplastic Disease, 4th ed. Philadelphia and London, Saunders, 1942, p 164
112. Stout AP: Fibrosarcoma: The malignant tumor of fibroblasts. Cancer 1:30, 1948
113. Stout AP: The fibromatoses. Clin Orthop 19:11, 1961
114. Stout AP: Mesenchymal tumors of the soft tissues. Trans Studies Coll Physicians, Philadelphia 31:91, 1963
115. Stout AP: Recent observations on mesenchymal tumors in adults and children. Canad Med Assoc J 88:453, 1963
116. Pack GT, Ariel IM: Fibrosarcoma of the soft somatic tissues: A clinical and pathologic study. Surgery 31:443, 1952
117. Kauffman SL, Stout AP: Congenital mesenchymal tumors. Cancer 18:460, 1965
118. Bruce KW, Royer RQ: Central fibromyxoma of the maxilla. Oral Surg 5:1277, 1952
119. da Silva Neto JB: Results of 22 cases of breast sarcoma over five years after surgery. Tumori 56:39, 1970
120. Malek RS, Utz DC, Farrow GM: Malignant tumors of the spermatic cord. Cancer 29:1108, 1972
121. Soft Tissue Tumors: Case 14, contributed by Hartney TX, discussed by Lattes R. Proc Amer Soc Clinical Pathologists, 1973 Annual Meeting, Chicago, 1973, p 75
122. Hajdu SI, Shiu MH, Fortner JG: Tendosynovial sarcoma: A clinicopathological study of 136 cases. Cancer 39:1201, 1977
123. O'Brien JE, Stout AP: Malignant fibrous xanthomas. Cancer 17:1446, 1964
124. Schwartz DT, Alpert M: The malignant transformation of fibrous dysplasia. Am J Med Sci 247:1, 1964
125. Balsaver AM, Butler JJ, Martin RG: Congenital fibrosarcoma. Cancer 20:1607, 1967
126. Exelby PR, Knapper WH, Huvos AG, Beattie EJ Jr: Soft-tissue fibrosarcoma in children. J Pediat Surg 8:415, 1973
127. Dahl I, Save-Soderbergh J, Angervall L: Fibrosarcoma in early infancy. Path Europ 8:193, 1973
128. Seel DJ, Booher RJ, Joel R: Fibrous tumors of musculoaponeurotic origin. Surgery 56:497, 1964
129. Mackenzie DH: Fibroma: A dangerous diagnosis. A review of 205 cases of fibrosarcoma of soft tissues. Br J Surg 51:607, 1964
130. Gould SE, Hinerman DL, Batsakis JG, Beamer PR: Diagnostic patterns: Lesions of fibrous tissue. Am J Clin Path 40:411, 1963
131. Pritchard DJ, Soule EH, Taylor WF, Ivins JE: Fibrosarcoma. A clinicopathological and statistical study of 199 tumors of soft tissues and trunk. Cancer 33:88, 1974
132. Werf-Messing BV, van Unnik JAM: Fibrosarcoma of the soft parts. Cancer 18:1113, 1965
133. Thorbjarnarson B: Sarcomas at the New York Hospital. Arch Surg 82:489, 1961
134. Hare HF, Cerny MJ: Soft tissue sarcoma: A review of 200 cases. Cancer 16:1332, 1963
135. Coran AG, Crocker DW, Wilson RE: A twenty-five year experience with soft tissue sarcomas. Am J Surg 119:288, 1970
136. Ferrell HW, Frable WJ: Soft part sarcomas revisited. Cancer 30:475, 1972
137. Solway HB: Radiation-induced neoplasms following curative therapy for retinoblastoma. Cancer 19:1984, 1966
138. Schoenberg MJ: Report on a case of bilateral glioma of the retina, cured in the non-enucleated eye by radium treatment. Arch Ophth 56:221, 1927
139. Pettit VD, Chamness JT, Ackerman LV: Fibromatosis: A fibrosarcoma following irradiation therapy. Cancer 7:149, 1954
140. Forrest AW: Tumors following radiation about the eye. Trans Am Acad Ophth Otol 65:694, 1961
141. Frezzotti R, Guerra R: Sarcoma following irradiated retinoblastoma. Arch Ophth 70:461, 1973
142. Fabrikant JI, Dickson RJ, Fetter BF: Mechanisms of radiation carcinogenesis at the clinical level. Br J Cancer 18:459, 1964
143. Regalson W, Bross ID: Hananiau J, Goryum N: The incidence of second primary tumor in children with cancer and leukemia: A 7-year survey of 150 consecutive autopsied cases. Cancer 18:58, 1965
144. Schwartz EF, Rothstein JD: Fibrosarcoma following radiation therapy. JAMA 203:296, 1968
145. Oberman HA, O'Neal RM: Fibrosarcoma of the chest wall following resection and irradiation of carcinoma of the breast. Am J Clin Path 53:407, 1970
146. Hatfield PM, Schultz MD: Post-irradiation sarcoma including 5 cases after x-ray therapy of breast carcinoma. Radiology 96:593, 1970
147. Hajdu SI: Pathology of Soft Tissue Tumors. Philadelphia, Lea & Febiger, 1979, pp 526
148. Vink M, Altman DA: Congenital malignant tumors. Cancer 19:967, 1966

149. Anderson DH: Tumors of infancy and childhood. I. In a survey of those seen in the pathology laboratory of the Babies Hospital during the years 1935–50. Cancer 4:890, 1951

150. Enzinger FM: Fibrous hamartoma of infancy. Cancer 18:241, 1965

151. Crawford M, Chung EB, Leffall LD, White JE: Soft part sarcoma in Negroes. Cancer 26:503, 1970

152. Bizer LS: Fibrosarcoma. Report of 64 cases. Am J Surg 121:586, 1971

153. Windeyer B, Dische S, Mansfield CM: The place of radiotherapy in the management of fibrosarcoma of the soft tissues. Clin Radiol 17:32, 1966

154. McNeer CP, Cantin J, Chu F, Nickson J: Effectiveness of radiation therapy in the management of sarcoma of the soft tissues. Cancer 22:391, 1968

155. Suit HD, Russel WO, Martin RG: Sarcoma of soft tissue. Clinical and histopathologic parameters and response to treatment. Cancer 35:1478, 1975

156. Castro B, Hajdu SI, Fortner JG: Surgical therapy of fibrosarcoma of the extremities: A reappraisal. Arch Surg 107:284, 1973

157. Lindberg RD, Martin RG, Romsdahl MM, Barkley HT: Conservative surgery and postoperative radiotherapy in 300 adults with soft tissue sarcomas. Cancer 47:2391, 1981

158. O'Day RA, Soule EH, Gores RJ: Soft tissue sarcoma of the oral cavity. Mayo Clin Proc 39:169, 1964

159. Andrews CF: Primary retroperitoneal sarcoma: Report of 28 cases. Surg Gynecol Obstet 30:480, 1923

160. Frank RJ: Primary retroperitoneal tumors: Report of 107 tumors. Int Abs Surg 4:383, 1938

161. McNamara WL, Smith HD, Boswell CS: Retroperitoneal tumors: Report of 8 cases. Am J Cancer 38:63, 1940

162. Donnelly BA: Primary retroperitoneal tumors. Report of 95 cases and review of literature. Surg Gynecol Obstet 83:705, 1946

163. Oberman HA: Sarcoma of the breast. Cancer 18:1233, 1965

164. Rissanen PM, Holsti P: A retrospective study of sarcoma of the breast and the results of treatment. Oncology 22:258, 1963

165. Treves N, Sunderland DA: Cystosarcoma phyllodes of breast, malignant and benign tumor—Clinicopathological study of 77 cases. Cancer 4:1286, 1951

166. Lester J, Stout AP: Cystosarcoma phyllodes. Cancer 7:335, 1954

167. Rix DB, Tredwell JJ, Forward AD: Cystosarcoma phyllodes (cellular intracanalicular fibroadenoma)—Clinicopathological relationship. Canad J Surg 14:31, 1974

168. Norris HJ, Taylor HB: Relationships of histologic features to behavior of cystosarcoma phyllodes. Cancer 20:2090, 1967

169. McDivitt RW, Urban JA, Farrow JH: Cystosarcoma phyllodes. Johns Hopkins Med J 120:33, 1967

170. Hajdu SI, Espinosa MH, Robbins GF: Recurrent cystosarcoma phyllodes: A clinicopathologic study of 32 cases. Cancer 38:1402, 1976

171. Kessinger A, Foley JF, Lemon HM, Miller DM: Metastatic cystosarcoma phyllodes: A case report and review of the literature. J Surg Oncol 4:131, 1972

172. Faraci RP, Schour L: Radical treatment of recurrent cystosarcoma phyllodes. Ann Surg 180:796, 1974

173. Shallow TA, Wagner FB: Primary fibrosarcoma of the liver. Ann Surg 125:439, 1947

174. Simpson HM, Baggenstoss AH, Stauffer MH: Primary sarcoma of the liver—A report of three cases. South Med J 48:1177, 1955

175. Steiner PE: Cancer of the liver and cirrhosis in Trans-Saharan Africa and the United States of America. Cancer 13:1085, 1960

176. Ojima A, Sugiyama T, Takeda T, Hazama F, Nakayki K, Uesugi Y, et al: Six cases of rare malignant tumors of the liver. Acta Path Jap 14:95, 1964

177. Snapper I, Schraft WC, Ginsberg DM: Severe hypoglycemia due to fibrosarcoma of the liver. Maandschr Kindergeneeskd 32:337, 1964

178. Totzke HA, Hutcheson JB: Primary fibrosarcoma of the liver—Case report. South Med J 58:236, 1965

179. Balouet G, Destombes P: Apropos of several apparently primary hepatic mesenchymal tumors—Trial classification and diagnosis of spindle cell tumors of the liver. Ann Anat Path (Paris) 12:273, 1967

180. Cavallo T, Lichewtiz B, Rozov T: Primary fibrosarcoma of the liver—Report of a case. Rev Hosp Clin Fac Med Sao Paulo 23:44, 1968

181. Smith D, Rele SR: A case of primary fibrosarcoma of the liver. Postgrad Med J 48:62, 1972

182. Walter VE, Bodner E, Lederer, B: Primary fibrosarcoma of the liver. Wien Klin Wachenschr 84:808, 1972

183. Alrenga DP: Primary fibrosarcoma of the liver. Cancer 36:446, 1975

184. Ali MY, Muir CS: Malignant renal neoplasms in Singapore. Br J Urol 77:792, 1964

185. Ashley DB: In Evans RW (ed): Histological Appearance of Tumor, vol 2, 3rd ed. Edinburgh, London and New York, Churchill Livingstone, 1978, p 813

186. Willis RA: The Borderland of Embryology and Pathology. London, Butterworth, 1958, p 506

187. Chesky VE, Hellwig CA, Welch JW: Fibrosarcoma of the thyroid gland. Surg Gynecol Obstet 111:767, 1960

188. Arlen M, Grabstald H, Whitmore WF: Malignant tumors of the spermatic cord. Cancer 23:525, 1969

189. Dehner LP, Smith BH: Soft tissue tumors of the penis. Cancer 25:1431, 1970

190. Bailey RV, Stribling J, Weitzner S, Hardy JD: Leiomyosarcoma of the inferior vena cava: Report of a case and review of the literature. Ann Surg 184:169, 1976

191. Melchior E: Sarcom der Vana Cava Inferior. Deutsch Z Chir 213:135, 1928

192. Cope JS, Hunt CJ: Leiomyosarcoma of the inferior vena cava. Arch Surg 68:752, 1954

193. Ornerheim WO, Tesluk H: Leiomyosarcoma of the inferior vena cava. Arch Surg 82:395, 1961

194. Allen J, Burnett W, Lee FD: Leiomyosarcoma of the inferior vena cava. Scottish Med J 9:352, 1964

195. Staley CJ, Valaitis J, Trippel OH, Franzblau SA: Leiomyosarcoma of the inferior vena cava. Am J Surg 113:211, 1967

196. Couinaud C: Tumerus de la Veine Cave Inférieure. J Chir (Paris) 105:411, 1973

197. Demoulin JC, Sambon Y, Bandinet V, et al: Leiomyosarcoma of the inferior vena cava: An unusual cause of pulmonary emboli. Chest 66:597, 1974

198. Dube VE, Carlquist JH: Surgical treatment of leiomyosarcoma of the inferior vena cava: Report of a case. Am Surg 37:87, 1971

199. Gue'don J, Mesnard J, Poisson J, Kuss R: Hypertension re'novasculaire par leiomyosarcoma de la Veine Cava Inf'erieure, Gue'rison de l'Hypertension et Survie de 2 ans apre's Intervention Chirurgicale. Ann Med Interne (Paris) 121:905, 1970

200. Hivet M, Poilleux J, Gastard J, Hernandez C: Sarcome de la Veine Cave Inf'erieure. Nouvelle Presse Med 2:569, 1973

201. Johansen JK, Nielsen R: Leiomyosarcoma of the inferior vena cava. Acta Chir Scand 137:181, 1971

202. Juraj MN, Midell AI, Bederman S, et al: Primary leiomyosarcoma of the inferior vena cava. Report of a case and review of the literature. Cancer 26:1349, 1970

203. Kalsbeek HL: Leiomyosarcoma of the inferior vena cava. Arch Chir Neerl 26:35, 1974

204. Kevorkian J, Cento DP: Leiomyosarcoma of the large arteries and veins. Surgery 73:390, 1973

205. Stuart FP, Barker WH: Palliative surgery for leiomyosarcoma of the inferior vena cava. Ann Surg 177:237, 1973

206. Wray RC, Dawkins H: Primary smooth muscle tumors of the inferior vena cava. Ann Surg 174:1009, 1971

207. Abell MR: Leiomyosarcoma of the inferior vena cava. Review of the literature and report of two cases. Am J Clin Path, 28:272, 1957

208. Lunning P: Flebosarcoom van de vena femoralis. Nederl, T Geneesk 112:713, 1968

209. de Vries WM: Primary sarcoma of the veins of left leg. Atlas of Selected Cases of Pathological Anatomy. Amsterdam, JG de Bussy Ltd., 1933, p 16

210. Salm R: Primary fibrosarcoma of aorta. Cancer 29:73, 1972

211. Brodowski W: Primares sarcom der Aorta thoracica mit Verbreitung des Neugebildes in der unteren Korperhalfte. Jahresb Leistung Fortschr Ges Med 8:213, 1873

212. Ali MY, Lee GS: Sarcoma of the pulmonary artery. Cancer 17:1220, 1964

213. Auffermann H: Primare Aortengeschwulst eigentumlichen Riesenzellen. Z Krebsforshc 11:298, 1912

214. Detrie P: Tumeur primitive intravasculaire de l'aorte. J Chir (Paris) 80:666, 1960

215. Miura M: Das primare Riesenzellensarcoma der Aorta thoracica. Int Beitr Wissensch Med Festschr R Virchow. 2:249, 1891

216. Nencki L: Zur Kenntnis der Primartumoren der gorssen Gefasstamme. Ueber einen Fall von Primarem Sarcom der Aorta abdominalis. Cardiologica 10:1, 1946

217. Karhoff B: Primartumor der Aorta. Zbl Allg Path 89:46, 1952

218. Kovaleva AN, Press BO: A case of primary sarcoma of the intima of the aorta (in Russian). Arkh Pat 21:62, 1959

219. Kaignodova PE, Berezovskaya EK: Endothelioma of the thoracic aorta (in Russian). Gudn Khun 5:88, 1963

220. Zeitlhofer J, Holzner JH, Krepler P: Primares fibromyxosarkom der Aorta. Krebsarzt 18:259, 1963

221. Smeloff EA, Reece JM, Masters JH: Primary intraluminal malignant tumor of the aorta. Am J Cardiol 15:107, 1965

222. Sladden RA: Neoplasia of aortic intima. J Clin Path 17:602, 1964

223. Bowles LT, Ring EM, Hill WT, Cooley DA: Haemangiopericytoma in a resected thoracic aortic aneurysm. Ann Thorac Surg 1:746, 1965

224. Blenkinsopp WK, Hobbs JT: Pedunculated hemangiopericytoma attached to the thoracic aorta. Thorax 21:193, 1966

225. Kattus AA, Longmire WP, Cannon JA, Webb R, Johnson C: Primary intraluminal tumors of the aorta producing malignant hypertension. N Engl J Med 262:694, 1960

226. Burns WA, Kanhonwa S, Tillman L, Saini N, Herman JB: Fibrosarcoma occurring at the site of a plastic vascular graft. Cancer 29:66, 1972

227. Geschieter CF, Copeland MM: Tumors of Bone, 3rd ed. Philadelphia, Lippincott, 1949

228. Cunningham MP, Arlen M: Medullary fibrosarcoma of bone cancer. Cancer 21:31, 1968

229. Dahlin DC, Ivins JC: Fibrosarcoma of bone. Cancer 23:35, 1969

230. Jaffe HL: Tumors and Tumorous Conditions of the Bones and Joints. Philadelphia, Lea and Febiger, 1958, p 298

231. Huvos AG: Primary fibrosarcoma of bone. A clinicopathologic study of 18 patients. NY State J Med 76:552, 1976

232. Weiss SW, Enzinger FM: Malignant fibrous histiocytoma. An analysis of 200 cases. Cancer 41:2250, 1978

233. Kempson RL, Kyriakos M: Fibroxanthosarcoma of the soft tissues: A type of malignant fibrous histiocytoma. Cancer 29:961, 1972

234. Kyriakos M, Kempson RL: Inflammatory fibrous histiocytoma, malignant fibrous histiocytoma, malignant histiocytoma, and epithelioid sarcoma: A comparative study of 65 tumors. Cancer 37:1584, 1976

235. Soule EH, Enriquez P: Atypical fibrous histiocytoma, malignant fibrous histiocytoma, malignant histiocytoma, and epithelioid sarcoma: A comparative study of 65 tumors. Cancer 30:128, 1972

236. Weiss SW, Enzinger FM: Myxoid variant of malignant fibrous histiocytoma. Cancer 39:1672, 1977

237. McCarthy EF, Matsuno T, Dorfman HD: Primary malignant fibrous histiocytoma of bone: A study of 35 cases. Human Path 10:57, 1979

238. Spanier SS, Enneking WF, Enriquez P: Primary malignant fibrous histiocytoma of bone. Cancer 36:2084, 1975

239. Solomon MP, Sutton AL: Malignant fibrous histiocytoma of the soft tissues of the mandible. Oral Surg 35:653, 1973

240. Ferlito A, Recher G, Polidro F, Rossi M: Malignant pleomorphic fibrous histiocytoma of the larynx (further observation). J Laryngol Otol 93:1021, 1979

241. Usher SM, Beckley S, Merrin CE: Malignant fibrous histiocytoma of the retroperitoneum and genitourinary tract. A clinicopathological correlation and review of the literature. J Urol 122:105, 1979

242. Raghavaiah NV, Mayer RF, Hagitt R, Soloway MS: Malignant fibrous histiocytoma of the kidney. J Urol 123:951, 1980

243. Williamson JC, Johnson JD, Lamm DL, Tio F: Malignant fibrous histiocytoma of the spermatic cord. J Urol 123:785, 1980

244. Sewell R, Levine BA, Harrison GK, Tio F, Schwesinger WH: Primary malignant fibrous histiocytoma of the intestine—Intussusception of a rare neoplasm. Dis Colon Rectum 23:198, 1980

245. Chen W, Chan CW, Mok CK: Malignant fibrous histiocytoma of the mediastinum. Cancer 50:797, 1982

246. Kern WH, Huges PK, Myer BW, Harley DP: Malignant fibrous histiocytoma of the lung. Cancer 44:1793, 1979

13

Tumors of the Muscle Tissue

Tapas K. Das Gupta

LEIOMYOMAS

Leiomyomas seldom occur in the soft somatic tissues but are relatively common in the gastrointestinal tract and uterus. Rare solitary cutaneous or subcutaneous leiomyomas have been found in most anatomic locations (Fig. 13.1). A conservative excision is usually curative.

Infrequently, a leiomyoma may occur in the retroperitoneum.[1-3] Pack and Ariel[4] reported one such instance in which the tumor was successfully excised. Vaginal leiomyomas occasionally appear to be hormone-dependent,[5-7] and there have been a number of case reports[5-6] describing a change in size and appearance of these polypoid lesions during pregnancy or under the influence of exogenous hormones.

Vascular leiomyomas are far more common than the cutaneous or subcutaneous varieties. As pointed out in Chapter 4, it is sometimes difficult to microscopically distinguish these tumors from angiomatous tumors. Occasionally they are painful; local excision is adequate.

Leiomyomas rarely occur as primary intraocular neoplasms,[8] and have often been mistaken for ocular malignant melanomas. Meyer and co-authors,[8] however, described seven cases of leiomyomas of the ciliary body from the Armed Forces Institute Registry of Ophthalmic Pathology, providing confirmatory data from their ultrastructural studies.

Visceral leiomyomas are common, especially those of the uterus and the gastrointestinal tract; in fact, uterine leiomyomas are one of the most common benign tumors encountered in women. Although only about one percent undergo malignant transformation, the possibility should be kept in mind. Aaro and associates,[9] in a review of Mayo Clinic material, found that, of 105 leiomyosarcomas, in 22 instances (21 percent) there was definite evidence of origin in a preexisting leiomyoma. This high incidence is probably skewed, since the Mayo Clinic is a referral center; but it emphasizes the possibility of malignant transformation. Rarely, some uterine leiomyomas metastasize, in spite of all the histologic criteria satisfying the benignity of the tumor.[10] Steiner[11] first used the term *metastasizing fibroleiomyoma* in a case report of a 36-year-old woman who died with bilateral lung involvement from an apparently benign tumor of the uterus. Spiro and McPeak[12] reviewed the literature and described seven additional cases of metastasizing leiomyoma, including one in the files of the Memorial Sloan-Kettering Cancer Center. In 1976, Pocock and co-workers[13] found a total of nine cases (Table 13.1).[11-18] It is obvious that the diagnosis of so-called metastasizing leiomyoma is retrospective and, whatever the histologic appearance might be, these tumors behave like leiomyosarcomas.

453

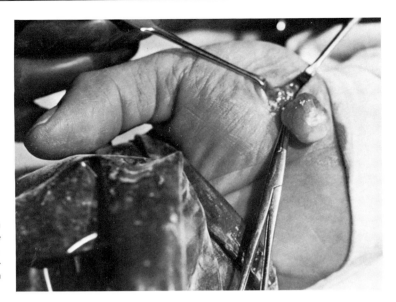

Figure 13.1. Operative specimen of a subcutaneous leiomyoma of the right hand in a 41-year-old man. Tumor was locally excised and patient has remained well for seven years (Fig. 4.41, Chapter 4).

Intravenous leiomyomatosis is a term used to describe a type of benign-appearing smooth muscle growth beyond the confines of the uterus. It is characterized by intravascular extension of cords and strands of benign myomatous tissue into the venous channels draining the pelvis. With the publications of Marshall and Morris,[19] Harper and Scully,[20] Thompson and co-workers,[21] and Steiner et al.,[22] at least 25 cases are now on record. Marshall and Morris[19] cited two instances in which death resulted from direct extension of the tumor up the inferior vena cava and into the right atrium, but metastasis has not been reported. With the exception of one patient who has survived 16 years without evidence of recurrence, the followup information on any of these cases has not exceeded four years. Although these tumors are intriguing and pose an intellectual challenge by their bizarre behavior in the presence of obvious histologic

TABLE 13.1. PULMONARY LEIOMYOMA ASSOCIATED WITH UTERINE LEIOMYOMA

Author	Patient Age	Duration of Chest X-Ray Changes	Solitary	Multiple	End Result
Steiner[11] (1939)	36	1½ yr		5 cm	Died of respiratory failure (autopsy)
Spiro and McPeak[12] (1960)	41	1 + yr	+		Alive and well at 10 + yr
Ariel and Trinidad[14] (1966)	40	2½ yr		+	Alive at 3 yr, but two new small pulmonary nodules
Konis and Belsky[15] (1966)	36	1 mo	+		No followup after thoracic surgery (1966)
Piccaluga and Capelli[16] (1967)	50	3 yr		+	Died of cardiac failure (autopsy)
Lefebvre et al.[17] (1971)	48	16 yr		+	Died with lung adenocarcinoma (autopsy)
Lefebvre et al.[17] (1971)	41	21 yr		+ 5 cm	Died of acute hemorrhagic pancreatitis (autopsy)
Barnes and Richardson[18] (1973)	25	1 yr		+	Omental leiomyoma noted 4 yr before chest x-ray changes noted
Pocock et al.[13] (1976)	41	21 yr		+	

benignity, clinically they are malignant and should be treated as such.

Leiomyomas of the Gastrointestinal Tract

Esophagus. Leiomyoma is the most common form of benign tumor found in the esophagus (Fig. 13.2), although compared to carcinoma it is still rare. Serematis and co-workers[23] reviewed the world literature and found 838 cases up to 1971, including 19 of their own. It occurs more frequently in men than in women, the ratio being 1.9 to 1.0. Over 50 percent of patients with leiomyoma of the esophagus are asymptomatic. Dysphagia and vague pain are the most common symptoms. Pyrosis is mentioned in the literature as being present in about 40 percent of cases, but it is considered mainly as a symptom of coexistent hiatal hernia. Diagnostic problems often arise, since smooth muscle tumors may mimic mediastinal neoplasms, cysts, or even aneurysms, or may complicate coexisting hiatal hernia and esophageal diverticulum. Transthoracic enucleation is the procedure of choice, although resection of the esophagus may be required in a few cases. Postoperative morbidity is minimal and results are excellent.

Stomach. Leiomyomas of the stomach usually are submucosal and located in the posterior wall. The majority of patients are older than 50 years. Both sexes and all races are affected. The diagnosis of leiomyoma of the stomach is usually incidental; however, as the tumor grows it can give rise to mucosal ulceration leading to either overt hemorrhage or occult bleeding. Sometimes it produces other gastric symptoms and the diagnosis is made by means of upper gastrointestinal x-rays. The treatment is local excision. If the tumor is large, partial gastrectomy might become necessary.

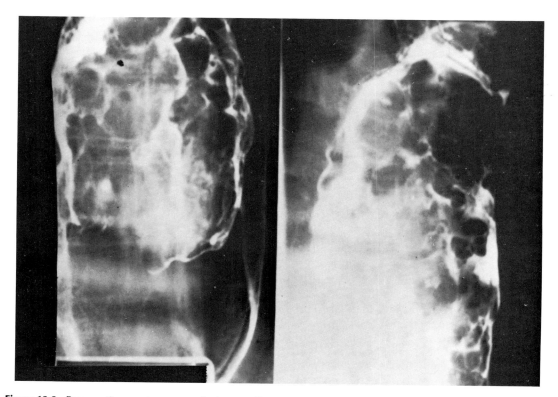

Figure 13.2. Preoperative roentgenogram (barium swallow) in a 59-year-old woman showing massive involvement of the intrathoracic esophagus with a polypoid mass consisting of both leiomyoma and leiomyosarcoma. A total esophagectomy was performed and the gastrointestinal continuity was accomplished by a left colon interposition. Patient refused any form of adjuvant treatment. One year later she was seen with metastatic leiomyosarcoma. (See also Fig. 4.43B, Chapter 4 for operative specimen.)

Small Intestine. Leiomyomas are second in frequency to adenomas among the benign intestinal neoplasms. Skandalakis and associates[24] comprehensively reviewed the subject in 1964 and found 713 cases of smooth muscle tumors of the small intestine. Leiomyomas are found in the duodenum, jejunum, and ileum, the majority being in the jejunum. These tumors are usually diagnosed by a long history of occult bleeding. Skandalakis and his co-workers[24] found that 72.6 percent of such patients had a history of gastrointestinal tract bleeding and 54.4 percent had pain as the predominant symptom. Occasionally the tumors were palpable. The treatment is excision of the tumor-bearing segment of the small intestine, with an end-to-end anastomosis.

Infrequently, leiomyomas occur in other viscera.[25-27] However, their rarity and the absence of symptoms frequently allow them to go unnoticed during the patient's lifetime.

TABLE 13.2. ANATOMIC LOCATION OF LEIOMYOBLASTOMAS AND SURVIVAL DATA ON PATIENTS AT MEMORIAL SLOAN-KETTERING CANCER CENTER*

Primary Site	No. Patients	Alive or Died of Other Disease	Died with Disease
Esophagus	1	—	1
Neck	1	1	—
Stomach	26	16	10
Duodenum	1	—	1
Jejunum	2	—	2
Ileum	2	1	1
Colon	2	1	1
Rectum	1	1	—
Retroperitoneum	1	—	1
Uterus	6	3	3
Vulva	1	1	—
Total	44	24	20 (45%)

Adapted from Lavin et al.,[30] 1972.

LEIOMYOBLASTOMA (EPITHELIOID LEIOMYOMA, BIZARRE LEIOMYOBLASTOMA)

Martin and co-workers[28] are credited with the first description of this clinicopathologic entity in 1960. In 1962, Stout[29] described a series of 69 cases of gastric leiomyoblastoma. Since Stout's paper, additional cases arising in the stomach and elsewhere have been reported.[30-34] Although these tumors can be malignant, the majority are benign. Lavin and associates[30] described 44 cases in the files of Memorial Sloan-Kettering Cancer Center. Table 13.2 shows the anatomic locations in these 44 patients, along with the survival data.

The stomach is the most common site of origin. In 1973, Abramson[34] collected over 190 cases of gastric leiomyoblastoma and added three of his own. The author has treated three cases at the University of Illinois and the West Side Veterans Administration Hospital. Gastric leiomyoblastoma is usually seen in patients above the age of 40 years and occurs about equally in both sexes. Gastric symptoms are similar to those of leiomyomas or any other gastric polypoid tumor. Abramson[34] found radiography to be the most valuable diagnostic aid. About 70 percent of the tumors are located in the antrum of the stomach, and in the majority of patients, a polypoid defect can be seen. Gastroscopy shows an umbilicated lesion, and a gastroscopic biopsy should provide a preoperative diagnosis with reasonable accuracy. Leiomyoblastomas are locally infiltrating lesions, a fact which should be taken into account when planning treatment. Additionally, some gastric leiomyoblastomas can metastasize and therefore should be treated as potentially malignant. Subtotal gastrectomy is the minimal acceptable form of therapy.

Abramson[34] described 23 cases of malignant gastric leiomyoblastoma. Lavin and co-workers[30] reported 10 cases, in 9 of which the patient died with metastatic disease on the average of three years after initial treatment and one year after clinical evidence of recurrence. Cornog[32] found 1 out of 10 cases of gastric leiomyoblastoma to be malignant. We have treated two cases of the malignant variety. Both patients are living apparently free of disease five years after subtotal gastrectomy.

Among the rare extragastric sites of leiomyoblastoma, the uterus appears to be the most common. Lavin et al.[30] found 6 such instances (14 percent) in a total series of 44 patients. Kurman and Norris[31] described the clinicopathologic features of 26 cases of uterine leiomyoblastoma in the files of the Armed Forces Institute of Pathology. Like their gastric counterparts, most of these tumors are benign, but on rare occasions they are known to metastasize.[31] In the series described by Lavin and co-workers,[30] three of six patients with uterine leiomyoblastoma died of metastatic disease at 1, 3, and 3.5 years, respectively, after undergoing abdominal hysterectomy. The three remaining patients were alive without evidence of disease 1, 21, and 40 years, respectively, after operation. In Kurman and Norris's[31] series of 26 patients, 25 were treated by hysterectomy. Followup information was available on 24. Nineteen of the 24 were free of disease at the time of the report in April 1976, the survival time ranging from 1 year, 9 months to 17 years, 8 months. Recurrence developed in three patients, and one died; the other two were treated successfully.

Leiomyoblastomas in other sites are so rare that a general guideline regarding their biologic behavior and principles of management is difficult to establish. Lavin, Hajdu, and Foote[30] found 12 patients with these tumors in unusual locations. The tumors in the two patients who died of the disease were located in the esophagus and retroperitoneum. Both tumors measured 10 cm. The patient with the esophageal primary survived nine years, and the one with retroperitoneal tumor died two years after palliative surgery. A leiomyoblastoma of the neck recurred locally six months after excision. Another patient with a vulvar primary was free of disease one year after wide local excision.

LEIOMYOSARCOMAS

Leiomyosarcomas of the soft tissue of the extremities are so rare that Pack and Ariel,[4] in a series of 717 cases of sarcoma of all types, did not encounter a single instance, although they observed a number in the viscera and retroperitoneum. Stout and Hill[35] reported 36 cases in the superficial tissues from 19 different institutions. Yannopoulos and Stout[36] added nine more cases found in patients younger than 16 years old, and in a later paper,[37] five in the mesentery and three in the omentum. Stout and Lattes,[38] on reviewing the files of the Laboratory of Surgical Pathology at Columbia University, found 75 cases in the retroperitoneum, one in the diaphragm, two in the mediastinum, and three in the orbit.

Leiomyosarcomas are found in many viscera, but most frequently they occur in the gastrointestinal tract[24,38-42] and the uterus.[9,43,44] They are encountered in connection with the smooth

TABLE 13.3. DISTRIBUTION OF LEIOMYOSARCOMA IN 57 PATIENTS, ACCORDING TO SITE OF ORIGIN (UNIVERSITY OF ILLINOIS SERIES, 1981)

Site	No. of Cases
Soft tissues of head and neck	2
Upper extremity (soft tissue)	4
Trunk	2
Lower extremity (soft tissue)	5
Soft tissues of pelvic wall	1
Stomach	7
Small intestine, including duodenum	11
Colon or rectum	2
Uterus	10
Vagina	1
Fallopian tube	1
Retroperitoneum	5
Kidney	1
Urinary bladder	1
Prostate	1
Round ligament	1
Inferior vena cava	1
Saphenous vein	1
Total	57

muscle coats of large veins and arteries.[45] In infants, they may arise in the prostate[46] and the urinary bladder.[47] Less often, they are reported in the respiratory tract[48-50] and, rarely, in the bone.[51,52] We have treated 57 cases of leiomyosarcoma in different sites at the University of Illinois (Table 13.3).

Leiomyosarcomas of the Soft Somatic Tissue

Of our 13 patients with leiomyosarcoma of the soft somatic tissues (Fig. 13.3A to 13.3D), 8 were female. Nine of the 13 tumors were in the extremities, a high incidence, since only occasional cases of leiomyosarcomas of the extremities have been encountered by most authors.[35-38] The majority of patients are women,[35] although this tumor has been reported in children.[36] Yannopoulos and Stout[36] described three female children with leiomyosarcomas of the superficial soft tissues and commented on two more from the literature. Botting, Soule, and Brown,[53] reviewing the files of Mayo Clinic, found five cases in children, three of whom were girls. The youngest of the nine patients at the University of Illinois Hospital was

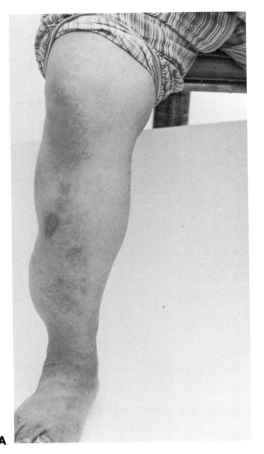
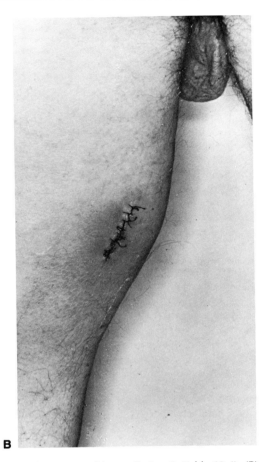

Figure 13.3. **(A)** Leiomyosarcoma of the lateral aspect of right leg of a 56-year-old man (Patient 2, Table 13.4). **(B)** Tumor of right medial thigh in a 57-year-old man.

a 15-year-old girl. Because of the rarity of leiomyosarcomas in the extremities, the data on all nine patients are briefly presented in Table 13.4.

The clinical data given in Table 13.4 and the information gleaned from published reports[35-38,53] can be used to develop some general guidelines for the management of leiomyosarcomas of the somatic tissues. Although the number of cases is few, it is appropriate to suggest that primary leiomyosarcomas in these locations probably should be treated by wide resection. The regional node-bearing areas should be taken into consideration when planning primary therapy. Patient 2 (Fig. 13.3A), refused a radical groin dissection, and inguinofemoral node metastases developed 14 months after an above-the-knee amputation. The five patients who survived five years or more without recurrence

underwent regional node dissection at the time of primary therapy (Table 13.4). Recently, one other patient was referred to us after the development of axillary node metastases from a cutaneous primary tumor in the lateral trunk. Weingrad and Rosenberg[54] analyzed the incidence of regional lymph node metastases in leiomyosarcomas and found that, in a collected series of cases, in all sites and at all stages the overall incidence was 11 percent. However, the data analyzed by these authors were somewhat confusing. Although it is difficult to quantitate the true incidence of regional node metastases, unless otherwise contraindicated we advocate a regional node dissection in extremity and truncal leiomyosarcomas of the soft tissues.

With the increasing use of adjuvant chemotherapy and radiation therapy, the need for

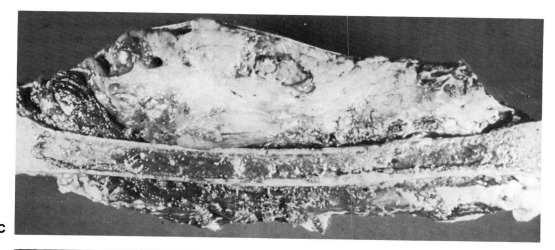

C

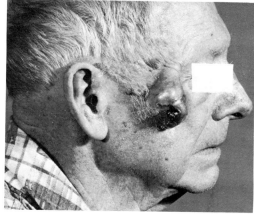

D

Figure 13.3. (C) Operative specimen of the thigh (Patient 3, Table 13.4) **(D)** Recurrent leiomyosarcoma of the skin of face of a 78-year-old man. Following wide excision he was treated with radiation therapy but died with pulmonary metastases 1.5 years later.

amputation in leiomyosarcomas of the extremities has considerably diminished. Our most recent experience suggests that malignant smooth muscle tumors are sensitive to chemotherapy. The judicious use of a multimodality treatment program after wide soft tissue resection and node dissection will adequately control most primary leiomyosarcomas and will improve the overall end result. Today Patient 1 in our series would not be subjected to a forequarter amputation without a trial of the above-mentioned treatment program.

Stout and Hill[35] found that in a series of 34 determinant cases only 12 (35 percent) survived with no evidence of tumor. Eleven (32 percent) died with tumor and another 11 (32 percent) were alive after either local recurrence or metastases, or both. Primary therapy failed in 22 (64 percent) of the patients in that collected series. A review of the treatment methods indi-

cates that in most instances the excision was inadequate. In a group of nine such patients at the University of Illinois Hospital, seven (77 percent) were living and well at the end of two years, and five (55 percent) at the end of five years (Table 13.4). Lindberg and co-workers[55] recently tried to evaluate the role of radiation therapy following conservative surgery in patients with leiomyosarcoma. Although the primary locations were not specified, the overall incidence of local recurrence in their series was 37.5 percent, considerably higher than in our series. Based on our own experience, we recommend a well-planned wide excision of the primary tumor, with appropriate regional node dissection when feasible. Along with this we strongly recommend adjuvant chemotherapy. Recently, without curtailing the extent of excision, we have initiated a program of additional preoperative intra-arterial infusion and radia-

TABLE 13.4 CLINICAL SUMMARY OF NINE PATIENTS WITH LEIOMYOSARCOMA OF THE EXTREMITIES (UNIVERSITY OF ILLINOIS SERIES, 1981)

Patient	Age	Sex	Location and Size of Primary Tumor	Status of Primary Tumor When First Seen at U of I	Regional Node Status	Type of Treatment	Recurrence (Local)	Metastases	End Result
1	15	F	L upper arm, 4-cm ovoid tumor	Referred after excision biopsy	–	Forequarter amputation	–	–	8 yr, N.E.D.†
2	56	M	R leg (Fig. 13.3A), 8-cm ovoid mass	Intact primary	Not enlarged at time of primary	Above-knee amputation	–	Regional node metastases	2 yr, Dead
3*	57	F	R medial thigh (Fig. 13.3C), 10 cm × 8 cm	Referred after a wedge biopsy	Not palpable	Radical groin dissection with hip joint disarticulation	–	Microscopic nodes in groin	6 yr, N.E.D.
4	55	F	R thigh, 6 × 5 cm	Referred after excision, radiated 6500 rads	+	Muscle group excision with node dissection	–	Nodes, liver, brain	2 yr, Dead
5	56	M	R upper arm, 6 × 5 cm	Intact primary	–	Muscle group excision with axillary dissection	–	–	5 yr, N.E.D.
6	48	F	R groin, original size of tumor, 5 × 4 cm, enucleated	Intact primary	–	Hemipelvectomy	–	–	5 yr, N.E.D.
7	46	M	R palm, 3 × 4 cm	Intact primary	–	Wide excision with axillary node dissection	–	1 Positive node	7 yr, N.E.D.
8	52	F	R medial arm, 8 × 12 cm	Intact primary	–	Intra-arterial infusion preop. RT, muscle group excision with axillary dissection	–	–	2½ yr, N.E.D.
9	48	F	Left posterior thigh, 5 × 6 cm	Recurrent tumor	+	Muscle group excision with groin dissection	–	2 Positive nodes	3 yr, N.E.D.

*Patients 3 and 6–9 received adjuvant chemotherapy (Table 8.17 Chapter 8).
†No evidence of disease.

tion therapy for Stage III extremity leiomyosarcomas (Chapter 8). We think this multimodality regimen will further curtail the need for amputation, without lowering the cure rate.

Gastrointestinal Tract

Twenty cases of leiomyosarcoma of the gastrointestinal tract constitute our present series, seven being in the stomach, one in the duodenum, six in the jejunum, four in the ileum, and two in the colon and rectum.

Stomach. Berg and McNeer[56] assessed the incidence of gastric leiomyosarcoma to be 1.3 percent of all gastric neoplasms. The clinical presentation of these tumors is similar to that of all other submucosal tumors. In large lesions a preoperative diagnosis either radiographically or by means of gastroscopy and biopsy is possible (Fig. 13.4). These tumors are commonly located in the posterior wall of the greater curvature of the stomach. The ideal treatment is partial or subtotal gastrectomy. Berg and McNeer[56] found that tumors smaller than 10 cm had a low incidence of regional metastases. Recurrence or regional node metastases is usually found in the omentum, mesentery, and liver.

Regional node metastases is less frequent than with leiomyosarcomas of the small intestine.

The results of treatment of gastric leiomyosarcoma are relatively good. In the 24 cases reported by Berg and McNeer,[56] 11 (46 percent) of the patients died, the crude survival rate being 54 percent. In 1971, Bergis and co-workers[57] found a five-year survival rate of 50 percent and a ten-year rate of 35 percent. In their study of 52 patients, those treated with a curative gastric resection had a 62 percent five-year survival rate. It appears that high histologic grade, large tumor size (>5 cm diameter), and invasion of adjacent organs adversely affect the prognosis. Of our seven patients, four had lower grade tumors without involvement of the adjacent organs and all four have been free of disease for five years or more.

Leiomyosarcoma of the stomach is also seen in children. Yannopoulos and Stout[36] found one case in the literature and described two cases of their own. One of these three patients died of metastasis to the liver and the other two were alive and well at two and seven years, respectively. Botting et al.[53] had four childhood cases in their files at the Mayo Clinic. Two patients were long-term survivors following gastric re-

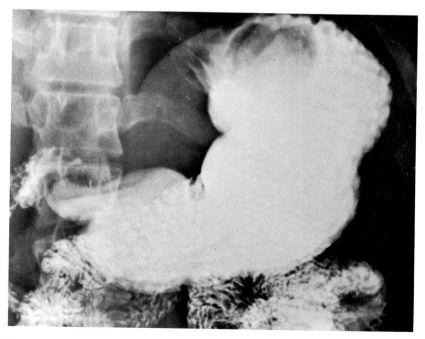

Figure 13.4. Leiomyosarcoma of the gastric fundus in a man 44 years old. A radical subtotal gastrectomy was performed. All the nodes were negative. Patient received adjuvant chemotherapy and is still disease-free after four years.

section. The third patient died 39 months after initial resection, with two instances of recurrence between initial operation and death. The fourth patient died of massive recurrence within three months.

Small Intestine. In 1955, Starr and Dockerty[58] reviewed the Mayo Clinic experience with 76 myomatous tumors of the small intestine, and an additional 230 cases reported elsewhere. In more than 60 percent of the Mayo Clinic patients the tumors were leiomyosarcomas. In 1964, Skandalakis et al.[24] reviewed the location of 259 reported cases of leiomyosarcomas in the small intestine and found the incidence to be as follows: duodenum, 66; jejunum, 77; ileum, 84. In 8 cases, the tumors involved both the jejunum and ileum, and in the remaining 24, the exact location could not be ascertained. Infrequently, these tumors are multicentric.[58] Leiomyosarcomas of the duodenum and small intestines are usually found in adults of both sexes. Neither Yannopoulos and Stout[36] nor Botting et al.[53] found any instance in children. Skandalakis and associates[24] reported that in their 259 cases fewer than 10 patients were under the age of 10 years. Of the 11 patients with leiomyosarcoma of the duodenum and small intestine in our series (Table 13.3), one was a 13-year-old boy with leiomyosarcoma of the jejunum.

The clinical presentation of small bowel leiomyosarcomas is not characterized by any particular symptom or constellation of symptoms. Melena or hematemesis is probably the most common associated symptom. Palpable tumors or pain due to intussusception are rarely encountered. Radiographic findings are positive in about 60 percent of patients and, when positive, confirm the presence of a small intestine tumor, characterized either by filling defects or by outlining the contour of a polypoid tumor.

Leiomyosarcomas of the small intestine metastasize to surrounding viscera, omentum, mesentery, liver, lung, and, in some cases, to the regional nodes.[24,42,59] About one third of all leiomyosarcomas have metastasized by the time they are operated upon.[24,42,58]

The ideal treatment is resection. Segmental resection should be done in jejunal and ileal tumors, but a duodenal leiomyosarcoma might require a pancreaticoduodenectomy. This author had one patient with duodenal leiomyosarcoma who successfully underwent pancreaticoduodenectomy at age 66, but died five years later of a cardiovascular accident. Five of 11 patients were treated by adjuvant chemotherapy. We think that for patients with large tumors or in whom there is evidence of regional extension, adjuvant chemotherapy (Chapter 8) is justified. If there is any doubt regarding adequacy of excision of the primary tumor, postoperative radiation therapy is also indicated. In their review, Skandalakis and associates[24] found that only 23 of their 259 patients were followed up for five years or longer. Of those for whom end result data were available, 82 percent had died of metastatic disease. In 1967, McPeak[42] reported that of the 16 patients treated at Memorial Sloan-Kettering Cancer Center, five (31 percent) survived for five years. Of this author's 11 patients (Table 13.3), five have been free of disease for five years, and one patient, as mentioned above, died after five years from unrelated causes, giving an overall tumor-free survival rate of 54 percent. The remaining five patients (45 percent) died with metastases within 36 months of initial surgery. In one, solitary metastasis to the right lung was found 14 months after resection, and a right lower lobe lobectomy was performed. The patient remained clinically free of disease for 18 months. Systemic metastases then developed and, in spite of multiple-agent chemotherapy, the patient died three months later.

Colon and Rectum. Leiomyosarcomas of the colon and rectum are rare. The most common symptoms are constipation, localized rectal pain, and rectal bleeding.[41,59] Quan and Berg[59] found that leiomyosarcomas constituted 0.1 percent of all smooth muscle tumors of the colon and rectum. The pattern of metastatic spread is similar to that of small intestine leiomyosarcomas. The treatment of choice for rectal lesions is still considered to be abdominoperineal resection,[59] although lesser procedures have been tried in some patients with apparently good results.[41,59] Our patient with rectal leiomyosarcoma was treated by abdominoperineal resection. In the past, the selection of the type of operation has not been based on any specific guideline. With increasing information on this disease, it appears that the smaller-sized tumors of the rectum can be treated with local resection and adjuvant radiation therapy.

Leiomyosarcoma of the Retroperitoneum

Retroperitoneal smooth muscle tumors are relatively uncommon.[3] In 1941, Golden and Stout[2] collected nine cases, six of which were malignant. Donnelly[60] reviewed 95 cases of retroperitoneal tumors without finding any instance of leiomyosarcoma. Pack and Ariel[4] described five cases in the retroperitoneum. In the files of the Laboratory of Surgical Pathology of Columbia University, Stout and Lattes[38] found 75 cases. We have treated five patients with retroperitoneal leiomyosarcoma (Table 13.5) (Fig. 13.5A and 13.5B).

Leiomyosarcomas of the retroperitoneal region are capable of reaching a large size, in contradistinction to the smaller lesions elsewhere, such as the superficial tissues or gastrointestinal tract. All five of our patients were seen initially because of abdominal pain and large intra-abdominal tumors. Because of their unimpeded growth potential, anatomic dissection of these tumors is difficult and in some instances almost impossible. Retroperitoneal leiomyosarcomas can locally infiltrate the surrounding viscera or can metastasize to the regional nodes and the liver. All our patients had visceral involvement. The incidence of lung metastases is similar to that for leiomyosarcomas in other sites. In one of our five patients, involvement of the right lobe of the liver necessitated partial resection of the liver (Patient 5).

The treatment of retroperitoneal leiomyosarcoma is complete excision with adjuvant chemotherapy and, when indicated, radiation therapy. However, the results of treatment will not substantially improve until the diagnosis of these tumors is made much earlier. Only two of our five patients remained well for three years, but later all had recurrent disease.

Leiomyosarcoma of the Mesentery

Yannopoulos and Stout[37] reported two cases of leiomyosarcoma and five cases of nonmalignant smooth muscle tumors of the mesentery. Paul and colleagues,[27] in 1968, reported an additional case. We have not come across any smooth muscle tumors in the mesentery or omentum, either benign or malignant.

Leiomyosarcomas of the Genitourinary Tract

Leiomyosarcomas of the genitourinary tract are also rare. Occasional cases of prostatic leiomyosarcomas have been reported in children.[46] Similarly, leiomyosarcomas of the kidney, bladder, spermatic cord, epididymis, and penis have also been described.[25,47,61-64] However, these are all rare instances and most reports are solitary case histories.

Male Genital Tract.

Prostate. Yannopoulous and Stout[36] described one instance of a 5-year-old boy with leiomyosarcoma of the prostate. The author has also treated one such case in an 8-year-old boy, who was first seen with dsysuria and a palpable suprapubic mass. The urologist in charge of the case performed a suprapubic cystostomy and intracystic removal of the tumor. When the histologic diagnosis was rendered, the child was referred to us for further management. After discussion with the operating surgeon, we treated the patient with irradiation. The family refused any further treatment and no followup data are available.

Spermatic Cord. Arlen, Grabstald, and Whitmore,[63] on reviewing the malignant tumors of the spermatic cord in the files of Memorial Sloan-Kettering Cancer Center, found only one case of leiomyosarcoma. They reported that only 18 such instances had appeared in the literature up to 1969. Buckley and Tolley[64] found a later case in the literature and added one of their own. The majority of patients were seen first with palpable tumors in the groin along the course of the spermatic cord. Diagnosis was established after excision of the tumor of the testis, with high ligation of the cord. Although no definitive guidelines for management are possible, it is recommended that these tumors, like leiomyosarcomas elsewhere, be treated by a multimodal management program.

Penis. Dehner and Smith[62] found three cases of leiomyosarcoma of the shaft of the penis in the files of the Armed Forces Institute of Pathology. One of the three patients had multiple local recurrences finally extending to the anterior abdominal wall, and the other two were living at the time the report was published.

Leiomyosarcoma of the scrotum is indeed rare. Recently, Johnson et al.[65] reported one case and upon review of the literature found only four additional cases.

Female Genital Tract.
Leiomyosarcomas of the female genital tract are not uncommon. Uterine

TABLE 13.5. SUMMARY OF CLINICAL FINDINGS IN FIVE PATIENTS WITH RETROPERITONEAL LEIOMYOSARCOMA TREATED AT THE UNIVERSITY OF ILLINOIS HOSPITAL

Patient	Age	Sex	Duration of Symptoms	Clinical Findings	Laboratory Findings	Primary Treatment	Patterns of Metastases	End Result	Comments
1	74	F	Two mo history of dull epigastric pain	Ill-defined nodular mass below liver edge, extending to umbilicus	All within normal limits angiogram refused	Resection of gross tumor	Lung, liver	Died at 57 mo with disease	—
2	40	M	Several mo	Palpable suprapubic mass (Fig. 13.5A and 13.5B)	Angiogram, retroperitoneal tumor (left)	Resection and postop radiation therapy	Lung, liver, brain	Died at 4 yr with disease	Recurrence 2 yr after primary resection, re-excised widespread metastases six months before death
3	37	F	Two mo chest pain abdominal pain	Icteric sclera, epigastric mass (liver met.), pelvic exam showed mass, cul-de-sac, ascites	Retroperitoneal mass with extreme pressure on all viscera	Exploratory laparotomy, mass totally unresectable, radiation therapy only	Widespread disease	Died at 4 mo with disease	Autopsy showed foci of adenocarcinoma in bile duct
4	65	F	Seven mo history of weight loss with change in bowel habits	Large retroperitoneal mass filling half of abdomen, 13 cm above pubic symphysis, pelvic masses	Venacavagram showed obstructed vena cava	Exploratory lap., unresectable, radiation therapy only	Widespread disease	Died at 8 mo with disease	No autopsy
5	64	F	Ten mo history of sacral pain	Palpable right abdominal mass	Angiogram outlined mass involving liver	Resected with partial resection of right lobe, adjuvant chemotherapy	—	Died at 2 yr with diffuse disease	—

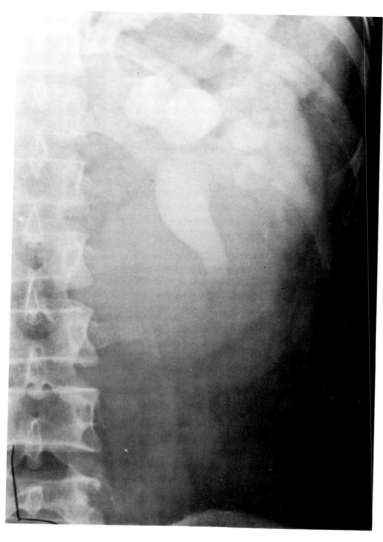

Figure 13.5. (A) Intravenous pyelogram showing the hydronephrotic displaced left kidney with a retroperitoneal tumor located inferiorly.

leiomyosarcomas[9,44,66-68] are the most frequent, but involvement of other parts has also been reported.[69-71] At the University of Illinois Hospital, we have come across 10 cases of leiomyosarcoma of the uterus, 1 of the fallopian tube, 1 of the vagina, and 1 of the round ligament.

Uterus. Leiomyomas, or fibroids, are the most common tumors encountered in the human uterus. Whereas the bulk of smooth muscle tumors occurring in other locations are malignant, those in the uterine musculature are benign in 99 percent of cases. Aaro, Symmonds, and Dockerty[9] reviewed the Mayo Clinic experience over a period of 26 years and found

105 cases of uterine leiomyosarcoma, constituting 59 percent of all the uterine sarcomas.

The majority of patients with uterine leiomyosarcomas are above the age of 40 years and there is no apparent relation to parity.[9,44,66,68] Aaro and co-workers[9] commented on the role of radiation therapy in the development of leiomyosarcomas. Instances have been reported in which uterine sarcomas developed years after irradiation for benign uterine bleeding. Of the 105 patients in the Mayo Clinic series,[9] seven had a history of previous roentgen or radium therapy to the pelvis for benign disease. Periods varying from 14 months to 33 years after irra-

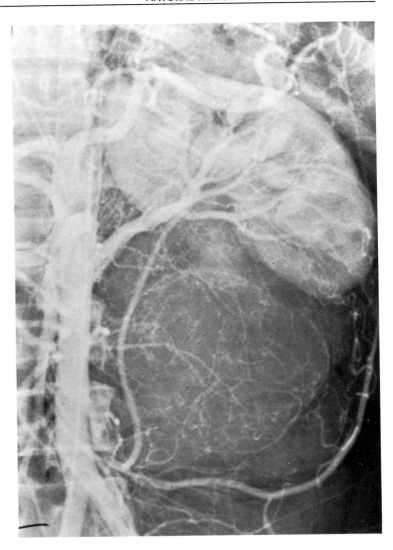

Figure 13.5. **(B)** Angiogram outlining the retroperitoneal tumor (Patient 2, Table 13.5).

diation elapsed before symptoms of malignancy developed. In recent years, however, such drastic treatment for functional uterine bleeding has been abandoned and radiation-induced leiomyosarcomas are not seen. We have no instance in the files of the University of Illinois Hospital.

Abnormal vaginal bleeding and abdominal or pelvic pain, along with a palpable tumor, constitute the most common presenting symptoms. In most instances, physical examinations of a pelvic mass with uterine localization is possible. Aaro and co-workers[9] found that three (2.8 percent) of 105 patients had an antecedent history of rapid growth of an apparent uterine fibroid. Montague et al.[68] documented a similar

case of leiomyosarcoma arising in a leiomyoma. In none of our patients was such the case.

The patterns of metastatic spread in uterine leiomyosarcoma are similar to those in other anatomic sites. Metastases to the lung and regional pelvic involvement are the most common forms of metastatic spread. Involvement of the liver, vagina, and other sundry sites is less common.

The clinical data on these patients are summarized in Table 13.6. In the Mayo Clinic series, of the 95 determinant patients, 30 (31.5 percent) survived for five years or longer. Of the ten patients in the University of Illinois group, two (20 percent) are disease-free after five years or

TABLE 13.6. SUMMARY OF CLINICAL FINDINGS IN TEN PATIENTS WITH UTERINE LEIOMYOSARCOMA TREATED AT THE UNIVERSITY OF ILLINOIS HOSPITAL

Patient No.	Age	Type of Treatment	Pelvic Recurrence	Metastasis	End Result	Remarks
1	56	Total abdominal hysterectomy and bilateral salpingo-oophorectomy	10 mo, mass in pelvis	Lung	Dead in 1 yr	Received pelvic radiation therapy and actinomycin D
2	58	Total abdominal hysterectomy, bilateral salpingo-oophorectomy	4 mo, mass in pelvis	Diffuse	Dead in 4 mo	Received actinomycin D
3	56	Total abdominal hysterectomy and bilateral salpingo-oophorectomy	Multiple pelvic and abdominal masses	Ascites	Died 9 mo later	Received postop irradiation when disease far advanced
4	66	Total abdominal hysterectomy and bilateral salpingo-oophorectomy	None	Liver and small intestine	Dead in 1 yr	Received postop radiation therapy
5	41	Total abdominal hysterectomy and bilateral salpingo-oophorectomy	None	None	Alive and well at 10 yr	Primary was small
6	59	Total abdominal hysterectomy and bilateral salpingo-oophorectomy; resection of abdominal wall	None	Lung, adrenals	Dead in $1\frac{1}{2}$ yr with disease	Tumor was large
7	62	Total abdominal hysterectomy and bilateral salpingo-oophorectomy (palliative)	None	Lung	Dead in 3 mo	Received adriamycin
8	55	Total abdominal hysterectomy and bilateral salpingo-oophorectomy	Regional nodes	Lung and liver	Dead in 11 mo	None
9	62	Total abdominal hysterectomy and bilateral salpingo-oophorectomy	None		Died of other causes	None
10	46	Total abdominal hysterectomy and bilateral salpingo-oophorectomy	—	—	Alive and well at 10 yr	—

more, and one patient died of unrelated causes. An overall survival rate of 30 percent has been reported by authors reviewing much larger series.[9,43,44]

Sixty of the 105 patients in the series reported by Aaro et al.[9] could be evaluated for correlation of the grade of malignancy of the primary tumor and the results of treatment. Of 18 with a grade 1 lesion, 13 survived for five years or more, as did 7 of 17 with grade 2, 3 of 12 with grade 3, and 2 of 13 with grade 4. When the gross anatomic extent of the lesion was correlated, these authors[9] found that, of 20 patients with malignancy limited to the myometrium, 14 survived five years. When the lesion involved the endometrium or the endocervix, 9 of 19 patients lived five years or more. However, only one of nine survived five years when uterine serosa was involved, and only 1 of 12 when the primary tumor showed extension beyond the uterus. Based on recent data on chemosensitivity of the tumor, it appears that patients with grades 3 and 4 uterine leiomyosarcomas should be treated with adjuvant chemotherapy.

Fallopian Tubes. Leiomyosarcoma of the fallopian tubes is indeed rare, as are all malignant tumors of this anatomic site. Because of its rarity,[72] no general guidelines regarding therapy can be devised. Only one such instance, in a 23-year-old woman, appears in our files. This patient was seen with a large tumor on the left side of the pelvis. A total abdominal hysterectomy and bilateral salpingo-oophorectomy was performed. The patient died with metastatic tumor within three years of diagnosis of the tumor.

Vagina. Like those of the fallopian tubes, leiomyosarcomas of the vagina are rare.[69,70] The largest series published was from the Mayo Clinic,[69] where eight cases were encountered from 1908 through 1961. No leiomyosarcomas of the vagina were reported in a 1971 study of vaginal cancers by Underwood and Smith.[71] Yannopoulous and Stout[36] reported one personal case of vaginal leiomyosarcoma in a girl of 13 and reviewed a case of vulvar leiomyosarcoma reported by Kelly.[73] The 13-year-old girl had a 7.5 × 5 × 4 cm lesion in the vagina, which was treated by local excision and irradiation. She has remained well for 17 years. Kelly's patient was 16 months old. After treatment by local excision and irradiation, local recurrence developed and she died 32 months after initial resection of the primary.

One patient with leiomyosarcoma of the vagina has been treated by this author. She is a 71-year-old woman who was first seen eight years ago with a polypoid mass in the posterior wall of the vagina about 4 cm from the outlet. A histologic diagnosis of leiomyosarcoma grade 3 was rendered and she was treated by posterior pelvic exenteration and vaginectomy. She is living disease-free eight years later.

Round Ligament. Leiomyosarcoma of the round ligament of the uterus is extremely uncommon. The same general guidelines can be used as for uterine or vaginal leiomyosarcomas. We have treated one such patient. She was first seen with a painful mass in the right groin. The tumor penetrated the periosteum of the pubis. A hemipelvectomy was done and she lived disease-free for 4.5 years.

Kidney. Until 1970, there were only 34 published cases of leiomyosarcoma of the kidney.[74] We have had only one such patient, and she was treated by radical nephrectomy (Fig. 13.6). However, within two years she had intra-abdominal recurrence along with a metastatic ulcerating tumor of the buttock. She was then placed on a CYVADIC regimen. After an indolent course for 13 months, the disease progressed rapidly and she died two months later.

Usually the most common symptom is pain on the side of the lesion, followed by hematuria and weight loss. Although the preoperative diagnosis of a renal neoplasm is straightforward, the histologic diagnosis is usually made after operation. The majority of patients described in the literature were found to have local recurrence or metastases, or both, following resection. In none of these cases, though, was there an adequate trial of adjuvant chemotherapy and radiotherapy.[74-76] Of the 17 patients on whom followup data are available, the longest survival time was 38 months.

Urinary Bladder. Leiomyosarcoma of the bladder is an extremely rare entity.[47,77] We recently saw such a case in a 32-year-old woman. She was treated by total cystectomy and construction of an ileal conduit. She refused adjuvant chemotherapy, which we had recommended.

Veins and Arteries

Smooth muscle tumors arising from the vasculature are relatively rare, although a number of instances of leiomyosarcoma arising from both large arteries[45,78-82] and veins[81,83-135] have been reported. There appear to be more case reports of venous leiomyosarcoma than of their arterial counterparts. The reason is unknown.

Major Arteries. Leiomyosarcomas originating in the major arteries are indeed rare.[45,78-82] The majority of reported cases have been in the pulmonary vasculature.[45,78-81] Even in this site, often the diagnosis is made at the operating table during thoracotomy performed for a suspected pulmonary embolus, or at postmortem examination. Because of the rarity of the tumor and absence of any characteristic clinical findings, guidelines for management cannot be drawn.

Veins. The rarity of these tumors is evident by the fact that in 1957, Abell,[86] in reporting two cases of leiomyosarcoma of the inferior vena

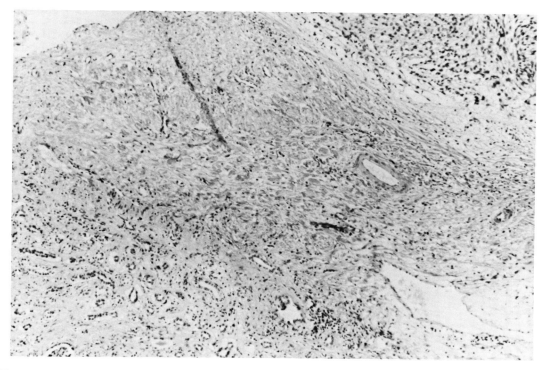

Figure 13.6. Micrograph of a leiomyosarcoma of kidney (H&E. Original magnification × 100). Patient died of massive intra-abdominal recurrence.

cava, could cull only six other cases, either benign or malignant, arising from the inferior vena cava. Nineteen years later, in 1976, Bailey and co-workers,[106] reviewing the literature on leiomyosarcomas of the inferior vena cava, found 46 cases, including two of Abell's and one of their own. Of interest is that 22 of the 46 were not diagnosed until autopsy. The reported incidence of tumors arising from other major veins is still rare. Stout and Hill[35] found only one instance in the superficial veins. In 1960, Thomas and Fine[110] found five cases of leiomyosarcomas of other veins, including one case of their own of the internal jugular vein, and also the case of the femoral vein already reported by Stout and Hill.[35] Szasz et al.[83] reviewed the literature in 1969 and found 19 cases of venous sarcoma, some of which probably did not represent true leiomyosarcomas.

Inferior Vena Cava. Of all the veins, the inferior vena cava is the most common site for the development of this rare tumor. We have treated only one such case (Fig. 13.7). After a preoperative diagnosis of a leiomyosarcoma of the

inferior vena cava, the patient was operated upon and the retroperitoneal tumor was excised. She remained well for 20 months. A solitary soft tissue metastatic lesion of the chest wall then developed, which was excised. Two months later she was found to have spinal cord metastases and, after multiple palliative procedures, she died three years after her initial operation. At no time was there any evidence of recurrence in the retroperitoneal area, the site of the primary leiomyosarcoma.

In 1966, Jonasson and co-workers,[107] from the U of Illinois, reported an additional case in which the extent of the disease was discovered only at autopsy (Fig. 13.8A to 13.8C).

Leiomyosarcoma of the inferior vena cava is primarily a disease of women, usually occurring in their 60s, although cases in younger patients have been reported.[87-95] Most frequently the tumor involves the middle third of the inferior vena cave[87,93,96,97] and both local spread and distant metastases are common.[95,107,108] Extensive local spread, with involvement of more than one segment of the inferior vena cava, the he-

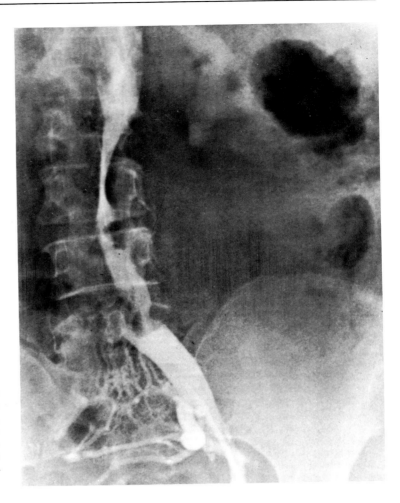

Figure 13.7. Inferior venacavogram showing the sarcomatous involvement of the inferior vena cava. The tumor was diagnosed preoperatively, one of the unusual instances of a preoperative cavogram outlining a leiomyosarcoma originating in the inferior vena cava.

patic veins,[106,111] the right atrium,[91] and the renal veins,[128,130] is not unusual. The most common sites of metastatic disease are the lung and liver. Associated leiomyomas of the uterus and esophagus have been reported,[95] as have primary carcinomas of the colon, breast, and lung.

Symptoms vary from those of our patient, with a palpable tumor, to those with rapidly progressive hepatic failure or massive edema from venous obstruction.[95,106-108,111] The signs and symptoms vary with the location of the tumor, the Budd-Chiari syndrome being found with the upper-third lesions,[111] renal vein thrombosis with the middle-third,[105] and isolated lower extremity edema with the lower-third.[105,129] In patients with no venous obstruction, the growth of the tumor is primarily extraluminal. Relatively few cases are operated upon with the hope of control of the primary tumor (Table 13.7).

Preoperative angiography, both arterial and venous, is of utmost importance. The local recurrence rate following surgery for the primary lesion has been reported to be 36 percent.[95] This high rate of local failure probably represents a lack of aggressiveness on the part of the operating surgeon at the time of initial operation. Additionally, the use of adjuvant therapy might alter the prognosis in a number of these patients. Of the 22 collected patients who were operated upon for cure (Table 13.7), seven (32 percent) lived for two years or more. This figure should improve with aggressive resection and the use of adjuvant chemotherapy and radiation therapy.

Veins Other Than Vena Cava. In a 1960 review of primary leiomyosarcomas of the veins, Thomas and Fine[110] found 13 cases, only five of which were in veins other than the inferior vena

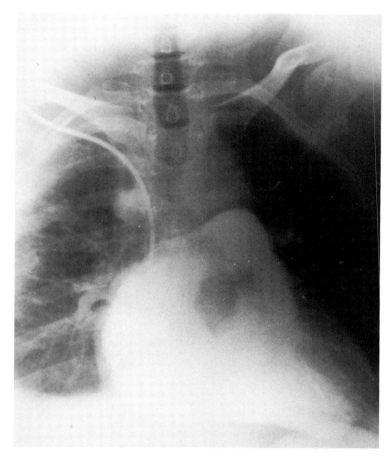

Figure 13.8. (A) Venous angiocardiogram. Note filling defect in venous outflow tract.

cava: one each in the femoral, inferior colic, internal jugular, antecubital, and saphenous.[110] Since then, only a few such case reports have appeared. In 1969, Szasz and associates[83] found a total of 19 cases. A recent review of the literature showed 29 cases, and the addition of one of our own brings the total to 30 (Table 13.8). Our patient had a leiomyosarcoma of the saphenous system of the left leg. Following an attempted vein stripping for what was erroneously thought to be varicosity of the long saphenous vein of the left lower extremity, this 63-year-old woman was referred to us for further management. The segment of the saphenous vein excised elsewhere showed leiomyosarcoma. Multiple subcutaneous nodules were still palpable along the course of the long saphenous vein. An en bloc wide soft tissue resection was performed, beginning at the medial malleolus and ending at the saphenofemoral junction, with in-continuity superficial groin

dissection. The nodes were negative. The patient is still disease-free ten years after excision of the primary leiomyosarcoma.

The major point to be emphasized in venous leiomyosarcomas is that, with proper excision, most patients can be salvaged.

Recently, primary leiomyosarcomas have been found to occur in various unusual anatomic sites.[49-52,136-138] Because of the rarity of this tumor in these locations, no guidelines regarding treatment can be developed. For the present, these cases should be recorded in detail so that further clinical data can be generated.

STRIATED MUSCLE TUMORS

Rhabdomyoma

An occasional benign tumor of the skeletal muscle has been described in the striated muscle of the somatic tissues, larynx, vulva, vagina, ton-

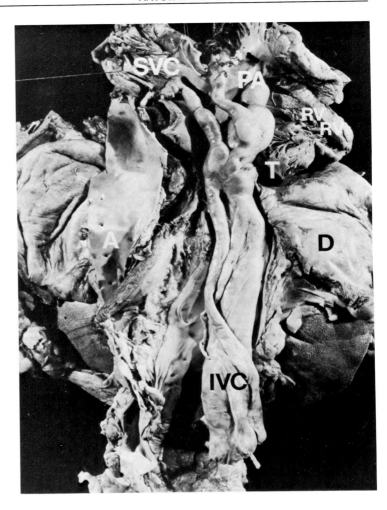

Figure 13.8. (B) Autopsy specimen. Posterior aspect of viscera; vena cava has been opened to show the intraluminal extension of the tumor. IVC—inferior vena cava; D—diaphragm; A—aorta; SVC—superior vena cava; PA—pulmonary artery; RV—right ventricle; and T—tricuspid valve.

gue, and nasal cavity.[139-142] Moran and Enterline[142] found only 11 acceptable cases and added one of their own. These tumors are benign and seldom grow to large size. The symptom usually depends on the location; for example, in the vulva a protruding grapelike mass arouses concern, and in the larynx, patients become hoarse. A diagnosis of rhabdomyoma is usually made after excision of the tumor. Excision is usually adequate.

Rhabdomyoma of the heart is found most often in neonates and children (Fig. 4.47A and 4.47B, Chapter 4). In 1939, LaBate[143] collected 51 cases, 46 of which were in children younger than 15 years. Batchelor and Maun[144] found that 52 percent died in the first year of life. Most likely these tumors represent a developmental malformation.[145] Pack and Ariel[4] noted that car-

diac rhabdomyomas were frequently associated with other congenital anomalies such as harelip, cleft palate, cystic kidneys, sebaceous adenomas, and tuberosclerosis.

Rhabdomyosarcoma

Rhabdomyosarcomas are usually classified into three different histologic types: embryonal, pleomorphic, and alveolar. The clinical features of each type will be discussed.

Embryonal Rhabdomyosarcoma (Sarcoma Botryoides).

Embryonal rhabdomyosarcomas are encountered in all parts of the human body, including the viscera.[4,38,146] For clarity of presentation, the discussion will be divided according to the three most common anatomic sites of presentation: the head and neck region, the trunk

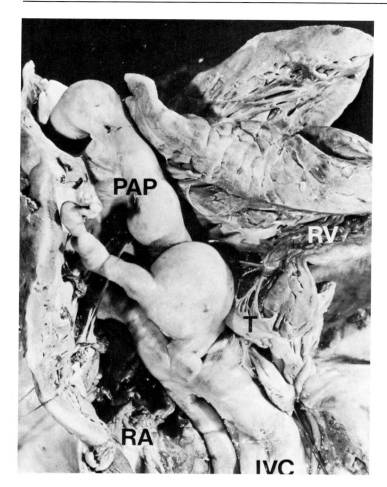

Figure 13.8. (C) Closeup of right heart chambers opened to demonstrate tumor coming from inferior vena cava (IVC) into right atrium (RA), crossing tricuspid valve (T) into right ventricle (RV) and protruding out the pulmonary artery (PA). (Courtesy of O. Jonasson, M.D., Cancer 19:1311, 1966, JB Lippincott.)

and the extremities. Certain other specific sites will also be discussed. Embryonal rhabdomyosarcoma in mucosal-lined cavities develop the gross appearance of a cluster of grapes, resulting in the clinical term botryoid sarcoma.

Head and Neck Region. Embryonal rhabdomyosarcomas of the head and neck region can probably be better subgrouped into those arising in the region of the orbit and those arising elsewhere within the head and neck region.

The orbit is a common site.[146-155] Jones and co-workers[148] found it to be the commonest primary malignant orbital tumor of childhood. Masson and Soule,[151] reviewing the Mayo Clinic material, found 88 cases of embryonal rhabdomyosarcoma from 1910 through 1964; 22 (25 percent) were in the orbit, most often originating in the upper inner quadrant and not infrequently involving the upper eyelid early in their clinical course. Sutow et al.,[156] in their review of the M. D. Anderson Hospital material, found the orbital variety in 19 percent of a total 78 patients with head and neck rhabdomyosarcomas. Our experience is similar: the primary tumor was in the orbit in 8 of 31 such patients (26 percent).

Although the orbital location is more common in infants and children, no age is immune. Masson and Soule[151] reported an age range from two weeks to 77 years. Of the eight patients with orbital rhabdomyosarcoma treated by the author (Table 13.9), six were male and two were female. Seven were between two and nine years of age, and one was a 45-year-old woman. This ratio reflects the overall high incidence in male children reported in most series.[147-151,153-156]

Exophthalmos is probably the most characteristic sign of true orbital rhabdomyosarcoma

TABLE 13.7. LEIOMYOSARCOMA OF THE INFERIOR VENA CAVA: A CLINICAL SUMMARY OF 22 PATIENTS TREATED WITH RESECTION OF THE PRIMARY TUMOR

Patient	Author(s)	Year	Age (Yr)	Sex	Size of Tumor	Extent of Primary Tumor	Recurrence	Metastases	End Result
1	Melchior[88]	1928	24	F	5 cm	?	—	—	Postop death
2	Cope and Hunt[84]	1954	33	F	6 cm	?	Yes	?	?
3	Allan et al.[89]	1964	67	M	20 cm	—	Yes	Pancreas	Living and well at 3 yr
4	Caplan et al.[90]	1966	72	F	20 cm	—	—	—	No data
5	Gariepy and Pope[91]	1967	47	F	15 cm	Stomach involved	Yes	Liver and lung	Living 5 yr after resection of recurrence
6	Nartowicz et al.[92]	1967	61	F	10 cm	—	—	—	Living and well, 3½ yr
7	Staley et al.[93]	1967	65	F	15 cm	—	Yes	Skin	Died after 1 yr w/CA of the breast
8	Hopson et al.[94]	1968	72	F	7 cm	—	—	—	
9	Gue'don et al.[95]	1970	43	F	"Large"	Renal vein	—	Lung	Dead at 2 yr
10	Jurayj et al.[96]	1970	66	F	—	—	Yes	Diffuse	Dead at 8 mo
11	Dube and Carlquist[97]	1971	61	F	4 cm	—	—	—	Alive at 9 mo
12	Wray and Dawkins[98]	1971	36	M	17 cm	—	—	Lung and kidney	?
13	Johansen and Nielsen[99]	1971	71	F	30 cm	—	—	—	?
14	Kevorkian and Cento[81]	1973	62	F	11 cm	—	—	Lungs	?
15	Couinaud[100]	1973	62	F	17 cm	Invaded uterus	Pelvis	Lungs	Died at 4 yr w/disease
		1973	73	F	19 cm	—	Yes	Liver	Died at 16 mo
16	Hivet et al.[101]	1973	62	F	10 cm	—	—	—	Postop death
17	Stuart and Barker[102]	1973	58	F	15 cm	Invaded pancreas and duodenum	Yes	Liver and muscles	8 yr ?
18	Demoulin et al.[103*]	1974	53	F	15 cm	To R atrium	—	—	?
19	Kapisnow and Brierre[104]	1974	71	F	17 cm	—	—	Omentum	2 yr
20	Kalsbeek[105]	1974	55	F	8 cm	—	—	—	Alive at 27 mo, sigmoid cancer
21	Bailey et al.[106]	1976	67	F	24 cm	—	—	—	Alive at 5 mo
22	Das Gupta*	1981	66	F	12 cm	Duodenum and inferior mesenteric artery	No	Anterior chest wall, dura of spinal cord, and mediastinum	Died 24 mo later

Patients 18 and 22 had preoperative angiograms. Patient 22 had resection of 14-cm segment of inferior vena cava.

TABLE 13.8. COLLECTED CASES OF LEIOMYOSARCOMA OF VEINS OTHER THAN INFERIOR VENA CAVA

Author(s)	Year	Age (Yr)	Sex	Tumor	Site	Operation	End Result
Brohl[112]	1897	56	F	Round cell sarcoma	Femoral	Excised	No data
Borchard[113]	1906	44	M	Sarcoma	Saphenous	Excised	No data
Ehrenberg[114]	1911	49	M	Giant cell sarcoma	S.V.C.	At autopsy	Metastases of pleura, heart, and retroperitoneum
van Ree[115]	1919	42	F	Leiomyosarcoma	Saphenous	Excised	No metastases 15 mo
Razzaboni[116]	1920	64	M	Sarcoma	Saphenous	Excised	
Ausbuttel[117]	1939	51	F	Sarcoma	Pulmonary	At autopsy	Heart metastases
Puig-Sureda et al.[118]	1947	61	F	Leiomyosarcoma	Inferior colic	Excised	
Haug and Losli[119]	1954	51	M	Leiomyosarcoma	Femoral	Excised	Lung metastases 3 yr later
Font and Noer[85]	1955	50	M	Leiomyosarcoma	Antecubital	Excised	
Johnston and Shands[120]	1955	67	F	Leiomyosarcoma	Femoral	Excised	Alive 9 mo later
DeWeese et al.[121]	1958	54	M	Leiomyosarcoma	Saphenous	Excised	
Light et al[108]	1960	42	M	Leiomyosarcoma	Femoral	Excised	No metastases 16 mo
Smout and Fisher[109]	1960	76	F	Leiomyosarcoma	Saphenous	Excised	
Thomas and Fine[110]	1960	27	M	Leiomyosarcoma	Internal jugular	Excised	Died 6 mo later
Stout[122]	1961			Sarcoma	Azygos		
Dorfman and Fishel[123]	1963	56	M	Leiomyosarcoma	Saphenous	Excised	Alive 1 yr later
Allison[124]	1965	3 yr, 9 mo	F	Leiomyosarcoma	Femoral	Wide local excision	
Cheek and Nickey[125]	1965	62	F	Leiomyosarcoma	L jugular	Excised	Alive 5 yr later
Lawrence et al.[126]	1966	59	F	Leiomyosarcoma	R iliac	Excised	No metastases 19 mo
Sakura et al.[127]	1966	54	M	Leiomyosarcoma	Femoral	Excised	No metastases 6 mo
Lopez-Varela and Garro[128]	1967	40	F	Leiomyosarcoma	Renal	Resected	
Szasz et al.[83]	1969	68	M	Leiomyosarcoma	Long saphenous	Excised	Dead 2 yr later
Leu and Nipkow[129]	1969	40	M	Leiomyosarcoma	Saphenous	Excised	Alive 2½ yr later
Bhathena and Vazquez[130]	1972	50	F	Leiomyosarcoma	Renal	L radical nephrectomy	
Larmi and Ninimaki[131]	1974	60	F	Leiomyosarcoma	Femoral	Excised	Recurrence 2 yr later
Nesbit and Rob[132]	1975	77	F	Leiomyosarcoma	Femoral	Radical resection	6 yr N.E.D.*
Gross and Horton[133]	1975	46	M	Leiomyosarcoma	Saphenous	Excised	Recurrence at 3 yr; 2 yr later N.E.D.
Jernstrom and Gowdy[134]	1975	64	M	Leiomyosarcoma	Long saphenous	Excised	4 mo postop N.E.D.
Gierson and Rowe[135]	1976	54	F	Leiomyosarcoma	Renal	Resected	Alive 12 mo postop
Das Gupta	1981	63	F	Leiomyosarcoma	Saphenous	L en bloc excision of saphenous vein w/groin nodes	10 yr N.E.D.

*No evidence of disease.

TABLE 13.9. CLINICAL SUMMARY OF EIGHT PATIENTS WITH EMBRYONAL RHABDOMYOSARCOMA OF THE ORBITAL REGION TREATED BY THE AUTHOR*

Patient	Age	Sex	Site of Primary	Stage	Treatment	Regional Node Status	Local Recurrence	Metastases	End Result
1	8	M	2.5 cm, inner canthus, invading surrounding structures	II	Orbital exenteration	−	−	−	8 yr, N.E.D.†
2	45	F	Large tumor upper eyelid	IIb	Excision, biopsy, and radiation therapy	−	−	Lung and liver	Dead at 18 mo with disease
3	8	M	1 cm, lesion lower eyelid	I	Excision and radiation therapy	−	−	−	8 yr, N.E.D.
4	6	M	2 cm, upper eyelid	I	Excision, biopsy, and radiation therapy	+	−	Developed neck node metastases Further radiation therapy	6 yr, N.E.D.
5	2	M	1 cm, upper eyelid	I	Excision, biopsy, radiation therapy, and chemotherapy	−	−	−	5½ yr, N.E.D.
6	4	M	2 cm, upper eyelid	II	Radiation therapy and chemotherapy	+	−	−	5 yr, N.E.D.
7	9	F	3 cm, started in upper eyelid (Fig. 13.9)	II	Biopsy, radiation therapy, and chemotherapy	−	+	−	−
8	7	M	2 cm, lower eyelid	II	Biopsy, radiation therapy, and chemotherapy	+	−	+	Dead at 1 yr

Four of these patients were seen by the author in consultation. The recommended treatment was actually given in the area hospitals. However, the patients have been followed by the author.
†No evidence of disease.

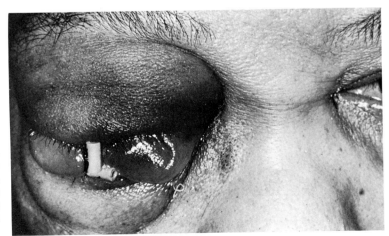

Figure 13.9. Embryonal rhabdomyosarcoma arising in right upper eyelid. The tumor progressed rapidly and the exuberant growth soon prevented vision. A tarsorraphy was done to prevent corneal ulceration (Patient 7, Table 13.9).

(Fig. 13.9). The rapid progression of the ex-ophthalmos is a striking feature. If the lesion starts in the eyelid, swelling and ptosis are frequently the presenting clinical features. Occasionally, children are first brought to the physician with a discrete mass.

The management of orbital rhabdomyosarcoma has undergone considerable modification in the last decade. It is generally agreed[156-165] that orbital exenteration, customarily resorted to in the past in all patients,[148-155,166] can be avoided in most instances without sacrificing the reported excellent end result. Liebner[157] has published good results with radiation therapy, even with apparently unresectable tumors (Chapter 7). Recent data on the results of treatment with a combination of surgery, chemotherapy, and radiation therapy[159-161,166] show that, in most instances, exenterative operations should be confined only to multimodality treatment failures.

The end result following appropriate management indicates that tumors of the orbit have the best prognosis among all types of rhabdomyosarcoma.[149-154,156-165] The National Combined Rhabdomyosarcoma Protocol studies[166] stage all patients with embryonal rhabdomyosarcoma (page 479). The primary tumors of the orbit and eyelids usually are recognized early and are treated at an early stage. This would explain the reason for the overall good prognosis. Six of our eight patients (75 percent) with orbital rhabdomyosarcoma lived for five years or more (Table 13.9). Two of the eight (25 percent) had clinically positive regional nodes at the time of initial therapy and in one (12 percent) a positive neck node subsequently developed. Two of the three with regional node involvement have survived for five years or longer (Table 13.9). One of the eight patients was treated by a radical operation. However, orbital exenteration is generally not indicated in primary orbital rhabdomyosarcomas.

Embryonal rhabdomyosarcomas of other sites in the head and neck region are relatively less common than the orbital variety.[147,149-154, 162-168] Masson and Soule[151] found that, after the orbit, the sites in decreasing order of frequency were the nasopharynx, nose, antrum, parotid area, mandible, tongue, soft palate, tonsil, larynx, temple, external auditory canal, mastoid, submaxillary area, cheek, and forehead. Twenty-three cases of extraorbital embryonal rhabdomyosarcoma in the head and neck region have been treated by the author. Table 13.10 shows

TABLE 13.10. DISTRIBUTION OF EMBRYONAL RHABDOMYOSARCOMA IN THE HEAD AND NECK REGION (EXCLUDING ORBIT)

Anatomic Site	Masson and Soule[151] (Mayo Clinic, 1965)	Das Gupta* (University of Illinois, 1981)
Nasopharynx	15	2
Nose	14	3
Antrum	7	1
Parotid area	6	1
Mandible	5	2
Tongue	3	—
Soft palate	3	3
Tonsil	2	—
Larynx	2	—
Temple	2	4
Ext. auditory canal	2	3
Mastoid	2	—
Submaxillary area	1	1
Cheek	1	2
Forehead	1	1
Total	66	23

*Eleven of these 23 patients were seen by the author in consultation; however, recommended treatment was followed by the area hospitals and adequate followup data were provided to make these cases determinant.

the anatomic distribution of these cases and a comparison with Masson and Soule's[151] series.

The patients were predominantly male and the peak incidence was between the ages of 2 and 8 and 13 and 15 years of age.[147,149-154,159,162-168]

The initial symptom is the presence of a painless tumor, usually of short duration. Patients with nasal or nasopharyngeal tumors frequently complain of nasal congestion, breathing difficulty, and nosebleed. Diplopia might be the only early symptom in some patients. Tumors in the parotid area occasionally infiltrate the facial nerve and give rise to facial nerve palsy. In some instances, the initial presentation is nodal enlargement alone. Although it is never possible to pinpoint the exact duration of the symptoms, in most instances the onset is sudden and the progression of symptoms rapid.

The incidence of regional node involvement in embryonal rhabdomyosarcoma of the head and neck region is high.[151,157,167,168] In our series, (Tables 13.9 and 13.10), four of our eight patients with orbital rhabdomyosarcoma had positive regional nodes. Of the 23 patients with nonorbital tumors, 5 (22 percent) had metastatic rhabdomyosarcoma in the regional nodes. Weingrad and Rosenberg[54] found that, in a combined total of 888 published cases of all types of rhabdomyosarcomas located in all anatomic sites, 108 patients (12.2 percent) had metastatic regional nodes. Therefore, treatment planning should include the regional node-bearing area.

Concepts in the management of extraorbital embryonal rhabdomyosarcomas have also undergone considerable change. From a therapeutic philosophy of nihilism, punctuated with instances of extensive surgical procedures and occasional case reports of a long-term survivor, the management programs in recent years have become standardized. The role of each mode of therapy has been more clearly identified, and extreme pessimism has given way to cautious optimism. The judicious use of limited excision, radiation therapy, and systemic chemotherapy has become the accepted mode of management.[157-166]

In our group of 23 patients, one case in the parotid area, one in the maxillary antrum, and two in the area of the temple were treated by wide excision and chemotherapy. A superficial parotidectomy with radical neck dissection for the tumor in the parotid area, a partial maxillectomy for that in the maxillary antrum, and wide excision (including the entire temporalis muscle with primary closure) for the two in the temporal area constituted the only means of local therapy. The remaining 19 patients were treated primarily with a combination of limited local excision, curative radiation therapy, and multi-agent chemotherapy. The most common drug regimen was a combination of cyclophosphamide, actinomycin D, and vincristine. Details of chemotherapy are given in Chapter 8.

Thirteen of the 23 patients (56 percent) survived five years or longer. It is evident that a judicious combination of all three modalities provides a better salvage rate than single-modality treatment. In 1973, Sessions and co-workers[147] reported that their five patients with localized disease showed an objective response. This was a remarkable difference from the end results reported in 1964 by Koop and Tewarson.[153] Similar spectacular results were attained by Donaldson and associates[164] in 19 patients treated at the M.D. Anderson Hospital. If the overall survival rates in localized head and neck embryonal rhabdomyosarcomas in recent years

TABLE 13.11 SURVIVAL RATE IN LOCALIZED HEAD AND NECK EMBRYONAL RHABDOMYOSARCOMAS (STAGES I AND II)*

Author	Year of Publication	No. Cases with Localized Tumors	5 Yr, N.E.D.†
Sutow et al.[156]	1970	20	34%
Ehrlich et al.[169]	1971	8	50%
Das Gupta	1981	22	62%

*For description of staging of embryonal rhabdomyosarcomas, see page 479.
†No evidence of disease.

are compared (Table 13.11), one finds that, in patients with localized tumor (stages I and II), the results of treatment are eminently satisfactory.

Trunk and Extremities. Although embryonal rhabdomyosarcomas in these anatomic locations are not encountered as commonly as in the orbit or elsewhere in the head and neck region, the incidence is frequent enough to merit careful separate consideration.

We have managed 21 patients with embryonal rhabdomyosarcoma of the trunk and extremities. The primary sites were as follows: superficial trunk, four; retroperitoneum and pelvis, three; perineal area, three; upper extremities, four; and lower extremities, including groin and buttocks, seven. Six of these patients were seen in consultation; however, they were treated as recommended and followup data were provided so that these six cases could be included in the present series.

AGE AND SEX. Three of the 21 patients in this series were adults aged 28, 37, and 46 years. Of the remaining 18 patients, five were adolescents between 13 and 17 years of age, and the other 13 were children between the ages of 1 month and 10 years. Fifteen of the 21 were males. The age distribution and male preponderance were similar to those in other published papers.[4,38,150-153,159,166,168-172]

The most common symptom in these patients was the appearance of a mass. Infrequently, pain was the first symptom. Lawrence and co-workers[152] found pain to be the initial symptom in seven of 48 patients. A detailed discussion of the nature of the associated pain can be found in Chapter 5.

REGIONAL NODE METASTASES. In 3 of our 21 patients the primary tumor was in the retroperitoneal and pelvic musculature, and therefore clinical evaluation of the regional nodes was possible in only 18 patients. Three of the 18 (16.6 percent) had both clinically and histologically positive node involvement at the time of initial therapy. Masson and Soule[151] found that regional nodes were affected in 37.5 percent of their cases. Lawrence and co-workers[152] had 8 (16.6 percent) of 48 patients with regional node involvement. In 1977, Lawrence and associates reviewed the incidence of regional node metastasis in 264 eligible entries in the Intergroup Rhabdomyosarcoma Study. These authors found the incidence as follows: extremities (17%), genitourinary sites (19%), head and neck region (3%), trunk (10%) and orbit (0%).[173]

The extent of the disease at diagnosis has a profound influence on the prognosis. Survival is longer with localized resectable tumors and no regional extension. Therefore, a clinical staging system has been developed to accurately assess the end results following various methods of management. Pratt and co-workers[159] proposed the following staging system, based on the resectability of the tumor at diagnosis:

Stage I: Localized. Recognized tumor completely resectable
Stage II: Adjacent structure, or local or regional lymph nodes involved, e.g., vagina and bladder, or vagina and pelvic lymph nodes; or a palpable tumor with involvement of neck, axillary, or inguinofemoral nodes
    A. Recognized tumor, completely resectable
    B. Recognized tumor, nonresectable or partly resectable
Stage III. Generalized
    A. Distant metastases with normal bone marrow
    B. Distant metastases with bone marrow infiltration

Although other schema have been advanced,[164,172] the Pratt staging system has been widely used and appears to provide important prognostic information.[159] For example, Jaffe and co-workers[165] reported their experience with 61 children staged according to Pratt: The survival rate was 46 percent, 19 percent, and 0 percent for stages I, II, and III patients, respectively.

GROUPING. Another method of classifying patients, especially those entered in clinical trials, has been recently developed. Patients are grouped according to the extent of disease at diagnosis and following surgery, and by the type of treatment they are to receive. This system, first used for Wilms' tumor,[174] has been adapted by the Intergroup Rhabdomyosarcoma Study[166,169,172,175] as follows:

Group 1. Localized tumor, completely resected
    A. Confined to the muscle or organ of origin
    B. Contiguous involvement with infiltration outside the muscle or organ of origin, as through fascial planes; microscopic confirmation of complete resection; no lymph node involvement
Group 2.
    A. Localized disease, grossly resected, but with residual microscopic disease; no lymph node involvement
    B. Regional disease, i.e., extension of tumor into an adjacent organ or regional lymph nodes, or both, completely resected without residual microscopic disease
    C. Regional disease with lymph node involvement, grossly resected but with residual microscopic disease
Group 3. Biopsy or incomplete resection of local or regional disease with gross residual tumor
Group 4. Distant metastatic disease present at the time of first diagnosis, i.e., to lung, liver, bones, bone marrow, brain, or lymph nodes beyond the regional echelon

TREATMENT AND END RESULTS. In the superficial trunk and extremities, if the primary tumor can be completely excised with concomitant regional node dissection, then this can be considered a successful form of primary therapy. Amputation of an extremity for embryonal rhabdomyosarcoma is generally not required, since in the majority of instances a wide soft tissue excision can control the primary tumor. For retroperitoneal tumors, removal of the tumor and regional node dissection is the ideal form of therapy, but in most instances the size of these tumors precludes adequate regional node dissection. As with embryonal rhabdomyosarcomas of the head and neck region, it is recognized that a judicious combination of excision, local radiotherapy, and systemic chemotherapy provides the best chance of cure. Twenty of the 21 patients in our series were treated with multimodal therapy.

Thirteen of the 21 (62 percent) lived two years or longer. One of the 13 died with metastatic disease after 2.5 years. Twelve (57 percent) survived five years or longer. Although the results of treatment in trunk and extremity rhabdomyosarcomas are not as good as those for the head and neck region, they still are much better than those reported during the era before combined modality treatment was initiated.[4,153,167,168] If the present clinical material is divided according to the staging proposed by Pratt and associates,[159] it is observed that 9 of 12 (75 percent) of the five-year disease-free survivors were in stages I and II (Table 13.12). These results are comparable to the end results for embryonal rhabdomyosarcoma of the head and neck region.[157-165]

Embryonal Rhabdomyosarcoma of Specific Sites. Embryonal rhabdomyosarcoma, or sarcoma botryoides, frequently arises in the genitourinary tract, and often in the abdominal viscera. Rarely, these tumors have been reported in still other sites, but most of those cases require further histologic proof before they can be accepted as embryonal rhabdomyosarcoma.

EMBRYONAL RHABDOMYOSARCOMA OF THE GENITOURINARY TRACT. Lesions of the genitourinary tract, commonly seen in children, should be further subclassified according to the patient's sex. In general, the tumors arising in the female genital tract carry a better prognosis than those in the male counterpart, with the urinary bladder occupying a middle position. Table 13.13 summarizes the clinical course of the embryonal

rhabdomyosarcomas of the genitourinary tract treated by the author.

EMBRYONAL RHABDOMYOSARCOMAS OF THE URINARY BLADDER. This tumor is relatively common in children of both sexes and when localized to the urinary bladder the results of treatment are good.

Patients with vesical rhabdomyosarcoma commonly complain of frequent urination, straining to void, acute urinary retention, and hematuria. Hydronephrosis and renal deterioration eventually ensue, owing to rapidly progressing urinary obstruction from tumor growth. The diagnosis usually is confirmed by excretory urography, cystoscopy, and cystography. Rarely, a polypoid tumor may be observed protruding through the urethral meatus (Fig. 4.48, Chapter 4). The tumor usually arises from the trigone or bladder base.

Extensive local tumor invasion may occur prior to the onset of symptoms. Early involvement of contiguous structures makes treatment by subtotal resection an unreliable method of therapy.[170] Radical cystectomy, prostatectomy, pelvic lymphadenectomy (since rhabdomyosarcoma frequently metastasizes to the lymph nodes), and urinary diversion in the form of an ileal conduit usually are necessary for all stage I and stage II cases. Since the bulbomembranous urethra is a common site of involvement and recurrence, resection of this area is also indicated.[170] However, if the tumor is diagnosed early and the location is such that a partial cystectomy and irradiation to the pelvic nodes are possible, then with additional use of adjuvant chemotherapy, a total cystectomy and the use of a long-term ileal conduit can be avoided. This multimodal treatment, when applicable, is ideal for preservation of a normal genitourinary tract and the prolongation of disease-free survival.

The common pitfall in the diagnosis and management of vesical embryonal rhabdomyosarcoma in infants is elaborated upon by briefly describing the problem in case 1, Table 13.13.

CASE REPORT

A four-month-old girl was sent to us with a presumptive diagnosis of embryonal rhabdomyosarcoma of the vulva. The mother stated that about six weeks previously she had noticed a small, cherry-shaped, dark-colored mass protruding from the child's vagina. Following a biopsy of the mass, she was told that this was a malignant tumor of the vagina. The in-

TABLE 13.12. SURVIVAL IN LOCALIZED EMBRYONAL RHABDOMYOSARCOMAS OF THE TRUNK AND EXTREMITIES (STAGES I AND II)

Authors	Year of Publication	No. of Localized Cases	5 Yr, N.E.D.*
Sutow et al.[156]	1970	5	60%
Ehrlich et al.[169]	1971	7	72%
Das Gupta	1981	12	69%

*No evidence of disease.

TABLE 13.13. CLINICAL SUMMARY OF SEVEN PATIENTS WITH EMBRYONAL RHABDOMYOSARCOMA OF THE GENITOURINARY TRACT (UNIVERSITY OF ILLINOIS SERIES)

Patient No.	Age	Sex	Primary Site	Status of Primary	Stage	Regional Extension	Regional Nodes	Surgery	Chemotherapy	Radiation Therapy	Survival	Comments
1	4 mo	F	Bladder	Recurrent tumor	II A	Urethra and vagina	+	Anterior exenteration	VAC regimen	800 rads preop	8 yr, N.E.D.*	
2	4 yr	M	Prostate	Recurrent after radiation therapy palpable suprapubic mass	II B	Bladder	+	Anterior exenteration	VAC regimen	–	8 yr, N.E.D.	Received curative course of radiation therapy and 22 mo of chemotherapy (see text)
3	9 yr	M	Spermatic cord	Untreated, 2 × 2 cm	II A	–	+	Orchiectomy excision of cord and retroperitoneal node dissection	VAC regimen	5,000 rads	5 yr	
4	4 yr	M	Spermatic cord	Recurrent tumors, 6 × 6 cm	II B	Surrounds soft tissue	+	Excision of bulk of the tumor	VAC regimen	6,000 rads	4 yr	
5	19 yr	M	Testis	Untreated, 6 × 6 cm	II B	Extension to spinal cord	–	Radical inguinoscrotal excision	Adriamycin and DTIC	–	5 yr, N.E.D.	Adriamycin and DTIC protocol is being used in adults
6	11 mo	F	Vagina	Untreated, 2 × 2 cm	II A	–	–	Hysterectomy and vaginectomy	VAC regimen	5,000 rads	5 yr, N.E.D.	
7	14 yr	F	Vagina	Recurrent tumor, filling vagina	II B	Urethra and bladder	+	Anterior exeneration	VAC regimen	5,000 rads	8 mo	Widespread metastases

No evidence of disease.

481

fant was operated upon, and part of the vulva and vagina excised. However, the tumor recurred within four weeks and she was referred to us for further management. The lesion was protruding through the urethra and a clinical diagnosis of embryonal rhabdomyosarcoma of the urinary bladder was made. She was investigated adequately and a procedure consisting of radical cystectomy, hysterectomy, and vaginectomy with an ileal conduit, was then performed. Following the operation she was treated with adjuvant chemotherapy. She is still free of disease after ten years. In retrospect, the added hysterectomy, vaginectomy, and vulvectomy could have been avoided if a proper diagnosis had been made prior to the original vulvectomy and contamination of the vulva and vagina.

Rarely, embryonal rhabdomyosarcoma of the bladder is seen in adults. In 1966, Joshi et al.[176] found only 13 cases and added one case of their own. Although little is known of the natural history of these tumors in adults, it is presumed that the general principles of management should be the same for all patients with embryonal rhabdomyosarcoma of the urinary bladder.

EMBRYONAL RHABDOMYOSARCOMA OF THE PROSTATE. Although prostatic rhabdomyosarcoma occurs at all ages, about 50 percent are found during infancy and childhood.[177,178] In the past, the average life expectancy after appearance of the first symptom was only seven months.[177-179] Prostatic sarcomas cause relatively late-appearing obstructive symptoms by displacing the urinary bladder, distorting the urethra, or compressing the rectum. Unlike the vesical rhabdomyosarcomas, the prostatic variety is aggressive and regional node metastasis occurs early, as does metastases to the lung. Local extension to the pubic bones and other pelvic bones is relatively common, even in the early stages of the tumor. Lemmon et al.[178] found that, of the 46 published cases of prostatic rhabdomyosarcoma, 39 (85 percent) had local extension to the bones. This early local involvement of the bone is a major reason for the high local recurrence rate reported in the past.[178]

The cure of prostatic rhabdomyosarcoma requires early diagnosis. Rectal examination of the prostate at the earliest hint of difficulty with micturition or defecation is the most informative diagnostic procedure. Cystography may demonstrate bladder displacement by a prostatic

neoplasm. A transurethral biopsy is often not possible because it is extremely difficult to perform cystoscopy with prostatic sarcoma displacing the urinary bladder. Perineal biopsy may be necessary to obtain a tissue diagnosis; however, the biopsy tract should be carefully treated.

In 1966, Lemmon and colleagues[178] reviewed the literature on rhabdomyosarcoma of the prostate and found a total of 46 cases, including one of their own, and only one instance of cure. Radical surgery was tried in only seven of these 46 cases. Reviewing the state of the art till the mid-1960s, these authors concluded that rhabdomyosarcomas were resistant to chemotherapy and radiation therapy and stressed early diagnosis and radical operation for cure of localized tumors. Grosfeld, Smith, and Clatworthy,[179] in a more recent review of their experience with all pelvic rhabdomyosarcomas, found six to be prostatic. Although these authors did not describe the treatment and end results specifically for the prostate, by using aggressive radical surgery with radiation therapy and chemotherapy, the three patients with stage I disease were salvaged. Pratt et al.[159] also described one patient with a stage II-B tumor who, after a perineal needle biopsy of the prostate, was treated only with radiation therapy to the perineum and para-aortic nodes. This treatment was combined with chemotherapy (vincristine, cyclophosphamide, and dactinomycin), with a resultant 23-month disease-free survival at the time of their report. One of our patients (Case 2, Table 13.13) also was originally treated with radiation therapy and chemotherapy, with apparent control of the local disease for about 22 months, at which time local recurrence developed, requiring an anterior exenteration. This patient is still disease-free eight years later. It is difficult to develop management guidelines based on individual case reports. However, it appears that in prostatic rhabdomyosarcoma initial aggressive radiation therapy and sequential chemotherapy can be tried for both local and systemic control of the disease. Radical prostatic surgery is kept in reserve for recurrent or uncontrollable primary tumors. It is emphasized, however, that if and when surgery is indicated, the procedure must be aggressive; otherwise, the rate of failure will be high.

TESTICULAR AND PARATESTICULAR EMBRYONAL RHABDOMYOSARCOMA. A groin or scrotal mass calls attention to these tumors, which most commonly arise from the structures of the spermatic cord.[63,179-180] Metastases to the lymph nodes are known to occur and appear to follow the spermatic vessels in patients with noninfiltrating lesions.[182-184] The para-aortic chain was positive in 3 of 11 boys who had routine retroperitoneal node dissection.[180] Of the three patients in our own series, two had positive retroperitoneal nodes (Table 13.13). The inguinal and external iliac chains can be affected when the sarcoma invades adjacent structures of the scrotum or inguinal canal.

Treatment consists of inguinal orchiectomy, with high ligation of the spermatic cord, and retroperitoneal lymph node dissection. The removal of the iliac nodes is restricted to the ipsilateral side.[172] Preservation of the branches of the contralateral sacral plexus avoids retrograde ejaculation, a troublesome complication that occurs following bilateral pelvic surgery. The margins of resection should be identified to assist the radiation therapist in planning treatment. The transscrotal route for biopsy or removal is contraindicated because of possible tumor implantation in the incision, as may occur with testicular cancers. In such cases, hemiscrotectomy is performed to avoid local recurrence. Our patient with testicular tumor (Case 5, Table 13.13) had a scrotal incisional biopsy prior to his visit here and required a hemiscrotectomy along with node dissection and excision of the spermatic cord.

All patients should be treated with adjuvant chemotherapy, and those with stage II-B tumors with microscopic disease should also be treated with postoperative radiation therapy. Patients with node involvement are treated with 4,000 to 6,000 rads in four to six weeks. Both kidneys should be shielded when the ipsilateral inguinal nodes, pelvic lymph nodes, and para-aortic nodes are irradiated. A biopsy of the scalene node is sometimes indicated and, if positive, the mediastinum should also be treated with radiation therapy.

The prognosis for patients with testicular or paratesticular rhabdomyosarcoma has been discouraging in the past.[180] As late as 1968,[180,181] the prognosis was dismal. In recent years, the prognosis has improved, as it has for embryonal types in other sites. Pratt et al.[159] provided a more optimistic picture. Of the three in our group, all have lived more than two years, and two, for five years or longer (Table 13.13). Although the prognosis in testicular and paratesticular rhabdomyosarcoma is probably worse

than for all other sites in the genitourinary tract, certainly this tumor is by no means beyond cure if properly diagnosed and treated while in stages I or II.

EMBRYONAL RHABDOMYOSARCOMA OF THE UTERUS AND VAGINA. These tumors present as fleshy outgrowths from the introitus.[4,159,183-187] The tumors become manifest because of a bloody, often foul-smelling discharge. In children they arise from the vagina rather than from the cervix, as is the case in adults,[185,187] and they infiltrate adjacent structures. Metastases to lymph nodes or more distant sites occur relatively late. In the present group of vaginal rhabdomyosarcomas (Table 13.13), a protruding tumor at the introitus was the initial clinical presentation. Hilgers et al.[185] reviewed the files from the Mayo Clinic and found ten instances of botryoid sarcoma of the vagina. These authors, after an extensive general review of the literature, described the results of treatment in these patients. From their own clinical material and other published cases they developed the following general guidelines for management: (1) Every genital tract lesion or episode of vaginal bleeding occurring in a young girl should be considered potentially malignant until proved otherwise. (2) Once the diagnosis has been established, a reasonable effort should be made to ascertain the extent of the disease. These authors[185] found that no patient with locally recurrent tumor due to inadequate initial treatment had ever been cured. (3) Finally, they concluded that initial radical pelvic surgery provides the patient with maximum opportunity for a cure, and that an anterior exenteration is the best initial radical procedure. A similar opinion regarding treatment has been expressed by Grosfeld et al.[170] Although Pratt and co-workers[159] advocated a somewhat less radical procedure, they agreed with the premise of adequate extirpation of the primary tumor. The author's personal experience rests on only two cases of vaginal rhabdomyosarcoma (Table 13.13). One of the two (Case 6) was staged II-A and was treated by hysterectomy, vaginectomy, pelvic inguinal node dissection, and adjuvant chemotherapy; the patient is still free of disease ten years later. However, Case 7 was a stage II-B recurrent tumor and this patient died within eight months. Recently, El-Mahdi et al.[187] reported a 25-year cure of vaginal rhabdomyosarcoma treated by irradiation only. According to these authors, at the time of their report in 1974 the 26-year-old patient was free of local or systemic disease, with hypoplastic external genitalia, hypofunction of the ovaries, an infantile vagina and uterus, but normal bowel and urinary function. It appears that, when a long-range view is taken, both aggressive radiation therapy and radical surgery have distressing sequelae. Therefore, a realistic appraisal of the type of sequelae, the methods of reconstruction, and the chance of maximum success in these reconstructive procedures is indicated prior to embarking on any method of management of the primary tumor.

Embryonal Rhabdomyosarcoma of Unusual Sites. Embryonal rhabdomyosarcoma has been reported in various unusual sites.[4,38,188–196] Their rarity in these sites arouses more interest in the embryogenesis of striated muscle fibers in these unusual locations than in the development of any logical management program. Hays and Snyder[188] reported two cases of rhabdomyosarcoma of the extrahepatic bile ducts. Both children were treated with resection and radiation therapy, but both died shortly after operation. In their review of the literature, these authors found only six such cases. All the patients died shortly after operative intervention. Goldman and Friedman[195] described two patients with embryonal rhabdomyosarcoma of the hepatic parenchyma. Recently Mihara and colleagues[197] described a case of rhabdomyosarcoma in the gallbladder of a six-year-old girl. After an extensive review of the literature, they concluded that there were 26 established and seven probable cases of rhabdomyosarcoma of the liver and the biliary system. These cases exemplify the rarity of this type of tumor. The presence of muscle tumors in the liver parenchyma or in the extrahepatic biliary system, where normally skeletal muscles are not observed, supports the concept that the normal hepatic blastema is derived from both endodermal and mesodermal elements (Chapter 3). The presence of rhabdomyosarcoma in the gastrointestinal tract also raises the intriguing question of the origin of skeletal muscle.

Pleomorphic Rhabdomyosarcoma. Pleomorphic rhabdomyosarcoma is predominantly a tumor of adult males (Fig. 13.10A to 13.10E). In our series, 3 of 32 patients (9.3 percent) were below the age of 20 years and one was 69 years old; the remaining 28 patients were between 20 and 60 years of age. A similar observation regarding the distribution of age and sex has been made by other authors.[198,199]

These tumors are found in all parts of the human body, but the preferred site of origin is the lower extremities (Table 13.14). In our series, 16 of 32 (50 percent) were found in a lower extremity and only one in the retroperitoneum. These tumors have also been reported in many other sites, such as those of apparent pulmonary origin,[193] the gastrointestinal tract,[188,189] the ovaries,[194] and the uterus.[200] However, some of these reports must be viewed with reservation, since absolute documentation has not been provided that these tumors were pleomorphic rather than embryonal.

The presenting complaint in most patients is of a painless mass of relatively short duration (Fig. 13.10A and 13.10B). In some instances the patient becomes aware of the tumor after minor trauma. Pain and discomfort are the presenting symptoms in about 25 percent of patients. Pain in the sciatic nerve distribution, as in other sarcomas of the buttock, is a relatively common symptom for tumors arising in that location.

The treatment of primary pleomorphic rhabdomyosarcoma is mainly operative. In contrast to treatment of the embryonal variety, radical excision has a better role. The type of radical excision, however, depends on the location of the primary tumor. In the present series, all 32 patients were treated with radical surgery (Table 13.15). In the series reported by Linscheid and associates,[199] 84 of 87 patients were treated by surgery and three by radiation therapy. It is our present practice to treat all primary pleomorphic rhabdomyosarcomas with adjuvant chemotherapy. The use of both preoperative and postoperative chemotherapy and radiation therapy is being evaluated in tumors of the lower extremities (Chapter 8).

The results of treatment in our 32 patients are shown in Table 13.16. Twelve received postoperative adjuvant chemotherapy. Of the 20 treated by resection alone, 65 percent survived five years with no evidence of disease. Of the 12 receiving adjuvant chemotherapy, 83 percent were disease-free at the end of five years (Chapter 8). These results, compared with the 45 percent and 32 percent five-year disease-free survival rates reported by Linscheid et al.[199] and by Keyhani and Booher,[198] respectively, are certainly an improvement. Although it is impossible to realistically compare the present end

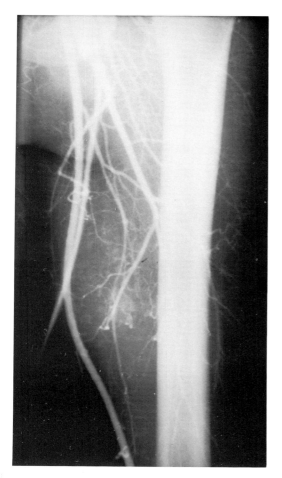

Figure 13.10. (A) Angiogram outlining a pleomorphic rhabdomyosarcoma in the left thigh of a 44-year-old man. This tumor was treated with our recent protocol of preoperative intra-arterial infusion with adriamycin, and by radiation therapy followed by a muscle group excision and groin dissection. After the wound healed, radiation therapy was completed and adjuvant therapy continued for one year. Patient is still disease-free after six years.

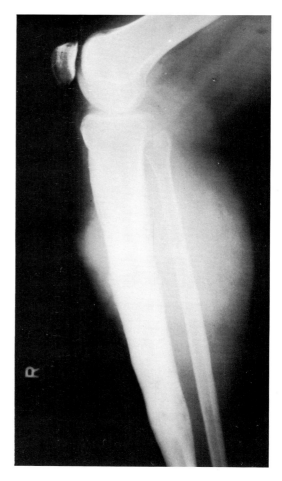

Figure 13.10. (B) Pleomorphic rhabdomyosarcoma of the leg. Note secondary involvement of the bone. Tibia was extensively involved. Patient underwent an above-knee amputation.

result data with previously published end results,[198,199] it seems that either adjuvant chemotherapy or multimodal limb salvage procedures are certainly additive factors in improving the prognosis. As with the embryonal variety, limb salvage procedures may effectively replace major amputations (Table 13.16). However, this does not imply an inadequate primary operation.

McNeer and associates[201] evaluated the role of radiation therapy in 109 patients with adult or pleomorphic rhabdomyosarcoma and found that adjunctive irradiation was ineffective, albeit only a small number of patients were treated by this method. From a review of the clinical material of Memorial Sloan-Kettering Cancer Center, these authors found that, of 12 patients treated solely with irradiation, 5 (42 percent) showed clinical response; however, only 2 (15 percent) showed "histological sterilization." They concluded that radical excision should be the mainstay of management of pleomorphic rhab-

486

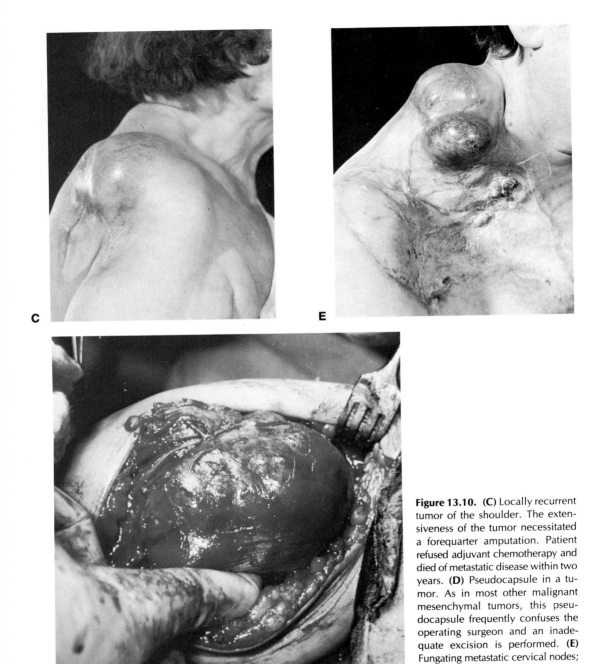

Figure 13.10. (**C**) Locally recurrent tumor of the shoulder. The extensiveness of the tumor necessitated a forequarter amputation. Patient refused adjuvant chemotherapy and died of metastatic disease within two years. (**D**) Pseudocapsule in a tumor. As in most other malignant mesenchymal tumors, this pseudocapsule frequently confuses the operating surgeon and an inadequate excision is performed. (**E**) Fungating metastatic cervical nodes; primary was located in the arm.

TABLE 13.14. SITES OF ORIGIN OF PLEOMORPHIC RHABDOMYOSARCOMA IN THREE SERIES

Site	Linscheid et al.*[199] (Mayo Clinic, 1965)	Keyhani and Booher[198] (Memorial Sloan-Kettering Cancer Center, 1968)	Das Gupta (University of Illinois, 1981)
Lower extremity	40	95	16
Upper extremity	47	59	10
Trunk	—	18	5
Head and neck	—	15	—
Miscellaneous	—	17	1
Total	87	204	32

*These authors reported only on tumors of limb girdles and extremities.

domyosarcomas. Similar conclusions were drawn by Linscheid et al.,[199] by Keyhani and Booher,[198] and others.[4,168,169,202–204] From our experience at the University of Illinois and from a review of the data from other larger series, it appears that radical operation should still be considered the best method for control of primary pleomorphic rhabdomyosarcoma.

In the author's series of 32 patients, local recurrence was found in 3 (9 percent) after initial surgical therapy and was associated with distant metastases in 2. The incidence of 3 percent local recurrence after adequate excision speaks well for the original treatment. Keyhani and Booher[198] reviewed their experience in the treatment of 75 locally recurrent operable rhabdomyosarcomas and found that adequate excision resulted in a salvage rate similar to that obtained for untreated primary tumors.

Our data are not adequate to evaluate the

TABLE 13.15. TYPES OF INITIAL SURGICAL TREATMENT IN UNIVERSITY OF ILLINOIS SERIES OF 32 CASES OF PLEOMORPHIC RHABDOMYOSARCOMA

Anatomic Site	Soft Part or Muscle Group Resection	Amputation	Total
Upper extremity	8	2	10
Trunk	5	—	5
Lower extremity	12	4	16
Miscellaneous sites	1	—	1
Total	26	6	32

exact role of postoperative radiation therapy in the management of primary pleomorphic rhabdomyosarcoma. However, the data from M. D. Anderson Hospital published by Suit and co-workers[205] suggest that, as in the embryonal variety, adjunctive radiation therapy may have a definite role in controlling the primary tumor. Recently, Lindberg et al.[55] updated the M. D. Anderson Hospital data on use of postoperative radiation therapy following conservative surgery in 17 patients with rhabdomyosarcoma. In this series, 5 of 17 patients (29 percent) had local recurrence. Based on our own clinical material, in which we have observed a marked improvement in the prognosis following adequate wide excision and adjuvant chemotherapy, we think wide primary soft tissue excision still constitutes the best method of controlling the primary tumor.

Pleomorphic Rhabdomyosarcoma of Unusual Sites. Pleomorphic rhabdomyosarcomas have been reported in various sites outside the body somite.[189–200] All are case reports of one or two patients. Consequently, no general guidelines regarding the natural history or management can be provided. Pleomorphic rhabdomyosarcomas have been reported in the esophagus, stomach, and duodenum,[189,191] as well as the gingiva,[206] uterus,[200] and ovaries.[194] If the case reports are any guide, then these patients should be treated by excision of the primary tumor. The results of treatment, however, have not been very satisfactory.

Pleomorphic rhabdomyosarcomas of the heart are extremely rare, with only about 33 such cases on record.[192,193] Rarely, these tumors are diagnosed antemortem. Matloff and co-

TABLE 13.16. COMPARISON OF FIVE-YEAR END RESULTS IN THREE SERIES OF PLEOMORPHIC
RHABDOMYOSARCOMAS, ACCORDING TO SURGICAL PROCEDURE*

Type of Operation	Linscheid et al.[199] (Mayo Clinic, 1965)	Keyhani and Booher[198] (Memorial Sloan-Kettering Cancer Center, 1968)	Das Gupta* (University of Illinois, 1981)
Soft part resection (muscle group)	6/8 (75%)	20/52 (38%)	11/16 (69%)
Amputation	19/47 (40%)	4/24 (17%)	2/4 (50%)
Total	25/55 (45%)	24/76 (32%)	13/20 (65%)

*The remaining 12 patients received adjuvant chemotherapy (Chapter 8).

workers,[192] reported one such case in which the diagnosis was made and the patient was operated upon. Following a second excision of the recurrence, she lived for a total of 34 months.

Alveolar Rhabdomyosarcoma. In 1956, a significant contribution toward the recognition of a sizable group of these neoplasms was provided by Riopelle and Theriault,[207] who demonstrated that certain "round cell sarcomas" with a peculiar pseudoglandular or pseudoalveolar pattern are actually malignant tumors of the rhabdomyoblasts. Today, alveolar rhabdomyosarcoma as an entity has become generally accepted.[208] It is agreed that the alveolar variant of rhabdomyosarcoma is a relatively frequent malignant neoplasm affecting patients under the age of 20 years. Enzinger and Shiraki[209] found that alveolar and embryonal rhabdomyosarcomas were the two most common soft tissue tumors in patients 20 years or younger in the files of the Armed Forces Institute of Pathology.

In 1969, Enzinger and Shiraki[209] reported the largest series on record of patients with alveolar rhabdomyosarcoma (110 patients from the files of the Armed Forces Institute of Pathology) and actually defined the general principles in the histologic diagnosis and the natural history of these tumors. We have treated 12 such patients.

The age at initial onset can range from a few months after birth to the sixth decade, although, as stated above, the majority occur in patients below the age of 20 years. The median age in Enzinger and Shiraki's group[209] was 15 years. In our series, the median was 18 years. There were eight males and four females in our group and a similar ratio has been found by other authors.[209-211]

These tumors, like other rhabdomyosarcomas, can arise in all parts of the human body. In the University of Illinois group of 12 patients, one tumor was in the neck, two were in the trunk, five in the upper extremities, and four in the lower extremities. In Enzinger and Shiraki's[209] series of 110 patients, the primary site could be determined in 109. The tumors were distributed as follows: head and neck, 20 patients; trunk, 30; upper extremities, 29; and lower extremities, 30.

The presenting feature usually is a tumor of relatively short duration. Associated pain or tenderness is rare. The diagnosis is usually reached after an adequate biopsy examination.

The treatment of primary alveolar rhabdomyosarcoma is mainly along the same lines as that of the embryonal type. The treatment plan should include judicious use of radiation therapy, excision of the primary with regional node dissection when indicated, and adjuvant chemotherapy.

Recently Hays and associates[212] reviewed the end-result data from the Intergroup Rhabdomyosarcoma Study. The period of follow-up ranged from 2.5 to 7.5 years after treatment of the primary tumor in all anatomic sites with the multimodal treatment protocols in operation. These authors observed an increased incidence of recurrence in extremity tumors as opposed to tumors arising in the head and neck or in the trunk. Further analysis of their data, based on histologic types, shows that the incidence of relapse is highest with alveolar rhabdomyosarcoma.[212] In clinical group 1, the recurrence rate with the alveolar subtype was 5 of 8, compared to 1 of 7 in embryonal and 1 of 6 in all other types. Similarly, in clinical group 2, the relapse rate in the alveolar type was 6 of 12, whereas in the embryonal it was 5 of 11, and 3 of 10 in all other types. These authors concluded that in their group of patients there was a clustering of the alveolar type of rhabdomyosarcomas in the extremities, and hence the worsening of the prognosis. The reason for this, however, is not immediately apparent.

Our experience with this histologic subtype of tumors is not as desolate as that of the Intergroup Rhabdomyosarcoma Study Group. Of the 12 patients in our series, 8 have been free of disease for five years or longer, and 4 died with widespread metastases. These survival data, compared with the report of a median survival of nine months by Enzinger and Shiraki[209] prior to institution of a well-designed plan of treatment, are certainly more favorable. Although the number of patients treated and followed by us is only 12, an overall five-year salvage rate of 66 percent is gratifying. The end result after radical operation followed by adjuvant chemotherapy certainly provides a better outlook than previously reported.[209–211]

In our present protocol, which is similar to that for embryonal rhabdomyosarcomas, amputation is avoided as often as possible. Our own observations of embryonal, pleomorphic, and alveolar rhabdomyosarcomas have led us to conclude that, in spite of histologic variations among these three types, all myogenic tumors arising from the skeletal muscles are responsive to both radiation therapy and chemotherapy, although the pleomorphic and alveolar types are not as sensitive as the embryonal type. Even then, we think that, for the pleomorphic type in adults and the alveolar type in adolescents and young adults, a concerted plan similar to that for the embryonal type in children should be instituted. This type of program should improve future end results and disease-free survival rates.

REFERENCES

1. Willis RA: The Borderland of Embryology and Pathology, London, Butterworth, 1958, p 411
2. Golden T, Stout AP: Smooth muscle tumors of the gastrointestinal tract and retroperitoneal tissue. Surg Gynecol Obstet, 73:784, 1941
3. Ranchod M, Kempson RL: Smooth muscle tumors of the gastrointestinal tract and retroperitoneum. Cancer 39:255, 1977
4. Pack GT, Ariel IA: Tumors of the soft somatic tissue. New York, Hoeber-Harper, 1958, p 535
5. Rywlin AM, Simmons RJ, Robinson MJ: Leiomyoma of vagina recurrent in pregnancy. South Med J 62:1449, 1969
6. Elliott GB, Reymonds HA, Fidler HK: Pseudosarcoma botryoides of cervix and vagina in pregnancy. J Obstet Gynecol Brit Comm 74:728, 1967
7. Norris HJ, Taylor HB: Polyps of vagina. A benign lesion resembling sarcoma botryoides. Cancer 19:227, 1966
8. Meyer SL, Fine BS, Font RL, Zimmerman L: Leiomyoma of the ciliary body: Electron microscopic verification. Am J Ophthalmol 66:1061, 1968
9. Aaro LA, Symmonds RE, Dockerty MB: Sarcoma of the uterus: A clinical and pathologic study of 177 cases. Am J Obstet Gynecol 94:101, 1966
10. Edelson MG, Davids AM: Metastasis of uterine fibroleimyomata. Obstet Gynecol 21:78, 1963
11. Steiner P: Metastasizing fibroleiomyoma of the uterus. Am J Path 15:98, 1939
12. Spiro R, McPeak CT: On the so-called metastasizing leiomyoma. Cancer 19:546, 1966
13. Pocock E, Craig JR, Bullock WR: Metastatic uterine leiomyomata. Cancer 38:2096, 1976
14. Ariel IM, Trinidad S: Pulmonary metastases from a uterine "leiomyoma." Report of a case: Evaluation of differential diagnosis and treatment policies. Am J Obstet Gynecol 94:110, 1966
15. Konis EE, Belsky RD: Metastasizing leiomyoma of the uterus: Report of a case. Obstet Gynecol 27:442–446, 1966
16. Piccaluga A, Capelli A: Metastasizing fibroleiomyomatosis of the uterus. A morphologic, histochemical and histomechanical study. Arch Ital Anat Istol Pathol 41:99, 1967
17. Lefebvre R, Nawar T, Fortin R, et al: Leiomyoma of the uterus with bilateral pulmonary metastases. Canad Med Assoc J 105:501, 1971
18. Barnes HM, Richardson RJ: Benign metastasizing fibroleiomyoma—A case report. J Obstet Gynecol Br Commonw 80:569, 1973
19. Marshall JF, Morris DS: Intravenous leiomyomatosis of the uterus and pelvis—Case report. Ann Surg 149:126, 1959
20. Harper RS, Scully RE: Intravenous leiomyomatosis of the uterus—A report of four cases. Obstet Gynecol 18:519, 1961
21. Thompson JW, Symmonds RE, Dockerty MB: Benign uterine leiomyoma with vascular involvement. Am J Obstet Gynecol 84:182, 1962
22. Steiner G, Warren JW, Judd AS: Intravenous leiomyomatosis—A case report. Am J Obstet Gynecol 87:166, 1963
23. Seramatis MG, Lyons WS, deGuzman VC, Peabody JW Jr: Leiomyomata of the esophagus: An analysis of 838 cases. Cancer 38:2166, 1976
24. Skandalakis JE, Gray SW, Shepard D: Smooth muscle tumors of the small intestine. Am J Gastroenterol 42:172, 1964
25. Clinton-Thomas CL: A giant leiomyoma of the kidney. Br J Surg 43:497, 1956
26. Aaxus T, Mylius E: Leiomyoma of the lung. Acta Chir Scand 124:372, 1962
27. Paul M, Attygalle D, Thambirajah M: The origins of leiomyomas. Br J Surg 55:9, 1968

28. Martin JF, Bazin P, Feroldi J, Cabanne F: Tumeurs myoides intramurales de l'estomac—Considerations microscopiques a propos de 6 cas. Ann Anat Pathol (Paris) 5:484, 1960

29. Stout AP: Bizarre smooth muscle tumors of the stomach. Cancer 15:400, 1962

30. Lavin P, Hajdu SI, Foote FW Jr: Gastric and extragastric leiomyoblastomas. Cancer 29:305, 1972

31. Kurman RJ, Norris HG: Mesenchymal tumors of the uterus. VI. Epithelioid smooth muscle tumors including leiomyoblastoma and clear-cell leiomyoma: A clinical and pathologic anlaysis of 26 cases. Cancer 37:1853, 1976

32. Cornog JL Jr: Gastric leiomyoblastoma: A clinical and ultrastructural study. Cancer 34:711, 1974

33. Abramson DJ: Gastric leiomyoblastoma: Report of three cases, one malignant. Ann Surg 179:625, 1973

34. Abramson DJ: Gastric leiomyoblastoma: Collective review. Surg Gynecol Obstet 136:118, 1973

35. Stout AP, Hill WT: Leiomyosarcoma of the superficial soft tissues. Cancer 11:844, 1958

36. Yannopoulos K, Stout AP: Smooth muscle tumors in children. Cancer 15:958, 1962

37. Yannopoulos K, Stout AP: Primary solid tumors of the mesentery. Cancer 16:915, 1963

38. Stout AP, Lattes R: Tumors of the Soft Tissues, Fasc 1. Washington DC, AFIP, 1967

39. Stout AP: Tumors of the Stomach. vol 6, pt 21. Washington DC, AFIP, 1953

40. Somervell JL, Mayer PF: Leiomyosarcoma of the rectum. Br J Surg 58:144, 1974

41. Stavorovsky M, Jaffa AJ, Papo J, Baratz M: Leiomyosarcoma of the colon and rectum. Dis Colon Rect 23:249, 1980

42. McPeak CJ: Malignant tumors of the small intestine. Am J Surg 114:402, 1967

43. Christopherson WM, Williamson EO, Gray LA: Leiomyosarcoma of the uterus. Cancer 29:1512, 1972

44. Vardi JR, Tovell HM: Leiomyosarcoma of the uterus: Clinicopathologic study. Obstet Gynecol 56(4):428, 1980

45. Henrichs KJ, Wenisch JH, Hofmann W, Klein F: Leiomyosarcoma of the pulmonary artery: A light and electron microscopical study, Virchows Arch Path Anat 383:207, 1979

46. Smith BH, Dehner LP: Sarcoma of the prostate gland. Am J Clin Path 58:43, 1972

47. Weitzner S: Leiomyosarcoma of urinary bladder in children. Urology 12:450, 1978

48. Pritchett PS, Fu YS, Kay S: Unusual ultrastructural features of a leiomyosarcoma of the lung. Am J Clin Path 63:901, 1975

49. Schanher PW Jr: Primary pulmonary leiomyosarcoma: Case report and review of literature. Ann Surg 181:20, 1975

50. Morgan PG, Ball J: Pulmonary leiomyosarcomas. Br J Dis Chest 74(3):245, 1980

51. Overgaard J, Frederiksen P, Helmig O, Jensen OM: Primary leiomyosarcoma of bone. Cancer 39:1664, 1977

52. Shamsuddin AK, Reyes F, Harvey JW, Toker C: Primary leiomyosarcoma of bone. Hum Path 11(5):581 (Suppl), 1980

53. Botting AJ, Soule EH, Brown AL: Smooth muscle tumors in children. Cancer 18:711, 1965

54. Weingrad DN, Rosenberg SA: Early lemphatic spread of osteogenic and soft-tissue sarcomas. Surgery 84:231, 1978

55. Lindberg RD, Martin RG, Romsdahl MM, Barkley HT Jr: Converative surgery and postoperative radiotherapy in 300 adults with soft tissue sarcomas. Cancer 47:2391, 1980

56. Berg J, McNeer G: Leiomyosarcoma of the stomach: A clinical and pathological study. Cancer 13:25, 1960

57. Bergis JN, Dockerty MB, Re Mino MT: Sarcomatous lesions of the stomach. Ann Surg 173:758, 1971

58. Starr GF, Dockerty MB: Leiomyomas and leiomyosarcoma of the small intestine. Cancer 8:101, 1955

59. Quan SHQ, Berg JW: Leiomyoma and leiomyosarcoma of the rectum. Dis Colon Rectum 5:415, 1962

60. Donnelly BA: Primary retroperitoneal tumors: Report of 95 cases and review of literature. Surg Gynecol Obstet 83:705, 1946

61. Hutcheson JB, Wittaker WW, Fronstin MH: Leiomyosarcoma of the penis: Case report and review of literature. J Urol 101:874, 1969

62. Dehner LP, Smith BH: Soft tissue tumors of the penis: A clinicopathologic study of 46 cases. Cancer 25:1431, 1970

63. Arlen M, Grabstald H, Whitmore WF Jr: Malignant tumors of the spermatic cord. Cancer 23:525, 1969

64. Buckley PM, Tolley DA: Leiomyosarcoma of the spermatic cord. Br J Urol 53:193, 1981

65. Johnson S, Rondell M, Platt W: Leiomyosarcoma of the scrotum. Cancer 41:1830, 1978

66. Bartsich EG, Bowe ET, Morre JG: Leiomyosarcoma of the uterus. A 50-year review of 42 cases. Obstet Gynecol 32:101, 1968

67. Hannigan EV: Uterine leiomyosarcoma. A review of prognostic clinical and pathological features. Am J Obstet Gynecol 134:557, 1979

68. Montague ACW, Swartz DP, Woodruff JD: Sarcoma arising in a leiomyoma of uterus. Am J Obstet Gynecol 92:421, 1965

69. Malkasian GD, Welch JS, Soule EH: Primary leiomyosarcoma of the vagina. Am J Obstet Gynecol 86:730, 1963

70. Tobon H, Murphy AI, Salazar H: Primary leiomyosarcoma of the vagina. Cancer 32:450, 1973

71. Underwood PB Jr, Smith RT: Carcinoma of the vagina. JAMA 217:46, 1971

72. Chalmers JA: Fibromyoma of fallopian tube. J Obstet Gynecol Br Emp 55:156, 1948

73. Kelly JA: Gynecologic cancer in children. Pediatrics 15:354, 1939

74. Islam MU, Tablibi MA, Boyd PF, Laughlin VC: Leiomyosarcoma of kidney. JAMA 212:2266, 1970

75. Weisel W, Dockerty MD, Priestly JT: Sarcoma of the kidney. J Urol 50:564, 1963

76. Bazaz-Malid C, Gupta DN: Leiomyosarcoma of kidney: Report of case with review of literature. J Urol 95:754, 1966

77. Papacharalambous AN, Pavlakis AJ: Leiomyosarcoma of the bladder. Br J Urol 51:321, 1979

78. Munk J, Giffel B, Kogan J: Primary mesenchymoma of pulmonary artery: radiologic features. Br J Radiol 38:104, 1965

79. Jacques JE, Barclay R: Solid sarcomatous pulmonary artery. Br J Dis Chest 54:217, 1960

80. Wolf PL, Kirsenman RC, Langston JD: Fibrosarcoma of the pulmonary artery masquerading as a pheochromocytoma. Am J Clin Path 34:146, 1960

81. Kevorkian J, Cento DP: Leiomyosarcoma of large arteries and veins. Surgery 73:390, 1973

82. Hernandez FJ, Stanley TM, Ranganath KA, Rubinstein AI: Primary leiomyosarcoma of the aorta. Am J Surg Path 3:251, 1979

83. Szasz IJ, Barr R, Scobie TK: Leiomyosarcoma arising from veins: Two cases and a review of the literature on venous neoplasms. Canad J Surg 170:415, 1969

84. Cope JS, Hunt CJ: Leiomyosarcoma of the inferior vena cava. Arch Surg 68:752, 1954

85. Font AJ, Noer HR: Primary leiomyosarcoma of antecubital vein: Report of case with review of literature. Grace Hosp Bull (Detroit) 33:35, 1955

86. Abell JR: Leiomyosarcoma of inferior vena cava: Review of literature and report of two cases. Am J Clin Path 28:272, 1957

87. Harland WA, Clamen M, Rodriguez VM: Leiomyosarcoma of inferior vena cava with clinical feature of Chiari's syndrome. Canad Med Assoc J 83:1964, 1960

88. Melchior E: Sarcom der Vana Cava Inerior. Deutsch Z. Chir 213:135, 1928

89. Allan J, Burnett W. Lee FD: Leiomyosarcoma of the inferior vena cava. Scott Med J 9:352, 1964

90. Caplan BB, Halasz NA, Bloomer WE: Resection and ligation of the suprarenal inferior vena cava. J Urol, 92:25, 1966

91. Gariepy JA, Pope RH: Leiomyosarcoma of the inferior vena cava. Conn Med 31:102, 1967

92. Nartowicz E, Domaniewaki J, Wiecko W: Leiomyosarcome de la Veine Cava Inférieure Traitement Errone de Cholécystite. Maroc Med 47:339, 1967

93. Staley CJ, Valaitis J, Trippel OH, Franzblau SA: Leiomyosarcoma of the inferior vena cava. Am J Surg 113:221, 1967

94. Hopson WB, Burlison PE, Sherman RT: Leiomyosarcoma of the inferior vena cava. Ann Surg 168:290, 1968

95. Gue'don J, Mesnard J, Poisson J, Kuss R: Hypertension renovasculaire par leiomyosarcoma de la veine cava Inférieure, Guerison del' hypertension et Survie de 2 ans après intervention chirurgicale. Ann Med Interne (Paris) 121:905, 1970

96. Jurayj NM, Midell AI, Bederman S, et al: Primary leiomyosarcoma of the inferior vena cava: Report of a case and review of the literature. Cancer 26:1349, 1970

97. Dube VE, Carlquist JH: Surgical treatment of leiomyosarcoma of the inferior vena cava: Report of a case. Am Surg 37:87, 1971

98. Wray RC, Dawkins H: Primary smooth muscle tumors of the inferior vena cava. Ann Surg 174:1009, 1971

99. Johansen JK, Nielsen R: Leiomyosarcoma of the inferior vena cava. Acta Chir Scand 137:181, 1971

100. Couinaud C: Tumerus de la Veine Cave Inférieure. J Chir (Paris) 105:411, 1973

101. Hivet M, Poilleux J, Gastard J, Hernandez C: Sarcome de la Veine Cave Inférieure. Nouvelle Presse Med 2:569, 1973

102. Stuart FP, Barker WH: Palliative surgery for leiomyosarcoma of the inferior vena cava. Ann Surg 177:237, 1973

103. Demoulin JC, Sambon Y, Bandinet V, et al: Leiomyosarcoma of the inferior vena cava: An unusual cause of pulmonary embolism. Chest 66:597, 1974

104. Kapsinow R, Brierre JT: Leiomyosarcoma of the inferior vena cava. J Louisiana State Med Soc 126:400, 1974

105. Kalsbeek HD: Leiomyosarcoma of the inferior vena cava. Arch Chir Neerl 26:35, 1974

106. Bailey RV, Stribling J, Weitzner S, Hardy JD: Leiomyosarcoma of the inferior vena cava: Report of a case and review of literature. Ann Surg 184:169, 1976

107. Jonasson O, Pritchard J, Lond D: Intraluminal leiomyosarcoma of the inferior vena cava: Report of a case. Cancer 19:1311, 1966

108. Light HG, Peskin GW, Ravdin IS: Primary tumors of the venous system. Cancer 13:818, 1960

109. Smout MS, Fisher JH: Leiomyosarcoma of saphenous vein. Canad Med Assoc J 83:1066, 1960

110. Thomas MA, Fine G: Leiomyosarcoma of veins: Report of two cases and review of the literature. Cancer 13:96, 1960

111. Beaird JB, Scofield GF: Budd-Chiara syndrome. Hepatic vein occlusion due to leiomyosarcoma primary in the inferior vena cava. Arch Intern Med (Chicago) 110:435, 1962

112. Brohl H: Sarcoma wenae femoralis dextra ligatura venae femoralis. (Abstr) Deutsche Wchnschr (Vereins-Beilage)23:30, 1897

113. Borchard: Ueber eine von Varicen des Unterschenkels ausgehende eigenthumliche Geschwulstdung (Angiosarkom). Arch Klin Chir 80:675, 1906

114. Ehrenberg L: Zwei Falle von Tumor in Herzen: ein Beitrag zur Kenntnis der Pathologie und symptomatologie der Herztumorch. Deutsches Arch Klin Med 103:293, 1911

115. van Ree A: Phlebosarcoma racemosum. Ned Tijdschr Geneesk 1:759, 1919

116. Razzaboni G: Sarcoma primitivo della vena safena interna (trombizzata). Arch Ital Chir 2:483, 1920

117. Ausbuttel F: Primares Lungensarkom. Franf Z Pathol 53:303, 1939

118. Puig-Sureda J, Gallart-Esquerdo A, Roca de Vinals R, Salleras V: Leiomiosarcoma de la vena colica izquierda inferior. Med Clin 8:104, 1947

119. Haug WA, Losli EJ: Primary leiomyosarcoma within the femoral vein. Cancer 7:159, 1954

120. Johnston JH Jr, Shands WC: Primary leiomyosarcoma of the femoral vein. Surgery 38:410, 1955

121. DeWeese JA, Terry R, Schwartz SI: Leiomyoma of the greater saphenous vein with preoperative

localization by phlebography. Ann Surg 148:859, 1958

122. Stout AP: Sarcomas of the soft tissue. Cancer 11:210, 1961

123. Dorfman HD, Fishel ER: Leiomyosarcoma of greater saphenous vein. Am J Clin Path 39:73, 1963

124. Allison MF: Leiomyosarcoma of the femoral vein: Report of a case in a child. Clin Pediat 4:28, 1965

125. Cheek JH, Nickey WM: Leiomyosarcoma of venous origin. Arch Surg 90:396, 1965

126. Lawrence MS, Crosby VG, Ehrenhaft JL: Leiomyosarcoma of the right iliac vein: Case report. Ann surg 164:924, 1966

127. Sakura O, Toda A, Morimoto K: Primary leiomyosarcoma within the femoral vein. Clin Orthop 44:197, 1966

128. Lopez-Varela EA, Peveira-Garro C: Leiomyosarcoma of the renal vein. Internat Surg 47:340, 1967

129. Leu HJ, Nipkow P: Malignant primary vein tumors. Angiologica 6:302, 1969

130. Bhathena D, Vasquez M: Primary renal vein leiomyosarcoma. Cancer 30:542, 1972

131. Larmi TKI, Ninimaki T: Leiomyosarcoma of the femoral vein. J Cardiovasc Surg 15:602, 1974

132. Nesbit RR Jr, Rob C: Leiomyosarcoma of a vein: Survival for six years. Arch Surg 110:118, 1975

133. Gross E, Horton MA: Leiomyosarcoma of the saphenous vein. J Path 116:37, 1975

134. Jernstrom P, Gowdy RA: Leiomyosarcoma of the long saphenous vein. Am J Clin Path 63:25, 1975

135. Gierson ED, Rowe JG: Renal vein leiomyosarcoma. Am Surg 42:594, 1976

136. Bloustein PA: Hepatic leiomyosarcoma: Ultrastructural study and review of the differential diagnosis. Hum Path 9:713, 1978

137. Kullman GL: Intranasal leiomyosarcoma. J Florida Med Assoc 67:931, 1980

138. Anderson WR, Cameron JD, Tsai SH: Primary intracranial leiomyosarcoma. Case Report with ultrastructural study. J Neurosurg 53(3):401, 1980

139. Cermsak RJ: Benign rhabdomyoma of the vagina. Am J Clin Path 52:604, 1969

140. Hanbury WJ: Rhabdomyomatous tumors of the urinary bladder and prostate. J Path Bacteriol 64:763, 1952

141. Misch KA: Rhabdomyoma purum: A benign rhabdomyoma of tongue. J Path Bacteriol 75:105, 1958

142. Moran JJ, Enterline HT: Benign rhabdomyoma of the pharynx. A case report and review of the literature and comparison with cardiac rhabdomyoma. Am J Clin Path 42:174, 1964

143. LaBate JS: Congenital rhabdomyoma of the heart. Am J Path 15:137, 1939

144. Batchelor TM, Maun ME: Congenital glycogenic tumors of the heart. Arch Path 39:67, 1945

145. Winstanley DP: Sudden death from multiple rhabdomyoma of the heart. J Path Bacteriol 81:249, 1961

146. Bizer LS: Rhabdomyosarcoma. Am J Surg 140:687, 1980

147. Sessions DG, Ragab AH, Vietti TJ, Biller HF, Ogura JH: Embryonal rhabdomyosarcoma of the neck in children. Laryngoscope 83:890, 1973

148. Jones IS, Reese AB, Kraut MD: Orbital rhabdomyosarcoma: An analysis of 62 cases. Am J Ophthalmol 62:203, 1959

149. Frayer WC, Enterline HT: Embryonal rhabdomyosarcoma of the orbit in children and young adults. Arch Ophthalmol 62:203, 1959

150. Pinkel D, Pickren J: Rhabdomyosarcoma in children. JAMA 174:293, 1961

151. Masson JK, Soule ED: Embryonal rhabdomyosarcoma of the head and neck: Report on eighty-eight cases. Am J Surg 110:585, 1965

152. Lawrence W Jr, Gegge G, Foote FW Jr: Embryonal rhabdomyosarcoma: A clinicopathological study. Cancer 17:361, 1964

153. Koop CE, Tewarson IP: Rhabdomyosarcoma of the head and neck in children. Ann Surg 160:95, 1964

154. Grossi C, Moore O: Embryonal rhabdomyosarcoma of head and neck. Cancer 12:69, 1962

155. Porterfield JF, Zimmerman LE: Rhabdomyosarcoma of the orbit. A clinicopathologic study of 55 cases. Virchow's Arch Path Anat 335:329, 1962

156. Sutow WW, Sullivan MP, Reid HL, Taylor HQ, Griffith: Prognosis in childhood rhabdomyosarcoma. Cancer 25:1384, 1970

157. Liebner EJ: Embryonal rhabdomyosarcoma of the head and neck in children. Cancer 37:2777, 1976

158. Horn RC, Enterline HT: Rhabdomyosarcoma: A clinicopathological study and classification of 39 cases. Cancer 11:181, 1958

159. Pratt CB, Hustu HO, Fleming ID, Pinkel D: Coordinated treatment of childhood rhabdomyosarcoma with surgery, radiotherapy, and combination chemotherapy. Cancer Res 32:606, 1972

160. Cassady RJ, Sagerman RW, Trelter P, Ellsworth RM: Radiation therapy for rhabdomyosarcoma. Radiology 91:116, 1968

161. Heyn RN, Holland R, Rewton WA, Tefft M, Breslow N, Harman JR: The role of combined chemotherapy in the treatment of rhabdomyosarcoma in children. Cancer 34:2128, 1974

162. Maurer HM: Current concepts in cancer. N Engl J Med 299:1345, 1978

163. Jaffe BF: Pediatric head and neck tumors. Laryngoscope 83:1644, 1973

164. Donaldson SS, Castro JR, Wilburn JR, Jesse RJ: Rhabdomyosarcoma of the head and neck in children: Combination treatment by surgery, irradiation and chemotherapy. Cancer 31:26, 1973

165. Jaffe N, Fitler RM, Farber S, Traggis D, Vawter GF, Tefft M, Murray JE: Rhabdomyosarcoma in children. Am J Surg 125:482, 1973

166. Heyn RN: The role of chemotherapy in the management of soft tissue sarcomas. Cancer 35:921, 1975

167. Pack GT, Eberhart WF: Rhabdomyosarcoma of skeletal muscle. Report of 100 cases. Surgery 32:1023, 1952

168. Stout AP: Rhabdomyosarcoma of skeletal muscle. Ann Surg 123:447, 1946

169. Ehrlich FF, Haas JE, Kieswelter WB: Rhabdomyosarcoma in infants and children—factors affecting long-term survival. J Pediat Surg 6:571, 1971

170. Grosfeld JL, Clatworthy HW Jr, Newton WA Jr: Combined therapy in childhood rhabdomyosar-

coma: An analysis of 42 cases. J Pediat Surg 4:637, 1969

171. Albores-Saavedra J, Martin RG, Smith JL: Rhabdomyosarcoma: A study of 35 cases. Ann Surg 157:186, 1963

172. Ghavimi F, Exelby PR, D'Angio, et al: Combination therapy of urogenital embryonal rhabdomyosarcoma in children. Cancer 32:1178, 1973

173. Lawrence W Jr, Hays DM, Moon TE: Lymphatic metastasis with childhood rhabdomyosarcoma. Cancer 39:556, 1977

174. D'Angio GJ: Management of children with Wilms' tumor. Cancer 30:1528, 1972

175. D'Angio GJ, Evans A: Soft tissue sarcomas. Chapter 18. In Bloom JC et al. (eds): Cancer in Children. Berlin and New York, Springer-Verlag, 1976

176. Joshi DP, Wessely Z, Seery WH, Neier CR: Rhabdomyosarcoma of the bladder in an adult: Case report and review of the literature. J Urol 96:214, 1966

177. McDougal WS, Persky L: Rhabdomyosarcoma of the bladder and prostate in children. J Urol 124:882, 1980

178. Lemmon WT Jr, Holland JM, Ketcham AS: Rhabdomyosarcoma of the prostate. Surgery 59:736, 1966

179. Grosfeld JL, Smith JP, Clatworthy HW Jr: Pelvic rhabdomyosarcoma in infants and children. J Urol 107:673, 1972

180. Alexander F: Pure testicular rhabdomyosarcoma. Br J Cancer 22:498, 1968

181. Tanimura H, Matsuhiro F: Rhabdomyosarcoma of the spermatic cord. Cancer 22:1215, 1968

182. Littmann R, Tessler AN, Valensi Q: Paratesticular rhabdomyosarcoma: A case presentation and review of the literature. J Urol 108:190, 1972

183. Tank ES: Treatment of urogenital tract rhabdomyosarcoma in infants and children. J Urol 107:324, 1972

184. Ghazali S: Embryonic rhabdomyosarcoma of the urogenital tract. Br J Surg 60:124, 1973

185. Hilgers RD, Malkasian GD Jr, Soule EH: Embryonal rhabdomyosarcoma (botryoid type) in the vagina: A clinicopathologic review. Am J Obstet Gynecol 107:485, 1970

186. D'Angio GJ, Teft M: Radiation therapy in the management of children with gynecologic cancers. Ann NY Acad Sci 142:675, 1967

187. El-Mahdi AM, Marks R, Thornton WN, Constable WC: Twenty-five-year survival of sarcoma botryoides treated by irradiation. Cancer 33:653, 1974

188. Hays DM, Snyder WH Jr: Botryoid sarcoma (rhabdomyosarcoma) of the bile ducts. Am J Dis Child 110:595, 1965

189. Yartid T, Nickels J, Hockerstedt K, Scheinin TM: Rhabdomyosarcoma of the esophagus. Light and electron microscopic study of a rare tumor. Virchows Arch Path Anat 386:357, 1980

190. Moses I, Coodley EL: Rhabdomyosarcoma of duodenum. Am J Gastroenterol 51:48, 1969

191. Templeton AW, Heslin DJ: Primary rhabdomyosarcoma of stomach and esophagus. Am J Roentgenol 86:896, 1961

192. Matloff JM, Bas H, Dalen JE: Rhabdomyosarcoma of the left atrium. J Thor Cardiovasc Surg 61:451, 1971

193. Makela V, Sjogren AL, Eisalo A: Rhabdomyosarcoma of the heart: a case report. Acta Path Microbiol Scand, Sect A 78:71, 1970

194. Payan H: Rhabdomyosarcoma of the ovary: Report of a case. Obstet Gynecol 26:373, 1965

195. Goldman RL, Friedman NB: Rhabdomyosarcohepatoma in an adult and embryonal hepatoma in a child. Am J Clin Path 51:137, 1969

196. Conquest HF, Thornton JL, Massie JR, Coxe JW: Primary pulmonary rhabdomyosarcoma: Report of three cases and literature review. Ann Surg 161:688, 1965

197. Mihara S, Matsumoto H, Tokunaga F, Yano H, Ota M, Yamashita S: Botryoid rhabdomyosarcoma of the gallbladder in a child. Cancer 49:812, 1982

198. Keyhani A, Booher RJ: Pleomorphic rhabdomyosarcoma. Cancer 22:956, 1968

199. Linscheid RL, Soule EH, Henderson ED: Pleomorphic rhabdomyosarcomata of the extremities and limb girdles: A clinicopathologic study. J Bone Joint Surg 47-B:715, 1965

200. Middlebrook LF, Tennant R: Rhabdomyosarcoma of uterine corpus. Obstet Gynecol 32:537, 1968

201. McNeer GP, Cantin J, Chu F, Nickson J: Effectiveness of radiation therapy in the management of sarcoma of the soft somatic tissues. Cancer 22:391, 1968

202. Thompson GCV: Rhabdomyosarcoma of skeletal muscle. Clin Orthop 19:29, 1961

203. Phelan JT, Juardo J: Rhabdomyosarcoma. Surgery 52:585, 1962

204. Purry H, Chu FCH: Radiation therapy in the palliative management of soft tissue sarcomas. Cancer 15:179, 1962

205. Suit HD, Russel WO, Martin RG: Management of patients with sarcoma of soft tissues in an extremity. Cancer 31:1247, 1973

206. Kaloyannides TM: Pleomorphic rhabdomyosarcoma of the gingiva. Oral Surg 27:150, 1969

207. Riopelle JS, Theriault JP: Sur une forme meconnue de sarcome des parties molles: Le rhabdomyosarcoma alveolaire. Ann Anat Path (Paris) 1:88, 1956

208. Enzinger FM: Recent trends in soft tissue pathology. In Tumors of Bone and Soft Tissue. Clinical Conference on Cancer, 1963. Chicago, Year Book Medical Publishers, 1965, p 315

209. Enzinger FM, Shiraki M: Alveolar rhabdomyosarcoma: An analysis of 110 cases. Cancer 24:18, 1969

210. Enterline HT, Horn RC: Alveolar rhabdomyosarcoma. A distinctive tumor type. Am J Clin Path 29:356, 1958

211. Mikulowski P, Thorbjorn B: Alveolar rhabdomyosarcoma. Acta Path Microbiol Scandinav 74:282, 1969

212. Hays DM, Soule EH, Lawrence W Jr, Gehan EA, Maurer HM, et al: Extremity lesions in the Intergroup Rhabdomyosarcoma Study (IRS-I): A preliminary report. Cancer 49:1, 1982

14

Tumors of the Peripheral Nerves

Tapas K. Das Gupta

BENIGN SOLITARY SCHWANNOMA

A benign solitary schwannoma (neurilemoma, perineural fibroblastoma, acoustic neuroma, etc.) may occur in any part of the body.[1-3] If the tumor arises from a large peripheral nerve it can easily be seen, but if it arises from an unnamed small nerve twig it is clinically indistinguishable from other types of soft tissue tumors.

Anatomic Distribution

Table 14.1 shows the anatomic distribution of benign solitary schwannomas in a series of 303 patients at Memorial Sloan-Kettering Cancer Center[4] and in a later series of 56 at the University of Illinois. It is clear that these tumors have a predilection for the head and neck region.

Although the symptoms and signs vary according to anatomic location, most patients are first seen with a painless mass of relatively long duration (Fig. 14.1). If the mass arises from a peripheral nerve, the patient may have pain along the course of the nerve before the mass is discovered. Some patients are initially seen solely because of pain along the radial, median, ulnar, or sciatic nerve.

Of the 303 patients in the Memorial Sloan-Kettering series,[4] 56.7 percent were female and 43.3 percent were male; 63 percent of the tumors

occurred in patients between the ages of 30 and 60 years. A similar sex and age distribution was observed in the 56 patients at the University of Illinois. No racial predilection was apparent in either series.

Head and Neck Region. Most commonly this tumor is seen as a fusiform mass in the lateral portion of the neck (Table 14.2), and frequently it poses a diagnostic and therapeutic problem (Fig. 14.2A to 14.2F). Although the primary objective should be excision only, occasionally some form of neck dissection is entailed. In all other areas of the head and neck region, simple enucleation is adequate.[4-9] Lesions in the scalp may require sequential excision, depending on the extent and local infiltration. Total extirpation of scalp lesions is often fraught with danger because of possible massive blood loss. Lesions of the face and parotid require exposure of the facial nerve.

A benign schwannoma of the vagus nerve is a rare, interesting clinical entity.[5,7,10,11] As of 1979 there were only 63 published cases.[11] To the best of our knowledge, no new patient has been added to this series. These tumors do not produce any symptoms of vagal insufficiency.

Acoustic neuromas arise from the sheath of the vestibular portion of the eighth nerve within the auditory canal; frequently they are

TABLE 14.1 ANATOMIC DISTRIBUTION OF SOLITARY BENIGN SCHWANNOMAS

Site	Das Gupta et al.[4] (Memorial Sloan-Kettering, 1969) No. of Cases	Das Gupta (University of Illinois, 1981) No. of Cases
Head and neck	136	15
Upper extremities	58	17
Trunk	26	6
Lower extremities	41	12
Mediastinum	28	2
Miscellaneous sites	14*	4†
Total	303	56

*Miscellaneous category from Memorial Sloan-Kettering Cancer Center includes eight in breast, one in hernial sac, one in pelvis, one in inguinal canal, two in retroperitoneal region, and one in sciatic nerve.

†Miscellaneous category from the University of Illinois includes two in retroperitoneum, one in inguinal region, and one in breast.

bilateral.[12,13] Early diagnosis is essential for maximum preservation of hearing. Approximately 33 percent of these tumors recur after subtotal intracapsular excision, but recurrence is rare after total excision.[12,13]

Upper Extremities. Table 14.3 shows the anatomic distribution in the series of cases at Sloan-Kettering Cancer Center and the series at the University of Illinois. Most patients seek medical advice because of a mass along the course of a nerve. Usually this mass enlarges slowly, creating a cosmetic defect. In a smaller number of patients, pain along the nerve is the initial symptom. Rarely, there may be pain because of

pressure of the mass on a bone, for example, a neurofibroma pressing on a phalanx (Fig. 14.3A and 14.3B).[4,9] In our series of 17 patients at the University of Illinois, 12 were initially seen because of a mass and 5 because of pain. If these tumors arise from a peripheral nerve, they can be enucleated with relative ease.

Lower Extremities. Table 14.3 shows the distribution of these tumors in the lower extremities. In our series of 12 patients at the University of Illinois, three had pain along the course of the nerve as the initial complaint. The pain occurred three to four months prior to recognition of the tumor. These tumors, like those in

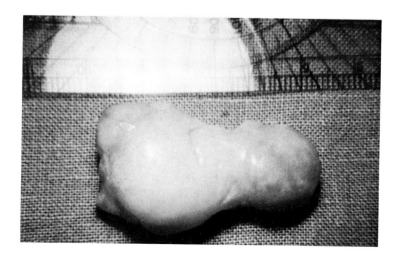

Figure 14.1. Benign schwannoma enucleated from the radial nerve. This patient, a 36-year-old woman, presented with an asymptomatic tumor at the posterolateral aspect of the right arm, requesting tumor be removed for cosmetic reasons.

TABLE 14.2. BENIGN SCHWANNOMAS OF THE HEAD AND NECK REGION

Site	Das Gupta et al.[4] (1969)	Das Gupta (1981)	Total
Scalp	7	1	8
Forehead	1	0	1
Face	2	1	3
Nose	4	0	4
Cheek	9	1	10
Tongue	8	1	9
Lip	3	0	3
Neck (lateral)	60	8	68
Parotid gland	10	1	11
Pharynx	8	0	8
Submaxillary gland	4	0	4
Hard palate	3	1	4
Soft palate	3	1	4
Miscellaneous sites*	14	0	14

One in eyelid, one in auditory canal, one in gum, one in floor of mouth, two in supraorbital region, one in infraorbital region, two in vagus nerve, one in vocal cord, one in pterygoid, two in preauricular area, and one in mastoid region.

the upper extremities, can be enucleated from the peripheral nerve.

Trunk. Usually a mass is the presenting symptom.[3,6,8] In our earlier series of 26 cases, 15 tumors were in various parts of the anterior, lateral, or posterior chest wall and 11 were in the anterior abdominal wall or lumbosacral region.[4] These tumors can be easily and successfully excised (Fig. 14.4).

Miscellaneous Sites. Benign solitary schwannomas also occur in the mediastinum[14,15] and various other miscellaneous sites.[8,9,16-23] In 1969 there were 28 benign neurogenic tumors of the mediastinum in the files of the Memorial Sloan-Kettering Cancer Center.[4] All these patients had been essentially asymptomatic and diagnosis was made after a routine chest roentgenogram showed a mediastinal mass. In the University of Illinois series, two patients were operated upon for a benign neurogenic posterior mediastinal tumor. Two retroperitoneal benign schwannomas have also been encountered (Table 14.1). In one, a large (21 × 20 × 12 cm) tumor was found at operation to lie posterior to the gastrocolic omentum (Fig. 14.5). It was

removed without difficulty. The specimen weighed 2.5 kg and had a dense fibrous capsule.

The patient remained well for three years, at which time a carcinoma of the left breast was diagnosed. She underwent a radical mastectomy elsewhere and died two years later, apparently of metastatic breast cancer. An autopsy was not done, and the status of the abdomen at the time of death is not known.

A benign solitary schwannoma is easily excised. Since the chance of malignant transformation is rare (Chapter 4 for detailed discussion), wide excisions are not advocated. When the tumor arises from a major nerve, it should be enucleated from the nerve trunk. Resection of the nerve is seldom required (Fig. 14.6). Benign peripheral nerve tumors are easily separated from the nerve trunk, which can and must be left intact.[24] Likewise, in the mediastinum and the peritoneal and pelvic cavities, the benign tumor can be enucleated.

Benign Solitary Schwannomas and Associated Tumors

In 1969, Das Gupta et al.[4] reported that 49 (16 percent) of 303 patients with benign solitary neurogenic tumors had an associated malignant tumor of some kind. Twenty-two had been treated for a malignancy prior to the development of the schwannoma, and 16 were found to have a simultaneous carcinoma. Seven were first seen because of the benign tumor and nine because of the malignancy. In 11 patients cancer developed after excision of the benign tumor.

The associated cancers seen most frequently in this study were epidermoid cancers of the skin (15), carcinoma of the breast (12), and carcinoma of the gastrointestinal tract (8). There were also carcinomas of the thyroid, uterine cervix, endometrium, and larynx, and three malignant melanomas. Of particular interest is the development of malignant melanoma and gastrointestinal tract cancers. In our present series of 54 patients, seven were treated for an associated cancer: two had cancer of the breast, three had cancer of the colon and rectum, and one each had malignant melanoma and cancer of the cervix. Assuming that a proportion of these are coincidental, it is still a relatively high incidence. Although no conclusions can be drawn regarding the association of benign schwannomas with other types of cancer, a careful study should be made of these so-called coincidences.

VON RECKLINGHAUSEN'S DISEASE (MULTIPLE NEUROFIBROMATOSIS)

Multiple neurofibromatosis has been observed in all races and in every part of the world.[25-27] The incidence was estimated by Prieser and Davenport[28] in 1918 as about 1 in 2,000 persons. Crowe and associates[26] estimated the incidence in the state of Michigan to be 1 in every 2,500 to 3,000 live births. Brasfield and Das Gupta[29] encountered an average of only five patients a year at Memorial Sloan-Kettering Cancer Center over a period of 20 years. At the University of Illinois there are approximately 10 new patients a year with von Recklinghausen's disease out of about 17,000 admissions.[30] Sexual distribution is probably equal, although early reports indicated a predilection for males. Crowe and associates[26] found that male patients constituted 52 percent of their series of 149. Fisher[31] reviewed the 466 cases reported up to 1927 and found that 64 percent of the patients were male. In a series of 110 patients from the Memorial Sloan-Kettering Cancer Center, combined with 60 patients from the University of Illinois Hospital, the percentage was 53 percent female.[29,30] Sergeyev[32] found a 52 percent female predominance in his series of 195 patients.

Because of the association of von Recklinghausen's disease with various benign and malignant soft tissue tumors and other cancers (Table 14.4),[29] some of the intriguing facets of the disease will be described in detail.

Genetic Aspects

The occurrence of this disease in multiple family members was reported by Virchow[34] as early as 1847, and again in 1862 by Hitchcock.[35] However, Thomson,[36] in 1900, was the first to point out that the condition was clearly hereditary. A year later, Adrian[37] reported that 20 percent of patients exhibited direct transmission. In 1918, Prieser and Davenport[28] established that the condition was not sex-linked and that it followed the mendelian law as a dominant trait.

Prieser and Davenport[28] noted that penetrance of the dominant gene is greater than 80 percent, which has been recently confirmed in other studies.[25,26,29] The penetrance of the gene in children of persons with sporadic cases is likewise greater than 80 percent, as attested to by the fact that approximately 40 percent of the children are affected. The expression of specific manifestations in multiple generations has been reported frequently, but as a rule the manifestations in a particular family are variable (Fig. 14.7).

The sporadic cases make up approximately half of those reported in the literature and it is impossible to clinically distinguish them from the familial types. It has not yet been established whether a sporadic case appears as the result of a new mutation or occurs in the child of a person possessing a nonpenetrant gene. Fifty percent of the patients are found to have affected relatives.[29,30] We have previously reported that in five families the disease could be traced through four generations.[29]

In monozygotic twins, concordance of clinical manifestations has been reported far more frequently than discordance.[38] As a rule there is marked phenotypic variation of the disease in a family, although Crowe and co-workers[26] found palmar and plantar neurofibromas to be an exception to this rule (Fig. 14.8). Another exception is bilateral acoustic neuroma, which appears to be a relatively consistent manifestation in affected families. It is not clear which genetic factors account for this departure from the general rule of variable expression in individual manifestation.

The basic genetic aspects of von Recklinghausen's disease are understood; however, the explanation of the penetrance and variable expression in individual manifestations remains to be discovered, as does the origin of sporadic cases.

Clinical Manifestations

The majority of patients manifest the physical signs before the age of 20 years.[29,30] In a study conducted at a pediatric hospital, Feinman and Yakovac[33] reported that 43 percent of their 46 patients had the stigmata at birth. The most common manifestation leading to diagnosis is multiple café-au-lait spots, along with subcutaneous and cutaneous neurofibromas.

Pigmentary Changes. The lesion classically identified with von Recklinghausen's disease is a brown macular pigmentation of the skin with definite, circumscribed geographic borders. This characteristic appearance has led to the use of the descriptive term of café-au-lait spot. These spots may be located anywhere on the body and

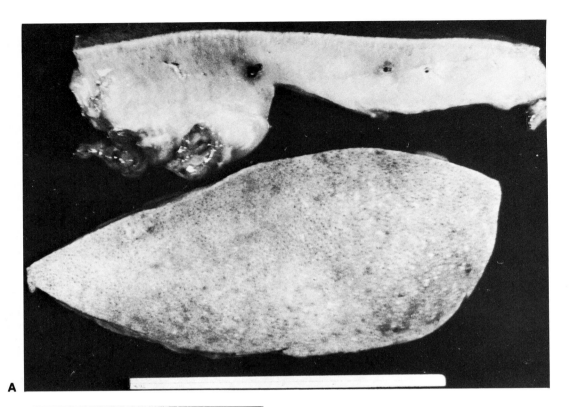

A

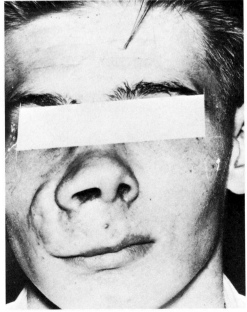

B

Figure 14.2. (A) Benign schwannoma of the scalp. Cut section shows infiltration of thickness of the scalp by glistening white neoplastic tissue. **(B)** Solitary schwannoma of the face, excised without residual deformity. **(C)** Benign schwannoma of the tongue. Patient complained of gradually increasing feeling of "heaviness" in the tongue. The tumor was excised with a rim of tongue tissue. **(D)** Solitary schwannoma of the right side of neck. Tumor arose from brachial plexus and was enucleated. **(E)** Benign schwannoma enucleated from soft palate of a 31-year-old man. **(F)** Benign schwannoma of the hard palate, left side. Note central ulceration (pressure necrosis) of the mucosa. This large mass required a subtotal maxillectomy. The orbital floor, however, could be saved.

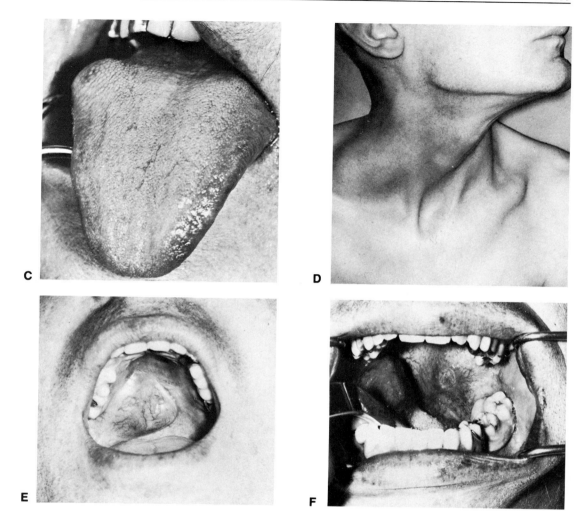

vary in size, configuration, and number (Fig. 14.9).

After Crowe and co-workers[26] investigated the genetic and clinical significance of these macular pigmentations, there was no question that these lesions were very much part of the disease. Their report in 1956 concluded that café-au-lait spots are pathognomonic findings of generalized neurofibromatosis. They suggested that any person with more than six café-au-lait spots larger than 1.5 cm must be presumed to have neurofibromatosis, even in the absence of a positive family history. In a number of patients, the only initial evidence of neurofibromatosis is macular pigmentation, with cutaneous tumors developing later in life.

In the series of 110 patients studied at Memorial Sloan-Kettering Cancer Center,[29] 108 had at least five café-au-lait spots larger than 1.5 cm distributed over the body. The majority were present at birth and in all patients were noticeable by nine years of age. In males, the color of these spots generally increases in intensity up to puberty and then remains stationary. In females, the areas become darker with pregnancy and remain dark throughout the gestational period. A return to their original light color does not occur uniformly and usually depends on the number of pregnancies. Whitehouse,[39] after evaluating 365 children younger than five years of age, stated that two or less café-au-lait spots are commonplace in childhood, that more than

TABLE 14.3. ANATOMIC DISTRIBUTION OF BENIGN
SCHWANNOMAS IN THE EXTREMITIES

Site	Das Gupta et al.[4] (1969)	Das Gupta (1981)	Total
A. Upper extremities			
Hand	20	4	24
Wrist	5	2	7
Forearm	8	5	13
Elbow	2	0	2
Arm	13	5	18
Shoulder girdle	10	1	11
B. Lower extremities			
Sole	0	1	1
Dorsum	0	3	3
Ankle	11	2	13
Leg	6	1	7
Calf	3	1	4
Knee	10	2	12
Thigh	6	1	3
Buttock	2	1	3
Groin	3	0	3

two spots occur in only 0.75 percent of normal children, and that five spots with a diameter of at least 0.5 cm should be considered diagnostic of von Recklinghausen's disease until proved otherwise.

A variation of the café-au-lait spots consists of numerous small spots in the axilla. This is referred to as "axillary freckling" (Fig. 14.10) and is probably diagnostic of neurofibromatosis. Crowe[40] found this pigmentation present in 20 percent of 523 neurofibromatosis patients he examined. He observed that axillary freckling is a pathognomonic sign of von Recklinghausen's disease. Hyperpigmentation may also be associated with neurofibromas, especially the plexiform type, resulting in the affected area taking grotesque shapes and sizes and frequently becoming elephantoid, with thick, loose, redundant hyperpigmented skin (Fig. 14.11A and 14.11B). Giant pigmented nevi (bathing trunk nevi) are sometimes associated either with underlying neurofibromatosis (Fig. 14.12),[26,29,41] or with malignant melanoma (Fig. 14.13).[42] We have encountered a similar case. An 11-year-old girl was referred to the University of Illinois with a history of metastatic brain tumor. The parents informed us she had been born with a bathing trunk nevus and had been seen by several dermatologists, only some of whom recommended sequential excision of the lesion. Because of the

controversy regarding excision, the parents delayed until the child was nine years old, at which time sequential excision was begun. However, after only three excisions in two years, she was admitted to the University of Illinois Hospital with evidence of a brain tumor. On exploratory craniotomy a left parietal lobe metastatic melanoma was noted. She received radiation therapy to the brain but died within three months. The primary site of the melanoma was never found, either in the excised skin or in the remainder of the integument. The possibility of a primary leptomeningeal melanoma was ruled out.

Sequential excision during childhood is recommended for all giant nevi (Fig. 14.14). The major reason for early excision is to eliminate the 10 percent chance of transformation into malignant melanoma or malignant transformation of the underlying plexiform neuroma. Early excision may also decrease the secondary psychologic effects of these cosmetically objectionable lesions. If melanoma supervenes, then the general principles of treatment for deep-level melanoma should be adhered to, that is, a careful workup followed by primary excision with in-continuity node dissection.

Benign Nerve Sheath Tumors Associated with von Recklinghausen's Disease

Cutaneous or subcutaneous peripheral nerve tumors (neurofibromas, schwannomas, or neurilemomas) vary in size from a few millimeters to about 20 cm and may be scattered over the body. Feinman and Yakovac[33] had 14 patients with cutaneous tumors at birth, although in Brasfield and Das Gupta's series[29] the majority initially appeared at puberty, the earliest occurrence being at six months of age and the latest at 18 years. The usual sequence is as follows: The neurofibromas are small, palpable, subcutaneous tumors; they can be found at birth or at infancy but usually become visible in the second and third decades of life (Fig. 14.15A and 14.15B). Some become pedunculated by the fourth decade (Fig. 14.15C), with an increasing number involving most of the body, including the areola in women, by the fifth decade (Fig. 14.15D). The plexiform neurofibroma (Fig. 4.60A to 4.60E, Chapter 4, and Fig. 14.11B), the characteristic feature of neurofibromatosis, is known to harbor a potential for malignant transformation. Even with this consideration aside, the plexiform neurofibroma still presents a myriad

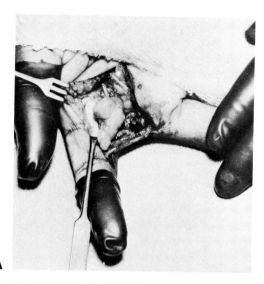

A

Figure 14.3. (**A**) Multilobulated neurofibroma being excised from the base of the index finger. (**B**) Roentgenographic appearance of the base of index finger as a result of bone absorption *(Courtesy of Cancer 24:355, 1969).*

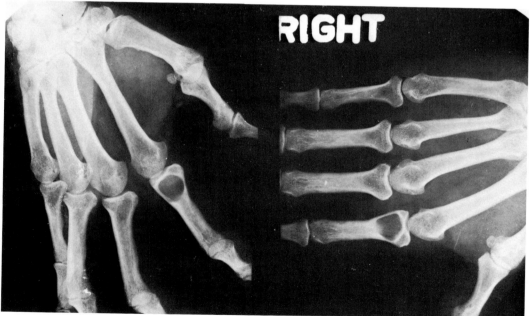

B

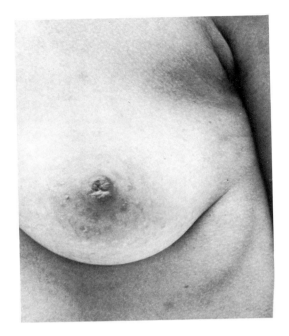

Figure 14.4. Benign solitary schwannoma arising from the sixth intercostal nerve. Lesion was excised with a free margin of intercostal nerve on both sides of the fusiform tumor. It was necessary to enter the chest cavity. Patient is still well five years later.

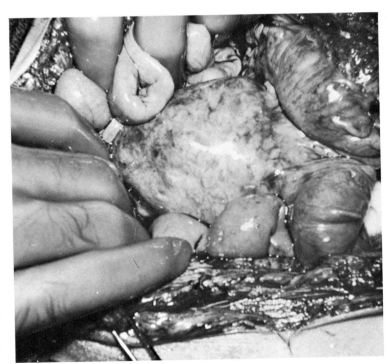

Figure 14.5. Intraoperative view of a retroperitoneal benign schwannoma. The entire tumor could be enucleated with little difficulty.

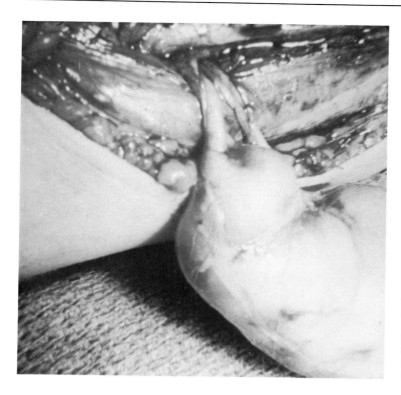

Figure 14.6. A relatively large schwannoma of the median nerve. It was tempting to perform a segmental excision of the nerve; however, a diagnosis of malignancy was not forthcoming. The tumor was thus dissected out from the main trunk of the median nerve. Final histologic diagnosis of a benign neurogenic tumor justified the time-consuming dissection. Patient is well six years later, without any functional deformity.

of difficult therapeutic problems. The extent of this lesion is difficult if not impossible to assess. Resection frequently leads to further recurrence. Whether the problem is cosmetic or whether it is an obstruction in the urinary, alimentary, or respiratory tract, radical treatment may be required to obtain a satisfactory result. Figure 14.16A to 14.16E demonstrates the frus-

TABLE 14.4. INCIDENCE OF ASSOCIATED COMPLICATIONS IN PATIENTS WITH VON RECKLINGHAUSEN'S DISEASE— TOTAL 110 PATIENTS

Associated Complications	No. Patients*	Percentage
Benign schwannomas	65	58.0
Osseous systemic involvement	52	47.2
Other types of cancer	16	14.5
Central nervous system involvement	13	12.0
Gastrointestinal tract involvement	12	11.0
Vascular lesion involvement	4	3.6
Miscellaneous cancers	5	4.5

*Some had more than one system involved.
Adapted from Brasfield and Das Gupta, 1972.[29]

tration that occurs with attempts at cosmetic excision of subcutaneous plexiform neurofibromas. Similar, apparently insurmountable cosmetic and orthopedic problems directly caused by the plexiform neurofibroma are frequently encountered. Figure 14.17 shows the effect of a large plexiform neuroma of the left thigh in a 23-year-old man with von Recklinghausen's disease. The local gigantism associated with elephantoid, hyperpigmented skin overlying the plexiform neuroma is relatively common.

Benign schwannomas are commonly seen in patients younger than 30 years of age, and a mass is usually the initial symptom. In Brasfield and Das Gupta's[29] series, 75 percent occurred in persons younger than 19, and 15 percent in those between the ages of 20 and 29 years. Treatment is greatly simplified by the absence of axons running through the tumor tissue. Meticulous dissection of the tumor from the major peripheral nerve is always possible, but in areas where the relation of the tumor to a named peripheral nerve cannot be demonstrated, a simple wide excision is adequate. Although attempts at total extirpation should always be made in patients with plexiform neuroma, a degree of conservatism should be used in the young of

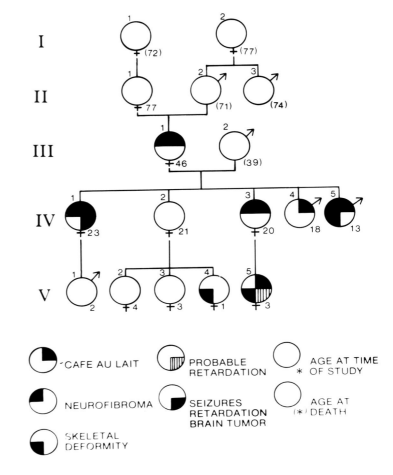

Figure 14.7. Pedigree of a family with von Recklinghausen's disease. Symbol III-1 is a patient with a sporadic case, representing either mutation or an instance in which one of the parents (II–1 and II–2) possessed a nonpenetrant gene. Symbol V–4 represents a patient with congenital bowed tibia; in this case either the mother (IV–2) possessed a nonpenetrant gene or the disease is late in being expressed and will become evident later in life *(Courtesy of Current Problems in Surgery, Ravitch MM et al. (eds). Vol XIV, Chicago, Year Book Medical Publishers, February, 1977).*

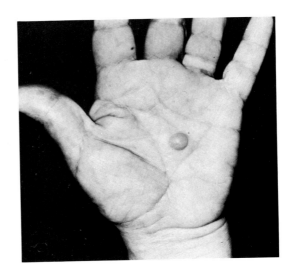

Figure 14.8. Palmar neurofibroma. This manifestation is rare even in florid cases of von Recklinghausen's disease, but is expressed frequently in families in whom it does occur. Patient had long family history of relatively uniform florid manifestations of von Recklinghausen's disease *(Courtesy of Current Problems in Surgery, Vol XIV, Chicago, Year Book Medical Publishers, 1977).*

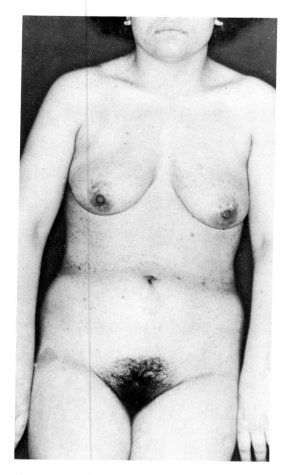

Figure 14.9. A 37-year-old woman with a large café-au-lait spot in the periumbilical region and in the inguinal crease. Also manifests small cutaneous neurofibromas.

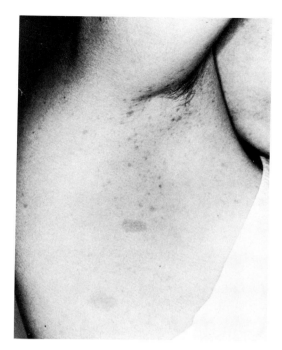

Figure 14.10. Axillary freckling in a 41-year-old woman. This is considered a pathognomonic sign of neurofibromatosis.

both sexes. It is extremely unusual to observe malignant transformation in a plexiform neuroma in children, adolescents, or young adults, and a major soft tissue resection is therefore seldom required.

Associated Clinical Manifestations of von Recklinghausen's Disease

The multifaceted clinical manifestations associated with von Recklinghausen's disease are extremely interesting, and a comprehensive study of these is of far-reaching clinical importance. Although detailed analyses of all these manifestations is beyond the scope of this book, a brief description of the more common associated conditions follows.

Central Nervous System (Table 14.5). Involvement of the central nervous system is basic to von Recklinghausen's disease. The incidence is so high and the clinical manifestations are so distinctive that some authors suggest that these manifestations be called the "central form" of the disease. Involvement of the central nervous system has been noted in 10 to 12 percent of patients.[26,29] A brief description of the more common involvements is given below.

Acoustic Neuroma. For the past 50 years bilateral acoustic neuroma has been considered to be associated with von Recklinghausen's disease. In Rodriguez and Berthong's[43] report, there were 40 cases of bilateral and 9 cases of unilateral acoustic neuroma. In 1916, Henschen[44] collected 245 cases of unilateral acoustic neuroma, of which only 5 were associated with von Recklinghausen's disease. But of 24 cases of bilateral acoustic neuroma, 19 were associated with von Recklinghausen's disease. Gardner and Frazier[45] reviewed 18 additional cases of bilateral acoustic neuroma reported between the years 1915 and

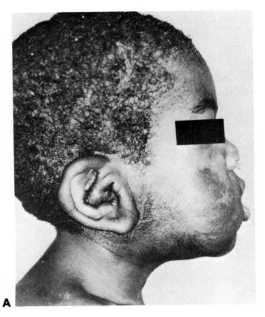
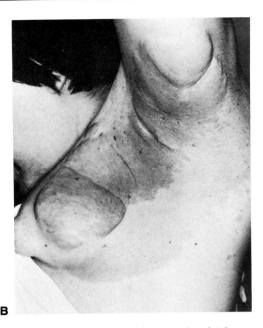

A   **B**

Figure 14.11. (**A**) A 7-year-old boy with area of hyperpigmentation of right side of face and hypertrophy of right ear. (**B**) Left axilla of 16-year-old girl with plexiform neurofibroma of breast and large area of hyperpigmentation (*Courtesy of Current Problems in Surgery, Vol XIV, Chicago, Year Book Medical Publishers, 1977*).

1930, and von Recklinghausen's disease was present in all. Crowe et al.[26] found a 4.5 percent incidence of acoustic neuroma in his large group of neurofibromatosis patients. Rarely are the symptoms manifest before the third decade of life; most commonly they are noted during the fifth decade. The tumors grow slowly with focal symptoms for years prior to increased intracranial pressure. Tinnitus is the usual presenting symptom, although some patients may first complain of progressive deafness or vertigo. If the tumor is small it may be difficult to identify the expansion radiographically, but in late stages the destruction of the walls of the internal auditory canal becomes obvious (Fig. 14.18).

The treatment of an acoustic neuroma is excision. Although intracapsular enucleation of the tumor is probably therapeutic, in about two-thirds of all cases it is advisable to attempt total excision, since it is more definitive and recurrence is unusual.[30,46] Unfortunately, operative injury to the facial nerve can be expected in about 50 percent of cases and is directly proportional to the size of the tumor. The five-year survival rate, according to Olivecrona,[46] is twice as high with total removal as with partial resection.

Glioma. One of the more common lesions is glioma of the optic nerve and the chiasma. In contrast, medulloblastomas are uncommon.[47] These tumors are usually found in younger patients, many in their second and third decades.[48] The gliomas described by Rubinstein[48] are the juvenile type of pilocytic astrocytomas of the third ventricle, and the ependymoma. The ependymomas are often multiple and are usually in the spinal cord. Exceptionally diffuse gliomas have been reported involving large areas of the central nervous system in about 45 percent of patients with von Recklinghausen's disease.[43] In gliomas affecting the optic nerve or the chiasm, gradual visual impairment is the rule. Radiographically, the usual finding is enlargement of the optic canal with retention of distinct cortical margins. Advanced cases may result in proptosis and blindness (Fig. 14.19A and 14.19B).

Meningioma. The occurrence of multiple intracranial tumors in von Recklinghausen's disease has been widely reported. In 1956, David and co-workers[49] reviewed 84 cases of multiple meningioma and found that 42 of the patients had von Recklinghausen's disease, acoustic neuromas, or both. In 1966, Rodriguez and

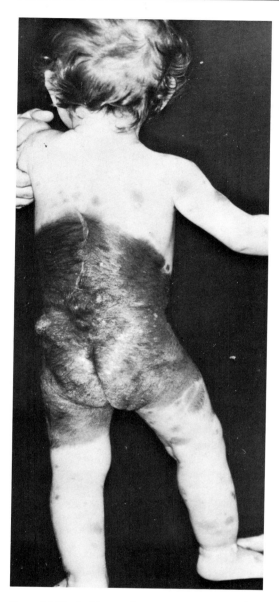

Figure 14.12. Bathing trunk nevus in a 1-year-old infant. Note abundance of hair, a characteristic feature. Nodular growths within the nevus are evident. Biopsy of these nodules showed them to be plexiform neurofibromas *(Courtesy of Current Problems in Surgery, Vol XIV, Chicago, Year Book Medical Publishers, 1977).*

Berthong[43] reviewed the published cases and found 49 instances of multiple meningioma in the following distribution: intracranial, 54 percent; intraspinal, 4 percent; intraspinal and intracranial, 42 percent; and orbital, 6 percent.

Multiple intracranial and spinal meningiomas associated with other tumors of the central nervous system are thought to be characteristic of the central form of von Recklinghausen's neurofibromatosis.[48] Radiographs show that intracranial meningiomas frequently cause localized hyperostosis, erosion, increased vascularity, or calcification (Fig. 14.20A and 14.20B). The meningiomas are attached to the inner aspect of the dura. The treatment is excision.

Spinal Lesions. Intraspinal meningiomas produce radiographic changes in only about 10 percent of cases, compared with 45 percent in patients with intraspinal neurofibromas.[38] Myelography is essential for diagnosis. In the group reported by Brasfield and Das Gupta,[29] there was spinal cord involvement only in those patients in whom the stigmata of multiple neurofibromatosis were observed after six years of age, with symptoms appearing between the ages of 20 and 25 years.

Syringomyelia. Syringomyelia was present in 20.5 percent of Rodriquez and Berthong's[43] patients with multiple intracranial tumors. The cavities were distributed throughout the spinal cord and the medulla oblongata. Poser,[50] in 1956, reviewed 234 cases of central nervous system neoplasms associated with syringomyelia. In 17 of his cases, syringomyelia was associated with von Recklinghausen's disease, and in 9, both von Recklinghausen's disease and meningioma were present.

Alimentary Tract. Recognition of involvement of the alimentary tract did not have to await sophisticated diagnostic studies to be appreciated as part of the disease. In his original paper, von Recklinghausen[51] described a patient with neurofibromas and malignant transformation in the stomach and jejunum. Most patients with neurofibromas of the gastrointestinal tract do not have associated von Recklinghausen's disease. River, Silverstein, and Topel[52] found that tumors of nerve sheath origin constituted 6 percent of the benign small bowel neoplasms in their series. They also found that 15 percent of the patients with neurofibroma of the gastrointestinal tract had von Recklinghausen's disease. Only 12 percent of the patients with von Recklinghausen's disease had gastrointestinal involvement in the combined series of 219 patients in studies by Ghrist,[53] Hochberg et al.,[54] and Brasfield and Das Gupta.[29] Hochberg and associates,[54] however, hypothesized that 50 per-

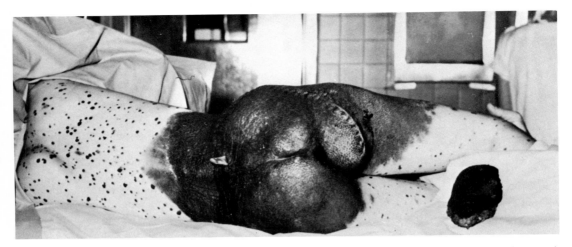

Figure 14.13. This 17-year-old girl was referred with a large nodular mass in the gluteal region of her bathing trunk nevus. Biopsy of the mass showed it to be malignant melanoma. Wide excision and in-continuity radical groin dissection were performed; the nodes contained both benign neval cells and metastatic malignant melanoma. She died of the metastatic melanoma within one year. Parents stated that while the girl was prepubertal they received conflicting opinions regarding the advisability of excising the nevus *(Courtesy of the late GP McNeer, MD, and Current Problems in Surgery, Vol XIV, Chicago, Year Book Medical Publishers, 1977).*

cent of von Recklinghausen patients may show hyperplasia of Auerbach's plexus throughout the entire gastrointestinal tract.

Involvement of the oral cavity is rare. Rappaport[55] found only seven cases reported between 1893 and 1946, but subsequent reports by Baden and co-workers,[56] Borberg,[25] Preston and associates,[57] and Chen and Miller[58] indicated an incidence in the range of 6 percent. The oral cavity is distinct from the remainder of the alimentary tract in that the mucosa is derived from the neuroectoderm. The oral area most commonly involved with neurofibroma is the tongue. As early as 1849, Smith[59] reported a case of multiple neurofibromatosis with oral manifestations, describing a tumor the size of a walnut on the left side of the tongue. Isolated neurofibromas lend themselves to local excision; multiple lesions present a more difficult management problem. The teeth do not appear to be primarily involved, except as part of congenital hemifacial hypertrophy in which there is uniform enlargement of the whole side or part of the face and similar enlargement of the underlying bone. Mandibular involvement is usually the result of a subperiosteal neurofibroma that has caused cortical erosion, or there may be irregular distortion by an adjacent plexiform neurofibroma.[60] One of the most distressing manifestations is secondary to cranial nerve in-

volvement, with impairment of the gustatory senses, coordination in swallowing, or the gag reflex.

The jejunum and the stomach are most frequently involved in von Recklinghausen's disease, followed by the ileum and duodenum.[61] Only rarely are the esophagus[62] or colon[63] affected (Fig. 14.21). This is contrary to the predominantly ileal location in isolated neurofibromas of the intestine not associated with the systemic disease. Hochberg et al.[54] reviewed 32 cases of gastrointestinal involvement in the literature and added seven cases of their own. The average age at diagnosis was 46 years. About one-third of the patients were asymptomatic, but others presented with bleeding, obstruction, intussusception, volvulus, or a mass. In some patients large segments of the jejunum require excision to control bleeding.[29] The most common origin of the neurofibromas is extraluminally in the subserosa, but submucosal and intramural locations are also encountered. Approximately 15 percent of the gastrointestinal tumors appear to be malignant, usually occurring in patients over 40 years of age (Fig. 14.22). Ulcerations, if present, are small and discrete in benign lesions. In malignant lesions they tend to be large and irregular. Multiplicity of gastrointestinal tumors occurs in approximately a third of those so affected.

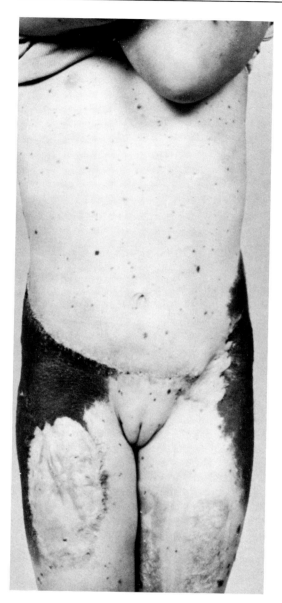

Figure 14.14. Bathing trunk nevus in an 8-year-old girl who is being treated by segmental excision. She was referred to us after several excisions were performed elsewhere.

The diagnosis can be made with careful upper gastrointestinal contrast studies. Since the lesions are hypervascular, intestinal angiography can be helpful in identifying the number and location of the tumors and in defining their blood supply.

Excision of these intestinal tumors is fa-

vored if possible. Malignant lesions require an en bloc resection, which may include other viscera or adjacent structures.

Genitourinary Tract. Involvement of the urinary tract with generalized neurofibromatosis was first reported by Gerhardt[64] in 1878. A 30-year-old patient had neurofibromas of the bladder neck, as well as cutaneous, intraspinal, intra-abdominal, and intrathoracic lesions. In 1932, Kass[65] first reported bladder involvement in a child. So far, there have been fewer than 40 cases of urinary tract involvement reported in patients with neurofibromatosis.[30]

One-third of all cases are reported in children, with involvement of males being twice as common. In general, the patients are either totally asymptomatic or complain of serious symptoms such as incontinence, retention, pain, or hematuria. Most male patients with urinary tract involvement are found to have a palpable mass above the prostate, and in a few instances a suprapubic mass can be felt. A submucosal mass may be visible on cystoscopy. The involvement may be localized and nodular; however, the usual picture is one of diffuse disease with ill-defined borders (Fig. 14.23).

The origin of the tumor appears to be the pelvic autonomic plexi,[66] which are located along the lateral aspects of the pelvic viscera, forming an extensive network of nerve fibers. The vesical and prostatic plexi are associated with the lower ureters and the bladder neck. This critical location accounts for the combined ureteral and vesical obstruction that occurs when the urinary tract is involved (Fig. 14.24A and 14.24B).

Treatment of plexiform neuromas of the bladder or other parts of the genitourinary tract depends on the symptoms the tumor produces. Although limited excision should initially be attempted, frequently the local extension of the tumor necessitates a radical operation, as described above.

Malignant transformation in the urinary bladder is rare. Ross's[67] case in 1957 probably represents the only undisputed case of neurofibrosarcoma of the urinary bladder in a patient with von Recklinghausen's disease.

Localized involvement of the ureter or renal pelvis with neurofibroma is extremely rare and is limited to a single report by Ravich[68] in 1935. This patient had an isolated neurofibroma of the left ureter but none of the stigmata of generalized neurofibromatosis.

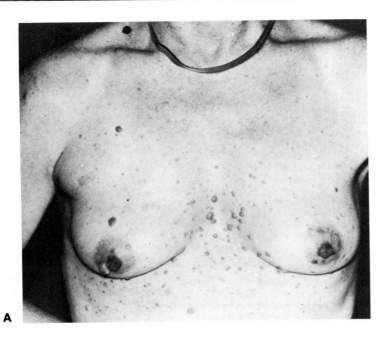

Figure 14.15. (A) A 23-year-old woman with cutaneous and subcutaneous nodules, not as yet unsightly *(Courtesy of Current Problems in Surgery, Vol XIV, Chicago, Year Book Medical Publishers, 1977).*

A

To this author's knowledge, genital involvement has never been reported in a male patient, and only rarely in a female patient. Brasfield and Das Gupta[29] reported one patient with vulvar involvement, and one other such patient was seen by the author at the University of Illinois.

Skeletal Involvement. The following assortment of skeletal involvements have come to be considered as part of neurofibromatosis: scoliosis, kyphosis, scalloping of vertebral bodies, enlarged vertebral foramina, long bone erosion, cysts, bowing, pseudoarthrosis, hypertrophy, and hypoplasia. Hunt and Pugh,[69] Brasfield and Das Gupta,[29] and Heard and Payne[70] in their large series found bony changes in about 50 percent of patients. About one-half of those so affected had vertebral abnormalities. Table 14.6 shows the clinical features of the common forms of osseous involvements and their treatments (Fig. 14.25A to 14.25C).

Malignant Tumors Associated with von Recklinghausen's Disease

There is a higher than normal incidence of associated malignant tumors in patients with von Recklinghausen's disease. Although the most common form encountered is a malignant tumor of peripheral nerve origin, several other apparently unrelated epithelial cancers are seen as well. A review of published works[71,72] shows that about half the malignancies of nerve sheath origin occur in patients with neurofibromatosis. The association of epithelial tumors, however, is of considerable interest. Brasfield and Das Gupta[29] found that in their series of 110 patients with von Recklinghausen's disease, 16 (14.5 percent) had nonneurogenic malignant tumors. Five of the 54 female patients (9 percent) were treated for carcinoma of the breast, six for malignant melanoma (Fig. 14.26), four for carcinoma of the thyroid, and one for cancer of the lung. Although there is one published case report of melanoma arising in a café-au-lait spot,[73] this author has never encountered such a case. An estimation of the true incidence of epithelial cancer in von Recklinghausen's disease is not available at this time.[47] To what extent the underlying neurofibromatosis influences the prognosis is unknown.

The relationship between pheochromocytoma or neuroblastoma with von Recklinghausen's disease has long been recognized. A detailed discussion regarding this association will be found in sections dealing with these entities.

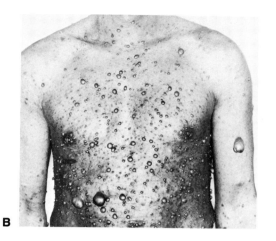

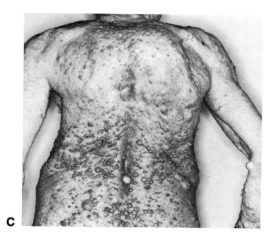

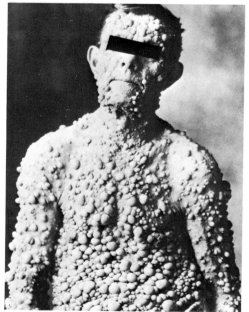

Figure 14.15. (**B**) Cutaneous and subcutaneous nodules are apparent in this 32-year-old man. (**C**) Same patient as in **B**, at age 49. Note progression of nodules and spinal deormity. (**D**) A 57-year-old man with extensive cutaneous involvement over entire body (*Courtesy of L. Solomon, Department of Dermatology, University of Illinois, and Current Problems in Surgery, Year Book Medical Publishers, 1977*).

SOLITARY MALIGNANT SCHWANNOMAS

Sex, Age, and Racial Distribution

These tumors are about equally divided between the sexes.[71,72,74,75] In the present series of 56, 30 (53.5 percent) were men and 26 (46.4 percent) were women. In our earlier series, 56 percent were men and 44 percent were women.[74] The tumor occurs in all ages; however, in one study[74] 42 percent of patients were between 30 and 50 years of age, and 15 percent were between 20 and 29 years of age. No racial predilection has been found in our two series.

Anatomic Distribution

Solitary malignant schwannomas can arise in the peripheral nerves in practically every anatomic region[72,74,75] (Table 14.7).

In the present group of 56 patients, seven tumors (12.5 percent) were in the head and neck region, 12 (21 percent) in the upper extremities, six (10.7 percent) in the trunk, and 24 (42.8 percent) in the lower extremities. Another seven

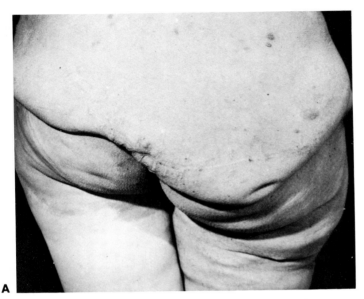

A

Figure 14.16. (**A**) to (**E**)—Shows the long-term effort required to obtain the semblance of a cosmetic result. This patient was 32 years old when she was referred with this huge plexiform neuroma of the lower back and buttock. Lateral view (**E**) is 11 operations and three and one half years later. One of the major problems encountered was the extensive microscopic involvement of the surrounding peripheral tissue, which is not usually recognized until recurrence in the margins of sequential excision.

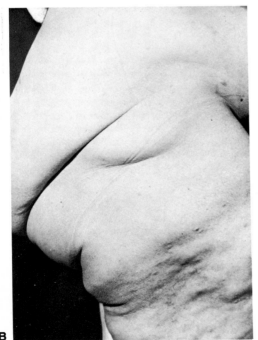

B

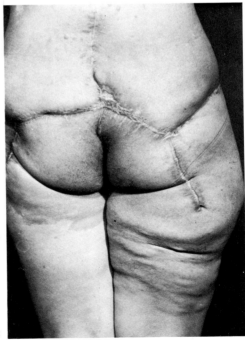

C

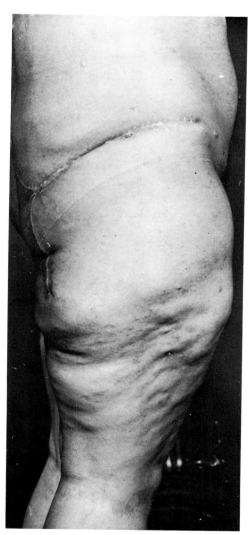

D

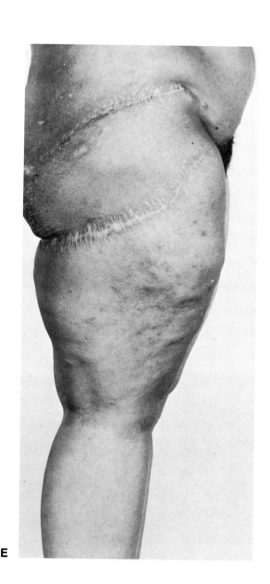

E

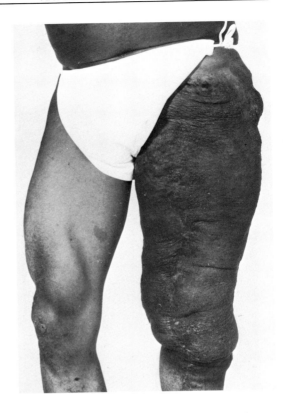

Figure 14.17. This 23-year-old man with known von Recklinghausen's disease came to our clinic with a history of café-au-lait spots present at birth and cutaneous neurofibromas developing at age 3 years. The plexiform neurofibroma that eventually involved his entire left thigh first became evident at age 7 years. It progressively enlarged, with the overlying skin becoming more pigmented, redundant, and thickened, and with concurrent overgrowth of the length and width of the femur. To retard growth of the bone, the distal femoral epiphysis was stapled when the patient was 10 years of age and the proximal epiphysis of the left tibia and fibula was stapled at age 15. This resulted in the legs being nearly equal in length at the completion of growth. By age 15, the patient had a thoracolumbar scoliosis and required spinal fusion. Pseudoarthrosis of the fusion developed and because of continued pain, a second fusion was performed when the patient was 22, by use of a Harrington rod. From age 10 until the present he has had numerous subcutaneous and cutaneous masses removed, all of which have been benign plexiform neurofibromas. *(Courtesy of Current Problems in Surgery, Vol XIV, Chicago, Year Book Medical Publishers, 1977).*

(12.5 percent) were in miscellaneous sites: three in the retroperitoneum, two in the pelvic wall, and one in the perineum (Table 14.7).

Patients with solitary malignant schwannoma are usually seen with a mass. In some instances, as in its benign counterpart, pain along the course of a peripheral nerve is the initial symptom (between 6 to 7 percent of patients). The size of the primary tumor is usually dependent on the duration of the tumor. In the present group of 56 patients, the largest tumor had a diameter of 20 cm and was located in the retroperitoneum.

Head and Neck Region. A diagnosis of malignant schwannoma in the head and neck region is primarily based on microscopic examination of the mass. The propensity of benign schwannomas to grow in the lateral portion of the neck has already been described. In contrast, solitary malignant schwannomas of the head and neck region are infrequent.[1-3,72,74,76] In the present series of seven patients, the distribution was two in the neck, one in the cheek, and four in the

scalp (Fig. 14.27A to 14.27C). A fusiform solid tumor in the lateral portion of the neck, which is movable from side to side but relatively immobile vertically, should be considered a schwannoma until proved otherwise. Microscopic examination will ascertain the malignancy or benignity of the lesion.

Upper Extremities. In our previous study of 69 patients,[74] 23 had tumor in the shoulder and axillae, 22 in the upper arm, 18 in the forearm, and one in the palm. In five, the tumor arose directly from the brachial plexus. In the present group of 12, three had tumor in the shoulder, five in the upper arm, three in the forearm, and one in the palm. In eight of the 12 the primary tumor appeared to arise from a peripheral nerve (Fig. 14.28A and 14.28B).

Trunk. This is a relatively rare site for a malignant schwannoma in patients who do not have von Recklinghausen's disease. However, in our 1970 report,[74] 38 were found to have this tumor in the soft tissue of the trunk. Eleven were in

TABLE 14.5. COMMON INVOLVEMENT OF THE CENTRAL NERVOUS SYSTEM IN VON RECKLINGHAUSEN'S DISEASE

Histologic Type	Age at Clinical Onset	Symptoms	Treatment
Schwannoma Cranial nerves			
VIII (acoustic neuroma)	30–50	Tinnitus, vertigo, deafness, facial nerve paralysis, ataxia	Observation for very early lesions, subscapular or total excision for all other lesions
V (trigeminal nerve)	30–50	Facial pain	Chemical or radiofrequency lesion of ganglion
Spinal nerve roots	20–50	Dermatone pain or paresthesia, cord compression with eventual paralysis	Excision of tumor and decompression of the nerve or cord
Neurofibroma Spinal nerve roots	20–50	As in schwannoma	As in schwannoma
Glioma Optic nerve and chiasmal glioma	1–15	Diminished visual field, proptosis, blindness	None (surgery and radiation no longer recommended)
Astrocytoma	10–30	Increased intracranial pressure or focal paralysis	Total or partial excision if possible; postoperative radiation if excision partial
Ependymoma	10–50	Cord compression, if intracranial symptoms are of increased intracranial pressure	Excision rarely possible; decompression followed by radiation is the usual therapy
Meningioma Orbital	20–40	Extremely variable symptoms dependent upon location (all meningiomas)	Excision; treatment augmented by radiation if excision is incomplete
Intracranial	20–50		
Intraspinal	20–40		
Syringomyelia	15–40	Slowly progressive sensory and motor loss with a bizarre pattern distribution	Radiotherapy may result in some pain relief, surgery is usually harmful, no therapy is probably best
Heterotopia of cortical architecture	Birth	Mental retardation	None

Courtesy of Current Problems in Surgery, Vol XIV, Chicago, Year Book Medical Publishers, 1977.

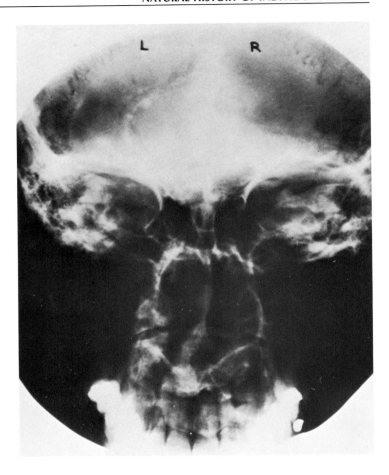

Figure 14.18. Skull film of a 53-year-old woman demonstrating erosion of left internal auditory canal by a large acoustic neuroma. She was known to have von Recklinghausen's disease and was seen because of pain in the tongue.

the anterior chest, nine in the lumbosacral region, and five in the anterior abdominal wall. The remaining 13 were distributed in the posterior and lateral trunk. In only 10 patients was the tumor associated with pain. In the present group of six patients, the tumor was located in the posterior trunk in four and in the anterior trunk in two.

Lower Extremities. The most frequent sites of origin of this tumor are the thigh and the buttocks (Fig. 14.29). Of the 24 patients in the present group, six tumors (25 percent) were in the buttocks and nine (37.5 percent) in the anterior and posterior thigh. The remaining nine tumors were located in the leg and region of the ankle. Das Gupta and Brasfield[74] described a series of 89 patients with tumor in the lower extremities: 42 were in the thigh, 17 in the legs, 10 in the buttocks, 9 in the area of the knee joints, 6 on the feet and ankles, and 5 in the groin. The

lesions in the buttocks frequently produce pain along the sciatic distribution resembling the pain of sciatica.

Miscellaneous Sites. In our present series, seven tumors (12.5 percent) were in miscellaneous sites: four in the retroperitoneum, two in the pelvis, and one in the perineum. A similar distribution was observed in our previous report.[74] An accurate diagnosis can be made only after histologic examination of the specimen.

Treatment

Management of this tumor is radical excision, based on location, shape, size, and local spread. The tumor plus its bed and any attached muscle, bone, fascia, or blood vessel, should be resected en bloc. If the nerve of origin is identified, it should be resected through a normal segment. The proximal margin of the resected nerve should be examined histologically at the

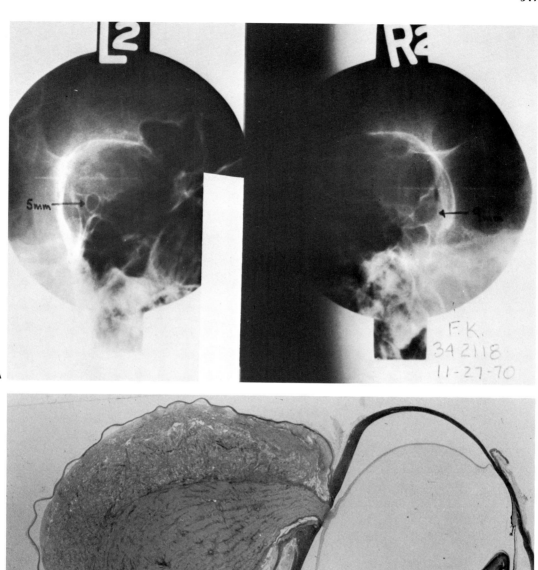

Figure 14.19. (**A**) Views of optic canals demonstrating a normal optic canal on the right with the left canal almost twice the diameter. (**B**) A large optic glioma that resulted in severe proptosis and blindness. Compression of the posterior globe is evident *(Courtesy of D Apple, MD, and Current Problems in Surgery, Vol XIV, Chicago, Year Book Medical Publishers, 1977).*

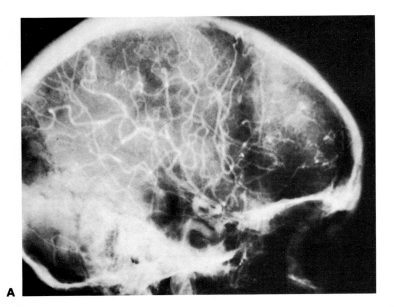

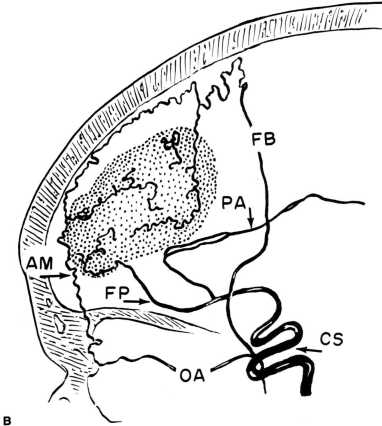

Figure 14.20. (A) Carotid angiogram showing a falx meningioma. (B) Line drawing of feeding vessels. CS, carotid sypnon; PA, pericallosal artery; FB, frontal branch of superficial temporal; AM, anterior meningeal artery; FP, frontopolar artery; OA, ophthalmic artery. *(Courtesy of Current Problems in Surgery, Vol XIV, Chicago, Year Book Medical Publishers, 1977).*

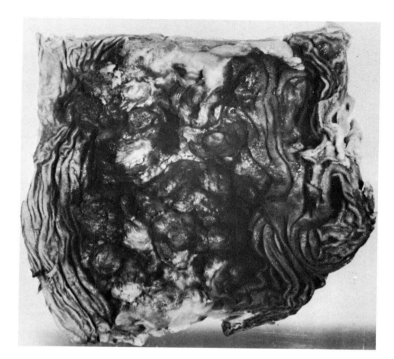

Figure 14.21. Unusual rectal involvement in a patient who died of pulmonary metastasis from a primary malignant schwannoma of a lower extremity. The only symptom the patient had of rectal neurofibroma was occasional bleeding from the anus *(Courtesy of Current Problems in Surgery, Vol XIV, Chicago, Year Book Medical Publishers, 1977).*

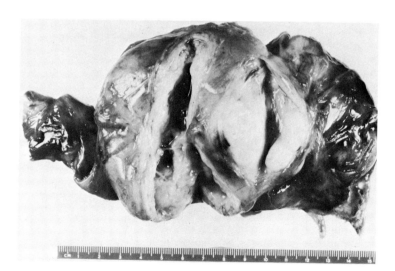

Figure 14.22. A polypoid neurofibrosarcoma in the jejunum of a 31-year-old man with neurofibromatosis. This tumor produced intussusception, causing small bowel obstruction *(Courtesy of Current Problems in Surgery, Vol XIV, Chicago, Year Book Medical Publishers, 1977).*

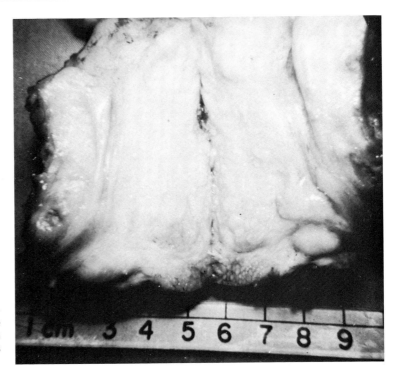

Figure 14.23. Urinary bladder; bisected specimen shows extensive involvement of the bladder wall with plexiform neuroma. Note thickness of the wall.

time of the operation. Regional node dissection is not indicated, since hematogenous spread is the primary route of metastases. When radical local excision is performed, restoration of nerve continuity is not always feasible. Since 68 percent of solitary malignant schwannomas arise in the peripheral nerves of the extremities, the feasibility of peripheral nerve grafting should be determined.

If the tumor is near the shoulder or hip joints or if there is nodular enlargement along the course of the affected major peripheral nerve, the logical primary treatment is major amputation. Limited local excisions are associated with local recurrences.

Radiation therapy alone as a curative form of management for primary malignant peripheral nerve tumors has been tried in the past.[76,77] McNeer and co-workers[77] reported that three of their four patients were long-term survivors. In our previous study,[74] 22 of 48 patients (46 percent) treated with radiation therapy alone survived for at least five years. Suit and co-workers[78] and Lindberg and associates[79] argued in favor of radiation therapy as a major mode of treatment (see Chapter 7). There is as yet no evidence that adjuvant chemotherapy plays a sig-

nificant role in the treatment of malignant schwannomas (Chapter 8).

End Results

In our present series of 56 patients, 44 (78.5 percent) were treated by radical excision alone, and 12 (21.4 percent) by surgery and postoperative irradiation. Forty (71 percent) have remained disease-free for at least five years (Table 14.8). In our previous study,[74] 201 of 232 patients were treated with intent to cure, 132 of the 201 being treated primarily by operation (Table 14.9). Of the 124 eligible for analysis, 37 (30 percent) were still disease-free after five years (Table 14.9). Of 12 patients who underwent major amputation, all had recurrent tumors and only three lived for five years or longer.

In an attempt to define in proper perspective the type of excision that should be used, the results of excision in our 1970 report[74] were compared with those in our present series (Table 14.10). Local limited excision alone[74] salvaged only 30 percent of the patients; therefore its continued use is not advisable. Comparison of soft tissue resection results between the two series is startling. In the 1970 report,[74] there was a 27 percent five-year disease-free survival,

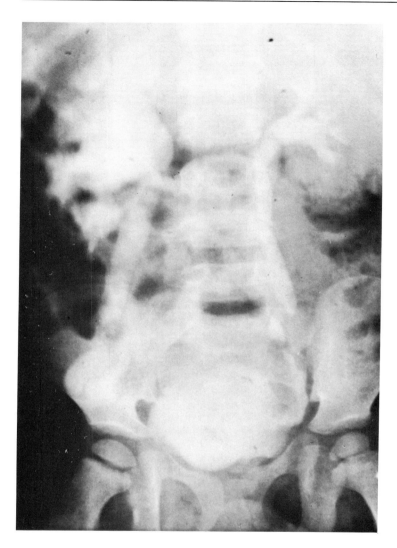

Figure 14.24. (A) Intravenous pyelogram of a 4-year-old boy with massive involvement of the urinary bladder. There is marked dilatation of the pelvis and ureter of the left side, with resultant thinning of the cortex *(Courtesy of Current Problems in Surgery, Vol XIV, Chicago, Year Book Medical Publishers 1977).*

whereas in the present series it is 81 percent. This vastly superior end result in the later series cannot be explained solely on the basis of technical considerations. It is probably related to the stage of the tumors. Analysis of the 56 patients in our present series, according to tumor size and grade, again confirms that the smaller the size and the more differentiated the tumor, the better the disease-free salvage (Table 14.11). Major amputation, if and when indicated, salvaged a number of patients. Nine of 17 (52 percent) in the present series have survived five years or longer. In our opinion, major amputations should be performed as a last resort, that is, when the patient cannot be salvaged by a

primary wide soft tissue resection alone or in conjunction with adjuvant use of radiation therapy. In certain anatomic locations, however, primary major amputation may be the initial therapy of choice.

Combined surgery and radiation therapy in 12 patients produced a cure rate of 58 percent in the Memorial Sloan-Kettering Cancer Center series.[74] In the University of Illinois group, radiation therapy was used only postoperatively and resulted in an overall salvage of 75 percent (Table 14.8). Six of our patients, following excision biopsy, were primarily treated by radiation therapy elsewhere, but we maintain their followup. Two (33 percent) are still disease-free

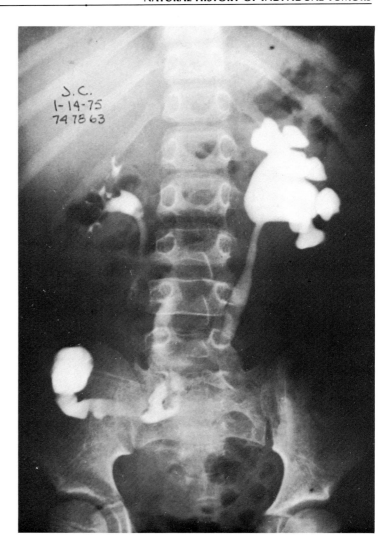

Figure 14.24 (B) Same child seven years after a cystectomy and ilieal conduit formation.

after five years. Lindberg and co-workers[79] recently reviewed the experience at the M. D. Anderson Hospital with 60 patients who had neurofibrosarcoma in various anatomic locations. With the use of conservative surgery and postoperative radical radiation therapy, these authors found a local recurrence rate of 33 percent and an absolute survival rate of 50 percent for five years. Evaluation of our present data shows that appropriate radical soft tissue resection produced a salvage rate of 81 percent in the 27 patients who underwent this procedure (Table 14.10). Therefore, substitution of this form of therapy for other modalities must be adequately justified.

Local Recurrence. Failure of initial therapy of the tumor is characterized by local recurrence. In Das Gupta and Brasfield's[74] series, 61 of 132 patients (46.2 percent) had local recurrence after initial operation. As expected, the local recurrence rate was highest with local excision: 40 (73 percent) of 55 patients, compared with only 10 (21 percent) of 48 patients who had wide soft tissue resection. Similarly, 9 (56 percent) of 16 patients had local recurrence after minor amputation. In the present series of 44 patients who were treated by operation alone, only 3 (6.8 percent) had local recurrence. This improvement is attributable to the abandonment of local excision and the expanded use of wide

TABLE 14.6. COMMON SKELETAL INVOLVEMENT

Histologic Type	Age at Clinical Onset	Symptoms	Treatment
Kyphoscoliosis	7–17	Deformity, back pain, dyspnea, paralysis	Milwaukee brace, skeletal traction, spinal fusion (Harrington rod)
Hypertrophy	2–20	Overgrowth usually associated with an adjacent plexiform neurofibroma	Resection of the plexiform neurofibroma is unlikely to be complete. Stapling of epiphysis at appropriate times may equalize growth
Vertebral scalloping	10–40	Usually none	None; may occur with no adjacent lesion causing erosion
Erosions	5–40	Usually none; however any bone is subject to deformity due to an adjacent neurofibroma	None, unless function or deformity dictates the need for therapy
Bowed tibia with pseudarthrosis	Birth–5	Bowed tibia, spontaneous fracture that does not heal	Long grafts spanning almost the entire diaphysis; casting very rarely successful
Cysts	10–40	Usually none; may palpate mass or sustain pathologic fracture	Usually none. If fracture occurs, removal of the offending neurofibroma in the bone is followed by a cast
Sphenoid bone dysplasias	Birth–15	Usually none; exophthalmos, orbital neurofibromas, pulsatile exophthalmos	No treatment to the bone defect; associated plexiform neurofibroma may be partially excised

Courtesy of Current Problems in Surgery, Vol XIV, Chicago, Year Book Medical Publishers, 1977.

soft tissue resection as the initial form of primary treatment.

MALIGNANT SCHWANNOMAS ASSOCIATED WITH VON RECKLINGHAUSEN'S DISEASE (FIGS. 14.30 to 14.34)

The association of malignant peripheral nerve tumors with von Recklinghausen's disease is well known.[27,30] Harkin and Reed,[3] D'Agostino et al.[71] and Hope and Mulvihill[47] found it impossible to establish the true incidence. Brasfield and Das Gupta[29] reported an overall incidence of 29 percent. Their conclusion was based on long-term observation of a large number of hospital-based patients. Of 18 patients observed until they were more than 50 years of age, malignant peripheral nerve tumors developed in nine. In other age categories the incidence was smaller. In a more recent study of 60 patients at the University of Illinois,[30] we found a similar high incidence of malignant peripheral nerve tumors. An increased incidence with advancing age is noted when the patients are followed up over a long period.

Whether the malignant nerve sheath tumor arises ab initio or is the product of malignant transformation of a preexisting benign nerve sheath tumor is a moot point.[80] D'Agostino et al.[71] found only two patients out of 21 in whom there was actual intermingling of the sarcomatous and neurofibromatous tissues. Harkin and Reed[3] argued that transformation of a benign schwannoma into a malignant variety rarely if ever occurs. In contrast, malignant nerve sheath tumors often are closely associated with a plexiform neurofibroma and transition to malignancy can be demonstrated (Patient 18, Table 14.12, Fig. 14.25C). A positive conclusion to this controversy may never be reached. The author has seen two patients in whom it is possible that a sarcoma developed at the site of a previously excised neurofibroma (Patients 10 and 17 in Table 14.12, Figure 14.30). This controversy, however, does not affect patient management, since therapy is not planned on the

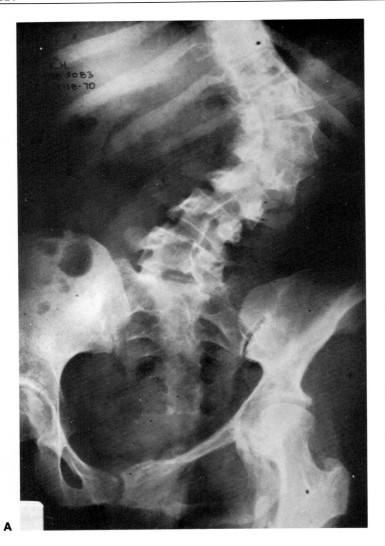

A

Figure 14.25. (**A**) An example of severe kyphoscoliosis in a young adult. This patient also had pseudoarthrosis of the tibia and fibula, which ultimately resulted in a below-knee amputation. Note dysplasia of hemipelvis. (**B**) Classical bowing of tibia with pseudoarthrosis in a child of 3 years. (**C**) An advanced case of von Recklinghausen's disease. Note the kyphoscoliosis, elephantiasis of localized skin, plexiform neurofibroma of the left gluteal area, and multiple cutaneous or subcutaneous neurofibromas. This 54-year-old man died of metastatic malignant schwannoma (see Fig. 14.34).

basis of whether the tumor arises ab initio or appears as a malignant transformation.

There is general agreement that malignant peripheral nerve tumors develop in relatively older patients. The peak age incidence in Heard's[81] series was between 20 and 30 years. D'Agostino and co-workers[71] reported a median age of 28. In Brasfield and Das Gupta's report,[29] 27 of 32 patients were over the age of 30 years. In Guccion and Enzinger's[80] review of cases, the median was 34 years. This information, combined with the knowledge that most benign nerve sheath tumors occur prior to the age of 20 years, suggests that nerve sheath tumors in the first

two decades of life should be considered benign, unless there is convincing pathologic evidence to the contrary.

The natural history of malignant schwannomas is similar, irrespective of when the stigmata of von Recklinghausen's disease are first observed. Pain, sudden enlargement of a preexisting mass, or the occurrence and rapid growth of a new tumor in an adult patient suggests malignancy. A biopsy of the mass should be done to determine malignancy. More than a single malignant primary lesion may occur in a patient with von Recklinghausen's disease.

The management of malignant schwan-

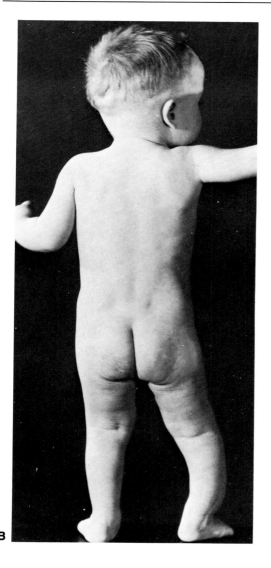

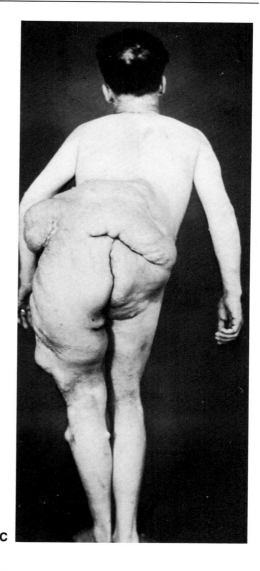

nomas associated with von Recklinghausen's disease is similar to that for the solitary variety. However, the prognosis is relatively poorer than with their solitary counterparts.[71,74,80,81] Of the 56 patients with solitary malignant schwannoma in the present study, 71 percent survived five years free of disease (Table 14.8); whereas in 18 patients with full-fledged stigmata of von Recklinghausen's disease in whom malignant schwannoma developed, only 22 percent had a disease-free five-year survival. Because of the paucity of available information, the clinical data on these 18 patients are summarized in Table 14.12.

TRAUMATIC NEUROMAS (AMPUTATION NEUROMAS)

The term *amputation neuroma* was first proposed in 1811 by Odier,[82] who believed these tumors to be of peripheral nerve origin. An accurate description of this entity, however, was first provided by Wood[83] in 1829. Although there was a definite lack of interest concerning this entity among the investigators of the early and middle nineteenth century, it was established that scar tissue was one of the contributing factors in the formation of amputation neuromas. In 1920, Huber and Lewis,[84] using rabbit pe-

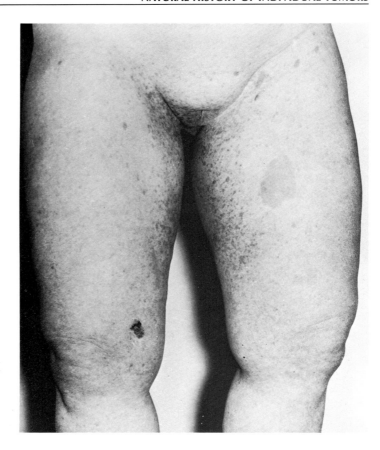

Figure 14.26. Large café-au-lait spot on left thigh, with melanoma in right distal thigh *(Courtesy of Current Problems in Surgery, Vol XIV, Chicago, Year Book Medical Publishers, 1977).*

ripheral nerves as their experimental system, described the histogenesis of amputation neuromas and popularized this term. A comprehensive clinical report of this entity in a large number of patients was reported by Cieslak and Stout[85] in 1946. At present, the terms amputa-

tion neuroma and traumatic neuroma are used interchangeably. Since the report by Cieslak and Stout,[85] several other studies dealing with the clinical and histopathologic features have been published.[86-89]

Neuromas arising at the end of a bisected

TABLE 14.7. ANATOMIC DISTRIBUTION OF SOLITARY MALIGNANT SCHWANNOMA

Sites	Das Gupta and Brasfield (1970)[74] Sloan-Kettering Cancer Center	Das Gupta (1981) University of Illinois Hospital	Combined Total
Head and neck	18	7	25
Upper extremities	69	12	81
Trunk	38	6	44
Lower extremities	89	24	113
Miscellaneous sites	18	7	25
Total	232	56	288

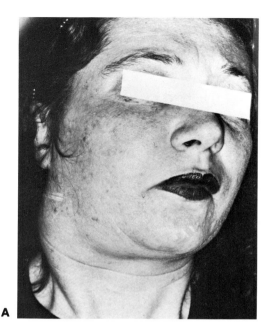

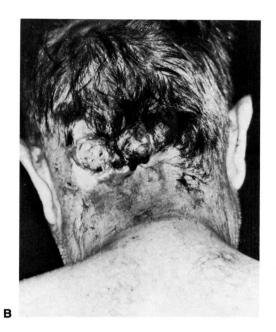

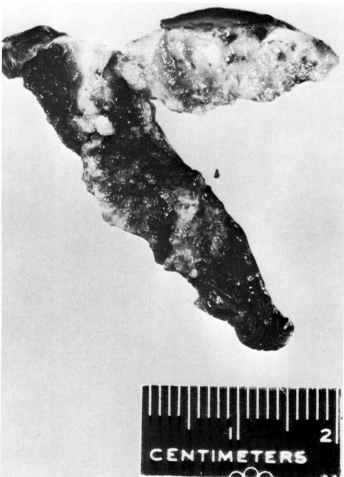

Figure 14.27. (A) Malignant schwannoma of the right side of neck. The nerve of origin could not be detected. Patient was treated with a standard radical neck dissection. (B) Recurrent malignant schwannoma of the scalp *(Courtesy of Annals of Surgery 171:419, J.B. Lippincott Co, 1970).* (C) Excised scalp showing extensive infiltration of the entire thickness.

527

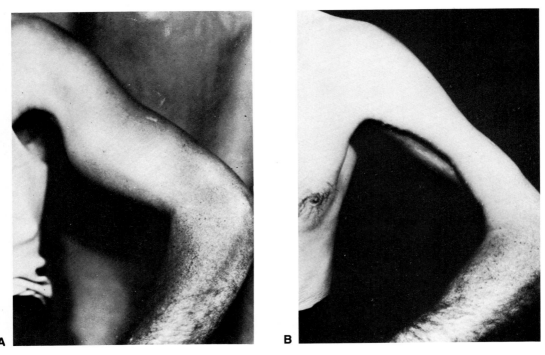

A   **B**

Figure 14.28. (**A**) A solitary malignant schwannoma of the arm. The tumor arose from the median nerve. The segment of nerve containing the tumor was excised. (**B**) Postoperative appearance of arm and forearm *(Courtesy of Annals of Surgery 171:419, J.B. Lippincott Co, 1970).*

Figure 14.29. Recurrent malignant schwannoma of the anterior thigh in a 50-year-old man. The recurrence under the scar (left) can be easily appreciated. In the right, the operative field shows the branches of the femoral nerve entering the tumor. Femoral vessels retracted laterally with a Penrose drain *(Courtesy of Annals of Surgery, 171:419, J.B. Lippincott Co, 1970).*

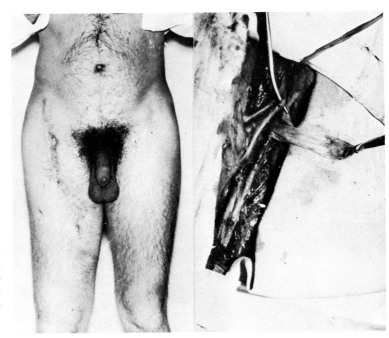

TABLE 14.8. SOLITARY MALIGNANT SCHWANNOMA: END RESULTS IN 56 PATIENTS ACCORDING TO TREATMENT

Type of Treatment	No. Patients	2 Yr, N.E.D.*	5 Yr, N.E.D.
Radical surgery only	44	34 (77.3%)	31 (70%)
Surgery and postop radiation therapy	12	9 (75%)	9 (75%)
Total	56	43 (77%)	40 (71%)

*No evidence of disease.

TABLE 14.9. MALIGNANT SCHWANNOMA—END RESULT IN 132 PATIENTS ACCORDING TO TYPE OF SURGICAL TREATMENT*

Type of Operation	No. Patients†	5 Yr, N.E.D.‡	10 Yr, N.E.D.
Local excision	55 (51)	15	11
Soft tissue resection	48 (45)	12	6
Minor amputation	16 (15)	7	5
Hemipelvectomy	2 (2)	1	1
Hip joint disarticulation	5 (5)	1	1
Interscapulothoracic amputation	5 (5)	1	0
Pelvic exenteration	1 (1)	0	—
Total	132(124)	37 (30%)	24 (19%)

*Courtesy of Annals of Surgery, J. B. Lippincott Co, 1970.[74]
†Numbers in parentheses represent patients eligible for 5-year end result analysis.
‡No evidence of disease.

TABLE 14.10. SOLITARY MALIGNANT SCHWANNOMA: 5-YEAR END RESULT ACCORDING TO TYPE OF RESECTION

Type of Operation	Das Gupta and Brasfield (1970)[74]	Das Gupta (1981)
Local excision	15/51* (29.4%)	—
Soft tissue resection	12/45 (26.6%)	22/27 (81%)
Minor amputation	7/15 (46.6%)	—
Hemipelvectomy	1/2 (50%)	3/6 (50%)
Hip joint disarticulation	1/5 (20%)	3/7 (42%)
Forequarter amputation	1/5 (20%)	3/4 (75%)
Pelvic exenteration	0/1	—
Total	37/124 (30%)	31/44 (70%)

*Number in denominator represents total number of patients and in the numerator, the 5-year survivors.

TABLE 14.11. DISEASE-FREE SURVIVAL, ACCORDING TO TUMOR SIZE AND GRADE OF 56 PATIENTS WITH MALIGNANT SCHWANNOMA (UNIVERSITY OF ILLINOIS SERIES)

Tumor Size	No. of Patients	Grades 1 and 2	5 Yr, N.E.D.*	Grades 3 and 4	5 Yr, N.E.D.
<5 cm	32	18 (94%)	17	14	11 (78.5%)
>5 cm	15	8	6 (75%)	7	5 (71%)
>5 cm and local infiltration to muscles and/or bones	9	3	1	6	0
Total	56	29	24 (83%)	27	16 (59%)

*No evidence of disease.

peripheral nerve following amputation for a benign disease, or after traumatic amputations, have been well described.[88-90] In 1969, Das Gupta and Brasfield[91] analyzed the clinicopathologic features of traumatic neuromas in 67 cancer patients in whom a neuroma developed after radical operation for a primary malignant tumor. They found that traumatic neuromas occurred at all ages, in both sexes, and in all anatomic sites. Almost all types of surgical procedures lead to the development of traumatic neuromas. However, they appear more frequently in the lateral portion of the neck, after a radical neck dissection or a forequarter amputation.

A swelling or mass of varying diameter in the surgical area is the common sign of a traumatic neuroma. Distinguishing a traumatic neuroma at the site of operation from local recurrence of the malignant tumor is often almost impossible (Fig. 14.35). In our previous study,[91] 7.5 percent of the neuromas were observed concomitantly with local recurrence. Furthermore, in 33 percent of the patients, local recurrence appeared after one or more traumatic neuromas

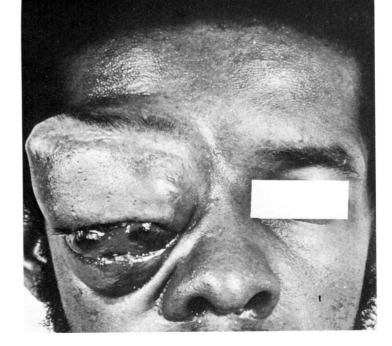

Figure 14.30. A 17-year-old boy with malignant schwannoma of the right upper eyelid developing on a plexiform neurofibroma that had been partially excised when the patient was 8 years old. In the intervening four years between first excision and development of malignant schwannoma, several other procedures were performed (Courtesy of Current Problems in Surgery, Vol XIV, Chicago, Year Book Medical Publishers 1977.)

it at a higher plane, and direct it away from the line of scar formation. During the initial operation, sharply resecting the nerve trunk and directing it away from the site of scar formation probably provides the best known protection against the development of neuromas.

TUMORS OF THE SYMPATHOCHROMAFFIN SYSTEM

Ganglioneuroma

Ganglioneuromas can occur along the entire sympathochromaffin axis (Fig. 4.66, Chapter 4). Although a benign ganglioneuroma is a relatively rare tumor, it is encountered often enough to merit discussion. The sites in which these tumors most commonly develop are the posterior mediastinum, retroperitoneum, pelvis, adrenal medulla, and neck, in order of decreasing frequency.[1,92] Multiple ganglioneuromas are uncommon and may be associated with the stigmata of von Recklinghausen's disease.[93-97] The symmetrical distribution of ganglioneuromas, as well as cutaneous presentation of these tumors, has also been described.[93,96,98,99] However, it appears that such presentations should be regarded as unusual manifestations of a neurocutaneous syndrome.[29,30,98,99]

These tumors are seen in all races and in both sexes. The incidence in females apparently predominates in a ratio of three to two.[100] Although 75 percent appear before the age of 20 years, they are seldom encountered in infants.[96,97,101,102]

Ganglioneuromas are usually recognized incidentally to some other ailment or on routine physical examination. Hamilton and Koop[101] found 12 of their 17 patients were asymptomatic. In the other five, the symptoms consisted of diarrhea, chest pain, abdominal distention, ptosis, and an altered gait. In our series of only four patients the diagnosis was made on routine physical examination. Three of the four tumors were located in the mediastinum and one in the retroperitonem. These are slow-growing tumors and often become quite large before detection. The symptoms are caused by pressure upon contiguous structures. In the mediastinum, the enlarging tumors might produce pressure on the trachea, resulting in persistent cough, dyspnea, or stridor.

Benign ganglioneuromas seldom are hormonally active.[101] Hamilton and Koop[101] found

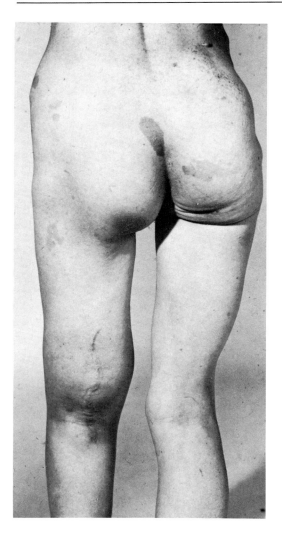

Figure 14.31. Large (12 × 15 cm) recurrent tumor of the posterior thigh and popliteal space in a 28-year-old woman (Patient 2, Table 14.12). Dissected sciatic nerve specimen from this patient is shown in Fig. 4.60 A, Chapter 4. *(Courtesy of Current Problems in Surgery, Vol XIV, Chicago, Year Book Medical Publishers, 1977).*

were excised. A diagnosis of traumatic neuroma in cancer patients must therefore be substantiated by histologic examination.

There is no known method of preventing the development of traumatic neuroma, especially in regions where a surgical procedure of necessity leads to the resection of a number of peripheral nerves. The plan of treatment of a traumatic neuroma is to identify the nerve stump, free it from the surrounding scar tissue, resect

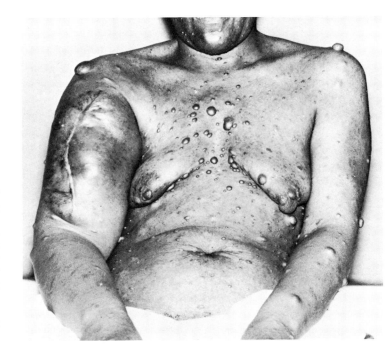

Figure 14.32. Obvious stigmata of neurofibromatosis with recurrent malignant schwannoma in right arm following inadequate local excision. Patient underwent muscle group excision and the local tumor was controlled at the time of her death, which was due to distant metastases (Patient 5, Table 14.12). *(Courtesy of Current Problems in Surgery, Vol XIV, Chicago, Year Book Medical Publishers, 1977).*

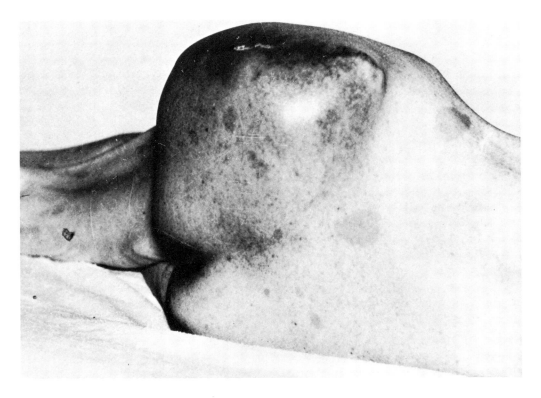

Figure 14.33. Large neurofibrosarcoma of the buttock *(Courtesy of Current Problems in Surgery, Vol XIV, Chicago, Year Book Medical Publishers, 1977).*

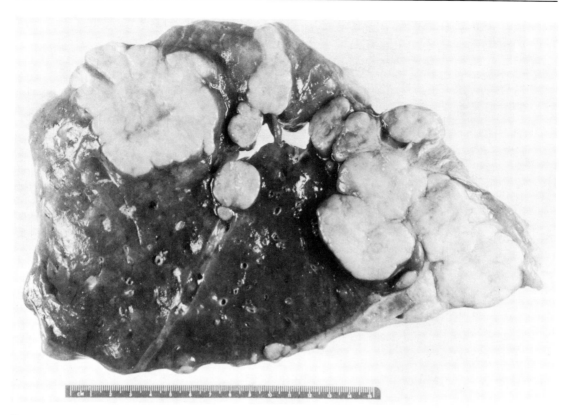

Figure 14.34. Metastatic malignant schwannoma to the liver. The primary site was on the back. The clinical photograph is shown in Figure 14.25C, Patient 18, Table 14.12.

that, in a relatively small number of patients, there is an increase in homovanillic and vanillylmandelic acid excretion levels. Serial determination of these levels both preoperatively and postoperatively can be used as biologic markers.

Since the most common site is the posterior mediastinum in children and young adults, the roentgenographic appearance of the chest is of clinical interest. A well-circumscribed mass may be evident and the adjacent vertebrae and ribs may show thinning and erosion. When the ganglioneuroma is of the so-called dumbbell or hourglass shape, x-rays may show a paravertebral mass, erosion of the pedicles, and enlargement of the paravertebral foramen. Calcification, when present, helps to distinguish a posterior mediastinal ganglioneuroma from congenital problems such as duplication of the foregut or bronchogenic cysts. Retroperitoneal ganglioneuromas have no specific x-ray findings, and an accurate preoperative diagnosis based on an intravenous pyelogram or an in-

ferior venogram or arteriogram is almost impossible. The routine use of CAT scans and ultrasonograms has as yet not increased the accuracy of preoperative diagnosis.

Treatment. The treatment of ganglioneuroma is excision. These tumors are well encapsulated and can be separated from their beds with remarkable ease. In the neck, careful dissection is needed from the surrounding structures. Frequently the tumor will be found to arise from a sympathetic ganglion, resection of which might lead to Horner's syndrome. In the hourglass variety, exploration of the vertebral canal is required as well.

Pheochromocytoma

Pheochromocytomas are rare tumors that produce a remediable form of hypertension, together with a wide spectrum of associated clinical manifestations. The locations of these tumors within the body follow the embryonic distri-

TABLE 14.12. CLINICAL SUMMARY OF MALIGNANT SCHWANNOMA ASSOCIATED WITH VON RECKLINGHAUSEN'S DISEASE (18 PATIENTS, UNIVERSITY OF ILLINOIS SERIES, 1981)

Patient	Age/Sex	Site of Primary	Type of Treatment	Recurrence or Metastases	End Result
1	40 F	Right gluteal cleft	Wide soft tissue resection	—	10 yr N.E.D.*
2	28 F	Posterior thigh	Hip joint disarticulation	Lung postop	Died 1 yr
3	45 F	Posterior thigh	Wide soft tissue and lung metastases	Local recurrence	Died 4 yr postop
4	40 M	Anterior thigh	Wide soft tissue resection	—	5 yr N.E.D.
5	47 F	Right arm	Same as above	Lung	Died postop 1 yr
6	56 F	Left arm	Forequarter	—	5 yr N.E.D.
7	45 M	Left leg	Mid-thigh amputation	—	10 yr N.E.D.
8	50 M	Gluteal area	Hemipelvectomy	Widespread	Died 1½ yr postop
9	55 M	Arm	Wide soft tissue resection	Widespread	Died 2 yr
10	65 M	Right neck	Two excisions with local recurrence	Lung	Died 2 yr postop
11	31 F	Thigh	Hip joint disarticulation	—	1 yr dead
12	50 M	Neck	Wide soft tissue resection	Lung	Died postop
13	40 F	Retroperitoneum	Wide soft tissue resection	Widespread	2½ yr dead
14	39 F	Anterior thigh	Same as above	Same as above	1½ yr dead
15	42 M	Back	Same as above	Same as above	3 yr dead
16	50 F	Gluteal region	Same as above	Lung	2½ yr dead
17	17 M	Right orbit	Same as above	Lung	1 yr dead
18	54 M	Back in an area of massive plexiform neuroma	Same as above	Lung	2½ yr dead

No evidence of disease.

TABLE 14.13. COMPARATIVE AGE DISTRIBUTION OF NEUROBLASTOMA IN FIVE LARGE SERIES

Age Distribution	Hospital for Sick Children, London[174] (129 cases)	Children's Hospital Columbus[170] (90 cases)	Children's Medical Center, Boston[175] (217 cases)	Tumor Registry California[171] (212 cases)	Memorial Sloan-Kettering Cancer Center[176] (133 cases)
0–11 mo	38%	30%	23%	32%	38%
12–13 mo	16%	20%	24%	14%	14%
2–6 yr	38%	38%	41%	37%	48%
7–19 yr	8%	12%	13%	17%	21%

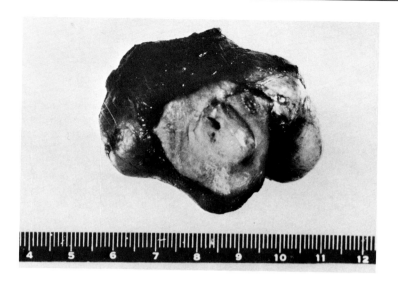

Figure 14.35. Traumatic neuroma removed from the lateral neck following radical neck dissection. Preoperatively, tumor was considered to be local recurrence.

bution of chromaffin tissue derived from the primitive neuroectoderm (Chapter 4). Many of the unique features of the disease are attributable to the pharmacologic effects of catecholamines, which the chromaffin tumors produce. Approximately 60 percent of pheochromocytomas occur in the adrenal glands and more than 90 percent lie between the diaphragm and pelvic floor.

Physiologic Considerations. In most respects the symptoms of pheochromocytoma stem directly from the excess production of catecholamines. In past decades many important advances were made toward understanding the pathways of biosynthesis and degradation of these compounds and the mechanisms that govern their storage and release.[103-105] These will be reviewed briefly, but the reader is referred elsewhere for more comprehensive reviews. The scheme of biosynthesis was first proposed in 1939[106] and has been confirmed by several workers in recent years.[103-105] The parent compound, tyrosine, is concentrated in body tissues by an active transport system and subsequently finds its way into several important metabolic pathways. The biosynthesis of catecholamines occurs in the adrenal medulla, in sympathetic nerve endings, in parts of the brain, and in enterochromaffinlike cells found in various parts of the gastrointestinal tract, lung, and various other organs.[105-107] The conversion of tyrosine to DOPA, catalyzed by the enzyme tyrosine hydroxylase,

takes place in the mitochondria of the cell. DOPA is subsequently converted to dopamine, which is then converted to norepinephrine in specialized granules within the sympathetic nerve endings and in the adrenal medulla. Most of the norepinephrine thus synthesized remains in situ until released by the action of sympathetic nerves. Norepinephrine is the principal catecholamine released by the sympathetic nerves.[105] The conversion of norepinephrine to epinephrine results from the action of an enzyme (phenylethanolamine N-methyl transferase) normally located only in certain cells of the adrenal medulla. This gland normally synthesizes and stores both norepinephrine and epinephrine.

In pheochromocytomas the biosynthesis of catecholamines proceeds along the same pathways as in normal tissue, although the rate of synthesis is more rapid. In many pheochromocytomas, only norepinephrine is formed. Others produce both norepinephrine and epinephrine. Those tumors that produce epinephrine usually arise within the adrenal medulla. Tumors that exclusively produce epinephrine are extremely rare. Catecholamines and other forms of biogenic amines are stored in the cells derived from the sympathochromaffin tissue. These intracytoplasmic storage sites have received considerable attention in recent years. The granules are specialized subcellular particles, identifiable in adrenergic nerves and chromaffin cells by electron microscopy. Similar granules have been identified in pheochromocytomas and in neuroblastoma tissue.[96,105,108] Norepinephrine and epinephrine are inactive as long as they remain within granules, but their full activity is manifested on release. The mechanisms by which the catecholamines are released from the granules have been extensively investigated.[106,107] Normally, small amounts of norepinephrine are released continuously and larger amounts in spurts, possibly representing phasic alterations in sympathetic nerve impulses. Following release at the effector site as a result of sympathetic stimulation, norepinephrine, which remains free, is again taken up by the granules and its physiologic action is terminated.

In patients with a pheochromocytoma, circulating catecholamines released from the tumor are taken up and stored in sympathetic nerve granules. Thus, even after removal of the tumor these patients may have increased stores of pressor amines and an increased excretion of norepinephrine and epinephrine, and their catabolites may occur in the urine for several days following successful surgery.

Inactivation or degradation of catecholamines is large effected by the enzyme catechol-O-methyl transferase (COMT). This enzyme is present in high concentrations in the liver and kidney and is principally responsible for inactivating released or circulating catecholamines, since the O-methylated catecholamine derivatives metanephrine (M) and normetanephrine (NM) are no longer physiologically active. The other enzyme principally involved in the metabolic destruction of the catecholamines is monoamine oxidase (MAO). This enzyme, which is present in most tissues, seems to play a major role in disposing of excessive stores of catecholamines by deamination in situ. The principal end products of catecholamine catabolism are those which are O-methylated (M and NM), and the final product of both O-methylation and deamination is 3-methoxy-4 hydroxymandelic acid or vanillylmandelic acid (VMA). The measurement of the urinary excretion of the catecholamines or their major catabolites is now recognized as a major means of establishing the diagnosis of pheochromocytoma.

Clinical Features. The initial manifestation of a pheochromocytoma may be a complicating vascular accident. The principal complications of an untreated pheochromocytoma stem from arterial hypertension, with findings similar to those in patients with sustained hypertension of comparable severity and duration. These include retinopathy, a cerebral vascular accident, myocardial infarction, congestive heart failure, or full-fledged malignant hypertension.[109-115] In addition, persistent high circulating catecholamine levels may result in cardiac arrythmias, particularly those of ventricular origin.[116] Pheochromocytomas occurring during pregnancy have sometimes produced symptoms of eclampsia.[117] Hyperglycemia and glycosuria often simulate diabetes mellitus.[109,114] The major cause is thought to be the catecholamine-induced inhibition of insulin secretion. Thomas and associates[110] found that patients with a pheochromocytoma have multiple symptoms: headaches (80 percent) and palpitation without tachycardia (64 percent) were among the major symptoms in a series of 100 patients.

Pharmacologic Tests. More than 20 years ago the histamine provocative test, the benzodioxane adrenolytic test, and the phenotolamine test came into widespread use for the diagnosis of pheochromocytomas. A provocative test with histamine has its chief value in patients having paroxysms of hypertension with intermittent normal pressure. This test has the hazard of being complicated by a cerebral vascular accident or myocardial infarction. Although a provocative test with tyramine[118] is supposedly free of side effects,[109] it is safer to rely on chemical methods of diagnosis.

Chemical Tests. The diagnosis of pheochromocytoma is generally made by chemical measurement of catecholamines and their degradation products.[109,114,119] Serum catecholamines can be measured accurately and the standarized methods for measuring urinary catecholamines are widely available. Over 90 percent of pheochromocytoma patients are identifiable by a single accurate determination of 24-hour urinary catecholamines. Interference may be caused by agents containing sympathomimetic amines. Therefore, extreme care should be used in the collection of the 24-hour urinary specimens. Methods for measurement of epinephrine and norepinephrine have been adequately developed and are routinely used in conjunction with examination of urinary catecholamines in the diagnosis of pheochromocytomas. Furthermore, with the use of vena cava catheters, samples of blood at different levels, with estimation of the levels of biogenic amines, have aided in the localization of these pheochromocytomas. History, physical examination, and chemical tests will usually confirm a diagnosis of pheochromocytoma. However, in some unusual cases, confusion with an intracranial tumor might occur.

Pheochromocytomas can be radiologically localized by means of intravenous pyelograms and tomograms. Angiography has become an extremely useful adjunct for diagnosis of these tumors.

Pheochromocytoma in Children. Pheochromocytomas have also been reported in children.[109,120] The ratio of males to females before puberty is two to one. However, with puberty there is a marked increase in incidence in females. The youngest patient on record with a symptomatic pheochromocytoma was one month old. The average age at diagnosis is 9.8 years.[109]

A high incidence of bilateral, multiple, and ectopic tumors, and a severe and stormy course are characteristic of this disease. In one series, 140 tumors were found in 100 children, including many in extra-adrenal locations.[120] In five children, a second tumor developed after initial surgery.

Common symptoms in children are headache, sweating, nausea, vomiting, weight loss, visual disturbance, seizures, weakness, and fatigue.[109,114,120] A peculiar reddish-blue mottling of the skin has also been reported. Polydipsia and polyuria are more common in children than in adults. Occasionally, obstructive uropathy or obstruction of a renal artery is the initial manifestation. Catecholamine excretion in children usually is predominantly norepinephrine, and sustained hyperexcretion is present in about 90 percent of patients. Since hypertension in children is uncommon, pheochromocytoma should always be considered.

The association of pheochromocytoma with cyanotic congenital heart disease has been reported in children.[111] It has been postulated that persistent hypoxemia could produce adrenal medullary hyperplasia and, eventually, an autonomously functioning pheochromocytoma. Hypertension and other signs and symptoms of catecholamine excess should be carefully considered in the evaluation of patients with congenital heart disease because of the risks associated with cardiac catheterization, angiography, and surgery. Some neuroblastomas and ganglioneuromas of childhood can produce catecholamines and thereby create confusion in the diagnosis. However, the natural histories of these tumors are entirely different and a diagnosis should not be difficult.

Familial Pheochromocytoma. Familial occurrence of pheochromocytoma has been known since the report of Calkins and Howard in 1947.[112] At least 16 kindreds have been studied and described. The mode of inheritance was autosomal dominant with a high degree of penetrance. Several features set these cases apart from the more common sporadic type. The instance of multiple tumors in familial patients is approximately 50 percent. The range of age at the time of onset of symptoms varies widely. Sustained hypertension has been more common than the intermittent type. Increased occurrence of familial thyroid neoplasms in patients with familial pheochromocytomas has also been reported,[121] as has the triad of familial bilateral pheochromocytomas, thyroid carcinoma, and hyperparathyroidism.[113,122]

Pheochromocytoma and Neurofibromatosis. The relationship between pheochromocytoma and neurofibromatosis was first noted by Suzuki[123] in 1910. MacKeith[124] reviewed the literature in 1944 and found that 165 cases of pheochromocytomas had been reported and that neurofibromatosis was present in nine. Davis and his co-workers[125] reviewed the literature up to 1950 and estimated the incidence of neurofibromatosis in patients with pheochromocytoma to be about 5 percent (10 of 203 patients).

In the two large series reported by Crowe and associates[26] and Brasfield and Das Gupta,[29] there was a low incidence of pheochromocytoma in patients with von Recklinghausen's disease (only one in each study). In the 60 patients studied at the University of Illinois Hospital, we have not encountered any case of pheochromocytoma associated with von Recklinghausen's disease.[30] Lynch and associates,[126] whose findings were similar, estimated the incidence of pheochromocytoma in von Recklinghausen's disease to be less than 1 percent. Tilford and Kelsch,[127] in 1973, reported a collected series of 57 neurofibromatosis patients with pheochromocytoma. The mean age of these patients was 41 years, and only three patients were under the age of 18. In adults with neurofibromatosis, hypertension is seven times more likely to be caused by pheochromocytoma than by renal artery stenosis. In children, however, the ratio is reversed, with renal artery stenosis being the more common cause.

In 1953, Glushien and co-workers[128] estimated that as many as 10 percent of patients with pheochromocytoma might have "neurocutaneous syndromes" and suggested that pheochromocytoma, neurofibromatosis, tuberous sclerosis, Sturge-Weber syndrome, and von Hippel-Lindau syndrome were all of common ectodermal origin and likely to appear in combination with significant frequency. These authors presented three cases—one of neurofibromatosis and pheochromocytoma, and two of neurofibromatosis and von Hippel-Lindau syndrome. In recent years an association has been observed between pheochromocytoma, the so-called neurocutaneous syndromes, and other disorders such as medullary thyroid carcinoma. Today, many agree that a 5 percent overall incidence of pheochromocytoma probably represents a reasonable estimate[129] in patients with all types of neurocutaneous syndromes.

Multiple Endocrine Adenomatosis II (MEA II).

A relationship between Sipple's syndrome and neurofibromatosis has been proposed because of the occurrence of pheochromocytomas and mucosal neuromas in Sipple's syndrome.[130] Since Sipple's report in 1961, the syndrome has undergone further clarification.[131,132] The mucosal tumor that occurs primarily in the lip should be classified as a true neuroma rather than a nerve sheath tumor or the "false neuroma" characteristic of von Recklinghausen's disease. Patients with these neuromas are now classified as having multiple endocrine adenomatosis (MEA IIb), which is characterized by medullary carcinoma of the thyroid, pheochromocytomas, multiple mucosal neuromas of the lips, tongue, and upper eyelids, plus *marfanoid habitus*. The only true overlap clinically with neurofibromatosis is the occurrence of pheochromocytoma. The C cell, which makes up the medullary carcinoma, belongs to the APUD series.[133] It is possible to attribute all the changes in Sipple's syndrome to the neural crest except hyperparathyroidism, which only rarely occurs in the MEA IIb form.

Pheochromocytoma of the Bladder.

The location of a pheochromocytoma in the bladder wall produces a distinct syndrome.[134] The unique situation of the tumor in a structure that changes dimensions in the physiologic process of micturition accounts for its different behavioral pattern. Typically, severe paroxysmal symptoms, especially throbbing headaches, occur with or shortly after micturition. Painless hematuria occurs in approximately 50 percent of cases.

In some cases, urinary metabolites of catecholamines have been normal, possibly because bladder tumors are symptomatic early in their existence, when hyperexcretion of catecholamines is present for very brief periods during contraction of the bladder. It is therefore important that the possibility of a pheochromocytoma of the bladder not be dismissed because of the absence of the usual biochemical findings, if this diagnosis is suggested from clinical evaluation.

Bladder pheochromocytomas are usually small and located in the muscular wall of the organ; therefore, cystoscopic findings and cystograms may be normal. The behavior of blood pressure during massage of the bladder and the adrenal region, and during distention of the bladder, may be of critical importance in confirming clinical suspicion.

Treatment. The treatment of pheochromocytoma is excision, irrespective of its location or the associated complicating factors. It is mandatory that preoperative evaluation be complete and that during the operation the patient be well monitored. The operative approach must take into consideration the fact that 10 to 15 percent of pheochromocytomas are bilateral. Since these tumors can occur anywhere within the sympathochromaffin axis, all patients should have an exploratory procedure.

CAROTID BODY TUMORS

These are among the rarest of the neoplasms in the cervical region.[135-137] Diagnosis can be established by biopsy, and once the diagnosis is established, the treatment is entirely dependent on the symptoms produced by the tumor. Excision must be undertaken with great caution. Small tumors can easily be dissected from the carotid vessels. Resection of the carotid artery is certainly not indicated in otherwise asymptomatic patients, but in symptomatic patients, if dissection of the tumor from the surrounding arteries is not possible, resection of the carotid vessels with reconstruction might be performed.

The simultaneous occurrence of a carotid body tumor and a pheochromocytoma is extremely rare; only five such cases have ever been reported.[138]

CHEMODECTOMAS

Chemodectomas (nonchromaffin paragangliomas) have been demonstrated to originate in the glomus jugulare,[139-142] the ganglion nodosum of the vagus nerve,[143,144] the auricular branches of the vagus nerve,[145] the tympanic ganglia of the glossopharyngeal nerve,[145] the ciliary ganglia,[145] the orbit,[146] the aortic bodies,[147-149] the mediastinum,[149,150] the retroperitoneum,[151-152] the lower extremities,[153,154] the cauda equina,[155] the muscular wall of the small intestine,[156,157]in rare instances in the pineal organ,[158] and in the lung.[159-161]

The majority are benign, showing only hyperplasia on microscopic examination, and usually occur in adults between the ages of 40 to 60 years.[151] It is suggested that these tumors are found more frequently in women. Brown[139] and Brown and Freyer[162] estimated that the occurrence in females is five times greater than in males. There is no outstanding racial incidence.

The symptoms produced are entirely dependent on the location of the tumor. In the glomus jugular tumors, when the eardrum is still intact, the most common presenting symptom is a conductive hearing loss accompanied by tinnitus and a feeling of fullness in the ear. As the tumor continues to grow, it becomes visible as a dark mass through the lower part of the drum. In advanced cases, bloodstained discharge from the ear and deafness are common findings. As its growth progresses, the tumor extends through the jugular foramen and spreads to the base of the skull. In about 40 percent of these patients the seventh cranial nerve is involved.[140]

In the ganglion nodosum of the vagal nerve, a cervical tumor is usually the presenting feature. In the mediastinum or in the retroperitoneum the mass produces all the symptoms of a space-occupying lesion and the histologic diagnosis is usually made after excision of the tumor. Smithers and Gowing[148] collected 28 cases of chemodectoma in the region of the aortic arch, including one of their own. They found that in all these cases the tumors were of long duration, and the mediastinal component with classic roentgenographic findings made preoperative diagnosis possible. Chemodectomas of the gastrointestinal tract can be diagnosed only after excision.

Smith, Hughes, and Ermocilla[158] reported a case of chemodectoma of the pineal body. Infrequently, chemodectomas may be hormonally active.[1,139,163-166] Instances of catecholamine-secreting nonchromaffin paragangliomas of the glomus jugulare, carotid body, and retroperitoneum are on record.[1,139-169] Levit and coworkers[141] suggested that, until the true frequency of functioning tumors is known, all patients with paragangliomas or chemodectomas should have routine preoperative determination of urinary catecholamines and their metabolites to decrease surgical morbidity and mortality.

Treatment

The treatment of choice for all chemodectomas is excision.[137,139,168,169] In certain instances, because of the location and extension of the tumor, adequate excision is difficult. In such cases, partial excision might be attempted, since these are extremely slow-growing tumors.

MALIGNANT GANGLIONEUROMA

Malignant ganglioneuroma probably occupies an intermediate position in the degree of histologic differentiation in the gamut of tumors designated as neuroblastomas, malignant ganglioneuromas, and ganglioneuroblastomas. By common usage, malignant ganglioneuroblastomas are those primary tumors that arise outside the retroperitoneum but histologically resemble neuroblastoma.

Malignant ganglioneuromas, infrequent as they are, usually occur in the lateral portion of the neck and, rarely, in the perineal region. Priebe and Clatworthy[170] found 3 of 92 (3 percent) consecutive cases of neuroblastoma in the neck, and all were in the one-year-or-under age group. Rosenfeld and Graves[6] reported that, of 32 primary neurogenic tumors of the lateral portion of the neck, only one (3 percent) was a malignant ganglioneuroma and three (9 percent) were benign ganglioneuromas. Oberman and Sullenger,[7] reviewing neurogenic tumors of the head and neck region at the University of Michigan, found that, over a period of 21 years, there had been 43 cases, of which two (4.6 percent) were neuroblastomas (malignant ganglioneuromas) of the neck.

The clinical presentation of these tumors is like that of any other lateral neck mass. Diagnosis is established by means of either an excision or an incision biopsy. In one of our patients, a 2-year-old child, the diagnosis was established after excision of an enlarged node. In children and young adults in whom there is difficulty in interpretation of the biopsy material from a neck tumor, chemical diagnostic tests for neuroblastoma are recommended (mentioned earlier in chapter).

The treatment of malignant ganglioneuroma is radical excision. Oberman and Sullenger[7] reported that one of their patients survived six years after partial excision and irradiation. In view of the rarity of these tumors, it is not possible to arrive at average survival figures. However, it is conjectured that if these tumors are treated as neuroblastomas, the results in the favorable age group would probably match those for neuroblastoma. Of the two patients in our files, one, a child who was two years old when operated upon, is alive and tumor-free three years later; the other, whose tumor was diagnosed at age eight years, died of metastatic disease.

NEUROBLASTOMA

Neuroblastomas are highly malignant tumors occurring predominantly in infancy and early childhood. In the California Tumor Registry, neuroblastomas constitute 5 percent of all childhood malignancies.[171] Several children's centers have reported the rate to be 10 to 12 percent.[98,172]

Age, Sex, and Race

This tumor occurs primarily in infancy.[173] In any large series, about 40 percent of the patients are between 2 and 6 years of age (Table 14.13). In about 17 percent, the tumors occur between the ages of 7 and 19 years.[170,171,174-176] Neuroblastomas are found with almost equal frequency in both sexes, and no racial predilection has been recorded. Rarely, neuroblastomas are found to be congenital.[177-179]

Anatomic Distribution

Neuroblastoma characteristically arises in any area along the distribution of the sympathetic chain, including the cranial ganglia. Primary in-

traspinal, intracranial, bone, and soft tissue tumors have also been described.[96] The majority, however, are located in the retroperitoneum, with the mediastinum the next most likely site of occurrence. Table 14.14 shows the anatomic distribution of primary neuroblastomas in five large series.

The early and widespread metastases resulting from the deep-seated primary tumor result in bizarre clinical expressions. The initial symptoms may be fever and anemia, with no localizing signs; but more frequently these symptoms accompany an abdominal mass. The most common clinical presentation may be enlarged cervical lymph nodes. An accurate diagnosis is established only after microscopic examination of the tissue with corroborative chemical examination.

The abdominal swelling that is frequently the presenting symptom must be differentiated from other space-occupying lesions. Wilms' tumor is probably the most common neoplasm from which neuroblastomas must be differentiated. The characteristic feature of an intra-abdominal mass containing calcific deposits is suggestive of neuroblastoma. The presence of osteolytic lesions along with a retroperitoneal tumor is almost diagnostic of neuroblastoma. Mediastinal lesions are usually diagnosed by means of routine chest x-rays.

Elevated urinary excretion of dopamine, VMA, and HVA in neuroblastomas has been adequately demonstrated.[172,180-183] Therefore, these chemical diagnostic tests (page 536) should be routinely used. If the levels of the biogenic amines and their breakdown products are lower after excision of the tumor, these data can be used as prognostic guides, since subsequent elevation might herald either local recurrence or metastases.

Treatment

Neuroblastoma must be diagnosed early and treated by radical excision and radiation therapy. Although the addition of chemotherapy was championed in the last decade, it is probably of little or no value in the ultimate outcome.[184,185]

End Results. The reported overall cure rate in the past varied between 9.7 percent and 36 percent.[171] The California Tumor Registry[171] found the overall cure rate to be directly related to age at diagnosis. For patients under 1 year of age,

TABLE 14.14. COMPARATIVE DISTRIBUTION OF ANATOMIC SITES OF PRIMARY NEUROBLASTOMA AS SEEN IN FIVE LARGE SERIES

Name of Center	Total Cases Reported	Year of Publication	Retroperitoneum	Mediastinum	Neck	Sacrum	Other	Unknown
Hospital for Sick Children (London)[174]	129	1959	70%	11%	5%	8%	—	6%
Children's Medical Center (Boston)[175]	217	1959	62%	13%	2%	5%	—	18%
Children's Hospital (Columbus, Ohio)[170]	90	1967	66%	17%	3%	3%	5%	6%
Memorial Sloan-Kettering Cancer Center (New York)[176]	133	1968	69%	8%	2%	4%	3%	14%
Tumor Registry (California)[171]	212	1969	63%	16%	2%	3%	5%	11%

it was 60 percent; for 1-year-olds it was 21 percent; between 2 and 6 years old, 10 percent; and between 7 and 19 years old, 8 percent.[170,171,174–186]

It has been well documented that survival of children with neuroblastoma is influenced by numerous factors: the extent or stage of the disease at diagnosis, the age of the patient, the site of the primary tumor, histologic evidence of tumor maturation (grading), and the presence or absence of lymphocytes in the tumor, bone marrow, or peripheral blood.[184,185,187-189]

The prognostic aspects of the clinical staging, and different forms of therapy, have been studied in a prospective fashion by the Children's Cancer Study Group (CCSG).[185] From their studies, it appears that the staging of the tumor as proposed by Evans and co-workers[188] is of considerable prognostic import. In this clinical staging system, stage I tumors are confined to the organ or structure of origin. Stage II tumors extend in-continuity beyond the organ structure of origin but do not cross the midline (regional lymph nodes on the homolateral side may be involved). If the tumor extends intradurally it is also stage II. Stage III tumors extend in-continuity beyond the midline (regional nodes may be involved bilaterally). The age of the patient at the time of diagnosis also has an influence on the overall prognosis. According to the CCSG therapeutic protocols, all eligible patients were treated by curative surgery, radiation therapy, or both, for localized stages I, II, and III tumors. On a randomized basis, half of these patients received cyclophosphamide for one year.[185] The results of treatment in 134 such patients showed that there were no relapses in stage I. In stages II and III the relapse rate was 13 percent and 38 percent, respectively. It was found that use of adjuvant cyclophosphamide for one year did not influence the prognosis either way. The survival, when computed according to age, was found to be 90 percent for children in the first and second years of life, falling to 47 percent for children 2 years of age or older. Similar age-related survival data have been published in the past from retrospective studies as well.[170,171,174,175,186] To what extent regional node involvement influences the prognosis is hard to define, since very few of the published reports have dealt with this facet adequately. The paucity of the data is evident even in the CCSG Study,[185] since information was available to the authors in only 46 of 134 patients. Twenty-seven of 32 patients

with stage II and 12 of 14 with stage III tumors had positive nodes. Eleven of 39 (28 percent) with positive nodes developed local recurrence and metastatic disease. There were no relapses in the six patients with no nodal metastases.

The prognostic influence of the site of the primary has been dealt with at length by various authors.[170,174,175] Whether above or below the diaphragm, it has little influence on the rate of recurrence or metastases, assuming that the tumor is adequately staged and is categorized according to the age of the patient.

Evans and co-workers[185] found that the end results have improved in recent years. This is certainly not due to the use of chemotherapy, since adjuvant cyclophosphamide does not appear to influence the prognosis. Probably the reason for this improvement is better staging, more aggressive resection, and radiation therapy. The aggressive attitude toward therapy is observed even in the management of metastatic neuroblastoma. Although the majority of these patients are treated by chemotherapy or radiation therapy, or both, in selected instances excision of the metastatic tumor is possible and is advocated.[101]

Maturation of Neuroblastoma

Although relatively rare, neuroblastomas and undifferentiated ganglioneuromas are known to mature into ganglioneuromas.[190-194] Cushing and Wolback,[191] in 1927, first reported the maturation of a neuroblastoma. Fox et al.[192] studied a patient 46 years after partial treatment and found no evidence of recurrence of the tumor. Since then several such cases have been reported.[186,190,193-195] All these case reports show the unique potential of an undifferentiated tumor in rare instances to become differentiated and spontaneously grow into mature ganglion cells. However, the factors responsible for such maturation still remain a matter of great puzzlement.

Relation to von Recklinghausen's Disease

A possible relationship between familial neuroblastoma and von Recklinghausen's disease was suggested by Knudson and Amromin[93] and Chatten and Voorhess,[196] who noted a high incidence of café-au-lait spots in their patients' families. Bolande and Towler[95] noted maturation of cutaneous lesions in familial neuroblastoma into ganglioneuromas and, finally, into lesions that closely resembled neurofibromas. After an extensive morphologic review, they were able to identify ganglion cells or ganglioneuromatous elements in von Recklinghausen's neurofibromas, ie, isolated ganglioneuroma resulting from the maturation of cutaneous lesions in familial neuroblastoma. According to Bolande and Towler,[95] the simultaneous occurrence of these two diseases in a single patient has been reported only twice in the literature. The common neural crest origin of the Schwann cell and the neuroblast led them to speculate on the embryologic and genetic relationships that may be shared by the two diseases. Additional embryologic information or greater evidence of a clinical association is necessary to consider their relationship significant.

Neuroblastoma in Unusual Sites

It has already been pointed out that primary neuroblastoma can occur in many unusual sites; for example, in the intraspinal space, intracranial locations, the orbit, buttock, the leg (Fig. 4.70A and 4.70B, Chapter 4), and the nares.[96] However, olfactory neuroblastoma (esthesioneuroblastoma) constitutes a truly unusual entity and therefore is briefly discussed.

Esthesioneuroblastoma The olfactory esthesioneuroblastoma is a rare malignant tumor arising in the region of the roof of the nasal cavity. Since Berger et al.[197] described the first case in 1924, about 105 additional cases have been reported.[198] In the files of the University of Illinois Hospital there are only two such cases, both occurring in males. Hutter et al.[199] reviewed the experience with 18 patients at Memorial Sloan-Kettering Cancer Center and concluded that esthesioneuroblastoma is a low-grade neuroblastoma; 3 of their 18 patients (17 percent) showed regional node metastases. Skolnick et al.[200] found cervical node metastases in 11 of 97 (11 percent) collected cases. These tumors are usually seen in the second decade and probably are more common in males. Multiple recurrences after excision or irradiation have been reported,[199,200] usually because adequate excision was not possible. However, with the combined craniofacial approach standardized in recent years, adequate excision can now be done and, combined with postoperative radiation therapy, should provide good salvage.[199-201]

MALIGNANT PHEOCHROMOCYTOMA

Malignant pheochromocytomas are rare tumors, and only a handful of cases have ever been documented.[96,202,203] It is almost impossible to clinically diagnose either a benign or malignant pheochromocytoma. If, at the time the tumor is excised, there is regional nodal metastases and these nodes are found to be chromaffin-positive, then a tentative diagnosis of malignant pheochromocytoma can be made. Otherwise the diagnosis should be based on the natural history of the tumor. If the patient dies of widespread metastases and the metastatic deposits are chromaffin-positive, then the diagnosis, of course, is certain.

MALIGNANT CHEMODECTOMA

Malignant carotid body tumors are extremely rare and most authors have personal experience with only one or two cases.[204-209] Frey and Karoll[169] described malignant carotid body tumors in three patients, all of whom died. One had brain metastases and the other two had locally untreatable tumors. Approximately 32 cases have been reported in which there was metastasis to the regional lymph nodes or to distant sites proven by microscopic examination.[204-211] Reported sites of distant metastases include lung, bone, liver, pancreas, thyroid, heart, trachea, orbit, and extradural space.[210-215]

The treatment of malignant carotid body tumors is difficult to outline. Suffice it to mention that, whenever possible, radical excision is in order, including excision of the carotid vessels with replacement by a prosthesis.

Malignant chemodectomas, like their benign counterparts, occur in the aortic bodies,[147-149] the ganglion nodosum of the vagus nerve,[143-145] glomus jugulare,[139-142] the ciliary ganglion,[145] the lungs,[160] the duodenum,[156,157] the middle ear,[140] and the retroperitoneum.[151] Olson and Abell[151] found the highest incidence of metastases in retroperitoneal chemodectomas (35 percent); next in order was the vagal body (20 percent) (Table 14.15). In all other sites, the incidence of distant metastases was negligible. Experience shows that of all the malignant chemodectomas (paragangliomas) the retroperitoneal variety is

TABLE 14.15. CLINICOPATHOLOGIC COMPARISON OF CHEMODECTOMAS (NONCHROMATTIN PARAGANGLIOMAS) ARISING IN VARIOUS SITES

Location	No. of Cases	Average Age	No. of Patients with Metastases	Percent of Patients with Metastases
Carotid body[212]	500	41	32	6
Glomus jugulare[213]	316	49	6	2
Vagal body[143]	20	44	4	20
Mediastinum[148,214]	20	40	0	0
Lung[160,215]	25	68	0	0
Duodenum[157]	9	52	0	0
Retroperitoneum[151]	23	33	8	35

the most lethal.[151] Our experience is limited to two male patients and both succumbed within three years of excision of the primary.

REFERENCES

1. Pack GT, Ariel I: Tumors of the Soft Somatic Tissues. New York, Hoeber, 1958
2. Russel DS, Rubinstein LJ: Pathology of Tumors of the Nervous System, 3rd ed. Baltimore, Williams & Wilkins, 1971
3. Harkin JC, Reed RJ: Tumors of the Peripheral Nervous System, series 2, fasc 3. Washington DC, AFIP, 1969
4. Das Gupta TK, Brasfield RD, Strong EW, Hajdu SI: Benign solitary schwannomas (neurilemomas). Cancer 24:355, 1969
5. Purney FJ, Moran JJ, Thomas GK: Neurogenic tumors of the head and neck. Trans Am Laryngol Rhinolog Otolog Soc, p 465, 1964
6. Rosenfeld L, Graves H Jr: Primary neurogenic tumors of the lateral neck. Ann Surg 167:847, 1968
7. Oberman HA, Sullenger G: Neurogenous tumors of the head and neck. Cancer 20:1994, 1967
8. Robitaille Y, Seemayer TA, El Deiry A: Peripheral nerve tumors involving paranasal sinuses: A case report and review of the literature. Cancer 35:1254, 1975
9. Das Gupta TK, Brasfield RD: Tumors of peripheral nerve origin: Benign and malignant solitary schwannomas. CA 20:229, 1970
10. Holland GW: Neurilemoma of the vagus nerve in the neck. Aust New Zeal J Surg 38:146, 1968
11. Pesavento G, Ferlito A, Recher G: Benign solitary schwannoma of the cervical vagus nerve: A case report with a review of the literature. J Laryngol Otol 93:307, 1979
12. Pool JL, Pava AA, Greenfield RC: Acoustic nerve tumors: Early diagnosis and treatment, 2nd ed. Springfield (Ill), Thomas, 1970
13. Pulei JL, House WF, Britton BH Jr, Hitselberger WE: A system of management of acoustic neuromas based on 364 cases: Trans Am Assoc Ophthalmol 75:48, 1971
14. Oberman HA, Abell MR: Neurogenous neoplasms of the mediastinum. Cancer 13:882, 1960
15. Ackerman LV, Taylor EF: Neurogenous tumours within the thorax: A clinico-pathological evaluation of forty-eight cases. Cancer 13:669, 1959
16. Sarot IA, Schwinner D, Schechter DC: Primary neurilemmoma of diaphragm. NY State J Med 69:837, 1969
17. Gore DO, Rankow R, Hanford JM: Parapharyngeal neurilemoma. Surg Gynecol Obstet 103:193, 1956
18. Dragh LV, Soule EH, Masson JK: Benign and malignant neurilemomas of the head and neck. Surg Gynecol Obstet 111:211, 1960
19. Lane N, Murray MR, Fraser GC: Neurilemoma of the lung confirmed by tissue culture. Report of a case. Cancer 6:780, 1953
20. Collins R, Gan G: Neurilemoma presenting as a lump in the breast. Br J Surg 60:242, 1973
21. Hart MS, Bason WC: Neurilemoma involving bone. J Bone Joint Surg 49(A):465, 1958
22. Fawcet JK, Dahlin DC: Neurilemoma of bone. Am J Clin Path 47:759, 1967
23. Ashley DJB: In Evans RW (ed): Histological Appearance of Tumors, 3rd ed. Edinburgh, London, Churchill Livingston, 1978
24. Cutler EC, Gross RE: Neurofibroma and neurofibrosarcoma of peripheral nerves unassociated with Recklinghausen's disease. Arch Surg 33:733, 1936
25. Borberg A: Clinical and genetic investigation into tuberous sclerosis and Recklinghausen's neurofibromatosis: Contribution to elucidation of interrelationship and eugenics of the syndromes. Acta Psychiatr Neurol (Suppl) 71:11, 1951
26. Crowe FW, Schull WJ, Neel JV: A clinical, pathological and genetic study of multiple neurofibromatosis. Springfield (Ill), Thomas, 1956
27. Thannhauser SJ: Neurofibromatosis (von Recklinghausen's) and osteitis fibrosa cystica localistata et disseminata (von Recklinghausen's). Medicine 23:105, 1944
28. Prieser SA, Davenport CB: Multiple neurofibromatosis (von Recklinghausen's disease) and its inheritance. Am J Med Sci 156:507, 1918
29. Brasfield RD, Das Gupta TK: Von Recklinghausen's disease: A clinicopathological study. Ann Surg 175:86, 1972

30. Wander JV, Das Gupta TK: Neurofibromatosis. In Current Problems in Surgery, vol 14, number 2. Chicago, Year Book Medical Publishers, February, 1977

31. Fisher GA: Recklinghausenshe kranheit und huttermaeler. Dermat Wchnshr 84:89, 1927

32. Sergeyev AS: On mutation rate of neurofibromatosis. Human Genet 28:129, 1975

33. Feinman NL, Yakovac WC: Neurofibromatosis in childhood. J Pediat 76:339, 1970

34. Virchow R: Uver die reform der Pathologischen und therapeutischen anschanngen durch die miakroskopischen untersuchungen. Virchows Arch Pathol Anat Phys Klin Med 1:207, 1847

35. Hitchcock A: Some remarks on neuroma, with brief account of three cases of anomalous cutaneous tumors in one family. Am J Med Sci 43:320, 1862

36. Thomson A: On Neuroma and Neurofibromatosis. Edinburgh, Turnbull and Spear, 1900

37. Adrian C: Uber Neurofibromatose und ihre Komplikationen, Beitr. Klin Chir 31:1, 1901

38. Vinken PJ, Bruyn GW: The Phakomatoses. In Handbook of Clinical Neurology, vol 14. New York, Elsevier, 1972

39. Whitehouse D: Diagnostic value of café-au-lait spot in children. Arch Dis Child 4:316, 1966

40. Crowe FW: Axillary freckling as a diagnostic aid in neurofibromatosis. Ann Intern Med 61:1142, 1964

41. Pack GT, Davis J: Nevus giganticus pigmentosus with malignant transformation. Surgery 49:347, 1961

42. McNeer GP: Treatment of melanoma (panel discussion) in 'The Pigment Cell'—Molecular, Biological and Clinical Aspects. Ann NY Acad Sci 100:166, 1963

43. Rodriguez HA, Berthong M: Multiple primary intracranial tumors in von Recklinghausen's neurofibromatosis. Arch Neurol 14:467, 1966

44. Henschen F: Zur histologic unit Pathogense der Kleinhimbrichen winkletumoven. Arch Psychiat Nervekr 56:21, 1916

45. Gardner WJ, Frazier GH: Bilateral acoustic neurofibromas: A clinical study and field survey of a family of five generations with bilateral deafness in 28 members. Arch Neurol Psychiat 23:266, 1930

46. Olivecrona H: Acoustic tumors. J Neurosurg 26:6, 1967

47. Hope DG, Mulvihill JJ: Malignancy in neurofibromatosis. In VM Riccardi, JJ Mulvihill (eds): Advances in Neurology, vol. 19. Neurofibromatosis (von Recklinghausen's Disease), Raven Press, 1981, p 39

48. Rubinstein LJ: Tumors of the Central Nervous System, fasc. 6. Washington DC, AFIP, 1972

49. David M, Hecaen J, Bonis A, cited by Wertheimer P, et al: Reflexions sur la Coexistence de neurinomes multiples, de miningiomes et de gliomes encephaliques dans la maladie nerveusede Recklinghausen: A propos deckitoneuromes. Neurochirugie 3:145, 1957

50. Poser CN: The Relationship between Syringomyelia and Neoplasm. Springfield (Ill), Thomas, 1956

51. von Recklinghausen FD: Ein herz von einem neugebornen welches mehrere theils nach aussen, theils nach den hohlen prominierende tumoren (Myomen) turg. Verhandl Ges Geburtsch 15, 1863

52. River L, Silverstein J, Topel JW: Collective review; Benign neoplasms of the small intestine. Int Abstr Surg 102:1, 1956

53. Ghrist TD: Gastrointestinal involvement in neurofibromatosis. Arch Intern Med 112:357, 1962

54. Hochberg FH, DaSilva AB, Goldabine J, Richardson EP Jr: Gastrointestinal involvement in von Recklinghausen's neurofibromatosis. Neurology (Minneap) 24:1144, 1974

55. Rappaport HM: Neurofibromatosis of the oral cavity. Oral Surg 6:559, 1946

56. Baden E, Pierce HE, Jackson WF: Multiple neurofibromatosis with oral lesions. Oral Surg 8:263, 1955

57. Preston FW, Walsh WS, Clarke TH: Cutaneous neurofibromatosis (von Recklinghausen's disease): Clinical manifestations and incidence of sarcoma in 61 male patients. Arch Surg 64:813, 1952

58. Chen AU, Miller AS: Neurofibroma and schwannoma of the oral cavity: A clinical and ultrastructural study. Oral Surg 4:522, 1979

59. Smith RW: A Treatise on the Pathology, Diagnosis and Treatment of Neuroma. Dublin, Hodges & Smith, 1849

60. Prescott GH, White RE: Solitary central neurofibroma of the mandible: Report of a case and review of the literature. J Oral Surg 28:305, 1970

61. Logan PJ: Visceral neurofibromatosis. Br J Surg 31:3060, 1964

62. Sturdy DE: Neurofibroma of the esophagus. Br J Surg 54:315, 1967

63. Raszkowski HJ, Hufner RF: Neurofibromatosis of the colon: An unique manifestation of von Recklinghausen's disease. Cancer 27:34, 1971

64. Gerhardt G: Zur diagnostk multiple neurobildung, Deutsches. Arch F Klin Med 21:268, 1878

65. Kass IH: Neurofibromatosis of the bladder. Am J Dis Child 44:1040, 1932

66. Pessin JL, Bodian M: Neurofibromatosis of the pelvic autonomic plexuses. Br J Urol 36:510, 1964

67. Ross JA: A case of sarcoma of the urinary bladder in von Recklinghausen's disease. Br J Urol 29:121, 1957

68. Ravich A: Neurofibroma of the ureter: Report of a case with operation and recovery. Arch Surg 30:442, 1935

69. Hunt JC, Pugh DG: Skeletal lesions in neurofibromatosis. Radiology 76:1, 1961

70. Heard GE, Payne EE: Scalloping of vertebral bodies in von Recklinghausen's disease of the nervous system (neurofibromatosis). Neurol Surg Psychiat 25:345, 1962

71. D'Agostino AN, Soule EH, Miller RH: Sarcomas of peripheral nerves and somatic tissues associated with multiple neurofibromatosis (von Recklinghausen's disease). Cancer 16:1015, 1963

72. D'Agostino AN, Soule EH, Miller RH: Primary malignant neoplasms of nerves (malignant neurilemomas) in patients without manifestations of

multiple neurofibromatosis (von Recklinghausen's disease). Cancer 16:1003, 1963

73. Perkinson NG: Melanoma arising in a café-au-lait spot of neurofibromatosis. Am J Surg 93:1018, 1957

74. Das Gupta TK, Brasfield RD: Solitary malignant schwannoma. Ann Surg 171:419, 1970

75. Ghosh BC, Ghosh L, Huvos AG, Fortner JG: Malignant schwannoma. A clinicopathologic study. Cancer 31:184, 1973

76. Hammond HL, Calderwood RG: Malignant peripheral nerve sheath tumors of the oral cavity. Oral Surg, Oral Med, Oral Path 28:97, 1969

77. McNeer GP, Cartin J, Chu F, Nickson J: Effectiveness of radiation therapy in the management of sarcoma of the soft somatic tissues. Cancer 22:391, 1968

78. Suit HD, Russel WO, Martin RG: Sarcoma of soft tissues: Clinical and histopathological parameters and response to treatment. Cancer 35:1478, 1973

79. Lindberg RD, Martin RD, Romsdahl MM, Barkley HT: Conservative surgery and postoperative radiotherapy in 300 adults with soft tissue sarcomas. Cancer 47:2391, 1981

80. Guccion JG, Enzinger FM: Malignant schwannoma associated with von Recklinghausen's neurofibromatosis. Virchow's Arch Path Anat 383:43, 1979

81. Heard G: Nerve sheath tumors and von Recklinghausen's disease of the nervous system. Ann Royal Coll Surg 31:229, 1962

82. Odier L: Mannual de Medicine practique. Geneva, JJ Paschond, 1811

83. Wood W: Observations on neuromas, with cases and histories of the disease. Trans Med-Chir Soc Edinburgh 3:68, 1829

84. Huber GC, Lewis D: Amputation neuromas, their development and prevention. Arch Surg 1:85, 1920

85. Cieslak AK, Stout AP: Traumatic and amputation neuromas. Arch Surg 53:646, 1946

86. Farley NH: Painful stump neuroma—treatment of. Minnesota Med 48:347, 1965

87. Klintworth GK: Axon regeneration in the human spinal cord with formation of neuromata. J Neuropath Exper Neurol 23:123, 1964

88. Tulenko JF: Cicatricial neuromas following neck dissection. Plast Reconst Surg 35:419, 1965

89. Gillesby WJ, Wu KH: Amputation neuromas of vagus nerves. Am J Surg 110:673, 1965

90. Swanson HH: Traumatic neuromas. A review of the literature. Oral Surg 14:317, 1961

91. Das Gupta TK, Brasfield RD: Amputation neuroma in cancer patients. NY State J Med 69:2129, 1969

92. Stout AP: Ganglioneuromata of the sympathetic nervous system. Surg Gynecol Obstet 84:101, 1947

93. Knudson AG Jr, Amromin GD: Neuroblastoma and ganglioneuroma in a child with multiple neurofibromatosis: Implications for the mutational origin of neuroblastoma. Cancer 19:1032, 1966

94. Smith J: A case of adrenal neuroblastoma. Lancet 2:1214, 1932

95. Bolande RP, Towler WF: A possible relationship in neuroblastoma to von Recklinghausen's disease. Cancer 26:162, 1970

96. Stowens D: Neuroblastoma and related tumors. Arch Pathol (Berlin) 63:451, 1957

97. Weller RO, Cervos-Navarro J: Pathology of Peripheral nerves. London, Butterworth, 1977

98. Dargeon MW: Tumors of Childhood. New York, Hoeber, 1960

99. Ashley DJB: In Evans RW (ed): Histological Appearance of Tumors, 3rd ed. Edinburgh, London, Churchill Livingstone, 1978

100. Carpenter WB, Kernohan JW: Retroperitoneal ganglioneuromas and neurofibromas. A clinical pathological study. Cancer 16:788, 1963

101. Hamilton JP, Koop CE: Ganglioneuromas in children. Surg Gynecol Obstet 121:803, 1965

102. Hauer GT, Andrews WD: The surgery of mediastinal tumors. Am J Surg 50:146, 1940

103. Iverson LL: The catecholamines. Nature 214:8, 1967

104. Wurtman RJ: Catecholamines. N Engl J Med 273:637, 1965

105. Paton DM (ed): The Mechanism of Neuronal and Extraneuronal Transport of Catecholamines. New York, Raven Press, 1976

106. Polashko H: Specific action of L-Dopadecarboxylase. J Physiol 96:50, 1939

107. Pearse AGE: The APUD Concept: Embryology, cytochemistry and ultrastructure of the diffuse neuroendocrine system. In Friesen SR (ed): Surgical Endocrinology. Philadelphia, Lippincott, 1978

108. Page LB, Jacoby GA: Catecholamine metabolism and storage granules in pheochromocytoma and neuroblastoma. Medicine 43:379, 1964

109. Page LB, Coopeland RB: Pheochromocytoma. DM, January 1968

110. Thomas JE, Rooke ED, Kvale WF: The neurologist's experience with pheochromocytoma. JAMA 197:754, 1966

111. Reynolds JL, Gilchrist TF: Congenital heart disease and pheochromocytoma. Am J Dis Child 112:251, 1966

112. Calkins E, Howard JE: Bilateral familial pheochromocytoma with paroxysmal hypertension: Successful surgical removal of tumors in two cases, with discussion of certain diagnostic procedures and physiological considerations. J Clin Endocrinol 7:475, 1947

113. O'Brien D: Pheochromocytoma with endocrinopathy. N Engl J Med 268:1365, 1963

114. Gifford RW, Kvale WF, Maher FT, Roth GM, Priestly JT: Clinical features, diagnosis and treatment of pheochromocytoma: A review of 76 cases. Mayo Clin Proc 39:281, 1964

115. Maier HC: Intrathoracic pheochromocytoma with hypertension. Ann Surg 130:1059, 1949

116. Samaan HA: Risk of operation in a patient with unsuspected pheochromocytoma. Br J Surg 57:462, 1970

117. El-Minawa MF, Paulino E, Cuesto M, Ceballos J: Pheochromocytoma masquerading as preeclamptic toxemia. Am J Obstet Gynecol 109:389, 1971

118. Engleman K: A new test for pheochromocytoma. JAMA 189:107, 1964

119. Gitlow SE, Mendlowitz M, Bertani LM: The biochemical techniques for detecting and establishing the presence of pheochromocytoma. Am J Cardiol 26:270, 1970

120. Stackpole RH, Myer MM, Uson AC: Pheochromocytoma in children. J Pediat 63:315, 1963

121. Nourok DS: Familial pheochromocytoma and thyroid carcinoma. Ann Int Med 60:1028, 1964

122. Schinke RN, Startmen WH: Familial amyloid producing medullary thyroid carcinoma and pheochromocytoma. Ann Int Med 63:1027, 1965

123. Suzuki S: Ueber zwei tumoren aus nebennierenmark-gewebe. Berlin Klin Wschr 47:1623, 1910

124. MacKeith R: Adrenal-sympathetic syndrome: Chromaffin tissue tumor with paroxysmal hypertension. Br Heart J 6:1, 1944

125. Davis FW Jr, Hull JG, Vardell JC Jr: Pheochromocytoma with neurofibromatosis. Am J Med 8:131, 1950

126. Lynch JD, Sheps SG, Bernatz PE, Remine WH, Harrison Jr EH: Neurofibromatosis and hypertension. Minnesota Med 55:25, 1972

127. Tilford DL, Kelsch RC: Renal artery stenosis in childhood neurofibromatosis. Am J Dis Child 126:665, 1973

128. Glushien PS, Mansuy MM, Littman DS: Pheochromocytoma: Its relationship to the neurocutaneous syndromes. Am J Med 14:318, 1953

129. Modlin IM, Farndon JR, Shepherd A, Johnson IDA, et al: Pheochromocytomas in 72 patients: Clinical and diagnostic features, treatment and long term results. Br J Surg 66:456, 1979

130. Sipple JH: The association of pheochromocytoma with carcinoma of the thyroid gland. Am J Med 31:163, 1961

131. Kairi MRA, Dexter RN, Burznyski NJ, Johston CC: Mucosal neuroma, pheochromocytoma and medullary thyroid carcinoma: Multiple endocrine neoplasia. Type 3. Medicine 54:89, 1975

132. Harrison TS, Thompson NW: Multiple endocrine adenomatosis, I and II. Current Problems in Surgery. Chicago, Year Book Medical Publishers, 50:51 (Aug.), 1975

133. Pearse AGE, Polak JM: Cytochemical evidence for the neural crest origin of mammalian ultimobranchial c cells. Histochemistry 27:96, 1971

134. Higgins PM, Tresidder GC: Pheochromocytoma of the urinary bladder. Br Med J 2:274, 1966

135. Krupski WC, Effeney DJ, Ehrenfeld WK, Stoney RJ: Cervical chemodectoma: Technical considerations and management options. Am J Surg 144:215, 1982

136. Shamblin WR, ReMine WH, Sheps SG, Harrison EG: Carotid body tumor (chemodectoma). Clinicopathological analysis of ninety cases. Am J Surg 122:732, 1971

137. Farr HW: Carotid body tumors: A thirty-year experience at Memorial Hospital. Am J Surg 114:614, 1967

138. Sato T, Saito H, Yoshinaga K, Shibota Y, Sasano N: Concurrence of carotid body tumor and pheochromocytoma. Cancer 34:1787, 1974

139. Brown JS: Glomus jugulare tumors. Methods and difficulties of diagnosis and surgical treatment. Laryngoscope 77:26, 1967

140. Lattes R, Waltner JG: Nonchromaffin paraganglioma of the middle ear (carotid body-like tumor; glomus-jugulare tumor). Cancer 2:447, 1949

141. Levit SA, Sheps SG, Espinosa RE, Remine WH, Harrison EG Jr: Catecholamine-secreting paraganglioma of glomus-jugulare region resembling pheochromocytoma. N Engl J Med 281:805, 1969

142. Duke WW, Roshell BR, Soteres P, et al: A norepinephrine-secreting glomus jugulare tumor presenting as a pheochromocytoma. Ann Intern Med 60:1040, 1964

143. Burman SO: The vagal body tumor. Ann Surg 141:488, 1955

144. Johnson WS, Beaher OH, Harrison EG: Chemodectoma of the glomus intravagale (vagal-body tumor). Am J Surg 104:812, 1962

145. Byrne JJ: Carotid body and allied tumors. Am J Surg 95:351, 1958

146. Fisher ER, Hazard JB: Nonchromaffin paraganglioma of the orbit. Cancer 5:521, 1952

147. Simons JN, Beahrs OH, Woolmer LB: Chemodectoma of an aortic body. Am J Surg 117:363, 1969

148. Smithers DW, Gowing NFC: Chemodectomas in the region of the aortic arch. Thorax 20:182, 1965

149. Olson JD, Salyer WR: Mediastinal paragangliomas (aortic body tumors). Cancer 41:2405, 1978

150. Mapp EM, Krouse TB, Fox EF, Voci G: Chemodectoma of the anterior mediastinum. Report of a case of probable aortic body origin with arteriographic findings. Radiology 92:547, 1969

151. Olson JR, Abell MR: Nonfunctional nonchromaffin paragangliomas of the retroperitoneum. Cancer 23:1358, 1969

152. Shimazaki M, Ueda G, Kurimoto H, Ito T, Imazumi R: Retroperitoneal nonchromaffin paraganglioma with hormonal activity. Acta Path Jap 15:145, 1965

153. Johnson RWP, Somerville PG: A malignant soft-tissue paraganglioma of the leg. Br J Surg 44:605, 1957

154. Carey JP, Bradley RL: Chemodectoma: a review with two new cases. Arch Surg 87:897, 1963

155. Horoupian DS, Kerson LA, Saiontz H, Valsamis M: Paraganglioma of cauda equina: Clinicopathologic and ultrastructural studies of an unusual case. Cancer 33:1337, 1974

156. Lukash WM, Hyams VJ, Nielsen OF: Neurogenic neoplasms of the small bowel: Benign nonchromaffin paraganglioma of the duodenum: Report of a case. Am J Dig Dis 11:575, 1966

157. Taylor HB, Helwig EB: Bengin nonchromaffin paragangliomas of the duodenum. Arch Path Anat 335, 1962

158. Smith WT, Hughes B, Ermocilla R: Chemodectoma of the pineal region, with observations on the pineal body and chemoreceptor tissue. J Path Bacteriol 92:69, 1966

159. Korn D, Bensch K. Liebow AA, Castleman B: Multiple minute pulmonary tumors resembling chemodectomas. Am J Path 37:641, 1960

160. Fawcett EJ, Husband FM: Chemodectoma of lung. J Clin Path 20:260, 1967

161. Ichinose H, Hewitt RL, Drapana T: Minute pulmonary chemodectoma. Cancer 28:692, 1971

162. Brown JB, Freyer MP: Carotid body tumors: Report of removal of tumor thought to be largest recorded. Surgery 32:997, 1952

163. Pryse-Davies J, Dawson IMP, Westbury G: Some morphologic, histochemical, and chemical observations on chemodectomas and the normal carotid body, including a study of the chromaffin reaction and possible ganglion cell elements. Cancer 17:185, 1964

164. Glenner GG, Crout JR, Robers WC: A functional carotid-body-like tumor secreting levarterenol. Arch Path 73:230, 1962

165. Hamberger B, Ritzen M, Wersall J: Demonstration of catecholamines and 5-hydroxytryptamine in the human carotid body. J Pharmacol Exp Ther 152:1966

166. Berdal P, Braaten M, Cappelan C Jr, et al: Nonadrenaline-adrenaline producing nonchromaffin paraganglioma. Acta Med Scand 172:249, 1962

167. Duke WW, Bashell BR, Soters P, Carr JH: A norepinephrine-secreting glomus jugulare tumor presenting as a pheochromocytoma. Ann Int Med 60:1040, 1964

168. Salyer KE, Ketchum LD, Robinson DW, Masters PW: Surgical management of cervical paragangliomata. Arch Surg 98:572, 1969

169. Frey CF, Karoll RP: Management of chemodectomas. Am J Surg 111:536, 1966

170. Priebe CJ, Clatworthy HWJ: Neuroblastoma: Evaluation of treatment of ninety children. Arch Surg 95:538, 1967

171. deLorimier AA, Bragg KJ, Linden G: Neuroblastoma in childhood. Am J Dis Child 118:441, 1969

172. Bill AH, Hartmann JR, Beckwith JB: The unique biology of childhood tumors with special reference to the biology of neuroblastoma. Pacific Med Surg 75:281, 1967

173. Miller RW, Fraumeni JF Jr, Hill JA: Neuroblastoma: Epidemiologic approach to its origins. J Pediat Surg 3:141, 1968

174. Bodian M: Neuroblastoma. Pediat Clin N Am 6:449, 1959

175. Gross RE, Farber S, Martin LW: Neuroblastoma sympathicum. A study and report of 217 cases. Pediat 23:951, 1959

176. Fortner J, Nicastri A, Murphy ML: Neuroblastoma: Natural history and results of treating 133 cases. Ann Surg 167:132, 1968

177. Vinik M, Altman DH: Congenital malignant tumors. Cancer 19:967, 1966

178. Wells HG: Occurrence and significance of congenital malignant neoplasms. Arch Path 30:535, 1940

179. Simpson TE, Lynn HB, Mills SD: Congenital neuroblastoma in the scrotum. Clin Pediat 8:174, 1969

180. Hinterberger H, Bartholomew EJ: Catecholamines and their acidic metabolites in urine and in tumor tissue in neuroblastoma, ganglioneuroma and pheochromocytoma. Clin Chim Acta 23:169, 1969

181. Voorhess ML: The catecholamines in tumor and urine from patients with neuroblastoma, ganglioneuroblastoma, and pheochromocytoma. J Pediat Surg 3:147, 1968

182. LaBrosse EH: 3-methocy-4-hydroxyphanylglycol in neuroblastoma. J Pediat Surg 3:148, 1968

183. Gitlow S, Bertani LM, Rausen A, Griebetz D, Dziedzik SW: Diagnosis of neuroblastoma by qualitative and quantitative determination of catecholamine metabolites in urine. Cancer 25:1377, 1970

184. Maurer HM: Current concepts in cancer: Solid tumors in children. New Engl J Med 299:1345, 1978

185. Evans AE, Albo V, Bangio GJ, Finklestein JZ, Leinkin S, Santulli T, Weiner J, Hammond D: Factors influencing survival of childhood neuroblastoma. Cancer 38:661, 1976

186. Swaen GJV, Sloof JL, Stoelinga GRA: A differentiating neuroblastoma. J Path Bacteriol 90:333, 1965

187. Beckurth JB, Martin RF: Observations on the histopathology of neuroblastoma. J Ped Surg 3:106, 1968

188. Evans AE, D'Angio GJ, Randolph J: A proposed staging system for children with neuroblastoma. Cancer 27:374, 1971

189. Lauder I, Aherne W: The significance of lymphocytic infiltration in neuroblastoma. Br J Cancer 26:321, 1972

190. Dyke PC, Mulkey DA: Maturation of ganglioneuroblastoma to ganglioneuroma. Cancer 20:1343, 1967

191. Cushing H, Wolback SB: The transformation of a malignant paravertebral sympathicoblastoma into a benign ganglioneuroma. Am J Path 3:62, 1927

192. Fox F, Davidson J, Thomas LB: Maturation of sympathicoblastoma into ganglioneuroma. Cancer 12:108, 1959

193. Fissane JM, Ackerman LV: Maturation of tumors of the sympathetic nervous system. J Fac Radiol (London) 7:109, 1955

194. Stewart FW: Experiences in spontaneous regression of neoplastic disease in man. Texas Rep Biol Med 10:239, 1952

195. Visfeldt J: Transformation of sympathicoblastoma into ganglioneuroma. Acta Path Microbiol Scand 58:44, 1963

196. Chatten JE, Voorhees ML: Familial neuroblastoma. Report of a kindred with multiple disorders. N Engl J Med 277:1230, 1967

197. Berger L, et Richard L: L'Esthesioneuroepithelioma olfactif. Bull de l'assoc franc du cancer 13:410, 1924

198. Kahn LB: Esthesioneuroblastoma: A light and electron microscopic study. Human Path 5:364, 1974

199. Hutter RVP, Lewis JS, Foote FW Jr, Tollefsen HR: Esthesioneuroblastoma: A clinical and pathological study. Am J Surg 106, 1963

200. Skolnick EM, Massari FS, Tenta LT: Olfactory neuroepithelioma: Review of the world literature and presentation of 2 cases. Arch Otolaryngol 84:644, 1966

201. Castro L, de la Paya S, Webster JH: Esthesioneuroblastoma: A report of seven cases. Am J Roentgenol 105:7, 1969
202. Sellwood RA, Wapnick S, Breckenridge A, Williams ED, Welbourn RB: Recurrent pheochromocytoma. Br J Surg 57:309, 1970
203. Campbell CB, Mortimer RH: A functioning malignant phaeochromocytoma occurring in a patient with neurofibromatosis. Aust Ann Med 17:331, 1968
204. Hamberger CA, Hamberger CB, Wersal J, et al: Malignant catecholamine-producing tumor of the carotid body. Acta Path Microbiol Scand 69:439, 1967
205. Cohen SM, Persky L: Malignant non-chromaffin paraganglioma with metastasis to the kidney. J Urol 96:122, 1966
206. Tu H, Bottomley RH: Malignant chemodectoma presenting as a miliary pulmonary infiltrate. Cancer 33:248, 1974
207. Coulson WF: A metastasizing carotid body tumor. J Bone Joint Surg 52-A:752, 1969
208. Pendergrass EP, Kirsch D: Roentgen manifestations in the skull of metastatic carotid body

209. tumor (paraganglioma) of meningioma and of mucocoele—A report of three unusual cases. Am J Roentgenol 57:417, 1947
209. Romanski R: Chemodectoma (nonchromaffin paraganglioma) of the carotid body with distant metasteses. Am J Path 30:1, 1954
210. Rangwala AF, Sylvia LG, Becker SM: Soft tissue metastasis of a chemodectoma. A case report and review of the literature. Cancer 42:2865, 1978
211. Say CC, Hori J, Spratt J Jr: Chemodectoma with distant metastases. Case report and review of literature. Amer Surg 39:333, 1973
212. Staats EF, Brown RL, Smith RR: Carotid body tumor: benign and malignant. Laryngoscope 76:907, 1966
213. Alford BR, Guilford FR: A comprehensive study of the tumors of the glomus jugulare. Laryngoscope 72:765, 1962
214. Patcher MR: Mediastinal nonchromaffin paragranuloma. J Thoracic Cardiovasc Surg 45:152, 1963
215. Zak FG, Chaber A: Pulmonary chemodectomatosis. JAMA 813:887, 1963

15

Tumors of the Synovial Tissue

Tapas K. Das Gupta

BENIGN TUMORS OF THE SYNOVIAL TISSUE

Synovioma

This is a rare tumor found around a joint in the extremities, typically the knee or ankle (Fig. 15.1), and around the flexor tendons of the hand and wrist. Generally the lesion is small and asymptomatic, and medical opinion is sought because of cosmetic problems. Infrequently, due to associated arthritis, patients complain of pain or difficulty in joint mobility. Routine excision is not mandatory; however, treatment of the underlying cause should be instituted.

Villonodular Synovitis

Villonodular synovitis is frequently seen in and around the flexor tendons of the fingers, wrist, and toes (Fig. 15.2 A and 15.2 B), and sometimes around the weight-bearing joints. It usually occurs in middle-aged persons of both sexes, but rare instances have been reported in children.[1] Bobechko and associates[1] reported pigmented villonodular synovitis in three children with cavernous hemangioma of the knee joint. Usually it is painless, although in some cases pain may be the presenting clinical feature. In general, the tumors are small and take the shape of the tendon over the joint around which they occur. Treatment of these cystlike swellings

consists of excision. Prior to excision, the extent of the tumor and the presence or absence of any associated systemic disease and local degenerative arthritic problems should be assessed.[2]

Giant Cell Tumor of the Tendon Sheath

This is a relatively common benign tumor encountered in the small joints of the extremities. Although these tumors are not derivatives of synovial tissue, for operational simplicity they are described in this section.

Most commonly they are found in middle-aged women, the average age being about 40 years. They occur frequently in the digits, on both the flexor and extensor aspects of the tendon sheaths (Fig. 15.3). These tumors may produce pressure erosion in the underlying bones and such an x-ray finding should not be taken as a sign of malignant transformation. There may be associated lipodystrophies, and although various theories regarding etiology have been forwarded,[3] none has yet been confirmed.

These tumors tend to grow as nodular overgrowths and their size is frequently determined by their location. Those of the fingers usually remain small and nodular, varying in size from 1 to 2 cm, whereas those occurring more proximally may grow as large as 6 to 7 cm. In fingers, the expanding tumor sometimes ruptures the tendon sheath and extends sub-

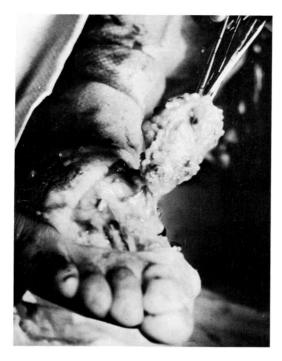

Figure 15.1. Synovioma of the dorsum of the foot in a 36-year-old man. The lesion was asymptomatic but was excised for cosmetic reasons. This lesion was incorrectly diagnosed as a neurofibroma in 1978.

cutaneously. Rarely, these tumors infiltrate the overlying skin.

Treatment of benign giant cell tumors of the tendon sheath is conservative excision although there is a possibility of recurrence. Pack and Ariel[3] found the recurrence rate reported in the literature varied from 7 to 44 percent. A meticulous dissection of the primary lesion reduces the incidence of local recurrence. Radical excision of the surrounding tendons or curettement of the underlying bone should be avoided.

Ganglion

Ganglions are cystic swellings in and around joint cavities and are not true neoplasms. The incidence is unknown, since most of them are not reported either by the physician or by the patient. Ganglions occur most frequently in the dorsum of the wrist (Fig. 15.4), arising from the tendon sheaths of the extensor tendons. Other sites of origin are the palmar aspect of the wrist, the fingers, the ankle, the dorsum of the foot, and, occasionally, the popliteal region. This is

usually a disease of adults and seldom is encountered in children.[3,4]

A ganglion forms a smooth round or ovoid mass over the affected joint. The cystic consistency and mobility along the course of the tendon sheath makes clinical diagnosis relatively simple.

In the past, a blow with a heavy book or other nonsurgical management was proposed, mainly to emphasize the nonneoplastic, nonmalignant and cystic nature of the lesion. If, however, these lesions are large and produce cosmetic problems, they should be dissectd out of the tendon sheaths. Most local recurrences following excision are the result of inadequate excision through a small incision.

MALIGNANT TUMORS OF THE SYNOVIAL TISSUE

Synovial Sarcoma (Malignant Synovioma)

Synovial sarcoma is a relatively rare malignant tumor. Sarcomas arising from synovial membrane were described in unillustrated communications by Hardie and Salter,[5] Marsh,[6] and Lockwood.[7] However, the tumor was adequately described for the first time in 1910 by Lejars and Rubens-Duvall.[8] By 1965, Cadman, Soule, and Kelly[9] estimated that a total of 519 cases existed in the literature. In 1966, Mackenzie[10] reported an additional 58 cases, bringing the total to 577. Rissanen and Holsti[11] added 13 cases in 1970. Van Andel,[12] reviewing the literature on treated cases, accepted a total of 450 and added 28 of his own. Gerner and Moore[13] found 34 cases in the files of Roswell Park Memorial Institute in 1975. Several other cases have also been documented.[14-28] At the University of Illinois Hospital, 34 such cases have been treated by the author. Based on the information derived from all these cases it is possible to define the natural history and develop general guidelines regarding its management.

Sex, Age, and Race. There is no predilection for either sex, although some authors have found a slight preponderance in males. Of the 34 patients in the University of Illinois series, 19 were men and 15 were women.

Synovial sarcoma is essentially a disease of young adults. Pack and Ariel[3,17] found that 60

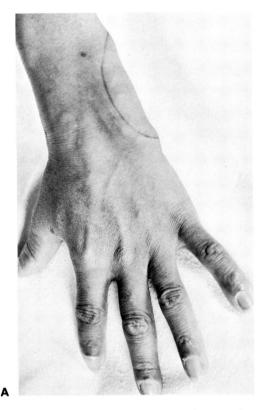
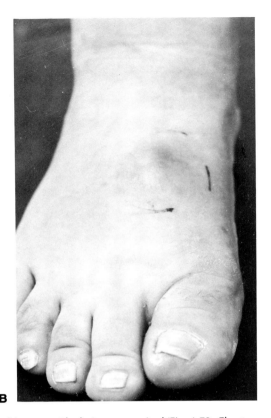

A   **B**

Figure 15.2. (**A**) Villonodular synovitis in the wrist of a 51-year-old woman. The lesion was excised (Fig. 4.73, Chapter 4) and she has remained well. (**B**) Villonodular synovitis in the dorsum of the foot. The lesion was deceptive, extending much further than could be seen or palpated.

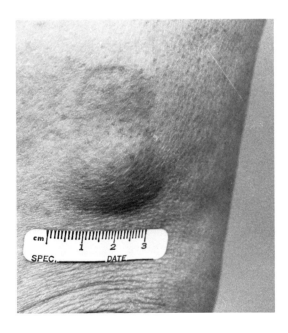

Figure 15.3. Giant cell tumor of the tendon sheath around the knee joint. The tumor was excised and has not recurred in the past seven years.

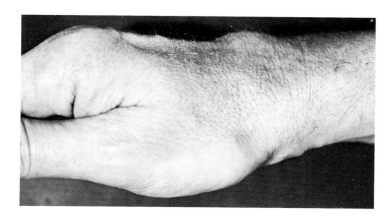

Figure 15.4. Ganglion of the dorsum of the wrist. This was excised only because the patient complained of various symptoms associated with this cystic swelling.

percent of their patients were between the ages of 15 and 40 years. In the author's series of 34 patients, the youngest was 14 years old and the oldest 79, the average age being 37 years.

Anatomic Location. Pack and Ariel[3] reported that synovial sarcoma occurs most frequently in the extremities. Most authors[9-13,16,17,23-30] have found that indeed this observation is correct, although as Cadman et al.[9] observed, only rarely is an obvious relationship found between the tumor and the synovial membrane. Instances of the tumor arising in the neck and trunk are also on record.[19-22,25] Table 15.1 shows the anatomic distribution in our series of cases, along with that in five other series. This tumor is encountered frequently in and around the knee joint: 28 percent in our series, and 21.6 percent in the series reported by Pack and Ariel.[3] In the remainder of cases in the lower extremities, the tumors seem to have no specific anatomic predilection (Fig. 15.5 A; Fig. 4.74, Chapter 4). In the upper extremities, the majority of cases occur in the wrist and hands. In our series, 7 of 11 (64 percent) occurred below the elbow (Fig. 15.5 B). The synovial sarcomas that arise in the tendons and bursae adjacent to the articular surfaces of a joint seldom involve the articular surfaces.

Synovial sarcomas rarely occur in the head and neck region (Table 15.1). In a total of 403 patients in six series, only four (0.9 percent) ases were recorded (Table 15.1). Because of this rarity, several authors have published case reports.[19-22] Golomb et al.,[20] in 1975, reported one case and found an additional 15 in the literature. Roth et al.[19] in the same years reviewed 24 cases from the files of the Armed Forces Institute of Pathology. Recently, Shmookler and associates[31]

pointed out that synovial sarcomas can also be found in the face and the oral cavity. From the files of the Armed Forces Institute of Pathology, these authors culled data on 11 cases: eight facial (four cheek, two parotid area, one intraorbital and one submental), and three intraoral (two tonsillar and one lingual). They also reviewed 22 similar case reports from the literature. It appears that the natural history of these tumors arising in the head and neck region is similar to that of tumors in other anatomic sites.

Clinical Features. The majority of patients with a synovial sarcoma present with a slow-growing, painless, mass. Pack and Ariel[3] reported that 58 percent of their patients had this initial symptom. In the author's series of 34 patients, 20 (59 percent) were initially seen with a painless mass. Three patients (9 percent) stated that a dull, aching pain preceded the appearance of a mass. Because of the mistaken notion that the pain is usually associated with arthritic or other degenerative disease, the diagnosis of sarcoma frequently is missed for several months, particularly in older patients. One of our patients, a 74-year-old man, had had pain around the left knee joint and the popliteal space for more than nine months before being referred to our clinic. He had been treated only with analgesics, and a slow-growing swelling in the popliteal space was missed. After the tumor became large enough to cause concern to the family, an aggressive diagnostic approach was undertaken.

Roentgenographic examination of the joints rarely helps in making an accurate diagnosis. A soft tissue shadow might be helpful in ascertaining the extent of the tumor, but there is no characteristic finding in x-rays. In recent years,

TABLE 15.1. ANATOMIC LOCATIONS OF SYNOVIAL SARCOMAS IN SIX SERIES

Anatomic Site	Haagensen and Stout[25] (1944)	Pack and Ariel[3] (1958)	Cadman et al.[9] (1965)	Mackenzie[10] (1966)	Rissanen and Holsti[11] (1970)	Das Gupta (1981)
Neck		—	1	—	—	3
Trunk		2	6	—	—	2
Upper extremities	22	24	32	22	4	11
Arm	(1)	(4)	(4)	(9)		(1)
Elbow	(9)	(2)	(6)	(6)		(3)
Forearm and hand	(12)	(18)	(22)	(7)	(4)	(7)
Lower extremities	82	34	95	36	9	18
Hip and thigh, groin	(12)	(8)	(39)	(7)	(1)	(6)
Knee	(49)	(13)	(21)	(15)	(7)	(5)
Leg, foot, ankle	(21)	(13)	(35)	(13)	(1)	(7)
Unknown				1		
Total cases	104	60	134	58	13	34

arthrography has also been tried, but the most reliable diagnostic method is microscopic examination of the tumor.

Regional Metastases. Synovial sarcoma has a tendency to metastasize to the regional nodes. In our series, the incidence was 18 percent. Pack and Ariel[3] reported a 16 percent incidence in their series, and Haagensen and Stout[25] an 11 percent incidence. Gerner and Moore[13] found about a 12 percent incidence. Weingrad and Rosenberg[32] found no instance of node metastases in their analysis of five cases from the files of the National Cancer Institute, but reported an overall incidence of 17 percent in a total of 535 published cases. The published incidence (Table 15.2) is difficult to interpret and even more difficult to apply in developing therapeutic guidelines. Although the true incidence of regional node metastases in stage I tumors is hard to define, for pleomorphic tumors (grades 3 and 4) we recommend regional node dissection along with resection of the primary. In locally advanced cases the incidence is much higher and treatment planning must incorporate the regional node-bearing area.

Treatment. The treatment of primary synovial sarcoma is wide soft tissue excision (Chapter 6). Infrequently, amputation of an extremity is indicated. Synovial sarcomas appear to be moderately sensitive to radiotherapy and chemotherapy, and under our present protocol the limb salvage procedures entail the routine use of the multimodal treatment programs for synovial sarcomas of the extremities (Chapter 8 for details). For synovial sarcomas located elsewhere in the body, we have embarked upon a program of wide excision of the primary tumor with adjuvant postoperative chemotherapy (Chapter 8). Recently, Lindberg and associates[29] published the M. D. Anderson Hospital data on the treatment of 24 patients with synovial sarcoma. These authors used a planned protocol of conservative surgery and radical radiation therapy, with a clinically acceptable result of 12.5 percent local recurrence.

If the regional node-bearing area is near the primary site it should be included in the therapeutic planning. If the primary tumor is larger than 5 cm and is pleomorphic, then a regional node dissection is advocated, irrespective of its distance from the tumor.

End Results. Of the 34 patients in our series, 13 were treated by operation alone, 13 received postoperative adjuvant chemotherapy, and the remaining 8 were treated by our present limb salvage protocol (Chapter 8). In this section, only the end results with the surgically treated patients are discussed. All 13 are eligible for five-year survival analysis. Nine (69 percent) are alive and well following primary therapy. One of the 13, a 27-year-old woman, had a remarkably indolent course. She was admitted to the University of Illinois Hospital in March 1968 with a recurrent tumor of the upper left thigh in the previous excision scar. About one year prior to this admission she had had a tumor excised and a diagnosis of synovial sarcoma was rendered. A review of the histologic material was found consistent with synovial sarcoma. She was treated by means of a left hemipelvectomy in April 1968. Pathologic examination of the specimen showed synovial sarcoma of the left upper thigh with invasion of the left hip joint. She was readmitted to the hospital in July 1968 for metastatic tumor to the left lung as well as an abdominal mass located in the left upper quadrant. She then underwent an exploratory procedure and a cystic mass was found in the body and tail of the pancreas. A resection of the body and tail of the pancreas, along with the spleen, was performed on July 24, 1968. Examination of the resected material showed both the cyst wall and the pancreatic bed to contain metastatic synovial sarcoma. She did well postoperatively and was discharged from the hospital. The patient was readmitted for the third time in October 1968, for resection of lung metastases. On November 6, 1968, a left upper lobe lobectomy with resection of portions of the third, fourth, and fifth ribs was performed. Examination of the specimen showed synovial sarcoma metastatic to the upper lobe of the left lung with extension to the parietal pleura and periosteal tissue, without actual invasion of the ribs. She did well postoperatively and was discharged on November 13, 1968.

She remained well for 21 months, at which time metastases to the right lower lung field was noted. A segmental resection of the right medial basilar segment was performed on August 19, 1970.

In September 1971, she began having severe headaches. Evaluation showed a left midtemporal and anterior parietal lesion. An exploratory craniotomy with enucleation of the metastatic tumor was performed October 21, 1971. She was discharged November 16, 1971. She received radiation therapy to the brain following enucleation of the tumor, although removal of the gross tumor had resulted in symptomatic relief of headaches and seizures.

She has remained well to date, that is, more than 12 years after resection of the fourth site of metastatic synovial sarcoma, and is leading an active life with a functional prosthesis.

The overall five-year survival rate in synovial sarcoma has been described as poor by most authors.[3,9,10,13-17,24,26] Table 15.3 summarizes the overall five-year end results in several series. In the past, when the reports consisted of a retrospective review of published cases, with a multitude of therapeutic modalities, the end results were poor. Pack and Ariel[3] were dealing with a group of patients with large tumors, and, frequently, with locally recurrent tumors after initial inadequate therapy. Haagensen and Stout[25] described the overall survival in a collected group of 104 patients. Among the more recent reports, Cadman, Soule, and Kelly[9] analyzed a large series of 134 patients from the files of the Mayo Clinic from 1905 through 1960 and found the disease-free survival rate to be 16.4 percent for two years and 10 percent for seven years. Although this is an excellent analysis of the clinicopathologic material, it suffers from the inevitable problem of a retrospective analysis, which has to deal with interpretation of multiple methods of treatment in vogue during five decades. In contrast, MacKenzie[10] found a five-year salvage rate of 51 percent in a relatively well-controlled group of patients. Gerner and Moore[13] reviewed the material from Roswell Park

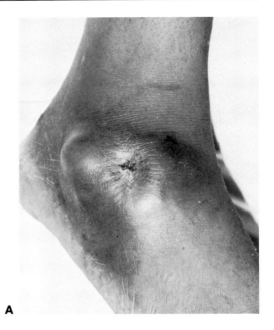

A

Memorial Institute and were unable to arrive at any guidelines regarding therapy. Analysis of the data in Table 15.3 shows a significant fall in the salvage rate between a two- and five-year period. This should be borne in mind when designing a prospective protocol.

In eight of our 13 patients treated by surgery alone, the tumor diameter was 5 cm or less, and in six of these, the histologic grade was between 2 and 3. All six lived disease-free for five years. In the other two the tumor was between grades 3 and 4, and one of these patients was a five-year survivor. In the remaining five, the tumor size was greater than 5 cm. In two

TABLE 15.2 COMPARATIVE INCIDENCE OF REGIONAL NODE METASTASES IN SYNOVIAL SARCOMA

Author(s)	Year of Publication	Total No. Cases Reported	No. Cases with Nodal Metastases
Haagensen and Stout[25]	1944	104	11 (10.57%)
Pack and Ariel[3]	1958	60	10 (16.6%)
Cadman et al[8]	1965	17 (134)*	4 (23.5%)
Rissanen and Holsti[11]	1970	13	0
Gerner and Moore[13]	1975	34	4 (11.7%)
Roth et al[19]	1975	8 (24)†	1 (4%)
Das Gupta	1981	34	6 (18%)

*Only 17 of 134 had node dissection.
†All 24 cases were in the neck, only 8 had neck dissection.

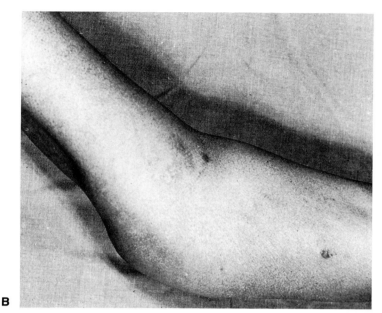

B

Figure 15.5. (**A**) Synovial sarcoma around the ankle joint in a 44-year-old man. He underwent a below-the-knee amputation and regional node dissection. One of 18 nodes contained metastatic tumor. He is still well three years later. (**B**) Synovial sarcoma in the ulnar aspect below the elbow. Patient was treated with wide soft tissue resection and adjuvant chemotherapy. She has been disease-free for six years.

of the five the histologic grades were 2 and 3 and both patients lived for five years or longer without any evidence of recurrence or metastases. The three remaining patients had histologic grades 3 and 4 tumors and all three died of metastatic disease. None of the 13 patients had local recurrence following primary wide soft tissue resection. As has been the general theme of this entire treatise, this result represents a planned surgical approach in the treatment of sarcomas.

In our group of 13 patients treated with postoperative adjuvant chemotherapy, seven of eight with high-grade synovial sarcoma sur-

vived five years or longer, ie, a cure rate of 87.5 percent was achieved (Table 8.17, Chapter 8). Therefore, it is reasonable to suggest that surgical treatment along with adjuvant chemotherapy, if used judiciously, can salvage at least 85 percent of the patients. However, systemic adjuvant chemotherapy is not needed for low-grade tumors.

Pack and Ariel[3] attempted to develop some prognostic criteria for patients with synovial sarcoma. From their series of 60 patients, they concluded that the overall prognosis is better for younger women with tumors arising in the fingers. Cadman and co-workers[9] found the in-

TABLE 15.3. COMPARATIVE STUDY OF END RESULTS IN SELECTED SERIES OF SYNOVIAL SARCOMAS

Authors	No. Cases	2 Yr, N.E.D.†	5 Yr, N.E.D.
Haagensen and Stout[25] (1944)	104	?	3 (2.8%)
Wright[15] (1952)	47	20 (42.5%)	9 (19%)
Pack and Ariel[3] (1958)	42	10 (24%)	8 (19%)
Vincent[16] (1960)	12	2 (16.6%)	1 (8.3%)
Anderson and Wildermuth[23] (1961)	27	16 (59%)	13 (48%)
Cadman et al[9] (1965)	134	22 (16.4%)	13 (9.7%)
Mackenzie[10] (1966)	49	?	25 (51%)
Gerner and Moore[13] (1975)	34	?	8 (26.6%)
Das Gupta (1981)	13*	11 (84%)	9 (69%)

*Only surgically treated cases are included.
†No evidence of disease.

cidence in fingers to be extremely low in their series of 164 cases. There are no definitive guidelines regarding sex or anatomic location in making a prognosis for synovial sarcoma patients. As with most other patients, if the diagnosis is made when the tumor is small and less pleomorphic, and all the treatment principles outlined above are applied, the prognosis will be improved. However, whether sex (ie, female hormones) plays any role is a moot point. Five of our nine surviving patients were women. A more vigorous endocrinologic investigation might yield some useful clinical data in the future.

Data on the treatment of synovial sarcoma by means of curative radiation therapy alone are sparse, and no definitive statement as to its efficacy can yet be made.[3,9,13,16,17,24,26] Roth et al.,[19] reviewing 24 cases in the files of the Armed Forces Institute of Pathology, found that four patients received either preoperative or postoperative radiation therapy. Of these, only one was living without evidence of disease after two years. McNeer et al.[30] found that two of five patients (40 percent) treated by radiation therapy alone survived for five years and that the addition of postoperative irradiation was useful in 47 percent of cases, whereas preoperative radiation therapy was unsatisfactory. The data on the role of radiation therapy found in the literature up to 1970 usually consisted of retrospective analyses of clinical material, and in most of these, the technical aspects were not sufficiently sophisticated and the conclusions should be viewed with caution. Suit and colleagues,[33] after a planned use of modern technology, obtained a 66 percent two-year salvage rate after local excision and radical radiation therapy. More recently, Lindberg et al.[29] obtained an absolute two- and five-year salvage of 75 percent and 58 percent, respectively. In our own patients, radiation therapy has been used mainly as a means of palliation (Chapter 7). The palliative value of radiation therapy is recognized and has been reported by other authors as well.[3,30] Although none of the patients in our present surgically treated group was treated with adjunctive radiation therapy, it appears that, in tumors of the extremities located distal to the elbow or the knee, it would be of immense value (Chapter 7).

The present University of Illinois program for the management of high-grade synovial sarcoma of the extremities consists of preoperative intra-arterial infusion with 200 mg of adriamycin. Preoperative radiation therapy of 3,000 rads is then followed by wide soft tissue resection. After the wound is healed, the patient receives another 2,000 rads, bringing the total to 5,000 rads. One month later, adjuvant therapy with adriamycin and DTIC is begun (Chapter 8). We expect this combination treatment will obviate the need for future amputations (Table 8.22, Chapter 8). It is emphasized that the extent of excision is not curtailed even if the tumor shrinks in size.

Varela-Duran and Enzinger[34] recently described a group of patients with synovial sarcoma in whom the primary tumor showed extensive calcification. Analysis of the histologic criteria and the natural history of 32 calcifying synovial sarcomas from the files of the Armed Forces Institute of Pathology led these authors to conclude that in this subset of patients the prognosis is better than with the commoner variety of synovial sarcomas. Of the 26 patients with followup information (average 8.9 years), 17 were alive and well and 6 died of disease. The five-year disease-free survival rate was 82.6 percent.

Clear Cell Sarcoma of Tendon Sheath

Clear cell sarcoma (Fig. 15.6) is a tumor of the extremities occurring in adults, with some preponderance in women.[35-41] Enzinger[40] concluded that, in civilian personnel, the tumor occurs probably twice as frequently in women as in men. No racial predilection has been reported.

The tumors are usually slow-growing and most commonly encountered in the extremities, especially near the ankle or the knee joints. In most instances, they are adherent to the underlying tendons and consequently are movable in only one axis, and are of firm consistency. The location of these tumors is shown in Table 15.4.

Clear cell sarcomas of the tendon sheath, like synovial sarcomas, metastasize to the regional nodes. However, the incidence of nodal metastases is unknown. Enzinger[40] found four of 21 patients (19 percent) and Mackenzie[38] reported four of six (66 percent) had regional node metastases. Only four cases have been treated by us, and in one there was metastasis to the regional nodes in the superficial groin.

It is not possible to develop guidelines for treatment on the basis of experience with so few patients. From an operational viewpoint it is

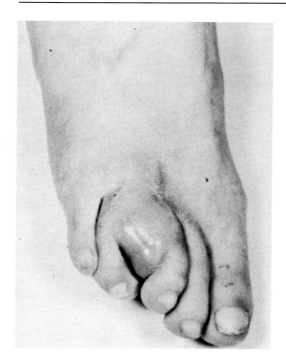

Figure 15.6. Clear cell sarcoma of the tendon sheath in a woman of 47 years. Apparently this tumor had been growing for three or four years before its present appearance.

logical to consider these tumors as variants of synovial sarcoma and treat them accordingly. This would imply a wide excision with concomitant regional node dissection.

The location of a clear cell sarcoma around the tendon of a joint frequently necessitates an amputation rather than a wide soft tissue excision. The role of curative radiation therapy for primary tumors and the efficacy of adjuvant chemotherapy in clear cell sarcoma awaits further trial.

The overall five-year survival in patients with clear cell sarcoma of the tendon sheath is hard to evaluate. From his collected material, Enzinger[40] suggested that patients with clear cell sarcomas have a somewhat better prognosis than do those with synovial cell sarcomas. However, he emphasized that after initial conservative excision most of these tumors recur and eventually metastasize, resulting in a uniformly grave prognosis. Hajdu and co-workers[35] had three of eight patients (37 percent) with clear cell sarcoma who survived five years. Of our four patients, three are eligible for five-year analysis. All three are living. In one, a locally recurrent tumor required re-excision 18 months after removal of the primary. The remaining patient died of widespread metastases within 16 months.

TABLE 15.4. ANATOMIC DISTRIBUTION OF CLEAR CELL SARCOMAS OF TENDON SHEATHS

Anatomic Location	Enzinger[40] (1965)	Dutra[36] (1970)	Mackenzie[38] (1971)	Hajdu et al.[35] (1977)	Das Gupta (1981)
Lower extremities	17	1	5	3	3
Achilles tendon	(4)				
Plantar surface	(4)	(1)			(1)
Ankle	(2)			(1)	(1)
Heel	(1)				
Patellar tendon	(2)				
Knee	(2)			(1)	
Buttock and thigh	(1)			(1)	
Toe	(1)				(1)
Upper extremities	4	2	1	5	1
Finger and palms	(2)	(1)		(1)	
Forearm	(1)			(2)	(1)
Arm	(1)	(1)		(2)	
Shoulder	—				
Trunk					
Back	—	—		1 (1)	
Total	21	3	6	9	4

TABLE 15.5. ANATOMIC LOCATIONS OF EPITHELIOID SARCOMA IN SIX SERIES

Anatomic Site	Enzinger[42] (1970)	Santiago et al.[46] (1972)	Soule and Enriquez[49] (1972)	Bryan et al.[53] (1974)	Pratt et al.[52] (1978)	Das Gupta (1981)
Head and Neck	2				1	
Trunk			1			1
Upper extremities	38	4	6	13	15	5
Finger and thumb	(13)	(1)		(5)	(4)	(1)
Hand	(8)			(5)	(10)	(1)
Wrist	(7)	(1)		(1)		
Forearm	(7)	(2)		(2)	(1)	(2)
Elbow	(2)					(1)
Upper arm	1					
Lower extremities	22	5			6	2
Buttock	(4)	(1)				
Thigh	(4)				(3)	(1)
Knee	(4)	(1)			(1)	
Lower leg	(7)	(2)				(1)
Foot	(3)	(1)			(2)	
Total	62	9	7	13	22	8

Epithelioid Sarcoma

Epithelioid sarcoma is a term introduced by Enzinger[42] in 1970 to designate a group of unusual sarcomas that are likely to be confused with synovial sarcomas or granulomatous processes and ulcerating squamous cell carcinomas. Since the definitive article by Enzinger, several other authors have described the clinicopathologic characteristics of epithelioid sarcoma.[33,43-54] Santiago et al.[46] suggested that probably in the past these tumors were recognized by other authors,[54-59] but under different names.

Epithelioid sarcoma is usually encountered in adult males.[41,51] Of Enzinger's[42] 62 patients, 49 were male and 13 were female. In the University of Illinois group, five of the eight pa-

TABLE 15.6. SUMMARY OF CLINICAL DATA ON EIGHT PATIENTS WITH EPITHELIOID SARCOMA
(UNIVERSITY OF ILLINOIS)*

Patient	Age	Sex	Location of Tumor	Status of Primary	Extent of Primary	Regional Node Metastases
1	64	M	Interscapular	Inadequately excised	Extensive infiltration	−
2	34	M	Forearm	Recurrent	Extensive infiltration	+
3	51	F	Forearm	Primary intact	Mobile, superficial	−
4	39	M	Hand	Locally recurrent	Extensive infiltration of the dorsal tendons	+
5	44	M	Wrist	Locally recurrent	Extensive infiltration	−
6	51	M	Thigh	Massive primary	Extensive infiltration	+
7	49	F	Leg	Intact primary	Mobile, superifical	−
8	11	M	Elbow	2 × 2 cm	Mobile, superfical	−

Patients 2, 3, 4, 7, and 8 are included in Table 8.17, Chapter 8.
†No evidence of disease.

tients were men. These tumors are most frequently seen in patients between the ages of 20 and 50 years, although both extremes in age have been reported.[41,46,48,51,52] The oldest patient in our group was 62 years old and the youngest was 11. No racial predilection has been observed.

Anatomic Location. These tumors occur predominantly in the extremities.[42,45,46,48,51–54] Enzinger noted that, with the exception of two of his 62 patients (in whom the tumors were in the scalp), the lesions were in the upper extremities in 38, and in the lower extremities in 22. Bryan et al.[53] reported that of 85 primary soft tissue sarcomas and 16 primary bone tumors involving the hand and forearm in the files of the Mayo Clinic, 13 were epithelioid sarcomas, making this entity third in frequency after fibrosarcoma and rhabdomyosarcoma. In the author's series of eight cases, one was in the posterior trunk, four were in the forearm and hand, one was in the elbow, and two were in the lower extremities (Table 15.5). Rarely, epithelioid sarcoma has been reported in the penis[44] and in bone.[47]

Patients with epithelioid sarcoma usually present with a small innocuous- looking lump in an extremity. These tumors are known for their relatively slow rate of growth. Nodules near the skin surface frequently become elevated and at a later stage of growth can become ulcerated, giving rise to the appearance of an ulcerating pyogenic granuloma. Deep-seated lesions fixed to the tendons or fascia are generally large and less well defined. Infrequently, these tumors are associated with pain or tenderness. They are relatively less common in the trunk (Table 15.5). The incidence of regional node metastases has been variously described by different authors. Enzinger[42] found metastasis in six of 62 patients (9.6 percent), and Santiago and co-workers[46] in three of nine (33 percent). Bryan et al.[53] observed metastases in three of 13 patients (23 percent). In our present series of eight patients, three (37 percent) had regional node metastases. In two of the three, the tumors were locally recurrent following inadequate excision (Table 15.6). This incidence of regional node metastases probably represents the incidence in advanced and locally recurrent tumors. In stage I primary tumors the true incidence is much lower, probably about 10 percent. However, because of this uncertainty it is recommended that the regional node-bearing area be taken into consideration during initial planning of therapy.

Treatment. The primary treatment for epithelioid sarcoma should be wide excision and regional node dissection. The major objective is

Surgical Treatment	Radiotherapy	Chemotherapy	End Result	Remarks
Wide excision	—	Yes (for metastatic tumor)	Dead of disease after 4 years	
Above elbow amputation	—	Adjuvant	6 years N.E.D.†	
Wide muscle group excision	—	Adjuvant	5 years N.E.D.	
Forearm amputation	—	Adjuvant	5 years N.E.D.	
Forearm amputation and axillary dissection	—	Yes (for metastatic tumor)	Dead of disease 3 years later	Autopsy showed lung, pancreas and other organ involvement
—	Yes	Yes (for metastatic tumor)	Dead within nine months	
Wide excision and regional node dissection		Adjuvant	5 years N.E.D.	
Wide excision and regional node dissection	Yes	Adjuvant	Living N.E.D. 3 years later	

to either eliminate or reduce the possibility of local recurrence. Most authors[39,43,44,49,50] have found that conservative local excision is associated with a high rate of local recurrence, resulting in poor prognosis and end results. In the University of Illinois material, an initial aggressive surgical approach, with adjuvant chemotherapy and, occasionally, radiation therapy, resulted in an excellent salvage rate of these patients (Table 15.6). Seven of the eight (87 percent) were disease-free at the end of two years. All four eligible for five-year end result analysis are alive with no evidence of recurrence or metastasis.

Primary curative radiation therapy alone has not been tried in our patients, and the published data are sparse. However, it appears that postoperative radiation therapy along with adjuvant chemotherapy might be a useful addition to the

TABLE 15.7. CHARACTERISTICS OF FOUR DIFFERENT MALIGNANT TUMORS PRESUMED TO BE OF SYNOVIAL TISSUE ORIGIN

	Synovial Sarcoma	Clear Cell Sarcomas Of Tendon Sheath	Epithelioid Sarcoma	Malignant Giant Cell Tumor of Soft Parts
Age	20–40 yr	30–50 yr	30–50 yr	40–80 yr
Sex	M:F 1:1	M:F 1:2	M:F 4:1	M:F 4:1
Common site	Extremities near major joints	Tendon sheaths over distal part of the extremities	Distal extremities	Extremities
Common clinical presentation	Painless tumor with relatively rapid increase in size	Small tumor usually attached to a tendon mobile in one axis	Painless tumor, slow-growing, frequently ulcerated, and resembling a pyogenic granuloma	Tumor is frequently associated with pain
Regional node metastases	10–25%	20–25%	10%	±
Roentgenographic findings	Nothing significant	Nothing significant	No specific findings	Frequent erosion of the superficial cortex of the adjacent bone
Histologic characteristics	Biphasic appearance	Lack of biphasic pattern and overall rarity of pseudoglandular clefts	An admixture of granulomatous and pseudocarcinomatous pattern	Pleomorphic and phagocytic multinucleated giant cells with occasional bone formation
Treatment	1. Wide excision with regional node dissection in pleomorphic types, adjuvant chemotherapy and radiation therapy	Same as synovial sarcoma. Because of location, frequently needs amputation	Same as synovial	Same as synovial
	2. For low-grade, wide excision alone is adequate	Same as synovial sarcoma. Because of location, frequently needs amputation	Same as synovial	Same as synovial
Local recurrence	+	±	±	±
Prognosis 5 yr N.E.D.*	69%	37 to 60%	80%	Superficial—50% Deep—20%

*No evidence of disease.

therapeutic armamentarium. Two of our patients received postoperative radiation therapy (Patients 6 and 8, Table 15.6).

We used adjuvant chemotherapy in five of our patients (Table 15.6). All five have been evaluated (Chapter 8). It appears to have a positive influence on prognosis (Table 8.17, Chapter 8). Three of the eight (Patients 1, 5, and 6, Table 15.6) were treated with multiagent chemotherapy for advanced disease, but no beneficial effect was observed.

End Results. The end results of treatment of epithelioid sarcoma, and the prognostic factors, are difficult to ascertain. Most of the published reports have been by pathologists,[42, 44–46,48,52] and the type of treatment described is based only on reported data in the charts, or from letters by clinicians. This author has found that definition of "wide" radical excision varies among surgeons. Patients have been referred to the University of Illinois with the notation that a wide excision had been performed when in reality it had been most conservative. Sometimes a tumor of the upper anterior leg has been treated with a below-knee amputation with a minimal margin of unaffected tissue, resulting in eventual failure of the primary treatment. Therefore the statement that epithelioid sarcoma continues to progress relentlessly after adequate excision should be viewed with caution.

In our material, 87 percent of the patients lived disease-free for two years and 75 percent for five years (Table 15.6). Soule and Enriquez[49] suggested that the prognosis is somewhat better for superficially located tumors, and this appears to be a tenable hypothesis. From a review of the published data,[35,42,44–46,48,52–54] it is difficult to arrive at an average number regarding five-year tumor-free survival. Enzinger,[42] who reviewed a large number of cases from the files of the Armed Forces Institute of Pathology, reported that of 62 cases, 54 had followup data ranging from one to 26 years. Forty-two of 54 patients were alive at the end of the followup period, although 12 (28.5 percent) had recurrence, 3 had metastases, and 2 had both recurrence and metastases. However, how many of these were free of tumor for five years cannot be ascertained from the paper. Mackenzie[45] reviewed nine cases and found two patients were free of disease for more than five years. Santiago et al.[46] reported three of nine patients living and well for five years. Soule and Enriquez[49] found only one patient out of a group of seven who

was free of disease after five years. The high frequency of local recurrence was described by all these authors.[42,45,46,49,52–54] None of the eight patients treated for cure at the University of Illinois had local recurrence (Table 15.6).

It appears that initial aggressive excision will certainly reduce the incidence of local recurrence and will improve the overall cure rate in patients with epithelioid sarcoma. It is likely that adjuvant chemotherapy and radiation therapy play a beneficial role; however, sufficient data are not yet available.

Malignant Giant Cell Tumor

Malignant giant cell tumor of the soft tissue is a rare tumor originally described by Berger[55] in 1938. Since then, several small series have been reported.[56–59] Although its histogenesis is still disputed, clinically this tumor is remarkably similar to malignant tumors arising from synovial tissues.

The tumor is commonly seen in adult males, and, like synovial sarcoma, frequently occurs in the extremities. It has a tendency for local infiltration, and involvement of adjacent bones is not uncommon.

From the limited number of cases studied to date, it appears that management should be similar to that of malignant tumors arising from synovial tissue. Although it is hard to describe the natural history of these tumors from such a small number of cases, it is evident that aggressive use of multimodality therapy probably will lead to improved prognoses.

Frequently, it is difficult to clinicopathologically distinguish between a synovial sarcoma, clear cell sarcoma of the tendon sheath, epithelioid sarcoma, and malignant giant cell tumor of the soft tissue. In Table 15.7 some of the more common features of each tumor type are summarized for ready reference.

REFERENCES

1. Bobechko WP, Kostuik JP: Childhood villonodular synovitis. Canad J Surg 11:480, 1968
2. Docken WP: Pigmented villonodular synovitis: A review with illustrative case reports. Semin Arthritis Rheum 9:1, 1979
3. Pack GT, Ariel IR: Tumors of the Soft Somatic Tissues. New York, Hoeber-Harper, 1958, p 494
4. Stout AP, Lattes R: Tumors of the soft tissues. Atlas of Tumor Pathology. Washington DC, AFIP, 1967

5. Hardie J, Salter SC: Primary sarcoma of the knee joint. Lancet 1:1619, 1894
6. Marsh HA: A case of sarcoma of knee joint. Lancet 2:1330, 1898
7. Lockwood CB: A case of sarcoma of synovial membrane of the knee joint. Lancet 2:1398, 1902
8. Lejars F, Rubens-Duvall H: Les Sarcomas primitifs des Synoviales articularies. Rev Chir 41:751, 1910
9. Cadman NL, Soule EH, Kelly PJ: Synovial sarcoma: An analysis of 134 tumors. Cancer 18:613, 1965
10. Mackenzie DH: Synovial sarcoma: A review of 58 cases. Cancer 19:169, 1966
11. Rissanen PM, Holsti P: Synovial sarcoma and its treatment. Oncology 24:108, 1970
12. Van Andel JG: Synovial sarcoma—A review and analysis of treated cases. Radiol Clin Biol 41:145, 1972
13. Gerner RE, Moore GE: Synovial sarcoma. Ann Surg 181:22, 1975
14. Aurich Von G: Uber maligne synovialome. Archiv fur Geschwulstforsch. 26:156, 1965
15. Wright CJE: Malignant synovioma. J Path Bact 64:585, 1952
16. Vincent RG: Malignant synovioma. Ann Surg 152:777, 1960
17. Ariel IM, Pack GT: Synovial sarcoma. Review of 25 cases. N Engl J Med 168:1272, 1963
18. Shiu MH, Castro EB, Hajdu SI, et al: Surgical treatment of 297 soft tissue sarcomas of the lower extremity. Ann Surg 182:597, 1975
19. Roth JA, Enzinger FM, Tannenbaum M: Synovial sarcoma of the neck: A follow-up study of 24 cases. Cancer 35:1243, 1975
20. Golomb HM, Gorny J, Powell W, Graff P, Ultmann JE: Cervical synovial sarcoma at the bifurcation of the carotid artery. Cancer 35:483, 1975
21. Batsakis JH, Nishiyama RH, Sullinger GD: Synovial sarcomas of the neck. Arch Otolaryngol 85:327, 1967
22. Kurgman ME, Rosin HD, Toker C: Synovial sarcoma of the head and neck. Arch Otolaryngol 98:53, 1973
23. Anderson KJ, Widlermuth O: Synovial sarcoma. Clin Orthop, No. 19. Philadelphia, Lippincott, 1961
24. Jacobs LA, Weaver AW: Synovial sarcoma of the head and neck. Am J Surg 128:527, 1974
25. Haagensen CD, Stout AP: Synovial sarcoma. Ann Surg 120:826, 1944
26. Kogstad O: Malignant synovioma. Acta Rheum Scand 16:81, 1970
27. Murray JA: Synovial sarcoma. Orthopaedic Clin North Am 8:963, 1977
28. Schiffman R, Chong TW: Vaginal bleeding as a presenting symptom of synovial sarcoma. Cancer 45:2428, 1980
29. Lindberg RD, Martin RG, Romsdahl MM, Barkley HT: Conservative surgery and postoperative radiotherapy in 300 adult soft tissue sarcomas. Cancer 47:2397, 1981
30. McNeer GP, Cantin J, Chu F, Nickson J: Effectiveness of radiation therapy in the management of sarcoma of the soft tissues. Cancer 22:391, 1968
31. Shmookler BM, Enzinger FM, Brannon RB: Orofacial synovial sarcoma: A clinicopathologic study of 11 new cases and review of the literature. Cancer 50:269, 1982.
32. Weingrad DN, Rosenberg SA: Early lymphatic spread of osteogenic and soft tissue sarcomas. Surgery 84:231, 1978
33. Suit HD, Russell WO, Martin RG: Sarcoma of soft tissues: Clinical and histopathologic parameters and response to treatment. Cancer 35:1478, 1975
34. Varela-Duran J, Enzinger FM: Calcifying synovial sarcoma. Cancer 50:345, 1982.
35. Hajdu SI, Shiu MH, Fortner JG: Tendosynovial sarcoma. A clinicopathological study of 136 cases. Cancer 39:1201, 1977
36. Dutra FR: Clear-cell sarcoma of tendons and aponeuroses: Three additional cases. Cancer 25:942, 1970
37. Kubo T: Clear-cell sarcoma of patellar tendon studied by electron microscopy. Cancer 24:948, 1969
38. Mackenzie DH: Clear-cell sarcoma of tendon and aponeuroses with melanin production. J Path 114:231, 1974
39. Hoffman GJ, Carter D: Clear-cell sarcoma of tendons and aponeuroses with melanin. Arch Path 95:22, 1973
40. Enzinger FM: Clear-cell sarcoma of tendons and aponeuroses: An analysis of 21 cases. Cancer 18:1163, 1965
41. Tsuneyoshi M, Enjoji M, Kubo T: Clear cell sarcoma of tendons and aponeuroses. A comparative study of 13 cases with a provisional subgrouping into the melanotic and synovial types. Cancer 42(1):243, 1978
42. Enzinger FM: Epithelioid sarcoma: A sarcoma simulating a granuloma or a carcinoma. Cancer 26:1029, 1970
43. Moore SW, Wheeler JE, Hefter LG: Epithelioid sarcoma masquerading as Peyronie's disease. Cancer 35:1706, 1975
44. Dehner LP, Smith BH: Soft tissue tumors of the penis. Cancer 25:1431, 1970
45. Mackenzie DH: Two types of soft tissue sarcoma of uncertain histogenesis. Br J Cancer 25:458, 1972
46. Santiago H, Feinerman LK, Lattes R: Epithelioid sarcoma: A clinical and pathologic study of nine cases. Human Path 3:133, 1972
47. DeLuca FN, Neviaser RJ: Epithelioid sarcoma involving a bone. Clin Orthopaed No. 107:168, 1975
48. Fisher ER, Hormvat B: The fibrocytic derivation of the so-called epithelioid sarcoma. Cancer 30:1074, 1972
49. Soule EH, Enriquez P: Atypical fibrous histiocytoma, malignant fibrous histiocytoma, malignant histiocytoma, and epithelioid sarcoma: A comparative study of 65 tumors. Cancer 30:128, 1972
50. Bloustein PA, Silverberg SG, Waddell WR: Epithelioid sarcoma: Case report with an ultrastructural review, histogenetic discussion and chemotherapeutic treatment. Cancer 38:2390, 1976
51. Males JL, Lain KC: Epithelioid sarcoma in XO/XX Turner's syndrome. Arch Path 94:214, 1972
52. Pratt J, Woodruff JM, Marcove RC: Epithelioid sarcoma: An analysis of 22 cases indicating prognostic significance of vascinlar invasion and regional lymph node metastases. Cancer 41:1472, 1978

53. Bryan RS, Soule EH, Dobyns JH, Pritchard DJ, Linscheid RL: Primary epithelioid sarcoma of the hand and forearm. J Bone Joint Surg 56-A:458, 1974

54. Tsuneyoshi M, Enjoji M, Shinohara N: Epithelioid sarcoma: A clinicopathologic and electron microscopic study. Acta Pathol Jap 30(3):411, 1980

55. Berger L: Synovial sarcomas in serous bursae and tendon sheaths. Am J Cancer 34:501, 1938

56. Black WC: Synovioma of the hand. Report of a case. Am J Cancer 28:481, 1936

57. De Santo DA, Tennant R, Rosahn PD: Synovial sarcomas in joints, bursae and tendon sheaths. Surg Gynecol Obstet 72:951, 1941

58. Bliss BO, Reed RJ: Large cell sarcomas of tendon sheath: Malignant giant cell tumors of tendon sheath. Am J Clin Path 49:776, 1968

59. Eisenstein R: Giant-cell tumor of tendon sheath: Its histogenesis as studied in the electron microscope. J Bone Joint Surg 50-A:476, 1968

60. Guccion JH, Enzinger FM: Malignant giant cell tumor of the soft parts. Cancer 29:1578, 1972

16

Tumors of the Vascular Tissue

Tapas K. Das Gupta

Tumors and tumorlike conditions of the vascular tissue comprise one of the most common groups of neoplasms of the soft somatic tissue. As already pointed out, the majority of hemangiomas, strictly speaking, are hamartomas rather than tumors, but operationally they are being considered as tumors. Although a strict categorization of vascular hamartomas, congenital malformations, and tumors is not always possible, a practical classification is provided (Table 16.1).

HEMANGIOMA

The growth of hemangiomas is inconsistent. They may remain constant in size or may grow pari passu with the child. The tumor inherits a certain momentum of growth that is usually uncertain but self-limited. Once the patient has achieved full size, the hemangioma generally stops growing, with the exception of the cirsoid or racemose type. The growth of vessels comprising the neoplasm is markedly affected by the element of mechanical pressure of the circulation. Therefore, the rate of growth and the architecture of the tumor are somewhat dependent on the factor of blood supply to the vessels of the hemangiomas.

The hemangioma is the most common tumor of infancy and childhood.[1] About 75 percent of these tumors are evident at birth and the greater part of the remainder appear in early infancy. In about one out of five patients, the hemangiomas are multiple, with as many as 25 observed in a single patient. No explanation is available for the preponderance in females, usually in a ratio of two to one. On occasion, hemangiomas have exhibited a startling acceleration in growth rate during pregnancy and, less frequently, at the onset of menstruation. There is no racial predilection. The majority are found in the skin and subcutaneous tissues, and at least 50 percent are located in the head and neck region. The location of the tumor in certain special regions such as the retro-orbital space, the breast, the scrotum, etc., calls for special consideration of treatment, which will be discussed later. Other hemangiomas, developing primarily in the tongue, liver, brain, retina, bone, and skeletal muscle, will also be separately reviewed.

Capillary Hemangioma
This most common of all hemangiomas occurs in the skin and mucous membranes and is congenital, although it may not be recognizable until variable periods after birth. The capillary hemangioma may grow rapidly, ranging in size from the minute "De Morgan" spots to the large,

TABLE 16.1. CLASSIFICATION OF VASCULAR HAMARTOMAS AND NEOPLASMS

Benign

1. Capillary hemangiomas
    Simple
    Port wine stain
    Spider angioma (nevus araneus, De Morgan's spots)
2. Infectious hemangioma—pyogenic granuloma
3. Cavernous hemangioma
    Superficial
    Hypertrophic
    Visceral
4. Cirsoid or racemose hemangioma—arteriovenous fistula
5. Special regional hemangiomas:
    Orbit and eye
    Brain
    Tongue
    Gastrointestinal tract
    Liver
    Skeletal muscle
    Bone
6. Systemic hemangiomatosis
    Congenital
    Acquired
7. Hereditary hemorrhagic telangiectasis (Rendu-Osler-Weber's Disease)
8. Congenital neurocutaneous syndromes associated with angiomatosis
    von Recklinghausen's neurofibromatosis and angiomas of the skin
    Tuberous sclerosis (Bourneville's syndrome)
    Pringle's disease and regional angiomas
    Encephalo-facial angiomatosis (Sturge-Weber's disease)
    Retinocerebral angiomatosis (von Hippel-Lindau's disease)
9. Hemangiopericytoma and glomus tumors (?)

Malignant

1. Angiosarcoma (malignant hemangioendothelioma)
2. Hemangiopericytoma (?)
3. Kaposi's sarcoma

flat, port wine stain. The common type, however, is a circumscribed, sessile, lobulated, and bright red tumor. The lumens of the vessels that comprise this tumor are either empty or contain a few immature-to-degenerate red blood corpuscles.

Port Wine Stain (Nevus Venosus; Nevus Flammeus). This pink-to-purplish, flat, superficial hemangioma is a congenital defect evident at birth and grows pari passu with the child. The superficial vessels of the dermis exhibit diffuse telangiectasia, but there are no proliferative masses such as are found with other hemangiomas. The purple patch blanches on pressure. In some cases, as the child grows older the color darkens rather than fades. Unfortunately, the face is the most common site, and the mucosa of lip, cheek, and oral cavity may be involved in continuity.

Treatment is disappointing and requires infinite patience and caution. It is important to emphasize to the parents that the majority of port wine stains disappear with age and that patience is essential. The feeding vessels are not large enough for injection therapy. Dermabrasion of the facial port wine stain provides excellent results. Sometimes tattooing of the stain is recommended. Suffice it to emphasize that tattooing is a cosmetic maneuver and should not be indiscriminately used in children. In adults the technique might be useful in instances in which the port wine stain is persistent and creates an embarrassment for the patient.

Spider Angioma (Nevus Araneus). The cutaneous arterial spider is a tiny red angioma that owes its descriptive name to its resemblance to a small red spider. It has been known by several synonyms, namely, spider nevus, vascular spider, spider angioma, spider telangiectasis, stellate hemangioma, nevus araneus, and nevus arachnoideus.

The arterial spider has a central point, bulb, or eminence from which many fine, hairlike, wavy strands radiate for 0.5 to 1.0 cm. The central point or body of the lesion may be so small as to be seen only by magnification or it may be a few millimeters wide, elevated, and palpable. The central point is often surrounded by a circular or star-shaped area of erythema, peripheral to which may be seen a contrasting halo. The fiery red color of the spider nevus is due to two factors, arterial blood and the thinness of the vascular walls. The spider angiomas are commonly located on the face, arms, fingers, upper trunk, and, less frequently, on the lower trunk and legs. Spiders of similar structure have been reported in the mucous membranes of the conjunctiva, tongue, lips, nasal mucosa, and gastrointestinal and genitourinary tracts. A congenital analog is to be found in Rendu-Osler-Weber's disease. Spider angiomas seldom occur in hairy skin such as the scalp, axilla, or pubis, and are related to hepatic cirrhosis.[2,3] The cutaneous spiders are also encountered in patients with gynecomastia; they do not need any active treatment.

Pyogenic Granuloma. This is an exuberant proud flesh that consists of multiple new capillaries, usually under the intact dermis or mucous membrane. Although the cause is obscure, it is usually seen after a small penetrating wound. It can arise anywhere in the body and usually is pedunculated. It appears infected and bleeds easily. The term pyogenic granuloma is a misnomer, since infection is seldom present. Excision results in cure.

Cavernous Hemangioma
The blood vessels become much more dilated in cavernous hemangioma than in the capillary type. This physical characteristic is due to an expanding connection between the general circulation and the channels of the fundamental capillary hemangioma, so that the capillaries become distended and form pools or sinuses. These spaces are limited by thin septa and form spherical sacculations or cul-de-sacs in which the circulation is sluggish. The efferent vessels are larger than in the capillary hemangioma. These tumors are soft and readily compressible, frequently extending into the subcutaneous tissues and presenting as grotesque-appearing masses. Depending on their vascular connections and location, visceral hemangiomas of the liver and gastrointestinal tract may reach enormous size and exhibit aggressive growth.

Cavernous hemangiomas of the subcutaneous tissues are frequently encountered in the extremities (Fig. 16.1A to 16.1C). In these anatomic locations the angiomas may be totally devoid of any cutaneous manifestation. McNeill and Ray[4] found that out of 35 patients with hemangioma of the extremities seen by the orthopedic department at the University of Illinois Hospital, only 12 (34 percent) had associated skin involvement. Most patients seek medical advice because of the painful swelling (Fig. 16.1D). Occasionally, large cavernous hemangiomas result in platelet consumption, due to mechanical trapping of platelets or congestive heart failure. Fortunately, these are rare clinical manifestations. Local gigantism is also encountered, but unilateral extremity enlargement in the absence of systemic angiomatosis is rare. In the series reported by McNeill and Ray,[4] 6 of 29

patients had systemic angiomatosis and all had extremity enlargement, whereas in the remaining 23 patients swelling and tenderness were the major complaints. Atrophy was noted in 12 patients.

Hypertrophic Hemangioma
This tumor is the benign analog of the malignant hemangioendothelioma. It is a solid, noncompressible tumor of variable hue, usually purplish-red (Fig. 16.2). The endothelial cell is the neoplastic unit, and the overgrowth of these endothelial cells tends to obliterate the lumens of the blood vessels. These neoplasms are often locally aggressive and tend to recur after operation. Although they are of hemangiomatous origin, they are solid tumors and never undergo spontaneous regression. The injection of sclerosing fluids is futile; complete excision is the treatment of choice.

Racemose Hemangioma or Cirsoid Aneurysm
The arterial racemose hemangioma develops de novo or through transformation of a preexisting quiescent hemangioma, such as the port wine stain. The essential or distinguishing feature is the size of the arteriovenous fistula, which may gradually become evident or have a surprisingly sudden onset, chiefly in adults. Most cirsoid hemangiomas are located on the face or neck and have close vascular connections with branches of the carotid artery. The tumor frequently resembles a pulsating mass of earthworms due to the clinical appearance of the dilated, tortuous, throbbing vessels. As with aneurysms, the constant pulsation of the tumor can erode adjacent bone. It may extend over the scalp, erode the skull, penetrate the cranium, and even communicate with the meningeal vessels. Excision after preliminary ligation of the arterial supply (in severe cases the external carotid artery) may be feasible. If the hemangioma is inoperable, the communicating artery must be ligated before attempting conservative therapy.

Spontaneous Regression of Hemangioma. Spontaneous cure of hemangiomas is possible and follows progressive diminution in the blood supply to the tumor by a stenosis of the afferent vessels, supplemented by progressive fibrous hyperplasia of the stroma. This retrogression of hemangiomas without any treatment is often accelerated at the period of first or second den-

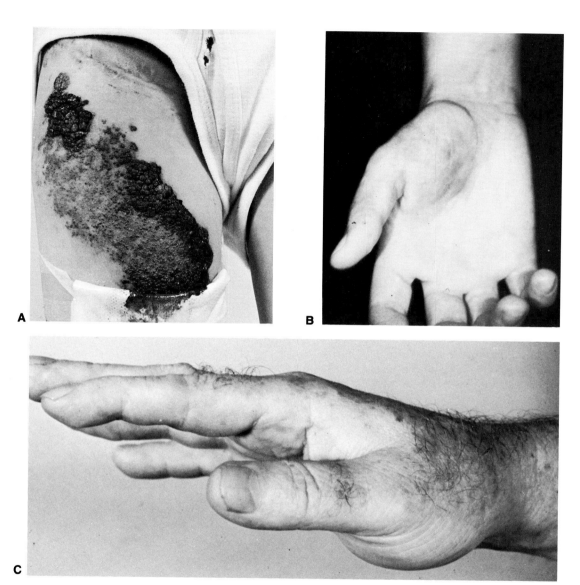

Figure 16.1. (A) Superficial spreading cavernous angioma of the right thigh in a 5-year-old boy. In certain areas, capillary elements were also present. Apparently, an excision was attempted (see scar in inguinal crease). The lesion was ulcerated and bleeding and was treated by wide excision two years ago; the child is growing normally. **(B)** Cavernous angioma of the thumb and thenar space in an 18-year-old boy. Note pigmentary change spreading through the skin of the thumb. He was treated conservatively with ligation of the feeding vessels and injection of sclerosing fluid with excellent cosmetic and functional end results. **(C)** Cavernous hemangioma of the thenar space extending to the remainder of the palm in a 44-year-old man. The hemangioma was tender and interfered with his livelihood (auto mechanic). However, extensive excision would have resulted in a nonfunctional hand. He has been treated by sequential excision and coagulation with cryotherapy. Although all the hemangioma has not been eradicated, he has a symptomless, functional, and cosmetically acceptable hand. **(D)** Cavernous angioma of the trunk in a 5-year-old boy. The child complained of pain and tenderness. The lesion was excised, with cure.

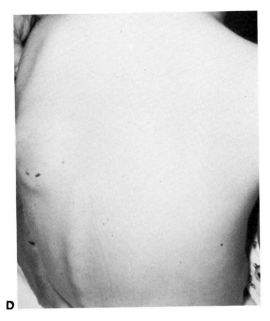

D

Figure 16.1 *Continued*

tition. Although the exact incidence of spontaneous regression is unknown, the frequency is high enough to justify a conservative attitude on the part of both the parents and the pediatrician.

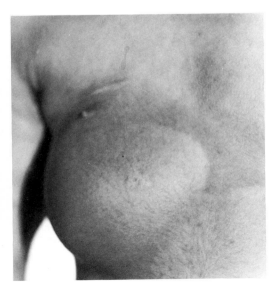

Figure 16.2. Hypertrophic hemangioma of the chest wall in a 24-year-old man. This had to be widely excised before all margins were found to be free of extension of the exuberative overgrowth of endothelial lining.

Treatment of Hemangiomas. Hemangiomas that ultimately require intervention can generally be treated by conservative methods. Although the role of steroids in hemangiomas is unclear, systemic administration of prednisone during the active growth phase of these lesions results in arrest of this process in 90 percent of patients.[5] A recommended therapeutic regimen is 40 mg (for a 15-pound baby) orally every alternate day for eight doses, with gradual tapering during a 60-day or 90-day period. Response to steroids becomes evident within 3 to 21 days. Once the accelerated growth phase is reversed, a plan for future therapy can be developed without any pressure.

Freezing or the production of artificial frostbite with carbon dioxide snow is still an effective method of treating superficial hemangiomas. In larger hemangiomas the appropriate area is selected and the cube of CO_2 snow is rubbed on for 10 to 20 seconds, care being taken to avoid contact of the snow with other areas. Sometimes several applications at two-to-three-week intervals are required before the effectiveness of this therapy is appreciated. Today, however, a cryogenic probe should supplement the use of CO_2 snow, achieving better cosmesis. Goldwin and Rosoff[6] concluded that cryosurgery is most useful in small, circumscribed saccular and superficial cavernous hemangiomas. Our experience is similar to that of Goldwin and Rosoff.[6] For extensive hemangiomas with multiple arteriovenous shunts involving the oral cavity, pharynx, and larynx, cryosurgery is not uniformly successful.[5]

The intravascular injection of sclerosing solutions is designed to cause thrombosis of the constituent vessels. This in turn produces sclerosis, atrophy, and absorption of the blood vessels with consequent regression and disappearance of the tumors. The needle must be introduced with great care and blood drawn prior to injection of any sclerosing fluid. The incidence of complications such as embolism are rare and usually not of any significant consideration. Nor is the type of sclerosing agent of any major import. Pack and Miller[2] used hot water, urethane, and sodium-morrhuate with satisfactory results. The use of sclerosing fluid is being replaced with intravascular clots or plugs in large hemangiomas with identifiable efferent vessels.

In large hemangiomas or in cirsoid aneurysms affecting an extremity or the head and neck region, a combination of ligation of the feeding vessels with clotting is useful (Fig. 16.3A).

Many hemangiomas of the skin and subcutaneous tissues are so well encapsulated and redundant that excision is the quickest and simplest method of treatment. (Fig. 16.3B). The fine linear scar is less conspicuous than the appearance of flat white skin that follows more conservative procedures. The exposure and double ligature of the entering vessels is easily accomplished by traction on the tumor after the circumferential incision has been made, making the operation relatively bloodless. McNeill and Ray[4] obtained good results by complete excision of the tumors. In 7 (20 percent) of their 35 patients, amputations were required (Table 16.2). From their analysis of treatment of extremity hemangiomas, these authors concluded that end results are poor in cases of overgrowth of the affected extremity. Amputation of an extremity should be resorted to only in patients in whom conservative means of therapy, including several attempts at excision, have failed.

The end results of treatment of hemangiomas are usually excellent. Their effective control frequently requires prolonged periods of treatment, taxing the patience of the clinician, the patient, and the family. Before treatment is initiated it is advisable to have a conference with all parties concerned regarding the protracted nature of the disease and the chronicity of the management program. The judicious, unhurried use of one method, or a combination of the methods outlined above, will result in satisfactory end results in most instances.

Specialized Regional Hemangiomas

Hemangiomas may occur anywhere in the body. A few distinctive hemangiomas occurring in locations that present specific problems will be described.

Orbital Hemangiomas. These hemangiomas may involve either the eyelid or conjunctiva or may develop in the retrobulbar fat, causing unilateral exophthalmos. Although it may be possible to dissect these tumors out, the operation is often uncertain, bloody, incomplete, and mu-

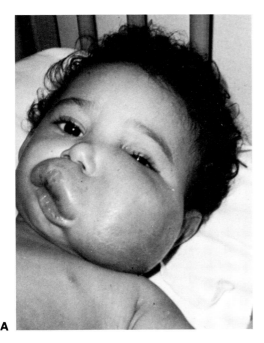

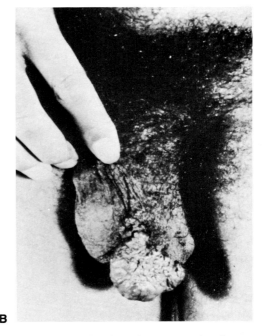

A **B**

Figure 16.3. (A) Large expanding hemangioma of the left cheek and neck in a male infant. This mass produced some respiratory distress and was infected. He was treated conservatively after ligation of the ipsilateral facial artery and vein with excellent results. (B) Scrotal hemangioma. The lesion was excised with excellent end result. *(Courtesy Ray B and Clark SS. Hemangioma of the scrotum. Urology 8:502, 1976)*

TABLE 16.2. AMPUTATION FOR EXTREMITY HEMANGIOMAS (SEVEN PATIENTS, UNIVERSITY OF ILLINOIS SERIES, MCNEILL AND RAY, 1974)[4]

No.	Age	Sex	Location	Complaint	Angiogram	End Result	Remarks
1	15	M	Calf	Pain and limp	No	Good with prosthesis	Apparently no recurrences
2	Birth	F	R lower extremity (diffuse)	Deformity and limp	No	Poor, recurrence in stump	Multiple local excisions; no evidence of disease
3	12	M	Arm (diffuse)	Pain and tender mass	No	Good after amputation	Results poor before amputation
4	Birth	M	Lower half body (diffuse)	Multiple masses	No	Good after hip disarticulation	Good results with prosthesis; received radiation therapy in infancy
5	Birth	M	Overgrowth	Mass and pain	Yes	Poor, even after amputation	Recurrence
6	Birth	M	Hypertrophy of foot	Enlarged foot	No	Transmetatarsal amputation	–
7	Birth	M	Arm	Swelling	No	Recurrence in amputated stump	Second amputation required

Courtesy Clinical Orthopaedics and Related Research 101:154, 1974.

tilating. Pack and Miller[2] and Pack and Ariel[7] suggested the use of nonoperative methods for the control of hemangiomas in this location.

Hemangiomas of the Brain. Hemangiomas of the brain can be solitary or can be a part of more generalized manifestations. The symptoms produced may not be solely due to the extent of involvement of the angioma, but perhaps are caused in part by hemorrhage within the tumor. Treatment of these lesions is based on the same general principles used for all other intracranial neoplasms.

Hemangiomas of the Mediastinum. Hemangiomas of the mediastinum are rare and are usually cavernous.[8] The clinical presentation can be that of any space-occupying tumor in the mediastinum, without any specific radiographic clue. The diagnosis is made after exploratory thoracotomy and excision of the tumor.

Hemangiomas of the Tongue (Fig. 16.4A and 16.4B). Lingual hemangiomas are usually the cavernous type and congenital in origin. The tip of the tongue is the most common site, but the entire tongue may be involved. With arterial communications, it may become an erectile organ of enormous dimensions, the *macroglossia angiomatosa*. Profuse hemorrhage can follow the slightest trauma from a minor bite or rough food.

The bulk of the tumor may interfere with mastication and speech. In most instances, repeated injection of sclerosing agents in small doses will produce fibrosis; occasionally, local fibrotic areas can be excised with an acceptable result.

Hemangiomas of the Gastrointestinal Tract. The stomach is seldom involved. Pack[9] described 16 cases in a collected series, but adequately documented cases are few. Probably, gastric hemangiomas are all congenital, although signs in newborns are rare. The symptoms and signs are similar to those in all other gastric neoplasms and the treatment is excision.

The small intestine and colon (Fig. 16.5) are occasionally the sites of multiple hemangiomas, usually associated with known superficial tumors. Cryptic intestinal hemorrhages herald the presence of these neoplasms. Intervention with resection and anastomosis is sometimes necessary, as repeated hemorrhage may be almost exsanguinating.

Hemangiomas of the Liver. Hemangiomas of the liver are quite common and the vast majority are small, presenting no clinical problems. In unusual instances they may attain large proportions and their removal is indicated. These are usually cavernous hemangiomas and may be single or multiple, usually lying just beneath or projecting from the surface of the liver. Nie-

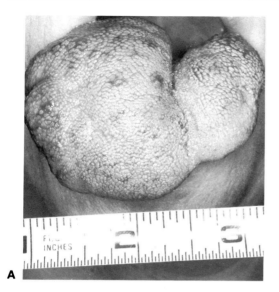
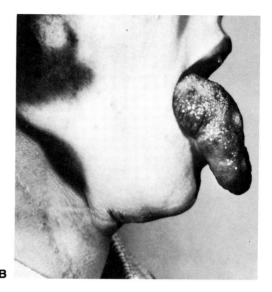

A   **B**

Figure 16.4. **(A)** Hemangioma of tongue in a 29-year-old woman. **(B)** Lateral view. Note the prominent cavernous area. Chewing chronically traumatized this area. Patient allowed injection of sclerosing fluid only. Although macroglossia has been a major problem, she refused any treatment. Size of tongue has not changed in last five years.

mann and Penitschka,[10] in their review of 103 cases collected from the literature, found that 81 percent of the patients were women, 11 percent men, and 8 percent infants and neonates. A similar observation has been made by other authors.[11-21]

A patient with a large hepatic angioma usually complains of an abdominal mass and nonspecific pressure symptoms such as abdominal pain, fullness, nausea, and vomiting. Infrequently, attention is directed to the upper ab-

domen due to rupture and bleeding from the hemangioma following blunt trauma. The operative mortality in such patients is high.[15,17,21]

Preoperative diagnosis of hepatic hemangiomas is difficult. Schumacker[11] reported that in only 2 of his 67 cases was a preoperative diagnosis possible. In hepatic angiograms, the characteristic features are areas of "cotton-wool-like" scattered pooling, which persists for a period, even in the venous phase (Fig. 16.6). Some authors[21] have found laparoscopy useful for

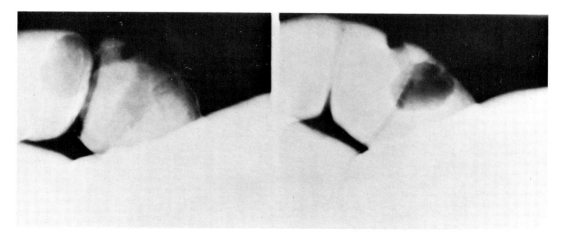

Figure 16.5. Polypoid hemangioma of the sigmoid colon. The lesion was treated by sleeve resection of the colon.

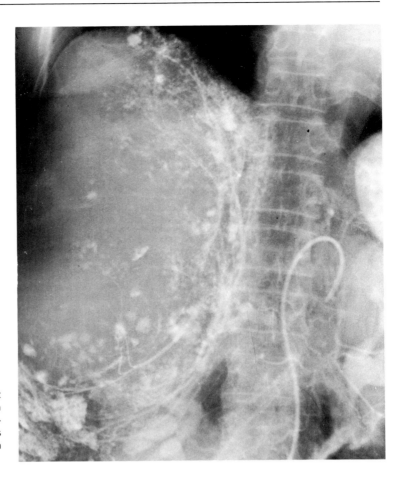

Figure 16.6. Hemangioma of right lobe of liver of a 57-year-old woman referred to us because of an expanding mass. Right lobectomy was performed and she is still well seven years later.

preoperative diagnosis, but it is difficult to ascertain the extent of liver involvement or the resectability of the tumor by means of laparoscopy alone. Ultimately, the correct diagnosis and the exact method of treatment suitable for a given patient can only be arrived at by means of an exploratory celiotomy. However, most of the diagnostic tests should be performed and all possible information obtained prior to an exploratory operation.

The treatment of large symptomatic hepatic hemangiomas, if technically possible, is excision. The resectability rate of hepatic angiomas cannot be accurately described, since most authors' experience is limited to only a handful of cases. A review of the literature[7,13,14,16,18,21] shows that the only curative form of treatment is excision, including right or left lobectomies, even in children and neonates.[20] We have operated upon one case of massive hemangioma of the

right lobe of the liver with good result (Fig. 16.6). The technical considerations for hepatic lobectomy for hemangiomas have already been described [10,13,18]

Hemangiomas of the Skeletal Muscles. Hemangioma of skeletal muscle may occur de novo as an isolated tumor in one muscle belly or group of muscles, or it may be part of a systemic hemangiomatosis involving an entire extremity.[22] In the former case, it is difficult to diagnose and to distinguish from other deeply situated somatic tumors, benign or malignant The following six diagnostic points are perhaps helpful: (1) diffuse tumefaction within the muscle proper, (2) temporary enlargement of the lesion after the application of a tourniquet above, (3) decrease in size of the tumor after elevation of the extremity, (4) pain and functional disability, (5) an aspiration biopsy that secures blood instead of identifiable solid tissue, and (6) roentgenographic localization of calcium deposits or phleboliths within the tumor.[23,24] The patients are generally under 30 years of age and the upper extremities appear to be the most common site.

Hemangiomas of Bone. Although a primary hemangioma of bone is rare,[2,4,7,24,25] it is likely that many such tumors remain undetected throughout life because the majority are slow-growing and asymptomatic. They may be discovered coincidentally at the time of radiographic examination for other lesions. The bones of the skull are most frequently involved, but other bones, namely, the vertebral column (especially the lumbar vertebrae), scapula, pelvic bones, rib, and phalanges may be sites of origin. The radiographic appearance of primary bone hemangiomas is usually characterized by their anatomic location.[26] For example, in the vertebral column the vertical striations are characteristic and diagnostic; in the flat bone, sunburst trabeculations of unusual size radiate usually from a common center and chiefly from the plane of the bone; in the cylindrical long bones, the usual loculations of the tumor are small and interspersed with a fine fibrillary framework. The cortex is usually destroyed but may extend into the center of the tumor. The periosteum may be elevated or expanded but is seldom ruptured. The x-ray appearance of a hemangioma of the bone may closely simulate giant cell tumor, fibrous dysplasia, or eosinophilic granuloma. A biopsy is necessary to establish the correct diagnosis. Hemangioma of the calvarium often erodes through the inner and outer tables and is difficult to distinguish from a dural endothelioma.

A cavernous hemangioma of a vertebra may provoke persistent backache, and thereby lead to discovery through x-ray examination. The inaccessibility of this tumor and its intimate incorporation into an irremovable structure, prohibit any attempt at complete excision. Occasionally the hemangioma progresses and destroys the body of the vertebra, resulting in its collapse, with a protruding tumor compressing the spinal cord. Whenever symptoms of spinal cord compression occur, laminectomy is indicated.

Accessible hemangiomas of bone may be suitable for a direct surgical attack. Curettage of the lesions in long bones with the help of cryoprobes, the implantation of bone chips, rib resection, trephine and removal of a table of calvarium, partial scapulectomy, segmental resection, and bone grafting, are all feasible measures under certain conditions.

Bone changes secondary to hemangioma in closely adjacent soft tissues follow four common patterns:

1. Local erosion and destruction of the bone: The hemangioma, by constant pressure and, in the case of cirsoid or arterial hemangiomas, by pulsating pressure, destroys the adjacent bone, leaving an irregular roentgenographic finding of combined destruction and regeneration.
2. Exostosis or osteoma: Bony outgrowths can develop at sites on the bones overlapped by deep hemangiomas. The similarity of sites of these two lesions speaks against coincidental occurrence. Probably the increased vascularity of the part causes the abnormality.
3. Local overgrowth or hypertrophy of the bone: The diameter of the bone is locally expanded, thickened, and hypertrophied.
4. Elongation of long bones of the extremity: In the presence of a systemic hemangioma involving an entire extremity it is not uncommon for the long bones of the affected site to lengthen sufficiently to cause a limp, because of the disparity in length with the normal side.

Systemic Hemangiomatosis

Systemic hemangiomas are those diffuse vascular tumors that usually occupy an entire extremity or portion of the head or trunk (Fig. 16.7). As much as the entire half of the body may be involved in this congenital process (Fig. 16.8). In the head and neck region, the hemangioma may follow the cutaneous distribution of some major nerve, eg, the trigeminal. In the extremities, the anlage of this tumor probably begins at the time of limb budding so that, as the arm or leg is formed, all of the tissues, namely, skin, muscle, bone, etc., become infiltrated by the tortuous vessels of the hemangioma. The extremity from the shoulder to the nailbeds or from the pelvis to the toes may be completely involved. With this increased blood supply, all the tissues of the extremity become hypertrophied and the long bones increase in length and diameter. The leg or arm is sometimes so heavy, bulky, and cumbersome that the unfortunate patient is functionally handicapped in addition to being disfigured (Fig. 16.9).

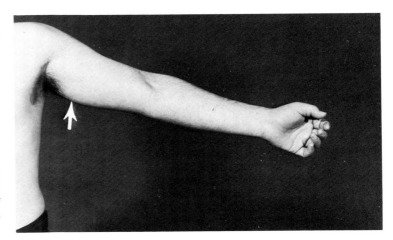

Figure 16.7. Overall involvement in the left arm of a 40-year-old man, extending from the palm (note the thenar eminence) to the axilla. A bulge in the upper medial aspect of the arm is obvious. Patient was treated with segmental resections.

Fundamentally, the systemic hemangioma is a congenital arteriovenous aneurysmal anomaly. There may be multiple communications between the arteries and veins. Blood vessels of all types take part in the process. The tumor may be partly capillary and partly cavernous in structure; or it may be a mixed hemolymphangioma. Other angiomatous lesions of visceral distribution, for example, in the liver, kidney, or brain, may coexist with these systemic hemangiomas.

The systemic hemangiomatosis is usually associated with some disturbance of the sympathetic nervous system of the portion of the body or the extremity involved. This is manifested either by hyperhidrosis or vasoconstriction. The extent of the arteriovenous shunt in the systemic hemangiomas varies greatly, depending on the size and number of the fistulous communications. In a few of our advanced cases the lesion was predominantly an arteriovenous communication. Various types of cardiovascular problems were associated with angiomatosis. In patients in whom the arteriovenous fistula could be identified, pressure proximal to the fistula resulted in the elevation of blood pressure and lowering of the pulse rate.

Treatment of systemic hemangiomatosis is difficult and unsatisfactory. Dissection of the main artery and vein, with ligation, sometimes provides reasonably good results. If the exact location of the fistula is identified, then the task becomes simple. Attempts have been made to ligate the subcutaneous vessels. A modified Kondoleon operation has also been attempted, but the results have been far from satisfactory. Amputation of the extremity is occasionally performed as a last resort.[4]

Systemic hemangiomatosis in some infants is perhaps representative of a basic defect in organization and development. It is frequently associated with neuroectodermal defects of diverse types, often identified by curious syndromes and symptom complexes bearing epon-

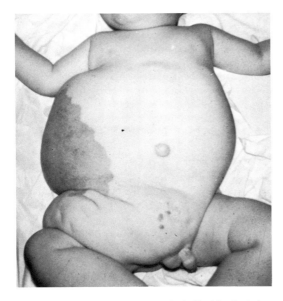

Figure 16.8. Angiomatosis of right half of body. Infant survived only two years after this photograph was taken. Angiomatosus malformation extended to the opposite side, and ulceration of the overlying skin with concomitant sepsis was the cause of death.

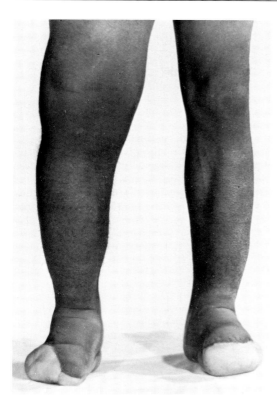

Figure 16.9. This 24-year-old man was born with systemic angiomatosis of both lower extremities. The diameter of the right leg and lower thigh is almost double that of the left. Involvement of the foot was so extensive that local hypertrophy (gigantism) interfered with walking. Tarsometatarsal amputation had to be performed on both sides.

yms. A description of some of these will be given in detail.

Hereditary Hemorrhagic Telangiectasia (Rendu-Osler-Weber's Disease). Hereditary hemorrhagic telangiectasia is an inherited maldevelopment of the minute blood vessels in localized areas, predisposing them to injury and serious bleeding. The requisite triad fulfilling the definition of this disease are (1) mucosal hemorrhages, usually epistaxis; (2) familial occurrence; and (3) the presence of telangiectatic small angiomas of the skin and mucosa, commonly in the oral and nasal cavities.

The disease is transmitted as a simple dominant gene, affecting both sexes and transmitted either through the male or female with the atavistic skipping of individuals or generations. Al-

though the anlage of the angiomas may be congenital, the minute tumors appear relatively late in the development of the individual. The onset of the disease may be heralded in children by nosebleeds, but the severe hemorrhages and clinically evident telangiectases usually start in the fourth or fifth decade of life.

The source of the epistaxis is usually in Kiesselbach's vascular plexus situated in the lower anterior segment of the nasal septum. Although the hemorrhages have been known to occur from the upper respiratory passages, the gastrointestinal tract, and even the kidney (hematuria), epistaxis is the most frequent expression and can follow simple sneezing. The intermittency and the severity of the bleeding may require repeated blood transfusions. The angiomas are usually tiny telangiectatic reddish-purple dots, seldom larger than 5 mm. It is a serious and crippling disease and is never relieved by spontaneous remission.

Congenital Neurocutaneous Syndromes Associated with Angiomatosis. Certain neuroectodermal defects involving the central nervous system and peripheral nerves are also frequently found in association with hemangiomatous lesions that may be intracranial, dermal, and visceral in distribution. Attempts have been made to lump many of these disorders under the headings of *phakomatoses*, *neurocutaneous syndromes*, or *neuroectodermal dysplasias*. The phakomatoses are tied together because they are congenital conditions of non-sex-linked dominant inheritance, with skin lesions, multiple tumors, and involvement of the central nervous system. They have variable widespread manifestations that occasionally overlap. Many of the reasons for forming such a group of diseases are artificial. The term phakomatoses is purely descriptive, and has no pathologic basis.[27] Bielschowsky[28] was the first to associate tuberous sclerosis with neurofibromatosis as dysplasia with a tendency toward the formation of blastema. In 1923, Van der Hoeve[29] coined the term phakomatosis to characterize the two disorders. He then added cerebral angiomatosis[30] and encephalofacial angiomatosis[31] to the phakomatoses. Since this original group of four maladies was grouped together under the term phakomatoses, several other entities have been added. The following better-known entities in the group of phakomatoses will be briefly described: (1) Bourneville's syndrome (tuberous sclerosis), (2) regional angiomas (Pringle's disease), (3) Sturge-Weber's disease (encephalofacial angiomatosis), and (4) von Hippel-Lindau's disease (retinocerebral angiomatosis).

Tuberous Sclerosis (Bourneville's Disease). Although one of the early reports of this entity was by von Recklinghausen,[32] this disease was first associated with neurofibromatosis in 1919. It is characterized by sebaceous adenomas, cutaneous angiomas, mental deficiency, and epilepsy. Hyperpigmentation may occur in the form of a single café-au-lait spot; however, multiple white macules are far more characteristic, histologically appearing to be secondary to a decreased amount of melanin in a normal number of melanocytes. Visceral organs are commonly involved with benign dysplasias, hamartomas, or cystic changes. These most commonly occur in the kidney, heart, and lung and are usually asymptomatic, but in later life progression may result in symptoms. The pulmonary cystic changes are very similar to those found in neurofibromatosis and may progress to respiratory failure. The brain characteristically has focal areas of disorganized cortical architecture (tubers) against a background of a distorted cortical pattern. Radiographically, intracerebral calcifications may be present after puberty. Retinal tumors and subungual fibromas occur in about 10 percent of these patients. Life expectancy in patients with significant cerebral involvement is less than two decades, but those with only cutaneous manifestations can expect near-normal longevity.

Pringle's Disease (Regional Angiomas). Scattered in a butterfly distribution over the skin of the nose, nasolabial folds, and cheeks are numerous nodules, pink, yellow, brown, and red, varying from 1 mm to 1 cm in size. This specific and symmetrical predilection has been explained as due to the distribution along the terminal filaments of the fifth cranial nerve. The terms "sebaceous adenoma" or "nevus multiplex of Pringle" have been found to be incorrect.[2] The nodules in fact are angiofibromas and analogous in many ways to von Recklinghausen's neurofibromas.

Encephalofacial Angiomatosis (Sturge-Weber's Disease). This syndrome was classified as one of the phakomatoses in 1936. It is usually present at birth and is characterized by a cutaneous telangiectatic hemangioma (port wine mark) in the distribution of the trigeminal nerve. On the ipsilateral side, meningeal angiomatosis extends into the depths of the sulci, with underlying cortical atrophy. After infancy, calcification develops in the affected cortex, resulting in epilepsy and mental retardation, with longevity greatly decreased. Rarely, pheochromocytoma has been reported to occur in these patients.

Retinocerebral Angiomatosis (von Hippel-Lindau's Disease). Von Hippel described the retinal changes in this disease in 1911, but it was not until 1926 that Lindau[27] made an extensive report of the visceral and central nervous system pathology. The most important lesion in this disease is the cerebellar hemangioblastoma, which can be either highly vascular or cystic. Angiomatosis may occur throughout the central nervous system and is especially diagnostic when present in the retina. The embryologic origin of most of the manifestations of this disease is primarily mesodermal. Pheochromocytoma is frequently associated with von Hippel-Lindau's disease and neurofibromatosis, the incidence being higher in von Hippel-Lindau's disease. The onset of symptoms of this disease is usually in middle age, being either neurologic or visual. No cases have been reported prior to puberty and no particular skin lesion is characteristic. Both Sturge-Weber's syndrome and von Recklinghausen's neurofibromatosis have been reported to occur in patients and families with von Hippel-Lindau's disease, resulting in a confusing picture but leading to interesting genetic speculation. It is doubtful that these reports represent any more than the chance synchronous occurrence of two distinct syndromes.

Benign Hemangiopericytoma

Hemangiopericytoma is considered benign if microscopically there is absence of any mitosis. In tumors in which only occasional mitotic activity is observed, the general tendency has been to consider them as more or less benign; however, on a long-term basis, their malignant potential becomes obvious with the development of local recurrence. Therefore, the treatment should be wide excision of the normal soft tissues surrounding the tumor. In our present group of patients, there are six in whom the tumors were classified as benign hemangiopericytoma. All six patients had subcutaneous tumors in the extremities and in none was the primary tumor larger than 3 cm. Unlike the situation with glomus tumors, none of the patients presented with unusual pain or tenderness related to the primary tumor. They all have remained free of disease for at least five years but will require further followup.

Glomus Tumor

Glomus tumors are usually small (3 to 5 mm) and are frequently encountered in the subungual region. Although they should fall under the category of smooth muscle tumors,[33-37] conventionally they are grouped with tumors arising from the vasoformative tissue.

They are usually single, but several instances of multiple tumors have been reported.[7,37] We have encountered five such instances. The tumor is found in adults of both sexes and has no specific racial predilection. Although most of the glomus tumors are superficial, ie, in the trunk or in the extremities, a few cases have been reported in the thoracic cavity,[38] the stomach,[39] and the vagina.[40]

The color of the visible tumors ranges from deep red to purple or blue, with the blue color more prominent. The tumor is usually well demarcated from the surrounding tissues. Pack and Ariel[7] described 20 patients with glomus tumors, the anatomic distribution being as follows: temple, one; thoracic wall, one; scapular region, one; hand, one; knee, two; arm, two; forearm, five; fingers, seven. Eleven patients with glomus tumors have been treated by the author, nine in the upper extremities and two in the lower. Of the nine in the upper extremities, seven were in the subungual region. Tsuneyoshi and Enjoji[40A] recently reviewed 63 cases of glomus tumors. These tumors were more common in young women (41), and the most common anatomic location was the fingers (35); 26 (74 percent) of the 35 were in the subungual region. All patients but one complained of pain. These authors histologically classified glomus tumors into three types: vascular (29 cases), myxoid (23 cases) and solid (11 cases). In keeping with recent observations, the presence of smooth muscle cells in these tumors was also observed.

The characteristic symptom of glomus tumor is pain, which occasionally is associated with localized vasomotor disturbance. The diagnosis of glomus tumor is made by the location and the accompanying pain. Infrequently, the pulsatile nature of the tumor can erode the terminal phalanx and a clear-cut destruction of the cortex of the terminal phalanx is seen. Clinical diagnosis is usually satisfactory and treatment can be initiated.

In most other locations, a glomus tumor produces symptoms characteristic of the site at which it arises. For example, Appelman and Helwig[39] reviewed the clinical features of 12 glomus tumors of the stomach from the files of the Armed Forces Institute of Pathology, plus 17 cases from the literature. They found that, of 29 patients, 11 were seen for ulcer symptoms and 12 for upper gastrointestinal bleeding. In the remainder, the glomus tumor was an incidental finding. The ideal treatment of a glomus tumor is excision.

MALIGNANT TUMORS

Angiosarcoma (Malignant Hemangioendothelioma)

Angiosarcomas are rare neoplasms. McCarthy and Pack[41] suggested that the true incidence was probably higher than the reported incidence. Pack and Ariel[7] reported that, in a 10-year period, 1,056 cases of benign angiomas were seen at Memorial Sloan-Kettering Cancer Center, but during that same period there were only 20 (1.8 percent) cases of angiosarcomas. During the same 10 years, the Pathology Department of Memorial Sloan-Kettering Cancer Center reviewed the microscopic materials from an additional 27 cases from all over the country.[7] Angiosarcomas of the skin,[42] head and neck region,[43,44] omentum,[45,46] trunk,[7,41,47] breast,[48-58] and viscera[7,59-68] have been described. Most of these represent reports of a few cases, and adequate guidelines for clinical management are not possible. Table 16.3 shows the anatomic distribution of 17 cases

TABLE 16.3. ANATOMIC DISTRIBUTION OF ANGIOSARCOMAS

Site	Pack and Ariel [7] (1958)	Das Gupta (1981)
Head and neck	7	3
Upper extremities	4	4
Lower extremities	7	2
Trunk	—	1
Breast	2	3
Retroperitoneum	—	1
Viscera	—	3
Total	20	17

of angiosarcoma encountered at the University of Illinois Medical Center.

Although primary angiosarcomas of the liver have been associated with polyvinyl chloride (PVC) and other agents,[69-82] little is known regarding their etiology in general.

Angiosarcomas are found in all ages, both sexes, and all races. The youngest patient in our group was 24 and the oldest 84 years of age.

Patients with angiosarcoma usually present with a moderately rapid-growing mass in the extremities, the scalp, or the trunk (Fig. 16.10A to 16.10C). The rapidity of the progression of the disease is sometimes the clue to the correct diagnosis of a given tumor.

Regional Node Metastases. Pack and Ariel[7] considered that the incidence rate of regional node metastases was as high as 45 percent. In the 11 patients in their series with extremity tumors, nine tumors were locally recurrent and the patients had been referred after a delay of more than a year. Weingrad and Rosenberg,[83] in their survey of the literature, did not come across any significant series other than that of Pack and Ariel's[7] for analysis of the incidence of regional node metastases. In our own series of six patients with extremity tumors, five had primary tumors, three of whom were sent to us after a wedge biopsy. Only one patient had metastatic disease to the regional nodes at the time of the primary operation.

Treatment. The treatment of angiosarcomas of the extremities has been unsatisfactory over the years.[7,41-44,84] In our series of six patients with extremity angiosarcomas, four (66 percent) are still disease-free five years or more after the primary operation. The other two were treatment failures (Table 16.4). Pack and Ariel[7] argued in favor of radical operation, including major amputations, in extremity angiosarcomas. It is apparent that some of the conclusions forwarded by these authors were based on their clinical material, a majority of which were large recurrent tumors of long duration.

Pack and Ariel[7] found that both primary and metastatic tumors were moderately radiosensitive. However, according to their estimate, radiation therapy is not curative and should be reserved for palliation only. McNeer et al.[85] found that of seven patients with angiosarcoma, three treated with surgery alone survived for five years, as did two who received postoperative irradiation.

Systemic chemotherapy as an adjuvant to surgery has been used in three patients with extremity angiosarcomas (Table 16.4). All three have survived five years free of tumor. Based on our own data and a published report,[86] it appears that adjuvant chemotherapy may have a place in the management of primary angiosarcomas of the extremities, but it is premature to draw any conclusions.

Angiosarcoma of the Breast. Angiosarcoma of the breast was first described by Schmidt.[87] However, Borrman[88] is credited with an adequate description of this entity in 1907. In 1969, Gulesserian and Lawton[55] presented a collective review of 42 cases of primary angiosarcoma of the breast. Since then, several other case reports have been published.[53,54,56-58] We have encountered three additional cases.

Of the three patients, two were initially seen with localized tumors of the breast and were treated by modified radical mastectomy. In both instances the regional axillary nodes were negative for any metastatic tumor. Both patients received adjuvant chemotherapy. One has remained disease-free for four years and the other died of diffuse metastases two and one-half years later. The third patient was initially referred with advanced disease (Fig. 16.11) and did not receive any treatment. She died within two months of her first visit to our clinic.

Angiosarcoma of the breast usually occurs in relatively young multiparous women. In four of the 51 cases, the patient was pregnant at the time of diagnosis.[49,58,89] In eight, the angiosarcoma developed after menopause.[58] Involvement of both breasts occurred in three patients,[51,57] However, in two,[57] the tumor probably was metastatic from the opposite breast.

The treatment is primarily excision and for all practical purposes a total mastectomy is adequate; however, in recurrent tumors, since there is some possibility of regional node metastases, a modified radical mastectomy is in order. The role of postoperative radiation therapy and chemotherapy is being evaluated.[56]

Angiosarcoma of the Head and Neck Region. Angiosarcomas of the head and neck region are curiously rare, considering the unusual frequency of hemangiomas in this region,[7,41,43,44,90] and it is therefore difficult to develop guidelines regarding their general management. Pack and Ariel[7] treated seven cases in the head and neck region. In 1968, Bardwil and co-workers[43] de-

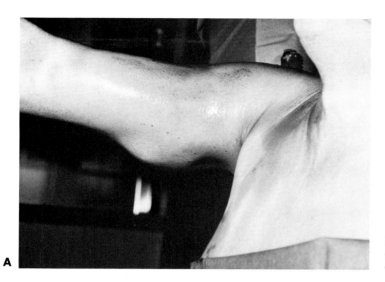

Figure 16.10. (A) An angiosarcoma of the upper arm in a 56-year-old man.

A

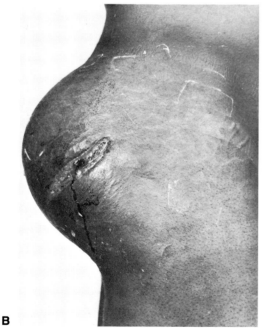

B

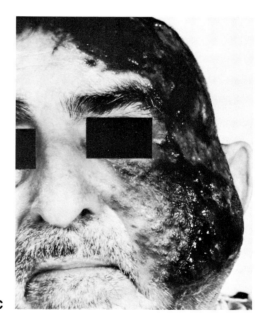

C

Figure 16.10. (B) Angiosarcoma of the buttock of a 24-year-old basketball player. After a minor trauma in the back, patient noticed gradual enlargement of the buttock. A diagnosis of gluteal abscess was made and the tumor incised. The drainage was sanguinous, with blood clots. When the drainage continued after five weeks, a biopsy was done, which showed angiosarcoma. A hemipelvectomy was performed and he survived for one and one-half years (Patient 3, Table 16.4). **(C)** Angiosarcoma of the scalp extending to the face. Treated with radiation therapy and systemic chemotherapy. The disease progressed relentlessly and within four months the patient died of diffuse metastases. *(Courtesy of Surgery Annual, 1975)*

TABLE 16.4. CLINICAL SUMMARY OF SIX PATIENTS WITH ANGIOSARCOMAS OF THE EXTREMITIES

No.	Age/Sex	Location	Status of Primary	Regional Nodes	Type of Treatment	Metastases	End Result (Length of Survival)	Remarks
1	65/F	R upper arm	3 × 4 cm tumor	—	Forequarter amputation	Lung, liver, neck nodes	6 months, dead with disease	Had widespread metastases prior to death
2	57/M	R thigh	4 × 5 cm	—	Hip joint disarticulation	—	6 yrs, N.E.D.*	Mass persisted for one and one-half yrs before patient sought medical advice (treated with adjuvant chemotherapy)
3	24/M	L buttock	15 × 10 cm	+	Hemipelvectomy with axillary dissection	Widespread	1½ yrs, dead	Patient seen after an incision biopsy of the lesion (five weeks' duration)
4	46/F	F forearm	2 × 2 cm	—	Wide excision	—	5 yrs, N.E.D.	Tumor apparently was of six months' duration, biopsied elsewhere. Treated with adjuvant chemotherapy
5	54/F	L hand	3 × 2 cm	—	Midarm amputation with axillary dissection	—	5½ yrs, N.E.D.	Sent here with local recurrence following conservative excision
6	34/M	L leg	2 × 2 cm	—	Above-knee amputation	—	5 yrs, N.E.D.	Treated with adjuvant chemothreapy

*No evidence of disease.

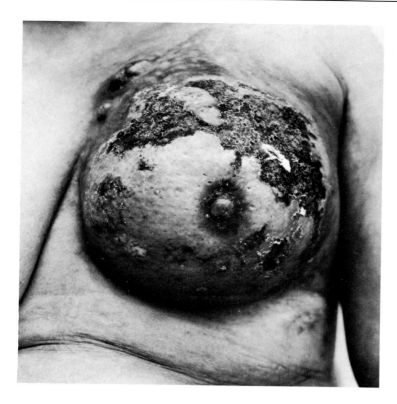

Figure 16.11. Angiosarcoma of the left breast of a 43-year-old woman. Note skin involvement. She was seen with far-advanced disease and was deemed incurable.

scribed 10 cases of hemangiosarcoma from the M.D. Anderson Tumor Institute, and in 1970 Farr et al.[44] published 10 cases from the files of the Memorial Sloan-Kettering Cancer Center. Only three cases have been encountered at the University of Illinois Hospital, all in the scalp (Fig. 16.10C). It appears that this is the most common site in the head and neck region. The majority of cases occur in the fifth decade, although these tumors have been reported in children. All three of our patients were more than 60 years of age.

In general, patients are first seen with an umbilicated dark lesion of the scalp. In untreated cases, satellite nodules are found surrounding the primary tumor. Initially the tumors appear vascular and often give the impression of a granuloma. Wide excision with adjuvant radiation therapy in this initial stage might provide up to 50 percent incidence of control of the primary tumor. However, in untreated or inadequately treated cases, there is a relatively high incidence of regional node metastases, and at this stage the results of treatment are unsatisfactory. Of the three patients in our group, all presented with advanced dis-

ease. Two died within a year, and the remaining patient is living with disease nine months after diagnosis and receiving multiagent chemotherapy.

In the primary treatment of angiosarcomas of the scalp, it is essential to recognize that there are deceptive horizontal and vertical extensions of the lesion that can only be recognized by microscopic examination of all the margins of the resected specimen. It is recommended that the primary excision of the scalp be full-thickness, including the pericranium and the outer table of the cranial vault. The margins should be wide (at least 5 cm) on all sides. Furthermore, the resected margin must be microscopically examined prior to covering the defect.

Angiosarcoma of the Viscera. Angiosarcomas of the intra-abdominal viscera, namely of the spleen and the liver, have been reported, but angiosarcomas of other viscera are extremely rare.

Angiosarcoma of the Heart. Of the 53 cases of angiosarcoma of the heart analyzed by Rossi and associates,[67] 34 were in males. The tumors most commonly originate in the right atrium. Most of the patients are adults, but a few cases have been reported in adolescents. Various treatment programs consisting of excision, radiation therapy, and chemotherapy have been tried. The median survival time from onset of symptoms is approximately three months. Recently, Bennett and co-workers[90A] emphasized that patients with primary angiosarcoma of the heart typically have signs of right-sided congestive heart failure. These authors suggested that an earlier diagnosis can be made by a nuclear cardiac scan which would show any filling defect.

Angiosarcoma of the Lungs. Angiosarcoma of the lungs is extremely rare, the first case being reported in 1931 by Wollstein.[59] Since then occasional case reports have appeared in the literature, but it is difficult to establish whether the lung was the primary site in these reports. It is not possible to make any generalization concerning pulmonary angiosarcomas. Suffice it to emphasize that all purported cases should be analyzed and published for future reference.

Angiosarcoma of the Liver. Alrenga[91] estimated that, up to 1975, 165 cases of angiosarcoma of the liver, with an autopsy frequency of

6 in 100,000, had appeared in the literature. Heath and co-authors[75] stated that the expected annual incidence of the tumor is 0.014 in 100,000, or 25 to 30 cases a year in the United States. Eight cases in 40,000 autopsies were encountered in Holland.[82] In contrast, 14 cases were noted in the population of 5,000 workers in PVC polymerization plants in the United States in a 15-year period.[74] Based on these data, it is suggested that polyvinyl chloride is an etiologic agent in the development of hepatic angiosarcoma. However, Fiechtner and Reyes[81] described four patients with hemangiosarcoma of the liver and all were from rural areas of Wisconsin with no known exposure to industrial pollutants.

The clinical manifestation of angiosarcoma of the liver in adult patients is not characterized by any specific presentation. In the majority of patients there is evidence of a hepatic tumor associated with liver failure of varying degrees. The diagnosis is established by angiography and finally by exploratory celiotomy (Fig. 16.12). Fiechtner and Reyes[81] noted that all their patients had symptoms of advanced liver disease: abdominal pain and distention of short duration. In adults, sudden unexplained enlargement of the liver with rapid liver failure should lead to a working diagnosis of angiosarcoma of the liver.

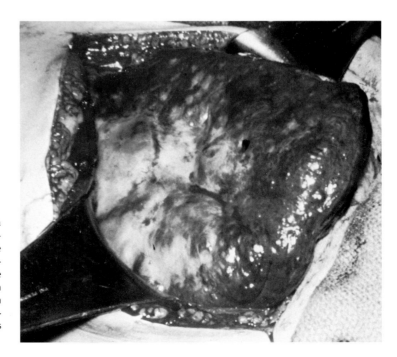

Figure 16.12. Hemangiosarcoma of the right lobe of the liver. Although involvement of the right lobe was known preoperatively, at operation it was found to also involve both lobes. Patient was treated with intra-arterial infusion and radiation therapy but died of extensive disease nine months after diagnosis was established.

The rarity of the tumors and the advanced stage at which diagnosis is made have resulted in a dismal prognosis after any form of therapy. Nagasue et al.[68] reported an eight-month control of a patient with angiosarcoma, using hepatic artery ligation and infusion of 5-FU through the portal vein for 27 days. These and other forms of innovative therapy must be attempted to control angiosarcoma of the liver in adults.

In our series of 17 cases of angiosarcoma, three were of the liver. Both lobes were involved in one patient, and she was treated with intra-arterial infusion and radiation therapy. She died nine months after diagnosis (Fig. 16.12). The remaining two patients had lobectomies and adjuvant chemotherapy (Table 8.15, Chapter 8). One was apparently disease-free three and one-half years after resection of the left lobe of the liver.

Juvenile angiosarcoma of the liver is rarer still. Blumenfeld et al.[63] found only 36 cases in the literature up to 1969 and added one of their own. Of these 37 patients, 32 had multiple and 5 had solitary lesions. Thirty of the patients with multiple tumors died. In one patient, the tumor metastasized to the lung and lymph nodes. Apparently two of the patients with multiple lesions survived.[63] All the patients with solitary lesions were living at the time of Blumenfeld and co-workers' report in 1969. Of interest is the statement that in one child the tumor spontaneously regressed, resulting in cure.[63]

Angiosarcoma of the Spleen. Angiosarcoma of the spleen is rare,[62,92] and only about 50 cases have been reported. Three of these 50 were encountered in children (two girls and one boy).[93] Of the three, one was 13,[94] one was 1.5,[95] and the other was 15 years old.[96] Of these three cases of childhood angiosarcoma, in only the one reported by Garlock[94] are details available. This child had a splenectomy for an intact tumor and lived for two years, after which the child was not followed.

Hemangiosarcoma of the spleen has been recorded in 47 adult patients.[62,92,97-103] Das Gupta, Coombes, and Brasfield[62] reported one of the first cases of an adult splenic angiosarcoma treated electively by splenectomy. This was in a 52-year-old woman who was admitted with a diagnosis of anemia and splenomegaly. At laparotomy, the spleen weighed 2,400 gm and measured 7 × 8 × 9 cm. A diagnosis of angiosarcoma of the spleen was made from the specimen. After splenectomy was done, the patient recovered and was discharged. She was readmitted four months later with diffuse metastatic involvement of the abdomen. She died within a month. A review of the published case reports in adults shows that in 23 (53 percent) of the 47 cases splenectomy was performed, and in the remaining cases the diagnosis was made at autopsy. Sixteen of the 23 (70 percent) required emergency splenectomy because of rupture of the spleen. None of the patients who were operated upon were long-term survivors.

Hemangiosarcoma of the spleen in adults is uncommon; however, the true incidence is probably not reflected in these 47 patients. It is therefore suggested that when the cause of splenic enlargement from disorders such as leukemia, lymphoma, and other hematologic abnormalities is ruled out, the possibility of hemangiosarcoma of the spleen should be considered. The prognosis for these patients is poor, and currently the only possible method of salvage is early diagnosis followed by splenectomy.

Primary hemangiosarcomas have been reported in other intra-abdominal locations.[45,46] Kalisher and co-workers[45] reported a case in the greater omentum. They concluded that tumors located in the mesentery, omentum, and retroperitoneum all had a similar clinical presentation and natural history, and could be treated in a similar fashion. One retroperitoneal hemangiosarcoma has been treated by the author. This was excised and the patient has been well for three years. Stein[104] reported the only case of hemangioendothelioma of the testes, and Ongkasuwan and associates[104A] found only eight instances of angiosarcoma of the uterus and only two in the ovary.

Hemangiosarcomas arising in peripheral nerves have always generated considerable interest, but the incidence is indeed rare.[105] Recently, Bricklin and Rushton[106] reported a case in the radial nerve and found only one other such instance in the literature.[105] Because of the extreme rarity in these locations, they are more of interest to the embryologist and morphologist than to the clinician.

Hemangiopericytoma

Malignant hemangiopericytoma was first described by Stout and Murray[107] in 1942. In 1949, Stout[108] described the natural history of 25 cases, thus firmly establishing the clinicopathologic features of this relatively new neoplasm. Although the etiologic factors of hemangiopericytoma are generally unclear, polyvinyl alcohol has been alluded to as a causative agent.[109] Prout and Davis[110] reported a case of hemangiopericytoma of the urinary bladder following exposure to polyvinyl alcohol.

Hemangiopericytoma may occur in any part of the human body (Table 16.5).[111-116] It has been described in the thorax,[117] a number of viscera,[110,118] the pelvis,[119,120] and several unusual sites.[121,122]

Of the 19 patients in our present series, ten were women and nine were men. A similar ratio has been reported by other authors.[111-113] The peak incidence appears to be in the middle decades.[111-115]

The tumor usually presents as a painless, slow-growing mass, which is often nodular and circumscribed. In some patients the presenting symptom is due to pressure on the adjoining structures (Fig. 16.13). In one of our patients with a presacral hemangiopericytoma, the pressure on the rectum simulated the symptoms of a cancer of the rectum.

Of the 19 hemangiopericytoma patients in this series, 14 presented with primary tumors and 5 with locally recurrent tumors. The size of the primary tumors varied. In six of the patients it was less than 5 cm; in four, between 6 and 9 cm; and in four it was almost 10 cm. Eight of the tumors were between grades 1 and 2, and the remaining 11, between grades 3 and 4.

Malignant hemangiopericytoma metastasizes via both the lymphatics and the bloodstream. Regional node metastasis in primary low-grade tumors is rare, but may be encountered either in high-grade primary tumors or in tumors recurring locally after initial excisions. In our series of 14 primary tumors, only two had metastatic regional nodes. Two of the five patients with locally recurrent tumors had regional node involvement.

The ideal treatment of malignant hemangiopericytoma is wide excision. In our series of 19 patients, three underwent major amputation. All three had local recurrence after initial excision elsewhere. Unfortunately, because of lack of appreciation of the malignant potential of this type of neoplasm, the majority of patients are initially treated with less than adequate excision. This results in repeated local recurrences and ultimately systemic extension and death. The following two case reports exemplify the existing confusion in the management of these patients.

CASE 1

A 24-year-old woman was referred to the University of Illinois Hospital with a diagnosis of recurrent hemangiopericytoma of the right groin. At the age of 23, she had noticed a "walnut-shaped" painless lump in the inner part of her right groin. Her physician recommended observation for three months. The size of the mass did not change. Although the physician wanted to continue observation, she insisted on excision. The tumor was excised and a diagnosis of hemangiopericytoma was made. She was told that the tumor had been adequately removed, that such tumors do not recur or metastasize, and that no further excision was indicated. The mass reappeared within three months, and another "wide" excision was performed. The tumor reappeared within six months, resulting in another excision. This time

TABLE 16.5. ANATOMIC LOCATION OF HEMANGIOPERICYTOMA

Site	O'Brien and Brasfield[113] (1965)	McMaster and Coworkers[112] (1975)	Enzinger and Smith[111] (1976)	Das Gupta (1981)
Head and neck	7	4	17	3
Trunk (including retroperitoneum, retropleural space, and perineum)	9	22	41	7
Upper extremities	2	9	11	3
Lower extremities	6	25	37	6
Total	24	60	106	19

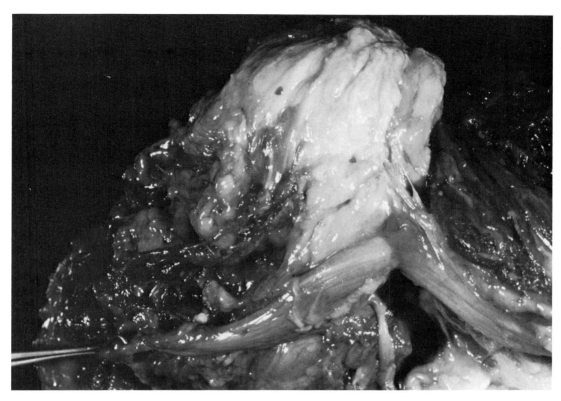

Figure 16.13. Resected hemipelvectomy specimen. Note the tumor is pressing on the sacral plexi. The plexi are separated in a V-shaped manner to show the relation of the tumor to the nerve roots. This 56-year-old woman complained of tense pain along the course of the sciatic nerve for one year before a pelvic and rectal examination was performed. Following hemipelvectomy she has remained well for six years.

the tumor recurred within two months and the patient started having pain in the anterior aspect of the thigh. Because of three recurrences within one year of primary excision, she was sent to the University of Illinois. Examination showed a 4 × 3 cm mass, located on the lateral margin of the femoral triangle about 2.5 cm below the anterior superior iliac spine. A muscle group excision of the anterolateral compartment of the thigh and excision of the anterior superior iliac spine with 3 cm of the anterior aspect of the iliac crest was then performed. The specimen showed the recurrent tumor infiltrating the anterior cutaneous nerve of the thigh. She has remained well for seven years. At age 31, she is active and has no residual deformity.

CASE 2

A 26-year-old man was sent to us with a diagnosis of recurrent hemangiopericytoma of the anterior abdominal wall and a bleeding duo-

denal ulcer. Three years previously he had noticed a small painless mass about two inches above the umbilicus on the right side of the abdominal wall. The tumor was locally excised and a diagnosis of hemangiopericytoma made. The tumor recurred in three months and a second excision was performed. He then received a total dose of 5,000 rads to the area of the tumor. After he recovered from the effects of radiation, he remained well for one and one-half years and completed his college studies. The tumor reappeared 20 months later and he was placed on a regimen of adriamycin, Cytoxan, and vincristine. In spite of the completion of a total dose of adriamycin, the tumor did not reduce in size and the patient started to lose weight. Approximately six months after chemotherapy was started, he had his first episode of upper gastrointestinal bleeding. Investigation suggested a bleeding gastric ulcer, and he was treated conservatively. Four weeks after the first episode he had a second episode of upper gastrointestinal bleeding, complicated by the appearance of gastric outlet obstruction. At this time he was transferred to the University of Ilinois.

On admission, he was dehydrated, emaciated, and febrile. A large epigastric mass was readily palpable, with skin changes over the mass. He was hydrated, given hyperalimentation, and investigated for evidence of extraabdominal extension of the tumor, following which he was operated upon, with excision of the anterior abdominal wall, partial gastrectomy, vagectomy, pancreaticoduodenectomy, and wedge excision of both lobes of the liver (Fig. 4.84, Chapter 4). Reconstruction of the gastrointestinal continuity was performed on classical lines. The anterior abdominal wall was repaired with bovine fascia lata and rotation of a skin flap from the chest. He remained free of tumor for four years (Fig. 6.13, Chapter 6). However, in the fifth year, he developed intraabdominal recurrence with extension to the posterior mediastinum. Another attempt at a massive excision was considered, but celiotomy showed the abdominal cavity to be replaced with tumor. He died soon after his last operation.

These two case reports illustrate the commonly held misconceptions regarding the management of patients with hemangiopericytoma: (1) that they are slow-growing tumors of low-grade malignancy, and (2) that they can be adequately controlled by means of primary irradiation and systemic chemotherapy, even with inadequate excision of the primary tumor. Long-term control of malignant hemangiopericytoma in any anatomic location can be accomplished only if the tumor is excised widely. Wide excision means a margin of normal soft tissue surrounding the tumor. However, in locations where an adequate margin is not possible, for example, in the retroperitoneum, either preoperative or postoperative radiation therapy might be considered.[123,124] Mira and co-workers[124] reported a relatively good response in large tumors after radiation therapy. However, these methods have not been tried sufficiently long to provide the reader with any guidelines.

End Results. In our present series of 19 patients with malignant hemangiopericytoma, of 16 patients eligible for two-year followup analysis, 14 (87 percent) were free of local recurrence or metastases. Of fourteen eligible for five-year analysis, 11 (79 percent) are still free of disease. Seven of these 14 had histologic grades 3 and 4 tumors and four are still disease-free after five years. None of the 19 patients was treated with adjuvant chemotherapy. In this small series, all histologic grades were treated similarly.

Backwinkle and Diddams[114] reviewed the literature in 1970 and found that, of the combined series of 177 cases treated by surgery alone, 95 patients (53.6 percent) survived for five years or more. Enzinger and Smith[111] found 67 percent of 106 patients collected from various sources were alive and 60 percent were without evidence of tumor at the time of their report in 1976. McMaster and co-workers[112] computed the results of treatment according to whether the tumors were histologically of borderline malignancy or were frankly malignant. In the borderline group of 16 patients, six (37.6 percent) were free of disease for five years or more. In the frankly malignant group, five (15.6 percent) of 32 patients survived without evidence of cancer. This striking difference in results of treatment reported in the collected series[112-114] can probably be explained on the basis of differences in the concept of wide excision. In any retrospective analysis spanning a long period and in which a number of investigators participate, frequently the same operation is performed differently by the different authors and the results cannot be compared.

The recurrence rate following primary operation is directly proportional to the inadequacy of the operation. Our two case reports show the problem of inadequate operation. In the present group of 14 patients with primary tumors, one (7 percent) had local recurrence following operation. In the series reported by McMaster et al.,[112] six of 16 (37.5 percent) in the borderline group and 15 of 32 (42 percent) in the frankly malignant group had local recurrence (Table 16.6). From all the available data, it is appropriate to recommend that all hemangiopericytomas with any mitotic figures in a high-power field be considered malignant. The true malignant potential of these tumors becomes evident only after some time has elapsed. The best treatment for malignant hemangiopericytomas is adequate wide excision. However, with the developing morphologic data indicating that these tumors probably are of smooth muscle cell origin, a vigorous trial with adjuvant chemotherapy and local radiation therapy is in order, especially to avoid limb ablation.

Pelvic Hemangiopericytoma. Hemangiopericytoma of the pelvis is relatively infrequent. In 1964, Spiro and associates[119] found 24 cases, 18

TABLE 16.6 LOCAL RECURRENCE AFTER PRIMARY OPERATION IN MALIGNANT HEMANGIOPERICYTOMA

Author	Year of Publication	Total No. of Cases	Incidence of Overall Local Recurrence
O'Brien and Brasfield[113] (Memorial Sloan-Kettering Cancer Center)	1965	24	50%
Backwinkel and Diddams[114] (collected from literature of cases of musculoskeletal and skin tumors)	1970	103	50.5%
McMaster et al.[112] (Mayo Clinic)	1975	48	43.75%
Enzinger and Smith[111] (AFIP)	1976	106	18%
Das Gupta (University of Illinois)	1981	14*	7%

*Only 14 patients had primary tumors.

uterine and six extrauterine. In 1976 Wilbanks et al.,[120] found 24 additional patients with the uterine variety and three with the extrauterine pelvic variety.

These tumors may present as a pelvic mass simulating either ovarian cancer or uterine enlargement, with menometrorrhagia simulating fibroids. Patients with uterine hemangiopericytomas have a better prognosis than those with the extrauterine variety. Wilbanks and co-workers[120] reviewed the literature and found that, in the 43 determinant cases of uterine hemangiopericytoma, four patients (11 percent) either died of their disease or had recurrence following primary excision. In contrast, of the seven patients with extrauterine hemangiopericytoma, only three survived.

Kaposi's Sarcoma

Kaposi's sarcoma was first described as a clinical entity in 1872.[125] Kaposi's original description of the entity is worth repeating. . . . "There develops on the skin, without known cause, either general or local, brown-red to blue-red nodules of the size of a grain of wheat, a pea or a hazelnut. Their surface is smooth, their consistency densely elastic. Often they are swollen like a sponge filled with blood . . . ." This accurate description of the initial presentation of this entity has not been bettered during the last hundred years.

Kaposi's sarcoma is most frequently encountered in patients from Eastern and Central Europe and certain parts of Northern Italy.[7,126,127] In the United States, most of the patients belong

to these ethnic groups. In the University of Illinois series of 25 patients, only one patient was a black woman and only one was of Northern European descent. It is indeed difficult to assess the actual incidence of Kaposi's sarcoma, since a number of these cases remain unrecognized and thus not reported. Although the disease is rare in American blacks, it occurs with great frequency among African blacks.[128-134] The frequency of the disease reported from various African centers varies (Table 16.7).[131,133-140] The condition appears to increase in frequency as one approaches the equator. The disease is infrequent in dry, sandy areas, the highest incidence being in moist, tropical areas.[132-134] Taylor and co-workers[129] found that Kaposi's sarcoma in the Congo Basin can be clinically divided into nodular, aggressive, and generalized types, with the clinical behavior varying from indolent (occasionally showing spontaneous regression) to fulminant (resulting in death). Because of the geographic and clinical similarities between Kaposi's sarcoma and Burkitt's lymphoma, the possibility of immune deficiency states as an etiologic factor in the development of Kaposi's sarcoma has been suggested.[129,141,142]

The most notable evidence in favor of an immune deficiency state is provided by the de novo appearance of Kaposi's sarcoma in renal transplant patients receiving prolonged immunosuppressive therapy.[143-147] Hardy and co-workers[143] reported one such case and reviewed the findings in five other patients. Two of the six eventually had visceral involvement, and one had reticulum cell sarcoma of the brain.[143] In the

TABLE 16.7. INCIDENCE OF KAPOSI'S SARCOMA IN AFRICAN CENTERS

Author	Year of Publication	Center	Incidence (%)
Elmes and Baldwin[135]	1944	Gold Coast (Republic of Ghana)	0.8
Edington[136]	1956	Nigeria	2.4
Thijs[137]	1957	Congo (Zaire)	9.1
Higginson and Oettle[138]	1960	Johannesburg	2.8
Timms[139]	1962	Durban	1.3
		Tanzania	4.0
Lothe[140]	1963	Uganda	3.4
		Kenya	2.4
Gordon[131]	1967	Salisbury	3.3
Slavin et al[133]	1969	Tanzania	4.0

first case, diagnosis was made at autopsy. In two cases,[146] discontinuation of all immunosuppressive agents led to complete regression of the skin nodules. In another case,[145] in which both prednisone and azathioprine were reduced but not discontinued, the lesions recurred and progressed without apparent visceral involvement. In one patient,[143] discontinuation of azathioprine led to the virtual disappearance of the skin nodules, leaving scars and persistent edema. Reynolds, Winkelman, and Soule[148] pointed out that in Kaposi's sarcoma there is not only a correlation with lymphoid and plasmacytic dyscrasias, but also the disease becomes manifest in patients with collagen disease treated with corticosteroids. Serial immunologic studies, both in vitro and in vivo have shown that normal blastogenic response to various mitogens and a positive reaction to purified protein derivative (PPD) are altered with the progression of the disease.[142,144,149]

The significance of the immune deficiency either demonstrated in vitro by lymphocyte responses, or in vivo by cutaneous anergy when there is clinical progression of the disease, is unclear and does not offer any etiologic explanation. However, if it is argued that, with immunosuppression, latent oncogenic viruses are activated,[150] leading to the development of Kaposi's sarcoma, then a clear role of a virus in the development of the disease can be hypothesized. Patients with Kaposi's sarcoma have been examined from the virologic viewpoint by Giraldo and co-workers.[150] These authors found herpes virus with the antigenicity of the Epstein-Barr virus in cultures derived from Kaposi's tumors. Hardy et al.[143] reported that four

of six allografted patients with Kaposi's sarcoma had documented herpes simplex infections prior to the onset of the tumor. In their own patients, Hardy et al.[143] found no apparent viral infection, but were able to demonstrate an elevated titer of Epstein-Barr virus (EBV) antibody in the serum. Recently, disseminated Kaposi's sarcoma syndrome was reported in an endemic cluster of young homosexual males in the United States.[151] The homosexual subpopulation has a well-documented high incidence of infection with gonorrhea, syphilis, condylomata acuminata, herpes simplex virus (HSV), cytomegalovirus (CMV), hepatitis A or B, etc. In the fulminant form of Kaposi's sarcoma seen in Africa, most of the patients show elevated serum antibody titers to CMV. These circumstantial evidences of a viral etiology are strong enough to justify further investigation.

Clinical Features.

Age. Although Kaposi's sarcoma occurs in all age groups, especially in young male homosexuals, in the United States most of the patients are older. The mean age at the time of diagnosis in the series reported by O'Brien and Brasfield was 70.[126] In the University of Illinois group, the mean age was 60, the youngest patient being 42 years old. Oettle[132] found that Kaposi's sarcoma is encountered in younger patients in Africa: all his patients were between 35 and 44 years of age. Slavin and co-workers[133] found that eight cases (7 percent) in a series of 117 were in children below the age of 16. Pediatric Kaposi's sarcoma has not been reported in the United States.[152]

Sex. Males predominate in all series. In Africa, Gordon[131] found 128 men in a total of 136 patients, and Slavin et al.[133] reported 108 males and nine females. A similar male preponderance is found in Europe and North America.[126,148,153-155] In the series reported by O'Brien and Brasfield,[126] 81 percent were men and 19 percent were women. In our series of 25 patients, 22 were men and three were women.

The initial presentation of a classic bluish-red macule can occur in the skin of all parts of the human body. However, the lower extremity constitutes the most common site (19 of 25 in our series). The lesions are usually small, 0.2 to 1 mm in diameter, lying in the dermis or subcutis and bulging the overlying epidermis (Fig. 16.14A to 16.14D). Closely continuous lesions sometimes coalesce and produce large conglomerate lesions (Fig. 16.14A). The more diffuse lesions give rise to plaquelike nodules (Fig. 16.14B). Although the lesions are principally in the subcutis or dermis, superficial ulceration is a frequent accompaniment of Kaposi's sarcoma of long duration (Fig. 16.14C).

The disease frequently involves symmetrical areas in the other extremity in a "stocking" or "glove" fashion and later extends centripetally to the trunk (Fig. 16.14A to 16.14C). As the subcutaneous tissues are diffusely infiltrated by the hemorrhagic, verrucous plaques, edema of the extremity ensues and the tumors ulcerate and bleed. Pain is not associated with this disease process, with the exception of tumors on the soles of the feet and of the penis. Variations to the classic macule, nodule, plaque, ulceration, and edema can also be encountered. In some patients the disease invokes intense fibrous tissue reaction and resembles some type of fibrous tissue tumor. Sometimes the lesions resemble a lymphangioma.

Regional lymphadenopathy is common in all phases of tumor growth. However, a majority of the patients with Kaposi's sarcoma do not have lymph node biopsies, and the extent to which the lymphadenopathy is due to associated infection, edema, or actual node involvement is hard to evaluate. Bhana et al.[156] suggested that regional node involvement from a locally aggressive tumor is more common in older patients.

The clinical presentation of Kaposi's sarcoma, therefore, can be summarized as being of four distinct types: The *nodular* variety is usually indolent and there is seldom regional node involvement; the *florid* form is locally aggres-

sive, with a tendency to fungation and ulceration; the *infiltrative* type invades muscles and bones; and the *lymphadenopathic type* is disseminated and virulent.

In the natural progression of the disease, about half of the patients ultimately have involvement of the submucosa of the gastrointestinal tract (Fig. 16.15A to 16.15C). From the gastrointestinal tract the disease progresses to both lungs, retroperitoneal nodes, thoracic nodes, and bones, in the terminal stages of the disease. Rarely, there is neurologic involvement in the terminal stages of Kaposi's sarcoma.[157]

Deviations from typical cutaneous onset are known to occur. However, prior to Dorffel's[158] monograph in 1932, it was generally believed that all extracutaneous lesions were metastatic, inasmuch as, up to that time, few cases had been described in which the skin lesions were absent or had been preceded by visceral lesions. Since then, several cases have been reported, apparently of primary tumors in the viscera[126,159-164] or other unusual locations.[126,155,164-169] Today, the trend of evidence suggests that Kaposi's sarcoma is a slow-growing, systemic, multicentric disease with long intervals between clinical manifestations in different sites.

Although the multicentricity of Kaposi's sarcoma is generally acknowledged, there are certain sites of clinical presentation that have always aroused considerable clinical interest, and these will be briefly elaborated upon.

Kaposi's Sarcoma of the Head and Neck. Kaposi's sarcoma may occur in the head and neck region, usually in conjunction with cutaneous lesions of the extremities.[126,131,133,153] However, in rare instances the initial manifestation of the disease might be a solitary lesion in the head and neck region. Table 16.8, developed from published reports,[126,148,149,154,166,170,171] shows the involvement of various anatomic sites within the head and neck region. In this series of 77 patients, only in 14 (18 percent) was the head and neck area the initial site of clinical presentation. In the remaining 82 percent, concomitant lesions elsewhere were present. Slavin et al.[133] found five head and neck cases in their series of 117 (4.2 percent). However, these authors cautioned that the incidence in their series might be underestimated because in African patients the only available method of diagnosis was biopsy of the cutaneous lesions. In the present series of 25 patients treated by the author, only

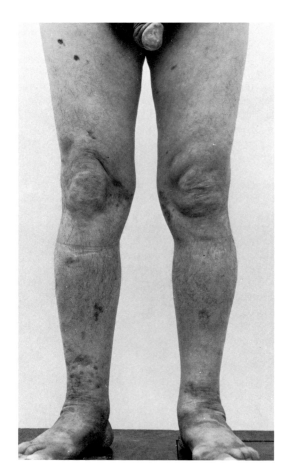

Figure 16.14. **(A)** Kaposi's sarcoma in a 69-year-old man. Note confluence on the anterior aspect of the leg in the ankle region. Several small umbilicated nodules can be seen in the thigh.

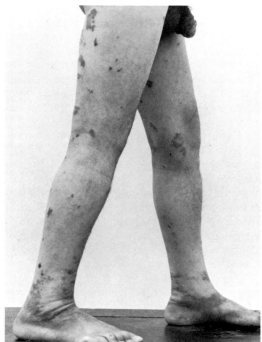

Figure 16.14. **(B)** Same patient; the lesions are progressing proximally. In the lateral aspect several small lesions have coalesced to form plaques.

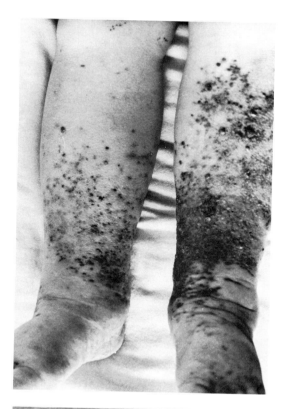

Figure 16.14. (C) Another patient, 65 years old, with extensive confluence of the cutaneous lesions producing "brawny" legs and skin ulcerations. *(Courtesy of Dr. B. Goldsmith, Augustana Hospital, Chicago, Illinois)*

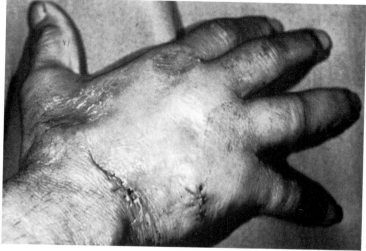

Figure 16.14. (D) Unusual instance of Kaposi's sarcoma involving the upper extremity. Note the flat pigmented lesion at the base of the thumb and index finger. Similar lesions were excised (incisions are seen) and provided the diagnosis.

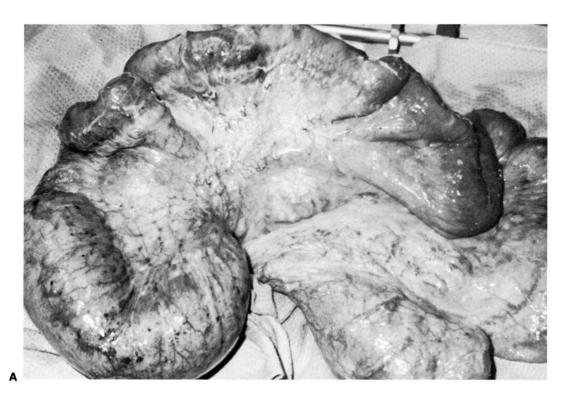

A

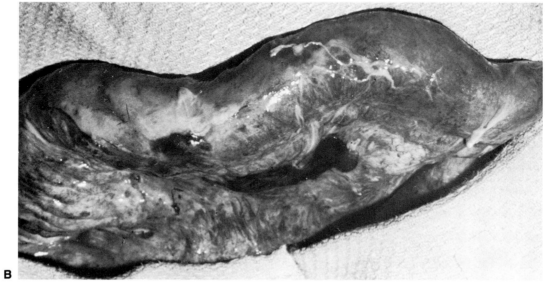

B

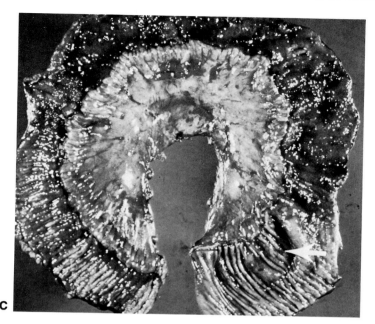

C

Figure 16.15. This 66-year-old man was admitted to the Division of Surgical Oncology of the VA West Side Hospital (Chicago) with evidence of lower gastrointestinal bleeding. Because he was being followed in our clinics for Kaposi's sarcoma, a diagnosis of gastrointestinal tract involvement was made preoperatively and he was operated upon. **(A)** Note the multiple punctate hemorrhagelike spots involving the serosa and the mesentery of the small intestine. On the right corner of the photograph a segment of the ileum appears to be dark with submucosal hemorrhage. **(B)** This segment was excised. The extensive plaquelike involvement of the mesentery is obvious. **(C)** Segment was cut open, showing the extensive segmental involvement of the mucosa and submucosa.

two (8 percent) had lesions in the head and neck region at the time of initial diagnosis. Both lesions were in the scalp and both patients had cutaneous manifestations elsewhere.

Intraoral primary Kaposi's sarcoma is extremely rare.[166] In 1975, Farman and Uys[166] reviewed the published reports and found eight cases and added one of their own. The locations included the palate, tongue, alveolar ridge, and lower lip. These authors[166] operated upon their patient, who died six months later, apparently of unrelated causes. At autopsy, there was no evidence of Kaposi's sarcoma anywhere in the body.

Kaposi's Sarcoma of the Lymph Nodes. In 1962, Ecklund and Valaitis[168] reviewed eight cases of apparent primary Kaposi's sarcoma of the lymph nodes and described one case of their own. Lee and Moore[169] added one more case from the

TABLE 16.8. KAPOSI'S SARCOMA OF THE HEAD AND NECK*

Site	No. Cases	Head and Neck Lesions Only	Coexistent Cutaneous Lesions of the Extremities	% Involvement of the Extremity Lesion
Skin of head and neck	13	—	13	100%
Cervical lymph nodes	4	2	2	50%
Oral cavity and oropharynx	15	1	14	93%
Tongue	4	2	2	50%
Tonsils	2	1	1	50%
Ear	12	4	8	66%
Nose	8	1	7	87%
Larynx	13	—	13	100%
Generalized lymphandenopathy	6	3	3	50%
Total	77	14	63	83%

This table was developed from the following published reports: References 126, 146, 147, 151, 163, 167, 168.

Memorial Sloan-Kettering Cancer Center. Bhana et al.[156] found that 16 (33 percent) of their 48 African patients had nodal disease. Dutz and Stout,[152] in 1960, reviewed 1,256 cases of so-called Kaposi's sarcoma in children under 16 years of age; they accepted 36 cases and added four of their own. In 9 (22.5 percent) of these 40 cases the patients presented with lymph node involvement. The known duration of disease in these nine cases varied from six months to 27 years. In our present series of 25, one patient was seen with initial node involvement, and in seven patients with advanced disease, concomitant lymph node metastases were observed. Bhana et al.[156] concluded that there are probably two main types of nodal involvement. One occurs predominantly in younger patients and involves many groups of lymph nodes. The sarcoma probably develops in situ and is associated with a poor prognosis. The other form is the result of metastases to nodes from an apparently aggressive tumor in the regional area. This type occurs more frequently in older patients and carries a better prognosis than that for generalized lymphadenopathy, though less favorable than that for patients without nodal involvement.

Kaposi's Sarcoma of the Gastrointestinal Tract. Although Kaposi's sarcoma in the late stage of the disease involves the submucosa of the gastrointestinal tract in about 50 percent of patients,[126,134,154,159,164] abdominal symptoms due to relatively localized segmental disease are rare. White and King,[159] in 1964, described two patients who were seen for intra-abdominal pain and intestinal obstruction. During operation, only segmental involvement with Kaposi's sarcoma was noted, and these segments were resected. Both patients required right hemicolectomy. They were apparently well and free of any obvious disease at the time of the report. Adlersberg,[160] in 1970, reported a case of Kaposi's sarcoma associated with ulcerative colitis and found only one other such case in the literature.[161] In our present series, one patient required resection for segmental Kaposi's sarcoma of the ileum and the cecum.

It is not appropriate to either recommend or perform an exploratory celiotomy in all patients with Kaposi's sarcoma who complain of abdominal symptoms. However, in patients in whom the disease is in remission, long-term palliation can be provided by a segmental re-section of the involved portion of the intestine. Preoperative diagnosis of visceral involvement with Kaposi's sarcoma in the absence of any cutaneous manifestation is impossible anywhere outside equatorial Africa.

Infrequently, Kaposi's sarcoma is encountered in the spleen,[158] heart,[170] adrenal,[158] and other unusual sites, but it seldom poses a clinical problem, as it does when occurring in the gastrointestinal tract.

Kaposi's Sarcoma Associated with Other Neoplasms. Since the original description of this entity,[125] reviews on the subject have clearly established the frequent association of Kaposi's sarcoma with other neoplasms, among which lymphomas are the most common.[126,127,131,132,148,153,167,169,170] O'Brien and Brasfield[126] found that 31 percent of their patients died of a second primary cancer.

The association of Kaposi's sarcoma with malignant lymphoma, and particularly with Hodgkin's disease, is well-documented.[126,141,167,172] In his review, Mortel[173] found that, of 54 cases of Hodgkin's disease associated with another tumor, 22 were in patients with Kaposi's sarcoma. Safai and co-workers[172] recently analyzed the data on patients with Kaposi's sarcoma treated at Memorial Sloan-Kettering Cancer Center between 1949 and 1975. By subjecting the data to extensive statistical analysis, they found that (1) 37 percent of patients with Kaposi's sarcoma had other primary malignancies; (2) there was a 20-fold increase in lymphoreticular malignancies after diagnosis of Kaposi's sarcoma; (3) in the Memorial Sloan-Kettering series of double primaries, lymphoreticular malignancies were involved in 8 percent of cases; for Kaposi's sarcoma alone, the corresponding figure was 58 percent.

In our series of 25 patients, three (12 percent) had associated lymphoma, two had Hodgkin's disease, and the third had lymphosarcoma of the stomach.

Although association with lymphoma is relatively well established, association with multiple myeloma is extremely rare.[148,162] Mazzaferri and Penn[174] argued that the low incidence of reported cases probably does not represent the true incidence of multiple myeloma in association with Kaposi's sarcoma. In support of their contention, these authors cited the reported description of moderate bone marrow plasmacytosis by a number of authors.

Primary cutaneous lesions in Kaposi's sarcoma frequently resemble malignant melanoma, but the concomitant appearance of melanoma and Kaposi's sarcoma is rare.[126] Rarely, thymomas have been reported in association with Kaposi's sarcoma.[175]

The association of other tumors, especially lymphomas, with Kaposi's sarcoma may suggest a susceptibility of the host's mesodermal anlage to some type of initiator of malignant change. Perhaps the inducing agent is chemical, viral, or immunosuppressive. One can only speculate whether this susceptibility is controlled genetically or acquired from the environment. It is essential that such patients be clustered and studied for a common denominator of tumor induction.

Treatment. Kaposi's sarcoma in initial stages is extremely radiosensitive, and radiation is the choice of therapy. In most instances the superficial macular lesions completely regress with a dosage of 1,000 to 2,000 rads. Radiation therapy is also effective in recurrent and/or confluent cutaneous lesions. Details of the methods of treatment are given in Chapter 7.

Systemic chemotherapy has been found to be useful in locally advanced cases of Kaposi's sarcoma and in patients with multiple site involvement.[175-179] Several instances are on record in which the use of systemic chemotherapy has produced long-term remission of the disease.

The prognosis for patients with Kaposi's sarcoma should be guarded. Although in the majority of patients the tumors are slow-growing and the disease remains localized for long periods of time, in a number of patients the tumor grows aggressively and centripetally, quickly, and proves fatal.

In the series of 25 patients, the followup has not been sufficiently long to make any definitive statements. Only 14 are suitable for eight-year analysis. Eleven of these are living apparently free of disease and three are living with disease. Two patients died of a second primary cancer, one of a cancer of the pancreas five years after diagnosis of Kaposi's sarcoma, and the other of cancer of the prostate six years after diagnosis of Kaposi's sarcoma. In the series reported by O'Brien and Brasfield[126] of 63 patients at Memorial Sloan-Kettering Cancer Center followed for a prolonged period, only eight were free of disease; 11 were living with Kaposi's sarcoma. These authors concluded that with longer followup the number of patients living free of disease will

likely be smaller. This probably is an accurate reflection of the prognosis for patients with Kaposi's sarcoma. Although long-term remissions can be achieved with the judicious use of radiation therapy and chemotherapy, absolute cure in most patients is perhaps not feasible.

REFERENCES

1. Matthews DN: Hemangiomata. Plast Reconstr Surg 41:528, 1968
2. Pack GT, Miller TR: Hemangiomas: Classification, diagnosis and treatment. Angiology 1:405, 1950
3. Patek AF Jr, Post J, Victor JC: The vascular spider associated with cirrhosis of the liver. Am J Med Sci 200:3417, 1940
4. McNeill TW, Ray RD: Hemangioma of the extremities: Review of 35 cases. Clin Orthopaed Relat Res 101:154, 1974
5. Edgerton MT, Hiebert JM: Vascular and Lymphatic Tumors in Infancy, Childhood and Adulthood: Challenge of Diagnosis and Treatment. Current Problems in Cancer, II, no. 7. Chicago, Year Book Medical Publishers, 1978
6. Goldwin RM, Rosoff CB: Cryosurgery for large hemangioma in adults. Plast Reconstr Surg 43:605, 1969
7. Pack GT, Ariel IR: Tumors of the Soft Somatic Tissues, Chapter 19. New York, Hoeber/Harper, 1958, p 384
8. Attar S, Cowley A: Hemangioma of the mediastinum: Collective review and case report. Am Surg 30:141, 1964
9. Pack GT: Unusual tumors of the stomach. Ann NY Acad Sci 114:985, 1964
10. Niemann F, Penitschka W: Die kavernosen Haemangiome "Kavernoma" der Leber. Bruns Beitr Klin Chir 195:257, 1957
11. Shumacker HB Jr: Hemangioma of the liver. Surgery 11:209, 1942
12. Hendrick JG: Hemangioma of the liver causing death in newborn infant. J Pediatr 32:309, 1948
13. Brunschwig A, Smith RR: Large hemangioma of the liver: Successful excision. Ann Surg 135:124, 1952
14. Wilson H, Tyson WT: Massive hemangioma of the liver. Ann Surg 135:766, 1952
15. Matsuo I: Hemangioma of the liver, complicated with massive intra-abdominal hemorrhage. Tokyo Med J 70:104, 1953
16. Henson SW Jr, Gray HK, Dockerty MB: Benign tumor of the liver. Surg Gynecol Obstet 103:327, 1956
17. Sewell JH, Weiss K: Spontaneous rupture of hemangiomata of the liver. Arch Surg 83:729, 1961
18. Krippaehne WW, Herr RH: Resection of massive hemangiomas of the liver. Surg Gynecol Obstet 116:761, 1963
19. Muehlbauer MA, Farber MG: Hemangioma of the liver. Am J Gastroenterol 45:355, 1966

20. Stone HH, Nielson IC: Hemangioma of the liver in the newborn: Report of a successful outcome following hepatic lobectomy. Arch Surg 90:319, 1965

21. Kato M, Sugawara I, Okada A, et al: Hemangioma of the liver: Diagnosis with combined use of laparoscopy and hepatic arteriography. Am J Surg 129:698, 1975

22. Backman L, Ohman U: Hemangioma of striated muscle: Report of a case. Acta Chir Scand 134:160, 1968

23. Jones KG: Cavernous hemangioma of striated muscle. J Bone Joint Surg 35-A:717, 1953

24. Heitzman E Jr, Jones B: Roentgen characteristics of cavernous hemangioma of striated muscle. Radiology 74:420, 1960

25. Unnik K, Ivins JC, Beabout JW, Dahlin DC: Hemangioma: hemangiopericytoma and hemangioendothelioma (angiosarcoma) of bone. Cancer 27:1403, 1971

26. Dahlin DC: Benign vascular tumors. In Bone Tumors. Springfield (Ill), Thomas, 1978, p 137

27. Lindau A: Studien uber Kleinhirncysten. Bau, Pathogenese und Beziehungen zur angiomatosis retinae. Acta Path Microbiol Scand (suppl) 1:1, 1926

28. Bielschowsky M: Entwurf eines Systems der Heyredodegene rationen des Zentrolnervens systems einsch liesslich der zugehorigen Striatumer Krankungen. J Physchol Neurol Leipz 24:48, 1918

29. Van der Hoeve T: Eye disease in tuberous sclerosis of the brain and in Recklinghausen's disease. Trans Ophthalmol Soc UK 43:534, 1923

30. Van der Hoeve T: Eye symptoms in phakomatoses: The Doyne Memorial Lecture. Trans Ophthalmol Soc UK 52:380, 1932

31. Van der Hoeve T: Eine vierte phakomatoses. Ber Keutsch Ophthalmol Ges 51:136, 1936

32. Von Recklinghausen FD: Ein herz von einem neugebornen welches mehrere theils nach aussen, theils nach den hohlen prominierende tumoren (Myomen) trug Ver handl. Ges Geburtsch 15, 1863

33. Murad TM, Von Haam E, Murthy MSN: Ultrastructure of a hemangiopericytoma and a glomus tumor. Cancer 22:1239, 1968

34. Battifora H: Hemangiopericytoma: Ultrastructural study of five cases. Cancer 31:1418, 1973

35. Tocker C: Glomangioma: An ultrastructural study. Cancer 23:487, 1969

36. Venkatachalan MA, Greally JG: Fine structure of glomus tumor: similarity of glomus cells to smooth muscle. Cancer 23:1176, 1969

37. Tarnowski WM, Hashimoto K: Multiple glomus tumors: An ultrastructural study. J Invest Derm 52:474, 1969

38. Brindley GV: Glomus tumor of the mediastinum. J Thor Surg 18:417, 1949

39. Appelman HD, Helwig EB: Glomus tumors of the stomach. Cancer 23:203, 1969

40. Banner EA, Winkelman RK: Glomus tumor of vagina: Report of a case. Obstet Gynecol 9:326, 1957

40A. Tsuneyoshi M, Enjoji M: Glomus tumor: A clinicopathologic and electron microscopic study. Cancer 50:1601, 1981

41. McCarthy WD, Pack GT: Malignant blood vessel tumors: A report of 56 cases of angiosarcoma and Kaposi's sarcoma. Surg Gynecol Obstet 91:465, 1950

42. Girard C, Hohnson WC, Graham IH: Cutaneous angiosarcoma. Cancer 26:868, 1970

43. Bardwil JM, Mocega EE, Butler JJ, Russin DJ: Angiosarcoma of the head and neck region. Am J Surg 116:548, 1968

44. Farr HW, Carandang CM, Huvos AG: Malignant vascular tumors of head and neck. Am J Surg 120:501, 1970

45. Kalisher L, Straatsma GW, Rosenberg BF, Vaitkevicius VK: Primary malignant hemangioendothelioma of the greater omentum. A case report. Cancer 22:1126, 1968

46. Stout APO, Hendry J, Purdie J: Primary solid tumors of the great omentum. Cancer 16:231, 1963

47. Gill W, McGregor JD: Malignant haemangioendothelioma. J Roy Coll Surgeons (Edin) 365:155, 1968

48. Stout AP: Hemangioendothelioma of the breast. Ann Surg 118:445, 1943

49. Enticknap JB: Angioblastoma of the breast complicating pregnancy. Br Med J 2:51, 1946

50. Mallory TB, Castleman B, Parris EE: Hemangiosarcoma of the breast. N Engl J Med 241:241, 1949

51. Batchelor GB: Haemangioblastoma of the breast. Br J Surg 46:647, 1959

52. Steingaszner LC, Enzinger FM, Taylor HB: Hemangiosarcoma of the breast. Cancer 18:352, 1965

53. Chen K, Kirkegaard D, Bocian J: Angiosarcoma of the breast. Cancer 46:368, 1980

54. Migliori E: Angiosarcoma of the breast. Tumori 63:199, 1977

55. Gulesserian HP, Lawton RL: Angiosarcoma of the breast. Cancer 24:1021, 1969

56. Antman KH, Corson J, Greenberger J, Wilson R: Multimodality therapy in the management of angiosarcoma of the breast. Cancer 50:2000, 1982

57. Kessler E, Kozenitsky IL: Haemangiosarcoma of the breast. J Clin Path 24:530, 1971

58. Dunegan LJ, Tobon H, Watson CG: Angiosarcoma of the breast: A report of two cases and a review of the literature. Surgery 79:57, 1976

59. Wollstein M: Malignant hemangioma of the lung with multiple visceral foci. Arch Path 12:562, 1931

60. Packard GB, Palmer HD: Primary neoplasms of the liver in infants and children. Ann Surg 142:214, 1955

61. Edmonton HA: Differential diagnosis of tumors and tumorlike lesions of the liver in infancy and childhood. Am J Dis Child 91:168, 1956

62. Das Gupta TK, Coombes B, Brasfield RD: Primary malignant neoplasms of the spleen. Surg Gynecol Obstet 120:947, 1965

63. Blumenfeld TA, Fleming ID, Johnson WW: Juvenile hemangioendothelioma of the liver: Report of a case and review of the literature. Cancer 24:853, 1969

64. Alpert LI, Benisch B: Hemangioendothelioma of the liver associated with microangiopathic hemolytic anemia: Report of four cases. Am J Med 48:624, 1970

65. Truell JE, Peck SD, Reiquam CW: Hemangiosarcoma of the liver complicated by disseminated intravascular coagulation. Gastroenterology 65:936, 1973

66. Strohl KP: Angiosarcoma of the heart. Arch Intern Med 136:928, 1976

67. Rossi NP, Kioschos JM, Achenbrener CA, Ehrenhaft JL: Primary angiosarcoma of the heart. Cancer 37:891, 1976

68. Nagasue N, Ogawa Y, Inokuchi K: Hemangiosarcoma of liver and spleen treated by hepatic artery ligation, intraportal infusion chemotherapy, and splenectomy. Cancer 38:1386, 1976

69. McMahon HE, Murphy AS, Bates M: Endothelial cell sarcoma of the liver following Thorotrast injection. Am J Path 23:585, 1947

70. da Silva HJ, Abbott JD, Cayolla da Mott L, et al: Malignancy and other late effects following administration of Thorotrast. Lancet 2:201, 1965

71. Regelson W, Kim U, Ospina J, et al: Hemangioendothelial sarcoma of liver from chronic arsenic intoxication by Fowler's solution. Cancer 21:514, 1968

72. Creech JL Jr, Johnson MN: Angiosarcoma of the liver in the manufacture of polyvinyl chloride. J Occup Med 16:150, 1974

73. Block JB: Angiosarcoma of the liver following vinyl chloride exposure. JAMA 229:53, 1974

74. Lloyd JW: Angiosarcoma of the liver in vinyl chloride/polyvinyl chloride workers. J Occup Med 16:809, 1974

75. Heath CW, Falk H, Creech JL: Characteristics of cases of angiosarcoma of the liver among vinyl chloride workers in the United States. Ann NY Acad Sci 246:1975

76. Lander JJ, Stanley RJ, Sumner HW, et al: Angiosarcoma of the liver associated with Fowler's solution (potassium arsenite). Gastroenterology 68:1582, 1975

77. Popper H: The heuristic importance of environmental pathology: Lessons from the vinyl chloride program. Arch Path 99:71, 1975

78. Thomas LB, Popper H, Berk PD, et al: Vinylchloride-induced liver disease: From idiopathic portal hypertension (Banti's syndrome) to angiosarcomas. N Engl J Med 292:17, 1975

79. Doll R: Discussion, Toxicity of vinyl chloride—polyvinyl chloride. Ann NY Acad Sci 246:320, 1975

80. Editorial: Vinyl chloride and cancer. Canad Med Assoc J 112:269, 1975

81. Fiechtner JJ, Reyes CN Jr: Angiosarcoma of the liver in a rural population: Four cases diagnosed in a 29-month period. JAMA 236:1704, 1976

82. Dalderup LM, Freni SC, Bras G, et al: Angiosarcoma of the liver. Lancet 1:246, 1976

83. Weingrad DN, Rosenberg SA: Early lymphatic spread of osteogenic and soft tissue sarcomas. Surgery 231, 1978

84. Theile FS: Uber Angiome und sarkomatose Angiome der Milz. Virchows Arch Path Anat 178:296, 1904

85. McNeer GP, Cantin J, Chu F, Nickson JJ: Effectiveness of radiation therapy in the management of sarcoma of the soft somatic tissues. Cancer 22:391, 1968

86. Pinedo HM, Kenis Y: Chemotherapy of advanced soft tissue sarcomas in adults. Cancer Treat Rev 4:67, 1977

87. Schmidt GB: Uber das Angiosarkom der Mamma. Arch Klin Chir 26:121, 1887

88. Borrman R: Metastasenaildung bei histologisch gutartign Geschwülsten. Beitr Path Anat 40:372, 1907

89. Shore JH: Hemangiosarcoma of the breast. J Path 74:289, 1957

90. Topuzlu C, Andrews WE, Trainer TK, Caccavo FA: Angiosarcoma of the carotid body. Am J Surg 117:400, 1969

90A. Bennett MT, Weber PM, Killebrew ET: Primary angiosarcoma of the heart detected by technetium-labeled erythrocyte cardiac imaging. Cancer 49:2587, 1982

91. Alrenga DP: Primary angiosarcoma of the liver. Int J Surg 60:198, 1975

92. Aranha GV, Gold J, Grage TB: Hemangiosarcoma of the spleen: Report of a case and review of previously reported cases. J Surg Oncol 8:481, 1976

93. Autry JR, Weitzner S: Hemangiosarcoma of spleen with spontaneous rupture. Cancer 35:534, 1975

94. Garlock JH: Primary angiosarcoma of the spleen. Mt Sinai J Med NY 6:319, 1940

95. Smith C, Rusk G: Endothelioma of the spleen. Arch Surg 7:371, 1923

96. Ferrara G, Shione R: L'Angiosarcoma primitivo della milza. Rass Fisiopat Clin 27:759, 1955

97. Bourne M, Cook T, Williams G: Hemangiosarcomatosis—Two cases presenting as hematologic problems. Br Med J 213:275, 1965

98. Wilkinson H, Lucas J, Foote T: Primary splenic angiosarcoma. Arch Path 85:213, 1968

99. Castrup HJ, Lennartz KJ: Haemangiosarkom der Milz. Zentrabl Allg Path 113:395, 1970

100. Donald D, Dawson D: Microangiopathic hemolytic anemia associated with hemangioendothelioma. J Clin Path 24:456, 1971

101. Toghill PJ, Rigby C, Hall G: Hemangiosarcoma of the spleen. Br J Surg 59:406, 1972

102. Stutz F, Tormey PC, Blom J: Hemangiosarcoma and pathologic rupture of the spleen. Cancer 31:1213, 1973

103. Hopfner C, Dufour M, Bluot M, Caulet T: Hemangioendotheliosarcoma splenique avec erythrophagocytose et angiopathie thrombotique. Virchows Arch Path Anat 356:66, 1975

104. Stein J: Hemangioendothelioma of the testes. J Urol 113:201, 1975

104A. Ongkasuwan C, Taylor JE, Tang C, Prempree T: Angiosarcomas of the uterus and ovary: A clinicopathologic report. Cancer 49:1469, 1982

105. Conway JD, Smith MB: Hemangioendothelioma originating in a peripheral nerve. Ann Surg 134:138, 1951

106. Bricklin AS, Rushton HW: Angiosarcoma of venous origin in radial nerve. Cancer 39:1556, 1977

107. Stout AP, Murray MR: Hemangiopericytoma: A vascular tumor featuring Zimmerman's pericytes. Ann Surg 116:26, 1942

108. Stout AP: Hemangiopericytoma: A study of twenty-five new cases. Cancer 2:1027, 1949

109. Maltoni C, Lefemine G: Carcinogenicity bioassays of vinyl chloride: Current results. Ann NY Acad Sci 245:175, 1975

110. Prout MN, Davis HL Jr: Hemangiopericytoma of the bladder after polyvinyl alcohol exposure. Cancer 39:1328, 1977

111. Enzinger M, Smith BH: Hemangiopericytoma: An analysis of 106 cases. Human Path 7:61, 1976

112. McMaster MJ, Soule EH, Ivins JC: Hemangiopericytoma: A clinicopathologic study and long-term followup of 60 patients. Cancer 36:2232, 1975

113. O'Brien B, Brasfield RD: Hemangiopericytoma. Cancer 18:249, 1965

114. Backwinkle KD, Diddams JA: Hemangiopericytoma: Report of a case and comprehensive review of the literature. Cancer 25:896, 1970

115. Angerval L, Kindblom LG, Nielsen JM, Stener B, Svendsen P: Hemangiopericytoma: A clinicopathologic, angiographic and microangiographic study. Cancer 42:4212, 1978

116. McCormack LJ, Gallivan WP: Hemangiopericytoma. Cancer 7:595, 1954

117. Ferguson JO, Clagett OT, McDonald JR: Hemangiopericytoma (glomus tumor) of the mediastinum—Review of literature and report of case. Surgery 36:320, 1954

118. Ernst CB, Abell MR, Kahn DR: Malignant hemangiopericytoma of the stomach. Surgery 58:351, 1965

119. Spiro RH, Brockunier A, Brunscwig A: Pelvic hemangiopericytoma. Obstet Gynecol 24:402, 1964

120. Wilbanks GD, Szymanska Z, Miller AW: Pelvic hemangiopericytoma: Report of four patients and review of the literature. Am J Obstet Gynecol 123:555, 1975

121. Baglio CM, Growson CN: Hemangiopericytoma of urachus: Report of a case. J Urol 91:660, 1964

122. Lenczyk JM: Nasal hemangiopericytoma. Arch Otolaryngol 87:110, 1968

123. Lal H, Sanyal B, Pant GC, et al: Hemangiopericytoma: Report of three cases regarding role of radiation therapy. Am J Roentgenol, Rad Ther, Nuclear Med 126:887, 1976

124. Mira JG, Chu FCH, Fortner JG: The role of radiotherapy in the management of malignant hemangiopericytoma. Report of eleven new cases and review of the literature. Cancer 39:1254, 1977

125. Kaposi M: Idiopathisches multiples pigmet Sarkom der Haut. Arch Derm Syph 4:265, 1872

126. O'Brien PH, Brasfield RD: Kaposi's sarcoma. Cancer 19:1497, 1966

127. Rothman S: Some clinical aspects of Kaposi's sarcoma in the European population. Acta Un Int Cancer 18:382, 1962

128. Lee FD: A comparative study of Kaposi's sarcoma and granuloma pyogenicum in Uganda. J Clin Path 21:119, 1966

129. Taylor JF, Smith PG, Bull D, Pike MC: Kaposi's sarcoma in Uganda—Geographic and ethnic distribution. Br J Cancer 26:483, 1972

130. Taylor JF, Templeton AC, Bogel CL, Ziegler J, Kyalwazi SK: Kaposi's sarcoma in Uganda—A clinical pathological study. Int J Cancer 22:122, 1971

131. Gordon JA: Kaposi's sarcoma: A review of 136 Rhodesian African cases. Postgrad Med J 43:513, 1967

132. Oettle AG: Geographical and racial differences in the frequency of Kaposi's sarcoma as evidence of environmental or genetic causes. Acta Un Int Cancer 18:331, 1962

133. Slavin G, Cameron HM, Singh H: Kaposi's sarcoma in mainland Tanzania: A report of 117 cases. Br J Cancer 23:349, 1969

134. Oettle AG: Geographical and racial differences in the frequency of Kaposi's sarcoma as evidence of environmental or genetic causes. In Symposium on Kaposi's Sarcoma. Monograph No. 2, African Cancer Committee of the International Union Against Cancer. New York, Karger, 1963, p 17

135. Elmes BG, Baldwin RBJ: Malignant disease in Nigeria: An analysis of a thousand tumors. Ann Trop Med Parasit 41:321, 1944

136. Edington GM: Malignant disease in the Gold Coast. Br J Cancer 10:595, 1956

137. Thijs A: Considerations sur les tumeurs malignes des indigenes du Congo Belge et du Ruande—Urundi. A propos de 2536 cas. Ann Soc belge Med Trop 37:295, 1957

138. Higginson J, Oettle A: Cancer incidence in the Bantu and "Cape Colored" races of South Africa: Report of a cancer survey in the Transvaal (1953 to 1955). J Nat Cancer Inst 24:589, 1960

139. Timms GL: Personal communication (1961) quoted by Oettle AG, 1962

140. Lothe F: Kaposi's sarcoma in Ugandan Africans. Oslo (Universitets-forlaget), 1963

141. Gilbert TT, Evjy JT, Edelstein L: Hodgkin's disease associated with Kaposi's sarcoma and malignant melanoma: Case report of multiple primary malignancies. Cancer 28:293, 1971

142. Master SP, Taylor JF, Kyalwazi SK, Ziegler JL: Immunological studies in Kaposi's sarcoma and malignant melanoma: Case report of multiple primary malignancies. Cancer 28:293, 1971

143. Hardy MA, Goldfarb P, Levine S, et al: De novo Kaposi's sarcoma in renal transplantation: Case report and brief review. Cancer 38:144, 1976

144. Dobozy B: Immune deficiencies and Kaposi's sarcoma (Letter). Lancet 1:625, 1973

145. Haim S, Shafir A, Better DS, et al: Kaposi's sarcoma in association with immunosuppressive therapy. Isr J Med Sci 8:1993, 1972

146. Myers BD, Kessler E, Levi J, Pick A, Rosenfield JB: Kaposi's sarcoma in kidney transplant recipients. Arch Inter Med 133:370, 1974

147. Taylor JF: Lymphocyte transformation in Kaposi's sarcoma (Letter). Lancet 2:883, 1973

148. Reynolds WA, Winkelman RK, Soule EH: Kaposi's sarcoma. Medicine 44:419, 1965

149. Mazzaferri EL, Penn GM: Kaposi's sarcoma associated with multiple myeloma. Arch Intern Med 122:521, 1968
150. Giraldo G, Beth E, Coeur P, Vogel CI, Dhru DS: A new model in search for viruses associated with human malignancies. J Nat Cancer Inst 49:1496, 1972
151. Friedman-Kien AE: Disseminated Kaposi's sarcoma in young homosexual men. J Am Acad Derm 5(4-6):468, 1981
152. Dutz W, Stout AP: Kaposi's sarcoma in infants and children. Cancer 13:684, 1960
153. Cook J: Kaposi's sarcoma. J Roy Coll Surg (Edin) 2:519, 1966
154. Bluefarb SM: Kaposi's sarcoma: Multiple Idiopathic Hemorrhagic Sarcoma. Springfield (Ill), Thomas, 1957, p 123
155. Ackerman LV, Murray JF: Symposium en Kaposi's sarcoma. Acta Un Int Cancer 18:311, 1962
156. Bhana D, Templeton AC, Master SP, Kyalwazi SK: Kaposi's sarcoma of lymph nodes. Br J Cancer 15:464, 1970
157. Gonzalez-Crussi F, Mossemen A, Robertson DM: Neurological involvement in Kaposi's sarcoma. Canad Med Assoc J 100:481, 1969
158. Dorffel J: Histogenesis of multiple idiopathic hemorrhagic sarcoma of Kaposi's sarcoma. Arch Derm Syph 26:608, 1932
159. White JAM, King MJ: Kaposi's sarcoma presenting with abdominal symptoms. Gastroenterology 46:197, 1964
160. Adlersberg R: Kaposi's sarcoma complicating ulcerative colitis: Report of a case. Am J Clin Path 54:143, 1970
161. Gordon HW, Rywlin AM: Kaposi's sarcoma of the large intestine associated with ulcerative colitis. A hitherto unreported occurrence. Gastroenterology 50:248, 1966
162. Gellin GA: Kaposi's sarcoma: Three cases of which two have unusual findings in association. Arch Derm 94:92, 1966
163. Stats D: Visceral manifestations of Kaposi's sarcoma. J Mt Sinai Hosp NY 12:971, 1946
164. Siegel JH, Janis R, Alper JC, et al: Disseminated visceral Kaposi's sarcoma: Appearance after human renal homograft operation. JAMA 207:1493, 1969
165. Gibbs RC, Hyman AB: Kaposi's sarcoma at the base of a cutaneous horn. Arch Derm 98:37, 1968
166. Farman AG, Uys PB: Oral Kaposi's sarcoma. Oral Surg 39:288, 1975
167. Rajka G: Kaposi's sarcoma associated with Hodgkin's disease. Acta Dermatovener 45:40, 1965
168. Ecklund RE, Valaitis J: Kaposi's sarcoma of lymph nodes: A case report. Arch Path 74:244, 1962
169. Lee SCH, Moore OS: Kaposi's sarcoma of lymph nodes. Arch Path 80:651, 1965
170. Cox FH, Helwig EB: Kaposi's sarcoma. Cancer 12:289, 1959
171. Gibbs R: Kaposi's sarcoma involving ears. Arch Derm 98:104, 1968
172. Safai B, Mike V, Giraldo G, Beth E, Good RA: Association of Kaposi's sarcoma with second primary malignancies; Possible etiopathologic implications. Cancer 45:1472, 1980
173. Mortel CC: Multiple primary malignant neoplasms, their incidence and significance. In Recent Results in Cancer Research, vol 7. New York, Springer-Verlag 1966, p 34
174. Mazzaferri EL, Penn GM: Kaposi's sarcoma associated with multiple myeloma. Arch Int Med 122:521, 1968
175. Maberry JD, Stone OJ: Kaposi's sarcoma with thymoma. Arch Derm 95:210, 1967
176. Scott WP, Voight JA: Kaposi's sarcoma: Management with vincaleucoblastine. Cancer 19:557, 1966
177. Vogel CL, Templeton CJ, Templeton AC, Taylor JF, Kyalwazi SK: Treatment of Kaposi's sarcoma with actinomycin D and cyclophosphamide: Results of a randomized clinical trial. Int J Cancer 8:136, 1971
178. Vogel CL, Primack A, Dhru D, et al: Treatment of a Kaposi's sarcoma with a combination of actinomycin D and vincristine: Results of a randomized clinical trial. Cancer 51:1382, 1973
179. Vogel CL, Clements D, Wanume DK, et al: Phase II clinical trials of BCNU (NSC-409962) and bleomycin (NSC-125066) in the treatment of Kaposi's sarcoma. Cancer Chemother Rep 57:325, 1973

17

Tumors of the Lymphatic Tissue

Tapas K. Das Gupta

Tumor and tumorlike conditions of the lymphatic tissue can be clinically divided as follows:

A. Benign
1. Lymphangiomas
   a. Papillary
   b. Cavernous
   c. Cystic hygroma
2. Lymphangiectasis
   a. Local
   b. Regional
3. Lymphedema
   a. Congenital
   b. Acquired
4. Lymphangiomyoma
B. Malignant
1. Lymphangiosarcoma
   a. Postmastectomy (Stewart-Treves syndrome)
   b. Not associated with mastectomy
2. Extranodal lymphomas
3. Extramedullary plasmacytomas

BENIGN TUMORS

Lymphangioma

Lymphangiomas are less common than hemangiomas but, although benign, they possess a remarkable power for continued growth, infiltration, and progressive extension over adjacent skin throughout childhood and adolescence, and occasionally even in adult life. Invariably, they are congenital malformations of the lymphatic system, and most are manifest in infancy. The condition of lymphangiectasis with edema due to lymphatic obstruction is not to be confused with the aforementioned lymphangiomas, which are hamartomatous growths. Nevertheless, lymphangiectasis or chronic lymphatic obstruction due to any cause should be considered in this relationship because it is sometimes a preneoplastic state resulting ultimately in lymphangiosarcoma.

Lymphangiomas can conceptually be viewed as blockage of lymphatic channels in any given location, with resultant ectasia of the channels and proliferation and infiltration of the surrounding structures. Their anatomic confines frequently determine their size, shape, and clinical characteristics. Because of this, lymphangiomas can be classified into three types: (1) simple or papillary, (2) cavernous, and (3) cystic hygroma.

Simple or Papillary Lymphangioma. The simple or papillary type is composed of agminated minute lymphatic cysts situated superficially in the skin and subcutaneous tissue and in the mucous membrane of the oral cavity.

Cavernous Lymphangioma. This type is usually more discrete, of greater bulk, situated subcutaneously, and compressible but not fluctuant (Fig. 17.1). It is supported by a fibrous tissue lattice, and interspersed between the lattice small multilocular cysts lined with smooth endothelial membrane containing lymph can be seen. The superadjacent skin may or may not be involved by tiny wartlike blobs which are pathognomonic of lymphangiomas. The cavernous variety is found in deeper locations where the anatomic boundaries prevent the development of large saccules, such as occurs in cystic hygromas. This type of lymphangioma is commonly encountered in the extremities, the trunk, the retroperitoneum, and the viscera.

Table 17.1 shows the incidence of cavernous lymphangiomas in different sites. Unlike cystic hygromas, they are relatively uncommon and sometimes are associated with hemangiomas. Eight (28.5 percent) of 28 patients in Fonkalsrud's[1] group had associated hemangiomas. In our series of six cases in the extremities, three were associated with hemangiomas.

Of the other locations of cavernous lymphangioma (Table 17.1), Bill and Sumner[2] found five in the mediastinum and one in the mesentery. In our present series one was in the pancreas, one in the retroperitoneum, and one in the pelvis. This tumor occurs with about equal frequency in both sexes.

The most common complaint is the presence of a gradually enlarging mass. Rapid expansion may be produced by hemorrhage or infection. In infancy, respiratory distress sometimes occurs if these lesions are located in the throat and neck, and may require emergency intervention. Although most of these lesions are diagnosed in infancy and childhood,[1-5] they occasionally are encountered in adult life, particularly in the viscera, retroperitoneum, and mediastinum.[2,6-15] In our present series, one retroperitoneal lymphangioma was encountered. This was in a 19-year-old boy with a history of a gradually enlarging abdomen for the previous three months. Clinical examination suggested ascites, but paracentesis revealed clear fluid, which yielded no clue regarding cytologic diagnosis. All the radiologic examinations were inconclusive as to the nature of the abdominal disease. He was operated upon and an enormous cyst was found completely filling the abdominal cavity. The cyst was excised in its entirety. The microscopic diagnosis was cystic and cavernous lymphangioma. Seven years later he is still free of any evidence of recurrence.

In general, cavernous lymphangioma requires complete excision in most anatomic sites. For infants, if possible, the operation should be delayed. In symptomatic and enlarging lesions, this luxury of waiting must sometimes be foregone and early operation becomes mandatory.[4] In some patients complete excision is not possible, and staged resections are necessary. Staged procedures become essential in large lymphangiomas of the head and neck region, for example, those involving the tongue,[16] the floor of the mouth, and the cheek. The need for staged

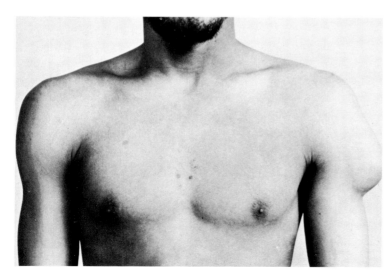

Figure 17.1. Simple papillary lymphangioma of the arm in a 29-year-old man. The lesion, 6 × 5 cm, was totally excised.

TABLE 17.1. ANATOMIC DISTRIBUTION OF CAVERNOUS LYMPHANGIOMAS IN FOUR SERIES*

Site	Harkins and Sabiston[4] (1960)	Bill and Sumner[2] (1965)	Fonkalsrud[1] (1974)	Das Gupta (1981)
Head and neck	14	35	9	3
Trunk	2	18	7	1
Lower extremity	8	3	9	4
Upper extremity	3	21	3	2
Other locations	–	6	–	3
Total	27	83	28	13

The areas involved are tabulated rather than the total number of cases. Thus a single extensive tumor involving the neck, axilla, and upper arm has been recorded three times.

excision of extensive lymphangiomas of the trunk and the extremities is relatively infrequent (Fig. 17.2A and 17.2B). Amputation of an extremity for extensive lymphangioma has been reported by Harkins and Sabiston,[4] but the need for such an operation is extremely rare and every effort should be made to avoid it. There is no evidence that a benign lymphangioma can become malignant, and therefore an aggressive surgical approach such as amputation must be tempered

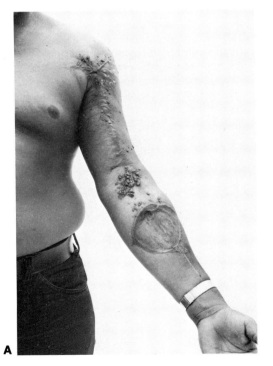
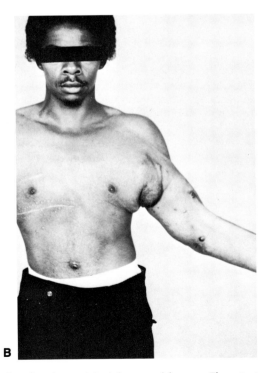

Figure 17.2. (A) A 46-year-old man with extensive cutaneous lymphangioma of the left arm and forearm. The extent of the skin involvement abruptly ends at the left shoulder. He sought medical opinion because of constant rupture of the cystlike spaces and persistent drainage complicated by recurrent episodes of infection. The skin graft area shows the area of first excision, which was performed two years prior to his visit to the University of Illinois Hospital. Since then, he has required four staged excisions, with gratifying results. **(B)** A 26-year-old man with extensive involvement of the left upper extremity with both cavernous and papillary lymphangiomas (anterior view).

with judicious conservatism. Rarely, a lymphangioma infiltrating the surrounding structure makes either a part or all of the extremity totally useless, and under these circumstances an amputation might be indicated. Radiation therapy for lymphangioma has been tried,[3,4] but it should be avoided in the management of a benign lesion.

A visceral lymphangioma certainly requires total extirpation. Rarely, lymphangiomas of the pancreas[10,12,14,17] and duodenum[15] have been described, but the exact incidence is impossible to assess. Usually, only larger lesions in certain unusual sites in the gastrointestinal tract are reported.

The author has encountered two instances of cavernous lymphangioma of the pancreas. One patient with involvement of the head of the pancreas was seen in consultation. After a pancreaticoduodenectomy performed elsewhere, she is doing well and apparently is back to normal activity. The second patient was an 18-year-old boy who was operated upon by the author (Fig. 17.3). Lymphangioma involved the body and neck of the pancreas. He was treated by subtotal pancreatectomy and is still well five years later.

Lymphangiomas of the Bone. The first case of lymphangioma of the bone was reported by Bickel and Broders[18] in 1947. The patient was a 5-year-old girl. Several additional cases in all age groups have since been reported.[19-26] The lesion in some instances progresses to multiple pathologic fractures and in other instances remains stationary for a long period of time. Similar to several other pathologic types, the lesion is seen in x-rays as a lytic defect in the shafts of the long bones. Therefore, the diagnosis is

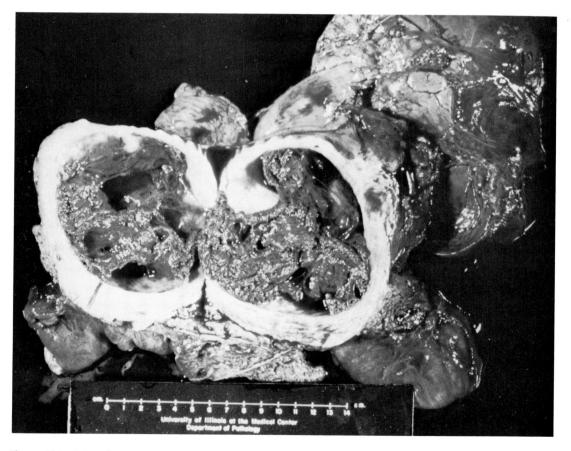

Figure 17.3. Subtotal pancreatectomy specimen showing a large lymphangioma of the body and tail of pancreas. Patient's mother first noticed a small epigastric mass when he was 6 years old.

always made after a biopsy. No specific form of therapy is known for this entity.

Cystic Hygroma. Cystic hygroma is the generally accepted term for a lymphangioma that arises in the posterior cervical triangle or supraclavicular fossa (Fig. 17.4). However, these lymphatic cysts also occur in other parts of the head and neck, axillae, and the groin as well.[1-5] In general, the larger lesions are found in close proximity to the large veins and lymphatic ducts.[1,2] Groups of hyperplastic nodes are frequently present.

The patient presents with a painless mass in the neck (Fig. 17.4). The cyst may become evident only after trauma or an upper respiratory tract infection. The natural history varies from progressive, static, or intermittent growth to rare regressive spontaneous disappearance.[1,4,27] Although congenital, these tumors are not always evident at birth, when perhaps 75 percent are noted.[1,4,5] Some 90 percent are found by age 2 years, although the age may vary from the newborn to the late thirties. Rarely, the lesion arises de novo in adults.

Signs and symptoms may include distortion of the face or neck; respiratory stridor with cyanosis by compression or mediastinal extension; dysphagia secondary to inflammation, infection, or compression; spontaneous infection with concomitant upper respiratory tract infection; sudden size increase by spontaneous hemorrhage, which may be fatal; and brachial plexus compression with pain or hyperesthesia.

These tumors are diffuse and poorly circumscribed. The overlying skin is usually normal, but if it is thinned by stretching, atrophy of the subcutaneous tissue may occur. Blue venous coloration and light transmission may result. On palpation, the tumors are soft, nontender, noncompressible, poorly delineated, cystic, and often adherent to the skin. Trabeculations or fibrotic areas may be palpable within the bulk of the mass. Usually located beneath the platysma muscle, they may penetrate deeply into the neck and perhaps extend into the mediastinum or axilla.

The treatment of cystic hygromas is excision as soon as it is feasible. However, keen judgment must be exercised to avoid injury to the nerves in the neck during resection of a tumor that in most instances is only cosmetically deforming. We have seen infants whose accessory nerve or hypoglossal nerve, or both, have been injured during operation for a cystic hygroma. Excision of hygromas must not be undertaken when the cyst is inflamed or in-

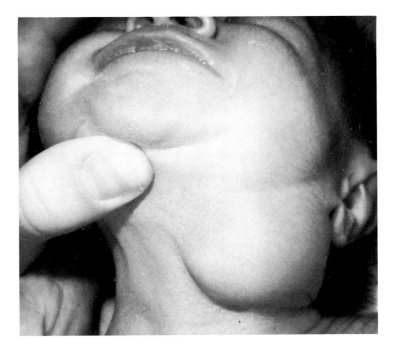

Figure 17.4. Cystic hygroma in a newborn. This was excised without any difficulty eight years ago.

fected. Recurrence is rare after adequate excision.

Lymphangiectasis

This disorder is an uncommon malformation of infancy and childhood resulting in chylous ascites or chylothorax. Fonkalsrud[1] described his experience with eight children, five boys and three girls. He found a variety of lymphatic involvements. Four children had multiple small lymphangiectatic cysts of the mesentery, three had similar cystic involvement of the mediastinum, and one had both mediastinal and intraabdominal lymphatic cysts. Chylous ascites was noted in two children and chylothorax in one. Treatment of these lesions is indeed problematic. Total excision of all the cysts is sometimes impossible. Frequently, partial resection and unroofing has to be resorted to, but this method results in recurrence of the ascites. Fonkalsrud[1] commented that, since lymphangiectasis without the complications is not a fatal disease, attempts should only be made to keep the expansion and compression of the vital structures in check. He also suggested that, in some instances, after the first year of life lymphangiectasis becomes less prominent and may be self-limiting.

Systemic lymphangiectasis. Infrequently, lymphangiomas are found to involve the entire extremity, extending from the shoulder to the fingertips or from the groin to the toes (Fig. 17.5A to 17.5C). This is a congenital deformity in which all the structures of the entire limb are involved with lymphangiectasis, resulting in a grotesquely swollen and deformed extremity. In certain instances the situation becomes such that the patient requests a major amputation, such as a hip joint disarticulation or forequarter amputation. These amputations should be avoided, but in some instances they might become necessary.

Lymphedema

Congenital lymphedema. Although the exact pathophysiologic factors of congenital lymphedema are not yet clear, it has been postulated to be due to underdevelopment of the superficial lymphatic system. In instances in which the congenital lymphedema of an extremity is encountered in the absence of a familial predilection, the term *lymphedema praecox* is generally used. In patients in whom a family history of edematous extremities is obtained, the term *Milroy's disease* has been used.

In the normal extremity, subcutaneous lymphatic channels accompany the main superficial veins to the lymph nodes in the groin or axilla. Similarly, deep lymphatic trunks accompany deep blood vessels of the extremities. The communications between these two systems in normal circumstances are found in the ankle, calf, popliteal fossa, and the adductor canal in the lower extremities; and in the epitrochlear area in the upper extremities. In congenital lymphedema, the hypoplastic or absent superficial lymphatic network of the involved extremity is unable to collect lymph, which then pools in subcutaneous fat until the hydrostatic pressure of the tissue exceeds the oncotic pressure of the superficial venous system, and venous decompression occurs. The deep lymphatic system of the extremities in patients with congenital lymphedema usually is normal, in contrast to lymphangiectasis of the extremities, in which both systems are involved.

The clinical manifestations of congenital edema (lymphedema praecox) are often evident only after adolescence, although the malformation is present from birth. Fonkalsrud[1] found that in 13 (33 percent) of 39 patients, the manifestations became apparent during adolescence. In some of the patients reported by Fonkalsrud[1] and Fonkalsrud and Coulson,[28] the edema was bilateral, and in some the extremity edema was associated with exudative enteropathy. The clinical features usually are characterized by the enlarged edematous extremity or extremities, resulting in cosmetic deformity, which in extreme cases might be functional as well.

Milroy[29] described familial lymphedema in a family of six generations comprising 97 persons, 23 percent of whom had congenital lymphedema. The basic factors related to the lymphedema, however, were similar to those in the more common nonfamilial congenital type of lymphedema.

Chronic obstructive lymphedema of the extremities in the adult is usually iatrogenically produced by either radical axillary or groin dissections. Infrequently, the lymphatic obstruction is secondary to infection. Parasitic infestation resulting in massive extremity edema with massive skin changes is still relatively common in some parts of the world.

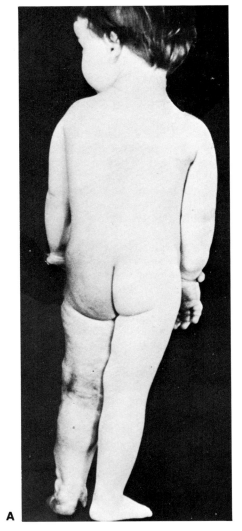 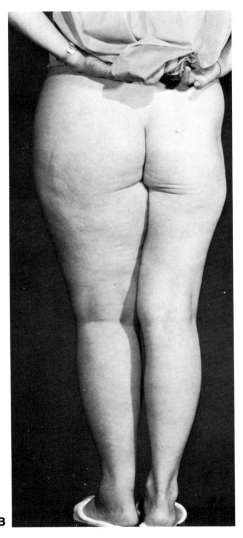

A   B

Figure 17.5. **(A)** Sixteen-month-old girl with extensive regional lymphangiomatosis of the left lower extremity. Posterior view shows involvement from the toes to the buttock. **(B)** Posterior view of extensive lymphangiomatosis of the left lower extremity in a 45-year-old woman. Note difference of circumference at the midthigh between the two extremities.

The chronically lymphedematous extremity poses a unique challenge in management.[1,2,4,6,27,28] However, the only relevance of this anomaly to the present discussion is the development of lymphangiosarcoma in such an extremity. The details of this aspect are discussed in the section on malignant tumors of the lymphatic system.

Lymphangiomyoma

Lymphangiomyoma is a rare benign disorder of the lymphatic system that was first recognized

and described in 1966 by Cornog and Enterline.[30] These authors reviewed 20 cases and concluded that the lesion occurred in a striking preponderance in women. The lesion often involves the thoracic duct, has a constant association with chylothorax, and a frequent association with pulmonary disease, consisting of lymphangiectatic honeycombing with the proliferation of smooth muscle and a typical lipid pneumonia, possibly of chylous origin. Following reappraisal of a previously published paper by Enterline and Roberts,[31] Cornog and Enterline[30]

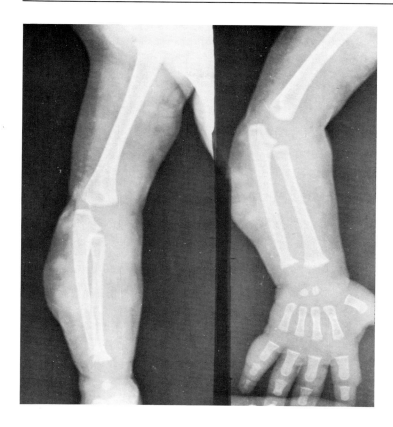

Figure 17.5. (C) Extensive lymphangioma of the right upper extremity in a male infant. There will be considerable deformity as the child grows older.

concluded that the term lymphangiopericytoma, used by Enterline and Roberts,[31] should be substituted by the term lymphangiomyoma. Based on their observations, Cornog and Enterline[30] suggested that the pulmonary cystic and muscular lesions associated with this entity are an independent expression of a tendency to malformation, as seen in tuberous sclerosis, but in part might be secondary to mediastinal lesions. These authors found no evidence of local infiltration or metastases in their 20 cases. They suggested that these lesions are not necessarily fatal and even chylothorax can be managed for prolonged periods.

Following Cornog and Enterline's[30] publication, several other reports have appeared.[30-34] It is apparent that, although this anomaly or hamartomatous malformation may occur in nodal and extranodal sites, the pulmonary involvement (being the most dramatic) receives most of the attention.[33-36] In 1975, Corrin and coworkers[33] published a comprehensive review of pulmonary lymphangiomyomatosis. To date, about 50 such cases have been reported, all of which have been in women in the reproductive

age group, the major complaint being breathlessness. This was usually progressive, and death from pulmonary insufficiency resulted within ten years. Functional changes in the lungs were obstructive or restrictive, or both. Pneumothorax, chylous effusions, and hemoptysis were frequent complications. Radiographically the lesions initially appear as fine, linear or nodular, predominantly basal densities, and progress to a pattern of bullous change, or honeycombing. Like eosinophilic granulomas, they involve all portions of the lungs, including the region of the costophrenic sinuses. There may be associated pleural effusion. A progressively increasing lung volume is characteristic. The lesions consist of an irregular nodular or laminar random proliferation of smooth muscle cells within all portions of the lung, with loss of parenchyma, leading to honeycombing. Proliferated muscle can obstruct bronchioles (with air-trapping and formation of bullae, often complicated by pneumothorax), venules (with pulmonary hemorrhage and hemosiderosis accompanied clinically by hemoptysis), and lymphatics (with chylothorax or chyloperitoneum). Both thoracic and abdominal lymph nodes and the thoracic duct can also be involved in the myoproliferative process, with formation of subsidiary minute channels and obstruction. Renal or perirenal angiomyolipomas can also occur.[37] Identical pulmonary lesions occasionally occur in tuberous sclerosis. The possibility of a relationship between tuberous sclerosis and lymphangiomyomatosis probably should be considered. One feature of note in pulmonary lesions of tuberous sclerosis is the presence of adenomatoid proliferations of epithelium. At present the question of whether lymphangiomyomatosis is a *forme fruste* of tuberous sclerosis[32,33,37] must be considered as unresolved. It may yield to further investigation, including chromosomal studies. As stated earlier, no malignant transformation in these cases has yet been documented.

MALIGNANT TUMORS

Lymphangiosarcoma

In 1948, Stewart and Treves[38] described an unusual tumor that developed in an edematous upper extremity following radical mastectomy long after the breast cancer was apparently controlled. After some initial confusion and controversy regarding the true identity of the tumor, it became apparent that this was a lymphangiosarcoma arising in an edematous extremity, not to be confused with recurrent or metastatic breast cancer. Since the original description by Stewart and Treves,[38] the occurrence of lymphangiosarcoma associated with chronic lymphedema due to any cause has become well recognized. Woodward and coworkers[39] found that through December 1970 there were 186 such cases reported in the literature, 162 of which occurred after radical mastectomy and 24 after other causes of edema. For the sake of clarity of presentation, discussion will be divided into lymphangiosarcomas associated with postmastectomy lymphedema and the sarcomas arising in other types of an edematous extremity.

Postmastectomy Lymphangiosarcoma (Stewart-Treves Syndrome). The average age of the patient at the time of onset of lymphangiosarcoma is about 63 years, although younger patients (44 years) and older patients (84 years) have been described.[39,40] We have treated three such cases in which the patients were 59, 65,

and 73 years of age. As expected, the overwhelming number of patients are women; however, Woodward and co-authors[39] found two instances in men in their review of the literature. No racial predilection has been noted for this cancer.

Lymphangiosarcoma usually appears in an edematous extremity several years after mastectomy. Although it is not possible to accurately pinpoint the exact time of appearance of the tumor, it is estimated that at least ten years elapse between the mastectomy and clinical manifestation of lymphangiosarcoma in the ipsilateral upper extremity. Apparently the tumor can be identified as early as one year after mastectomy and as late as 26 years.[39] In the 151 cases in which the interval was recorded, lymphangiosarcoma first appeared at a median interval of 10 years, 4 months (Fig. 17.6).

Lymphangiosarcoma first became clinically apparent in the upper arm in two of our patients and in the forearm in the remaining patient (Fig. 17.7A and 17.7B). Woodward et al.,[39] in their review of 90 reported cases, found that in 68 (75.5 percent) the lesion was initially recognized in the arm, in the elbow, and the forearm.

Usually the arm, which is the site of tumorigenesis, is swollen and hypertrophied, with brawny, atrophic, hyperkeratotic, suffused, purplish skin. There is limitation of function, with accompanying pain in some instances. Initially a blue or purplish macular or nodular lesion is seen, the lesion enlarges, and with time a confluence of a number of these lesions makes the diagnosis simple (Fig. 17.7B).

Treatment. Various modalities of treatment have been tried for postmastectomy lymphangiosarcoma.[3,38,39] Herrmann and Ariel,[40] in 1967, reviewed the results of treatment in 91 reported cases and concluded that the prognosis was poor in this disease and that neither surgery nor radiation therapy influenced the end result in any appreciable manner. However, after this pessimistic report, several comprehensive reviews were published[39,41] showing that the results of treatment were not as depressing as had been thought. Woodward et al.,[39] reviewing the Mayo Clinic experience in 21 patients, found that initial treatment consisted of primary amputation in ten patients, irradiation in six, local excision in two, irradiation and chemotherapy in one, and chemotherapy in one. One patient with advanced disease received no treatment. Of the ten patients treated with amputation, there were

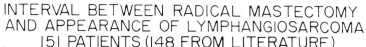

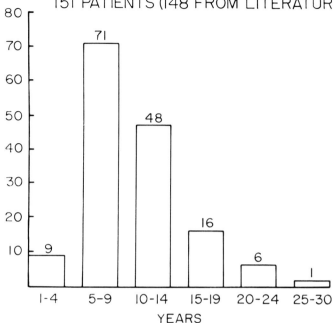

INTERVAL BETWEEN RADICAL MASTECTOMY
AND APPEARANCE OF LYMPHANGIOSARCOMA
151 PATIENTS (148 FROM LITERATURE)

YEARS

Figure 17.6. Histogram showing the interval of appearance of lymphangiosarcoma after radical mastectomy.

four five-year survivors (40 percent); one of the four had metastases after five years. In contrast, none of the six patients treated with radiation therapy alone survived for five years, nor did either of the two patients treated with local excision, both of whom had local recurrence. These authors[39] found no beneficial effect from chemotherapy as a primary form of treatment. In our series of three patients with postmastectomy lymphangiosarcoma, two patients were treated by forequarter amputation, one of whom is still disease-free at the end of five years. The remaining patient, who was treated with combined radiation, systemic chemotherapy, and immunotherapy, lived for 18 months.

In 129 of the 162 cases of lymphangiosarcoma collected by Woodward and co-workers,[39] the median survival rate was 19 months. Woodward and his co-workers[39] compared the published survival rates of 61 patients treated either by forequarter amputation or by shoulder disarticulation with those of the 48 patients treated by radiation therapy alone and found that those subjected to amputation had a slightly better prognosis. The difference was significant at two years (P = 0.05), but of borderline significance

at one year (P = 0.06). There are too few patients treated by either method to allow comparisons of survival rates. Of the 11 patients who survived for more than five years, seven were treated by amputation (four by forequarter amputation and three by shoulder disarticulation), two by wide excision, and one by radiation therapy (17-year survival). The remaining patient received intra-arterially administered radioactive yttrium.[40]

The incidence of local recurrence following a major amputation is lower than that in patients treated by radiation therapy. The failure of amputation is usually metastatic disease, whereas in the irradiated group local failure precedes distant disease. Based on our limited experience and the experience of other authors[38,39,40] it appears that radical ablative operation probably offers a better opportunity for cure.

Lymphangiosarcoma Not Associated with Mastectomy. As pointed out earlier, lymphangiosarcoma can occur in any chronically edematous area (Fig. 17.8). Lymphangiosarcoma of the anterior abdominal wall has been reported in the edematous anterior abdominal wall fol-

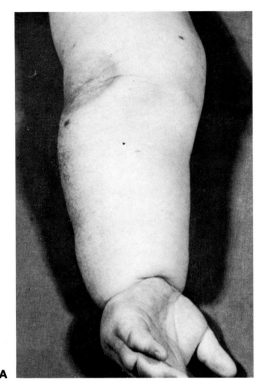
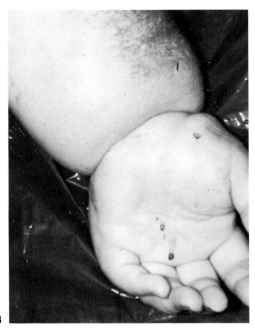

A   **B**

Figure 17.7. **(A)** A small pigmented lesion in the posterolateral aspect of the arm was the first sign of a lymphangiosarcoma that developed in a lymphedematous extremity following radical mastectomy eight years earlier. Careful scrutiny shows several minute lesions on the arm and another lesion below the skin graft. An apparent attempt for control of the initial lesions was made by wide local excision when the tumor recurred, before the patient was referred to us. **(B)** Postmastectomy lymphangiosarcoma showing confluence of multiple cutaneous lesions in the forearm and the wrist, a sign of advanced stage of the disease.

lowing bilateral lymphadenectomy for carcinoma of the penis.[42] Approximately 27 patients have been found with lymphangiosarcoma in a chronically edematous extremity not associated with the aftermath of radical mastectomy (Table 17.2),[43-64] eight of whom had a congenitally edematous extremity. In the remaining 19 patients edema was either idiopathic or due to various other causes. As in the postmastectomy variety the results of treatment are not encouraging; however, extremity amputation probably provides some long-term cures.

It is probably appropriate to evaluate the role of regional perfusion in lymphangiosarcoma arising in any chronically edematous extremity. However, because of the rarity of the lesions, definitive statements cannot be made. It is expected that, with the decreasing number of radical mastectomies performed, the future

incidence of postmastectomy lymphangiosarcoma will be much lower. Consequently, the few cases of chronically lymphedematous extremity that could develop into lymphangiosarcoma might be too few to design any form of study protocol.

Extranodal Lymphoma

A malignant lymphoma occasionally may be encountered in the somatic tissues and may mimic a soft somatic tissue neoplasm (Fig. 4.89, Chapter 4). For example, the initial presentation of malignant lymphoma may be an anterior abdominal wall tumor resembling a lipoma. In other instances, the tumors might be encountered in the gastrointestinal tract, conjunctiva, maxillary antrum, breast, and various other locations. The diagnosis is established by means of microscopic examination of the biopsy specimen. Once

TABLE 17.2. TWENTY-SEVEN REPORTED CASES OF LYMPHANGIOSARCOMA NOT ASSOCIATED WITH MASTECTOMY

Author(s)	Year of Publication	Age	Site	Cause of Lymphedema	Duration of Lymphedema (yr)	Treatment	Comments
Lowenstein[43]	1908	56	L arm	Traumatic	6	Amputation	Alive, 2 yr
Kettle[44]	1918	44	R leg	Idiopathic	40	Hip disarticulation	Alive, 3 yr
Nather[45]	1921	59	R leg	Traumatic	11/12	Amputation	Alive, 1 yr
Aegerter and Peale[46]	1942	40	R leg	Idiopathic	29	Amputation	Dead, 6 yr
Martorell[47]	1951	44	R leg	Infection	$\frac{1}{2}$	Radiation therapy and amputation	Dead, 4 yr
Raven and Christie[48]	1954	56	L arm	Extensive nevus	?	Excision and forequarter amputation	Dead, postop
Aird et al[49]	1956	60	R leg	Idiopathic	8	Amputation	Dead, 3 yr
Liszauer and Ross[50]	1957	28	R leg	Congenital	28	Excision	Dead, 8 mo
Whittle[51]	1959	31	R leg	Idiopathic	11	Chemotherapy	Dead, 6 mo
Francis and Lindquist[52]	1960	52	L thigh	Fibrosarcoma of the proximal femur	5	Hemipelvectomy	Dead, postop
Scott et al[53]	1960	46	L hand	Congenital	46	Amputation	Dead, 4 yr
Taswell et al[54]	1962	18	L arm	Congenital	18	Shoulder disarticulation	Dead, 11 mo
Ibid	1962	65	L leg	Idiopathic	37	Amputation	Alive, 15 yr
De Jager[55]	1963	43	R leg	Chondroma of tibia	?	Amputation	Dead, 2 yr
Ibid	1963	64	R forearm	Abscess of second rib	22	Radiation therapy	Alive, 3 yr
Ibid	1963	44	R thigh	Tuberculosis	?	?	Dead
Vandaele et al[56]	1963	35	R leg	Idiopathic	26	Amputation	Alive, 10 mo
Gray et al[57]	1966	65	L arm	Axillary node dissection; radiation therapy	8	Forequarter amputation	Dead, 9 mo
Prudden and Wolarsky[58]	1967	28	R thigh	Congenital	Intermittently for years	Hemipelvectomy	Alive, 10 mo
Danese et al[59]	1967	26	L hand	Idiopathic	17	None	Dead, 4 mo
Huriez et al[60]	1968	35	R leg	Idiopathic	26	Amputation	Alive, 10 mo
McBride et al[61]	1969	—	R thigh	Carcinoma of cervix	—	—	—
Bunch[62]	1969	13	L axilla	Congenital	13	Forequarter amputation	Dead, 3 mo
Finlay-Jones[63]	1970	34	L thigh	Congenital	34	Excision, radiation therapy	Dead, $2\frac{1}{2}$ yr
Merrick et al[64]	1971	52	L arm	Congenital	52	Forequarter amputation	Dead, $2\frac{1}{2}$ yr with metastases
Das Gupta	1981	36	R arm	Congenital	36	Forequarter amputation	$2\frac{1}{2}$ yr, N.E.D.*
Das Gupta	1981	54	L lower extremity	Congenital	53 (?)	Midthigh amputation and adjuvant chemotherapy	$1\frac{1}{2}$ yr, N.E.D.

*No evidence of disease.

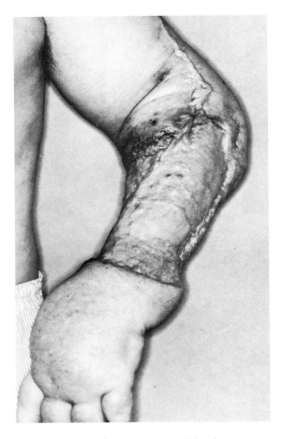

Figure 17.8. Lymphangiosarcoma arising in an apparently congenitally lymphedematous left upper extremity. Several attempts at local excision failed and this 46-year-old man was then referred to us. A forequarter amputation was performed, resulting in a five and a half-year disease-free survival (Table 17.2).

of this entity resembles a soft tissue sarcoma. A palpable tumor or a lesion that can be seen in x-rays of the skeletal system automatically means the disease is of several years' duration. If the treatment reduces the mass the prognosis is improved, although most patients will eventually die of the disease. The presence of M-protein in a patient with a soft tissue tumor is diagnostic of myeloma.

In general, the treatment is nonsurgical and consists of treatment of symptoms, as well as use of systemic chemotherapy with melphalan, cyclophosphamide, or chlorambucil. In an apparently localized plasma cell tumor, if there is no indication of systemic disease, the tumor should be treated primarily by means of radiation therapy, eg, in solitary lesions of the nose or nasopharynx. In rare instances, the local lesion can be excised with good response. We have had two patients in whom local excision was performed. One was a 51-year-old woman whom we followed up for five years without any evidence of progression of disease, after excision at another medical center of an apparently solitary plasmacytoma located at the medial end of the left clavicle. The second one, whom we treated, was a 66-year-old woman with a large (15 × 12 cm) left scapular mass causing extreme difficulty of motion. A biopsy showed a plasma cell tumor and elevated M-protein. A subtotal scapulectomy was performed. Immediately following the operation there was a fall of M-protein levels and she improved. She received localized radiation therapy and has remained well for five years without any evidence of spread of disease.

the diagnosis of malignant lymphoma is made, the treatment is based on the histologic type and the extent of disease.

Extramedullary Plasmacytoma

These uncommon tumors usually originate in the nose, nasal sinuses, oropharynx, bronchi,[65] gastrointestinal tract,[65-72] and even in the meninges.[73] They tend to remain localized for long periods before spreading to other sites. Plasma cell tumors may also originate in the intestine. Since the normal plasma cells in the nasopharynx and intestine mainly synthesize IgA, it is not surprising that most of the plasma cell tumors that develop in these sites likewise produce IgA. In rare instances, local manifestation

REFERENCES

1. Fonkalsrud EW: Surgical management of congenital malformations of the lymphatic system. Am J Surg 128:152, 1974
2. Bill AH, Sumner DS: A unified concept of lymphangioma and cystic hygroma. Surg Gynecol Obstet 120:79, 1965
3. Pack GT, Ariel IR: Tumors of the Soft Somatic Tissues. New York, Hoeber/Harper. 1958, p 472
4. Harkins GA, Sabiston DC: Lymphangioma in infancy and childhood. Surgery 47:822, 1960
5. Woodring AJ: Cervical cystic hygroma. A review of the literature and report of an unusual case. Ann Otol Rhin Laryngol 77:978, 1968
6. Beahrs OH: Chylous cysts of the abdomen. Surg Clin N Am 30:1081, August 1950
7. Eliason EL: Perforated chylous cyst of mesentery. Ann Surg 101:1452, 1935

8. Harrow BR: Retroperitoneal lymphatic cyst (cystic lymphangioma). J Urol 77:82–89, 1957
9. Handelsman JC, Ravitch MM: Chylous cysts of the mesentery in children. Ann Surg 140:185, 1954
10. Farrel WJ: Intra-abdominal cystic lymphangioma. Am J Surg 108:790, 1964
11. Lynn RB: Cystic lymphangioma of the adrenal associated with arterial hypertension. Canad J Surg 8:92, 1965
12. Sturim HS: Intra-abdominal cystic lymphangiomas. Am J Surg 109:807, 1965
13. Sarrias BA: Two cases of cystic lymphangioma of the mesentery. Bull Soc Int Chir 30 (Sept-Dec):519, 1971
14. Pack GT, Trinidad SS, Lisa JR: Rare primary somatic tumors of the pancreas. Arch Surg 77:1000, 1958
15. Elliot RL, Williams RD, Bayles D, Griffin J: Lymphangioma of the duodenum. One report with light and electron microscopic observations. Ann Surg 163:1,86, 1966
16. Litzow TJ, Lash H: Lymphangiomas of the tongue. Proc Staff Meetings Mayo Clinic 36:229, 1961
17. Gonzales LE, Zapatero AH, Fernandez EP: Lymphangioma of the pancreas. Chir Ghastroent 10:225, 1976
18. Bickel WH, Broders AC: Primary lymphangioma of the ilium. Report of a case. J Bone Joint Surg 29-A:517, 1947
19. Harris R, Prandoni AG: Generalized primary lymphangiomas of bone: Report of case associated with congenital lymphedema of forearm. Ann Intern Med 33:1302, 1950
20. Cohen J, Graig JM: Multiple lymphangiectases of bone. J Bone Joint Surg 37-A:585, 1955
21. Falkmer S, Tilling G: Primary lymphangioma of bone. Acta Orthop Scandinavica 26:99, 1956
22. Hayes JT, Brody GL: Cystic lymphangiectasis of bone. J Bone Joint Surg 45-A:107, 1961
23. Shopfner CE, Allen RP: Lymphangioma of bone. Radiology 76:449, 1961
24. Rosenquist CJ, Wolfe FC: Lymphangioma of bone. J Bone Joint Surg 50-A:158, 1968
25. Brower AC, Culver JE Jr, Keats TE: Diffuse cystic angiomatosis of bone: Report of two cases. Am J Roentgenol 118:456, 1973
26. Asch MJ, Cohen AH, Moore TC: Hepatic and splenic lymphangiomatosis with skeletal involvement: Report of a case and review of the literature. Surgery 76:334, 1974
27. Ravitch MM: Radical treatment of massive mixed angiomas (hemolymphangiomas) in infants and children. Ann Surg 134:228, 1951
28. Fonkalsrud EW, Coulson WF: Management of congenital lymphedema in infants and children. Ann Surg 177:280, 1973
29. Milroy WF: An undescribed variety of hereditary oedema. NY Med J 56:505, 1892
30. Cornog JL, Enterline HT: Lymphangiomyoma. A benign lesion of chyliferous lymphatics synonymous with lymphangiopericytoma. Cancer 19:1909, 1966
31. Enterline HT, Roberts B: Lymphangiopericytoma. Cancer 8:582, 1955
32. Wolff M: Lymphangiomyoma: Clinicopathologic study and ultrastructural confirmation of its histogenesis. Cancer 31:988, 1975
33. Corrin B, Liebow A, Friedman PJ: Pulmonary lymphangiomyomatosis. Am J Pathol 79:347, 1975
34. Gray ER, Carrington CB, Corong JL: Lymphangiomyomatosis: Report of a case with ureteral involvement and chyluria. Cancer 35:490, 1975
35. Vazquez JJ, Fernandez-Cuervo L, Fidalgo B: Lymphangiomyomatosis. Morphogenetic study and ultrastructural confirmation of the histogenesis of the lung lesion. Cancer 37:2321, 1976
36. Kreisman H, Robitailler Y, Dionne P, Palayew N: Lymphangiomyomatosis syndrome with hyperparathyroidism (a case report). Cancer 42:364, 1978
37. Montforet WJ, Kohnen PW: Angiolipomas in a case of lymphangiomyomatous syndrome. Relationships to tuberous sclerosis. Cancer 34:317, 1974
38. Stewart FW, Treves N: Lymphangiosarcoma in postmastectomy lymphedema: A report of six cases in elephantiasis chirurgica. Cancer 1:64, 1948
39. Woodward AH, Ivins JE, Soule EH: Lymphangiosarcoma arising in chronic lymphedematous extremities. Cancer 30:562, 1972
40. Herrmann JP, Ariel IM: Therapy of lymphangiosarcoma of the chronically edematous limb. Am J Roentgenol 99:393, 1967
41. Tragus ET, Wagner DE: Current therapy for postmastectomy lymphangiosarcoma. Arch Surg 97:839, 1968
42. Calnan J, Cowdell RH: Lymphangioendothelioma of the anterior abdominal wall: Report of a case. Br J Surg 46:375, 1959
43. Lowenstein S: Der Atiologische Zusammenhand zwischen akutem einmaligem. Trauma und Sarcom: ein Beitrag zur Aetiologie der malignen tumoren. Beitr Klin Chir 48:780, 1906
44. Kettle EH: Tumors arising from endothelium. Proc Roy Soc Med 11:19, 1918
45. Nather K: Uber ein malignes Lymphangioendotheliom der Haut des Fusses. Virchows Arch Path Anat 231:540, 1921
46. Aegerter EE, Peale AR: Kaposi's sarcoma: A critical survey. Arch Path 34:413, 1942
47. Martorell F: Tumorigenic lymphedema. Angiology 2:386, 1951
48. Raven RW, Christie AC: Hemangiosarcoma: A case with lymphatic and hematogenous metastases. Br J Surg 41:483, 1954
49. Aird I, Weinbren K, Walter L: Angiosarcoma in a limb the seat of spontaneous lymphoedema. Br J Cancer 10:424, 1956
50. Liszauer S, Ross RC: Lymphangiosarcoma in lymphoenhdema. Canad Med Assoc J 76:475, 1957
51. Whittle RJM: An angiosarcoma associated with an oedematous limb: A case report. J Fac Radiol 10:111, 1959
52. Francis KC, Lindquist HD: Lymphangiosarcoma of the lower extremity involved with chronic lymphedema. Am J Surg 100:617, 1960
53. Scott RB, Nydick I, Conway H: Lymphangiosarcoma arising in lymphedema. Am J Med 28:1008, 1960
54. Taswell HF, Soule HH, Conventry MB: Lymphangiosarcoma arising in chronic lymphedematous extremities. J Bone Joint Surg 44-A:277, 1962
55. De Jager H: Oorspronkelijke Stukken: Secundair lymfangiosarcoom. Ned Tijdechr Geneeskd 107:1344, 1963

56. Vandaele R, Van Craeynest W, Haven E, Dupont A: Lymphangiosarcome sur lymphangiosarcome sur lymphoedeme primitif du bras. Bull Soc Fr Dermatol Syphiligr 70:722, 1963

57. Gray GF Jr, Gonzales-Licea A, Hartman WH, Woods AC: Angiosarcoma in lymphedema: An unusual case of Stewart-Treves syndrome. Bull Johns Hopkins Hosp 119:117, 1966

58. Prudden JF, Wolarsky ER: Lymphangiosarcoma of the thigh: Case report. Arch Surg 94:376, 1967

59. Danese CA, Grishman E, Oh C, Brieling DA: Malignant vascular tumors of the lymphedematous extremity. Ann Surg 166:245, 1967

60. Huriez C, Desmons F, Agache P, Bombart M, Benoit M: Lymphangiosarcome sur elephantiasis monstrueux de la jambe chez une femme agee 35 ans. Bull Soc Fr Dermatol Syphiligr 75:10, 1968

61. McBride CM, Reeder JW, Smith JL: Angiosarcoma in the lymphaedematous limb. South Med J 62:378, 1969

62. Bunch GH: Discussion, Lymphangiosarcoma following post-mastectomy lymphedema (Barnett WO, Hardy JD, Hendrix JH). Ann Surg 169:968, 1969

63. Finlay-Jones LR: Lymphangiosarcoma of the thigh: A case report. Cancer 26:722, 1970

64. Merrick TA, Erlandson RA, Hajdu SI: Lymphangiosarcoma of a congenitally lymphedematous arm. Arch Path 91:365, 1971

65. Stout AP, Kenney FR: Primary plasma cell tumors of the upper air passages and oral cavity. Cancer 2:261, 1949

66. Ahmed N, Ramos S, Sika J, LeVeen HH, Piccone VA: Primary esophageal plasmacytoma. Cancer 38:943, 1976

67. Douglass HO Jr, Sika JV, LeVeen HH: Plasmacytoma—A not so rare tumor of the small intestine. Cancer 28:456, 1971

68. Godaro JE, Fox JE, Levinson JJ: Primary gastric plasmacytoma—Case report and review of literature. J Digest Dis 18:508, 1973

69. Hellwig CA: Extramedullary plasma cell tumors as observed in various locations. Arch Path 36:95, 1943

70. Line DH, Lewis RH: Gastric plasmacytoma. Gut 10:233, 1969

71. Carson CP, Ackerman LV, Maltby JE: Plasma cell myeloma. A clinical, pathological and roentgenologic review of 90 cases. Am J Clin Path 25:849, 1955

72. Hampton JM, Gandy JR: Plasmacytoma of gastrointestinal tract. Ann Surg 145:415, 1957

73. Mancilla-Jemenez R, Tavassoli FA: Solitary meningeal plasmacytoma: Report of a case with electron microscopic and immunohistologic observations. Cancer 38:798, 1976

18

Heterotopic Bone and Cartilage

Tapas K. Das Gupta

BENIGN

Localized Myositis Ossificans

Solitary myositis ossificans is a rare clinical entity probably related to chronic minimal trauma. A common example is the bony hard mass that develops in the medial aspect of the thigh of horseback riders, which has been termed "rider's bone." A localized hard tumor along the long axis of a muscle, which on routine roentgenographic examination shows the presence of osseous tissue, suggests a diagnosis of myositis ossificans. If the patient provides a history of chronic trauma, this diagnosis becomes more likely. In a number of instances, however, there is no such history of chronic trauma (Fig. 18.1). For example, a diagnosis of osseous metaplasia of the breast[1-3] must be established by histologic examination. Treatment of symptomatic solitary myositis ossificans is local excision.

In rare instances this tumor can develop into an osteogenic sarcoma. Pack and Ariel[4] described one such case. In 1956, Fine and Stout[5] made an extensive study of the published cases and those in the files of Columbia University's Department of Surgical Pathology and found a total of 46. In two of their own cases and in ten published cases malignant change in a benign tumor could be suggested. However, in only one of these 12 cases was a histologic diagnosis of solitary myositis ossificans made in a preex-

isting tumor and this had been left untreated. In all other instances the diagnosis of a malignant change in a preexisting myositis ossificans was made on the basis of the history of a preexisting tumor of long duration. Using long intervals as the criterion for accepting the hypothesis that malignant transformation can occur in a preexisting site of ossification, Fine and Stout[5] found that in seven (15.2 percent) of their 46 cases, extraskeletal osteogenic sarcoma developed in a preexisting solitary myositis ossificans.

Progressive Myositis Ossificans

This entity is extremely rare and is distinctly different from the localized or solitary form.[6] Rosenstein[7] noted a group of characteristic symptoms that sharply differentiate this condition from the localized form. These are (1) ossification of a muscle without any apparent cause; (2) manifestation of the disease at birth or in early life; (3) progressive and unrelenting course, unaffected by any treatment; and (4) association with several congenital anomalies, especially of the fingers and toes. Rosenstein[7] collected 119 cases and added one of his own. Pack and Braund[8] described one patient with progressive myositis ossifications in whom osteogenic sarcoma developed in the back muscles.

In general, progressive growth with asso-

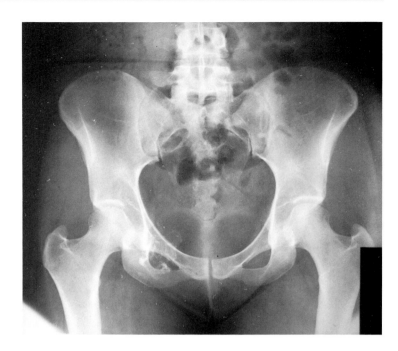

Figure 18.1. Heterotopic bone formation within right side of pelvis in a 22-year-old woman. She was operated upon and the bone was removed.

ciated ossification of muscles continues until most of the muscles from the skull to the feet are involved. It occurs most frequently in boys, but the disease is so rare that no sex or race ratio can be established. This author has never encountered a patient with progressive myositis ossificans.

Chondroma of Soft Parts

Benign extraskeletal chondroma is rare.[9] Most cases occur in the hands and feet[9,10] but a few have been observed in such sites as the tongue[11] or cheek.[12] These are essentially benign tumors,

although Chung and Enzinger[10] reported that in 10 of 56 (18 percent) patients the tumor recurred once. These tumors should be treated by excision with a satisfactory margin, and any attempt at a major excision should be avoided.

MALIGNANT

Extraskeletal or Extraosseous Osteogenic Sarcoma

Although extraskeletal bone formation under a variety of different stimuli is not uncommon, the occurrence of osteogenic sarcoma outside

TABLE 18.1. EXTRAOSSEOUS OSTEOGENIC SARCOMA ARISING IN A SITE OF PREVIOUS IRRADIATION

Author(s)	Year of Publication	Type of Primary Tumor	Total Radiation Therapy Dose	Interval after Radiation Therapy (in months)
Auerbach and co-workers[32]	1951	Seminoma in a 23-year-old man	4,000 rads, skin dose	50
Kaufmann and Stout[22]	1963	Retinoblastoma in an 8-month-old infant	14,387 rads tissue dose in three courses	132
Boyer and Navin[25]	1965	Seminoma in a 29-year-old man	4,500 rads, skin dose	49
Ibid[25]	1965	Teratocarcinoma of testis in 37-year-old man	5,400 rads, skin dose	121

the skeletal system is rare. The first documented case was reported by Boneti[13] in 1700, followed by case reports by Morgagni[14] in 1763, Muller[15] in 1838, and Cooper[16] in 1845. In the early part of this century Coley,[17] Rhoades and Blumgart[18] and Mallory[19] further described this entity. After Wilson's[20] report in 1941, Schaffer,[21] in 1952, collected 44 patients from the literature who were presumed to have had extraosseous osteogenic sarcoma. Fine and Stout[5] found only one case in a review of 147 cases of osteogenic sarcoma and reports of 864 surgical specimens and 9,065 autopsies. They made a critical study of published cases and were reluctant to accept several as genuine extraosseous osteogenic sarcomas. They did,[5] however, obtained clinical and microscopic data on 12 acceptable cases and added these to the 34 previously established cases. Kauffman and Stout,[22] in 1963, reported two additional cases of this tumor in children.

With the establishment and acceptance of this tumor as a firm clinicopathologic entity, several additional case reports appeared in the literature.[23-26] In 1968, Das Gupta, Hajdu, and Foote[27] described the natural history of nine cases of extraosseous osteogenic sarcoma treated at Memorial Sloan-Kettering Cancer Center. Subsequently, Allan and Soule,[28] Wurlitzen and co-workers,[29] and Rao et al.[30] reported the experience at the Mayo Clinic, M.D. Anderson Tumor Institute, and the Roswell Park Memorial Institute, respectively. In 1978, Dahn and associates[31] reported the only instance of extraskeletal osteosarcoma arising in the soft tissues of an organ (larynx).

The etiologic factors in extraosseous osteogenic sarcoma, as in all other sarcomas, are still unknown. The relationship of localized myos-

itis ossificans to extraosseous osteogenic sarcoma has already been discussed, but even though it is possible to have malignant transformation of a preexisting solitary myositis ossificans, the incidence is extremely rare and does not require serious clinical consideration. However, as with fibrosarcomas and osteogenic sarcomas, radiation-induced extraosseous osteogenic sarcomas have been reported, albeit rarely.[22,25,32] To date, only four such cases have been documented (Table 18.1). A review of these four cases shows that once an extraskeletal osteogenic sarcoma develops in an irradiated area, the prognosis is grave. Considering the large number of patients with seminoma, retinoblastoma, and several forms of malignant lymphoma treated solely by radiation therapy, remarkably few cases have been reported.

Extraskeletal osteogenic sarcoma occurs in all age groups. Although in the review of Fine and Stout[5] the disease was seen most often in elderly men, in our experience there has been no age, sex, or race predilection. Our youngest patient was a 31-year-old woman.[27] In the four radiation-induced cases, the ages of the patients were lower than the average age reported in the literature.[22-24,32] We have treated five cases of extraskeletal osteogenic sarcoma at the University of Illinois Hospital. The ages of the patients were 45, 47, 69, 58, and 82 years, respectively (Table 18.2). The location of the tumors corresponded generally with that of osteogenic sarcoma of the extremities, especially the lower. A similar preponderance in the lower extremities has also been reported by other authors.[27-30] In our group of five patients, two tumors were located in a lower extremity, one in the chest wall, one arose in the right pleura, and one in an upper ex-

Location of Extraosseous Sarcomas	Treatment for Sarcoma	End Results
Lumbar soft tissue	Excision	Death in 3 years with local recurrence and lung metastases
Soft tissue of floor or the orbit	Local excision	Death in 10 months with local recurrence and extension
Lumbar soft tissue	Inadequate excision	Alive with local recurrence and paraplegia at the time of report, presumed dead of disease by now
Anterior abdominal wall	Excision	Death in 13 months with local recurrence and intestinal obstruction

TABLE 18.2. CLINICAL SUMMARY OF FIVE PATIENTS WITH EXTRAOSSEOUS OSTEOGENIC SARCOMA TREATED AT THE UNIVERSITY OF ILLINOIS HOSPITAL

Patient No.	Age/ Sex	Primary Site	Status of Primary	Treatment at U of I	Local Recurrence	End Results
1	47 M	Posterior thigh	Intact primary 5 × 6 cm (Fig. 18.2 A)	Muscle group resection	−	Living and well 6 yr after treatment
2	58 M	Pleura	Exploratory thoractomy elsewhere and diagnosis established	Radiation therapy and chemotherapy	−	Died of diffuse disease 18 mo after diagnosis
3	69 F	Soft tissue of lateral chest wall	Intact primary, 4 × 5 cm tumor	Chest wall resection	−	5½ yr, N.E.D.*
4	82 M	Medial aspect of left thigh	Primary treated with 6,000 rads prior to U of I admission with a large 5 × 5 cm persistent ulcer	Wide soft tissue resection; residual tumor (microscopic only)	−	Died 2 mo later of unrelated cause
5	42 M	Lateral aspect of left arm	Intact primary 4 × 5 cm	Wide soft tissue excision	−	2 yr, N.E.D.

*No evidence of disease.

tremity (Fig. 18.2A to 18.2D). The clinical histories of the nine patients from Memorial Sloan-Kettering Cancer Center reported by Das Gupta and co-workers[27] are summarized in Table 18.3. It is difficult to draw guidelines for diagnostic criteria in these patients. In the soft somatic tissues, a tumor showing intrinsic calcifications along with elevated serum alkaline phosphatase levels should arouse clinical suspicion of an ex-

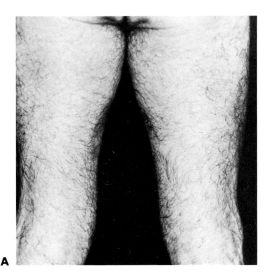

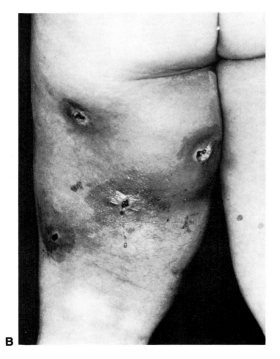

A　　　　　　　　　　　　　　　　**B**

Figure 18.2. **(A)** Extraskeletal osteosarcoma in a 47-year-old man (Pt. 1, Table 18.2). Living disease-free six years later. **(B)** Locally recurrent tumor in a 50-year-old woman. She has been treated too recently to be included in Table 18.2.

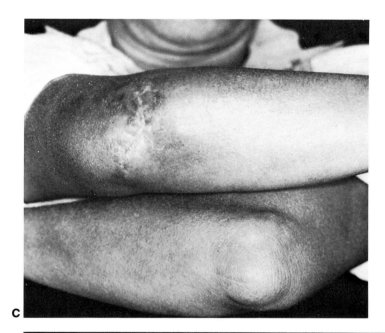

Figure 18.2. **(C)** Scar induration and swelling in the right elbow. **(D)** Pre-operative x-ray of right elbow showing bone destruction in ulna (Pt. 1, Table 18.3). (*Courtesy of Annals of Surgery*)

C

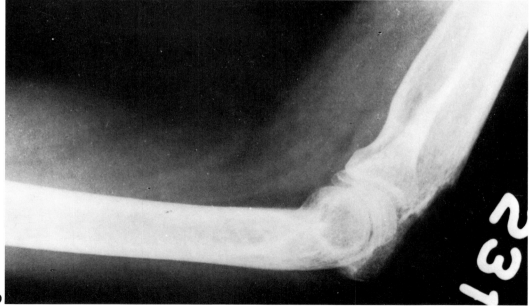

D

TABLE 18.3. CLINICAL SUMMARY OF NINE PATIENTS WITH EXTRASKELETAL OSTEOGENIC SARCOMA REPORTED BY DAS GUPTA ET AL. 1968[27] (MEMORIAL SLOAN-KETTERING CANCER CENTER SERIES)

Patient No.	Age/Sex	Primary Site	Initial Therapy	Status of Primary	First Treatment at Memorial Hospital	Local Recurrence After First Therapy at Memorial Hospital	End Results
1	48 F	Multiple local excisions	Recurrent tumor	Excision of right elbow joint	None		2 yr, N.E.D.*
2	68 M	Thigh	None	9 cm oval tumor in infragluteal fold	Wide excision	Yes, multiple recurrence	16 mo, dead with diffuse metastases
3	53 F	Lateral wall	Multiple local excisions	Recurrent ulcerating tumor	Chest wall resection	None	17 mo, dead with pulmonary and hepatic metastases
4	31 F	Buttock	Multiple local excisions	6 cm oval tumor in the region of the previous scar	Wide excision	Yes	2 mo, dead with pulmonary metastases
5	50 F	Thigh	Multiple local excisions	Recurrent 18 cm	Hemipelvectomy	None	1 yr, dead with pulmonary metastases
6	33 F	Thigh	Primary tumor locally excised for biopsy	No obvious primary tumor	Groin dissection and hip joint disarticulation	None	16 mo, N.E.D.
7	41 M	Zygomatic region	None	3 cm tumor	Wide excision	None	12 yr, N.E.D.
8†	64 F	Thigh	Multiple local excisions	Recurrent 6 × 8 cm tumor	Wide excision	Yes	5 yr, dead of disease
9	44 F	Thigh	None	20 × 15 cm primary tumor	Refused any form of operation at first; later hemipelvectomy	None	6 mo, dead of disease

*No evidence of disease.
†Patient 8 had a subtrochanteric amputation at a later date.
Courtesy of Annals of Surgery.

traosseous osteogenic sarcoma. However, this should be distinguished from malignant fibrous histiocytoma with bone and cartilage formation.[33] Bhagavan and Dorfman,[33] suggested that malignant fibrous histiocytomas with osteoid and chondroid elements are less aggressive than extraskeletal osteosarcomas or chondrosarcomas. The final diagnosis, of course, is dependent on the histologic findings. Although general guidelines regarding management cannot be formulated on the basis of the small number of cases reported, probably wide excision, when possi-

ble, is the ideal method of management (Fig. 18.3A to 18.3C).[27,30-32] Radiation therapy does not seem to have been beneficial in the cases reported thus far. The role of chemotherapy has not been ascertained.

Of the 14 patients in the combined group from Memorial Sloan-Kettering Cancer Center and the University of Illinois, only four (29 percent) survived five years or longer, one being a 12-year survivor at the time of the report in 1968 (Table 18.3). Of the remaining ten patients, eight died at various intervals after initiation of pri-

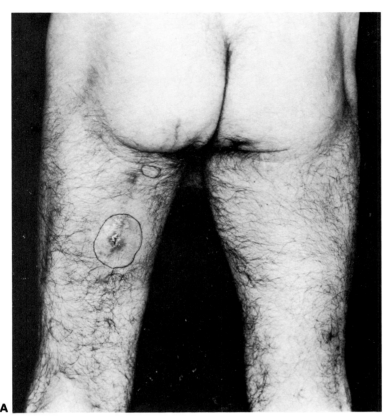

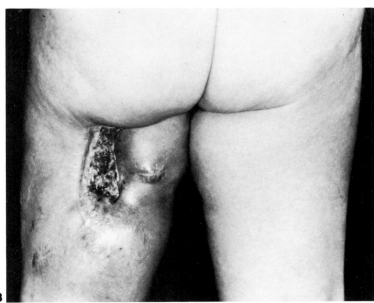

Figure 18.3 **(A)** Although the primary excision appeared to be adequate, this 57-year-old man was recently sent to us with a recurrence in the middle of the scar. During reoperation it was observed that the original excision was not as wide as was thought. He is doing well one year after second excision. **(B)** Ulcerating recurrence after inadequate multiple excisions and radiation therapy. Patient refused hemipelvectomy, treated only palliatively (too recent for inclusion in Table 18.2). **(C)** Second local recurrence in a 68-year-old man (Pt. 2, Table 18.3). *(Courtesy of Annals of Surgery)*

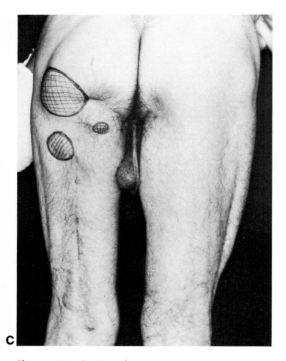

C

Figure 18.3. Continued

mary treatment and two lived disease-free for two years or more (Tables 18.2 and 18.3). One patient died of unrelated causes. A review of the cases gleaned from the published case histories shows that the overall five-year disease-free survival rate is only 17 percent (Table 18.4). Although the incidence of local recurrence reported in the past is high,[27-30] in the present group of five patients, four were treated with wide local excision (Table 18.2) and none had locally recurrent tumor. Therefore, it appears

that initial adequate wide excision might change the dismal results reported thus far (Table 18.4).

The role of radiation therapy for these tumors has not been adequately evaluated. In the few cases in which it has been used, the results have not been satisfactory. Patient 4 in Table 18.2 received curative radiation therapy, but excised specimens contained microscopic foci of tumors. In one of the nine cases reported by Das Gupta et al.[27] the use of preoperative radiation therapy improved the prognosis. Systemic chemotherapy has not been found to be useful. In our patient with pleural osteogenic sarcoma, various combinations were found to be of no value.

Extraskeletal Chondrosarcoma

Extraskeletal chondrosarcoma is a rare tumor described in 1953 by Stout and Verner,[33A] who collected a series of seven such cases. Subsequently, additional cases have been recognized and reported.[34-42] In 1972, Enzinger and Shiraki[43] reviewed 34 cases of extraskeletal chondrosarcoma from the files of the Armed Forces Institute of Pathology, constituting the largest documented series in the literature.

Extraskeletal chondrosarcoma occurs in all age groups, is equally prevalent in both sexes, and seems to have no racial predilection. The etiologic factors are not known. Of interest is a case of chondrosarcoma of the chest associated with lucite spheres used as a plombage for compression of the tuberculous cavity, reported by Thompson and Entin.[37]

In most instances the neoplasm occurs as a single, slow-growing, firm, superficial or deep nodule, or localized soft tissue swelling. Like extraosseous osteogenic sarcoma, this tumor

TABLE 18.4. CLINICAL FINDINGS AND END RESULTS IN SIX SERIES OF EXTRASKELETAL OSTEOGENIC SARCOMA

Authors	Year	No. of Patients	Sex		Average Age (yr)	5 Yr Disease-free
			M	F		
Fine and Stout[5]	1956	12	6	6	51.3	1
Das Gupta et al[27]	1968	9	2	7	48.0	2
Allan and Soule[28]	1971	26	14	12	47.5	5
Wurlitzen et al[29]	1972	9	4	5	58.7	0
Rao et al[30]	1978	8	4	4	52.7	2
Das Gupta (present series)	1981	5	4	1	64.0	2
Total		69	34	35	54.0	12 (17%)

most frequently occurs in a lower extremity. Enzinger and Shiraki[43] found that in 29 (85 percent) of 34 patients the primary tumor was in a lower extremity. These tumors have also been described in the tongue,[44] thoracic wall,[22,35] and urinary bladder.[22,35] We have encountered three patients, in all of whom the lesions were in the lower extremities. Because of the rarity of these tumors, the clinical histories of these three cases are summarized in Table 18.5.

Adequate wide excision appears to be the best form of treatment for extraskeletal chondrosarcomas. Radiation therapy and chemotherapy probably have little effect.

Enzinger and Shiraki[43] pointed out that, although the clinical behavior of these sarcomas may vary considerably, there is no doubt that extraskeletal chondrosarcomas are far less aggressive than chondrosarcomas of the bone.[34] This observation has been echoed by Smith and his co-workers.[42] Patient 2 (Table 18.5) underwent excision of the gluteal muscles with subsequent good functional quality and satisfactory end results, whereas in a similar patient reported by Stout and Verner[33A] a hemipelvectomy was performed. If an initial approach of aggressive wide excision is taken, amputations can often be avoided. With this type of wide excision little or no functional deformity results and additional radiation therapy or chemotherapy can be avoided.

Extraskeletal Ewing's Sarcoma

In 1975, Angervall and Enzinger[45] described the pathologic features and clinical behavior of 39 small, round, or oval sarcomas occurring in the soft tissues. These tumors are histologically indistinguishable from Ewing's sarcoma of the bone. The tumors chiefly affect young adults (median age 20 years) and most commonly involve the soft tissues of the lower extremities and the paravertebral region. Followup data ranging from one month to 14 years were available in 35 of the 39 patients (93 percent). Of these, 13 (37 percent) were alive at the time of the report.[45] In the majority of fatal cases, the clinical course was rapid, with metastatic lesions developing within a few months after excision of the primary tumor. From this study,[45] guidelines regarding therapy are impossible. A number of these patients were treated with different types of excision, radiation therapy, and, finally, a variety of chemotherapeutic agents. However, based on the histologic features, which resembled those of Ewing's sarcoma of the bone, it is appropriate to assume that this tumor should show a good response to combination radiation therapy and sequential chemotherapy, as reported for Ewing's sarcoma of the bone.[46,47]

Only two such patients have been treated by the author. The primary tumor was in the rectosacral space in one, a 35-year-old man, and in the forearm of the other, a 29-year-old man. The sacral tumor was diagnosed after a nine-month delay. The initial symptom was pain in both instances. In the first patient, a partial resection of the sacrum and gluteal muscles was done, followed by local radiation therapy of 5,000 rads. The patient then received a one-year course of multiagent chemotherapy (cyclophospha-

TABLE 18.5. CLINICAL SUMMARY OF THREE PATIENTS WITH EXTRASKELETAL CHONDROSARCOMA TREATED AT THE UNIVERSITY OF ILLINOIS HOSPITAL

Patient No.	Age	Sex	Primary Site	Status of Primary	Treatment at U of I	Local Recurrence	End Result
1	47	M	Left posterior thigh	Two recurrences, excised and irradiated, 5,000 rads	Muscle group excision	None after operation at U of I	7 yr, N.E.D.*
2	35	M	Right buttock	5 × 7 cm mass	Excision of gluteal muscles	Negative	4½ yr, N.E.D.
3	26	F	Right thigh	Enucleated 7 × 5 cm tumor	Anterolateral compartment muscle group excision	Negative	3½ yr, N.E.D.

*No evidence of disease.

mide, vincristine, and adriamycin). He remained disease-free for three years but pulmonary metastases developed. There was no evidence of local recurrence. The second patient was treated with a wide excision and similar multimodal treatment program.

In a preliminary review of 26 cases encountered in the Intergroup Rhabdomyosarcoma Study, Soule et al.[48] found that these lesions were more common in the extremities, and that 17 (65 percent) of 26 patients were apparently disease-free at the time of their report. All 26 patients were treated by wide local excision, radiation therapy, and systemic chemotherapy.

REFERENCES

1. Willis RA: The Borderland of Embryology and Pathology, chap 14. London, Butterworth, 1958, p 506
2. France CJ, O'Connell JP: Osseous metaplasia in the human mammary gland. Arch Surg 100:238, 1970
3. Ling HW, Stewart IS: A bony tumor of the breast. Br Med J 2:364, 1955
4. Pack GT, Ariel IM: Tumors of the Soft Somatic Tissues: A Clinical Technique. New York, Hoeber/Harper, 1958, p 332
5. Fine G, Stout AP: Osteogenic sarcoma of the extraskeletal soft tissue. Cancer 9:1027, 1956
6. Ryan KJ: Myositis ossificans progressiva: Review of the literature and report of a case. J Pediat 27:348, 1945
7. Rosenstein J: A contribution to the study of myositis ossificans progressiva. Ann Surg 68:485, 1918
8. Pack GT and Braund RR: The development of sarcoma in myositis ossificans: Report of 3 cases. JAMA 119:776, 1942
9. Dahlin DC, Salvador AH: Cartilaginous tumors of the soft tissues of the hand and feet. Mayo Clinic Proc 49:721, 1974
10. Chung EB, Enzinger FM: Chondroma of soft parts. Cancer 41:1414, 1978
11. Bamachandran K, Viswannthan R: Chondroma of the tongue. Report of a case. Oral Surg 25:487, 1968
12. Hankey GT, Waterhouse JP: A calcifying chondroma in the cheek. Br J Oral Surg 5:239, 1968
13. Boneti T: De ventris tumors, in Sepulchretum, sive anatomia practica excadaveribus morbo denatis. Geneva, Cramer et Parachon, Vol 3, Sect 21, Obs 61, 1700, p 522
14. Morgagni JB: The Seats and Causes of Diseases. Translated by B. Alexander. London, A. Miller and T. Cadell. Vol 3, letter L, Obs 41, 1763, p 63
15. Müller J: Uber den feinern Bau der Drankhaften Gesehwulste. Berlin, G. Reimer, 1838, p 48
16. Cooper A: The Anatomy and Diseases of the Breast. Philadelphia, Lea and Blanchard, 1845, p 47
17. Coley WB: Myositis ossificans traumatica: A report of three cases illustrating the difficulties of diagnosis from sarcoma. Ann Surg 57:305, 1913
18. Rhoades CP, Blumgart H: Two osteoblastomas not connected with bone, histologically identical with osteogenic sarcoma and clinically benign. Am J Path 4:363, 1928
19. Mallory TB: A group of metaplastic and neoplastic bone and cartilage containing tumor of soft parts. Am J Path 9:765, 1933
20. Wilson H: Extraskeletal ossifying tumors. Ann Surg 113:95 1941
21. Schaffer LW Jr: Extraskeletal osteochondrosarcoma—Review of literature and report of a case. Am Surg 18:739, 1952
22. Kauffman SL, Stout AP: Extraskeletal osteogenic sarcomas and chondrosarcomas in children. Cancer 16:432, 1963
23. Lowry K Jr, Doyle-Hanes C: Osteosarcoma of extraskeletal soft tissue: A case report. Am Surg 30:97, 1964
24. Yannopoulos K, Bom AF, Griffiths CO, Crikelair GF: Osteosarcoma arising in fibrous dysplasia of the facial bones: Case report and review of the literature. Am J Surg 107:556, 1964
25. Boyer CW Jr, Nawin JJ: Extraskeletal osteogenic sarcoma: A late complication of radiation therapy. Cancer 18:628, 1965
26. Lewis RJ, Lotz MJ, Beazley RM: Extraosseous osteosarcoma: Case report and approach to therapy. Ann Surg 40:597, 1974
27. Das Gupta TK, Hajdu SI, Foote FW Jr: Extraosseous osteogenic sarcoma. Ann Surg 168:1011, 1968
28. Allan CJ, Soule EH: Osteogenic sarcoma of the somatic soft tissue: A clinicopathologic study of 26 cases and review of the literature. Cancer 27:1121, 1971
29. Wurlitzen F, Ayala A, Ronsdahl M: Extraosseous osteogenic sarcoma. Arch Surg 105:691, 1972
30. Rao U, Cheng A, Didolkar MS: Extraosseous osteogenic sarcoma; Clinicopathological study of eight cases and review of the literature. Cancer 41:1488, 1978
31. Dahn LJ, Schaffer SD, Carder HM, Vellios F: Osteosarcoma of the soft tissue of the larynx: Report of a case with light and electronmicroscopic studies. Cancer 42:2343, 1978
32. Auerbach O, Friedman M, Weiss L, Amory HI: Extraskeletal osteogenic sarcoma arising in irradiated tissue. Cancer 4:1095, 1951
33. Bhagavan BS, Dorfman HD: The significance of bone and cartilage formation in malignant fibrous histiocytoma of soft tissue. Cancer 49:480, 1982
33A. Stout AP, Verner EW: Chondrosarcoma of the extraskeletal soft tissue. Cancer 6:581, 1953
34. Dahlin DC, Henderson ED: Chondrosarcoma—a surgical and pathological problem. Review of 212 cases. J Bone Joint Surg 38-A:1025, 1956
35. Goldenberg RR, Cohen P, Steinlauf P: Chondrosarcoma of the extraskeletal soft tissues. J Bone Joint Surg 49-A:1487, 1967
36. Korns ME: Primary chondrosarcoma of extraskeletal soft tissue. Arch Path 83:13, 1967
37. Thompson JR, Entin SD: Primary extraskeletal chondrosarcoma: Report of a case arising in con-

junction with extrapleural lucite ball plombage. Cancer 23:940, 1969

38. Angervall L, Enerback L, Knutson H: Chondrosarcoma of soft tissue origin. Cancer 32:507, 1973
39. Steiner GC, Mirra JM, Bullough PG: Mesenchymal chondrosarcoma—A study of the ultrastructure. Cancer 32:926, 1973
40. Yao-Shi F, Kay S: A comparative ultrastructural study of mesenchymal chondrosarcoma and myxoid chondrosarcoma. Cancer 33:1531, 1974
41. Pittman MR, Keller EE: Mesenchymal chondrosarcoma: Report of a case. J Oral Surg 32:443, 1974
42. Smith MT, Farinacci CJ, Carpenter HA, Bannayan GA: Extraskeletal myxoid chondrosarcoma: A clinicopathological study. Cancer 37:821, 1976
43. Enzinger FM, Shiraki M: Extraskeletal myxoid chondrosarcoma: An analysis of 34 cases. Hum Path 3:421, 1972
44. Vassar PS: Chondrosarcoma of the tongue: A case report. Arch Path 65:261, 1958
45. Angervall I, Enzinger FM: Extraskeletal neoplasm resembling Ewing's sarcoma. Cancer 36:240, 1975
46. Dahlin DC: Ewing's sarcoma and malignant lymphoma (reticulum cell sarcoma) of bone. In Tumors of Bone and Soft Tissue. Chicago, Year Book Medical Publishers, 1965, p 179
47. Rosen G, Wollner N, Tan C, et al: Disease-free survival in children with Ewing's sarcoma treated with radiation therapy and adjuvant four-drug sequential chemotherapy. Cancer 33:384, 1974
48. Soule EH, Newton W, Moor TE, Tefft M: Extraskeletal Ewing's sarcoma. A preliminary review of 26 cases encountered in the Intergroup Rhabdomyosarcoma Study. Cancer 42:259, 1978

19
Undetermined Histogenesis
Tapas K. Das Gupta

Although the list of benign and malignant tumors of uncertain histogenesis is becoming smaller, there are still some in which the correct histogenetic type is difficult or almost impossible to determine. In the absence of such classification, the clinical features of these diverse groups are described in this section.

BENIGN

Granular Cell Myoblastoma

Although an uncommon tumor, granular cell myoblastoma is seen in all age groups. Strong et al.,[1] reviewing the Memorial Sloan-Kettering experience, found that their youngest patient was 11 months old and the oldest 68 years, the average age being 38.1 years. Vance and Hudson,[2] in their series, found the average age to be 29 years, the youngest being 10 and the oldest 72.

In the University of Illinois material, the tumor occurred predominantly in women. Similar observations have been made by Strong et al.[1] and by Vance and Hudson.[2]

Although Vance and Hudson suggested a greater propensity for these tumors to grow in American blacks, our own observations, as well as those of others,[1-7] do not seem to substantiate

this. In our series of 32 patients, the tumor was found in 20 white and 12 black patients, and in Strong and co-workers'[1] series of 95 patients, 86 were white and 9 were black.

Granular cell myoblastoma occurs in all parts of the human body. The tongue is overwhelmingly the predominant site for this neoplasm.[1,3,7-9] The incidence was 28.2 percent in the series reported from Memorial Sloan-Kettering Cancer Center[1] and 25 percent in the series reported by Vance and Hudson.[2] Table 19.1 shows the comparative incidence of tumors in different anatomic locations. In Vance and Hudson's series[2] there were 50 tumors in 42 patients. In the series reported by Strong and co-authors,[1] there were 110 tumors in 95 patients, and in our series, 36 tumors in 32 patients. No organ or tissue of the body is free from development of this entity.[1,2] Various reports have included origin in the middle and external ear,[10] breast,[7,11] larynx,[12] parotid,[13] esophagus,[14,15] tracheobronchial tree,[16-18] gastrointestinal tract (including cystic duct, pancreas, and common bile duct),[19-24] urinary bladder,[25] and female reproductive tract.[26-28] Stout and Lattes[29] considered congenital epulis as a congenital granular cell tumor.

The majority of our 32 patients sought medical opinion for a slow-growing, asymptomatic tumor (Fig. 19.1). Only four patients complained of associated pain or a tingling sensa-

628

TABLE 19.1. ANATOMIC LOCATION OF GRANULAR CELL MYOBLASTOMA IN THREE SERIES

Site	Vance and Hudson[2] (1969)	Strong et al.[1] (1970)	Das Gupta (1981)
Eyelid	–	1	–
Lip	–	2	1
Tongue	13	39	7
Neck	2	3	2
Larynx	1	4	0
Shoulder	0	1	1
Breast	7	6	6
Chest wall	1	9	7
Back	3	9	3
Abdominal wall	5	2	3
Perineum	7	2	2
Upper extremity (including axilla)	7	18	3
Lower extremity (including groin)	2	7	1
Miscellaneous sites (eg, viscera)	2	7	–
Total	50	110	36

tion. In most series[1-3] the initial presentation was an asymptomatic lump. However, in some instances, certain specific symptoms have been noted, depending on the location of the tumor. For example, patients with tumors in the vocal cords complained of hoarseness,[12] those with tumors in the gastrointestinal tract were seen for bleeding,[19,20] and those with tumors of the biliary tract have had symptoms of acute cholecystitis.[23,24] In a number of instances the tumor has been identified only at autopsy.[14,22] These unusual locations of granular cell myoblastomas are interesting and provide an insight into the histogenesis of the tumor. However, from a clinical viewpoint antemortem diagnosis of these tumors in locations such as the biliary tract or the pancreas is impossible. These tumors are usually small, nonulcerated, nodular lesions arising from the dermis or subdermal or submucosal tissue. Rarely, larger tumors have occurred deeper in the somatic tissues.[1,2]

The treatment of granular cell myoblastoma is wide local excision. In the past, owing to lack of information concerning the histogenesis and natural history of these tumors, various other forms of treatment were tried,[1,2] resulting in less than optimum results. There is no place for radiation therapy or chemotherapy in the treatment of these benign tumors. Most of the local recurrences are directly related to inadequate

excision. Based on our experience and on a review of the literature, a 3-cm margin on all sides is sufficient in most instances. In lesions located in the viscus, excision sometimes must be radical because of the location. For example, granular cell myoblastoma of the stomach or cecum might require a partial gastrectomy or right hemicolectomy.

The patients in our series have all been followed up for at least five years, and all have remained free of the problem for which they were initially treated.

In our series, there were 4 of 32 patients (12.5 percent) with multiple primary tumors. The incidence was 14.2 percent and 8.4 percent in the series reported by Vance and Hudson[2] and Strong et al.,[1] respectively. Early reports implied that multiplicity is a rare occurrence; however, with increasing information it appears that multiple primary granular cell myoblastomas are not uncommon. Various theories regarding this multiplicity have been forwarded[5,20] but none have been substantiated.

The association of granular cell myoblastoma with other neoplasms, both benign and malignant, has been observed. In our present series of 32 patients, two (6.25 percent) were treated for carcinoma of the breast. Strong et al.[1] found that 11 (11.6 percent) of their patients had a second primary tumor. Three of the 11

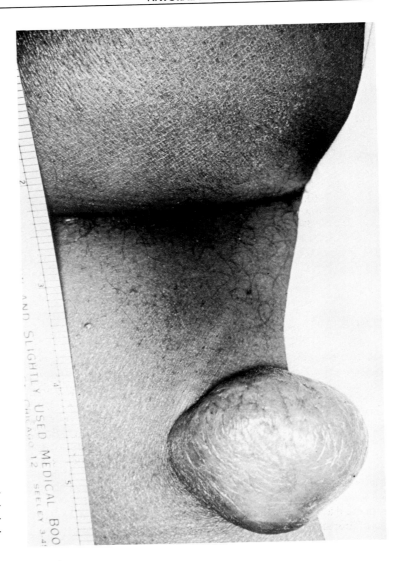

Figure 19.1. A slow-growing pedunculated tumor of five years' duration in the posterior thigh of a 48-year-old woman. Following excision, she has remained well.

had breast cancer, and one each had adenocarcinoma of the lung, lymphosarcoma, carcinoid of the colon, carcinoma of the esophagus, melanoma, carcinoma of the cervix, osteochondroma, and thyroid adenoma.

Benign Mesenchymoma

In 1938, Tauber and colleagues[30] used the term mesenchymoma to describe an unusual tumor of the scalp composed of undifferentiated cells of possible mesenchymal origin. Stout, in 1948,[31] applied this term to designate a group of tumors composed of at least two differentiated mesenchymal elements not ordinarily found together in a given tumor. He reported eight such cases. Since that time a few additional case reports have appeared in the literature.[32,33] A clinicopathologic diagnosis of benign mesenchymoma must be made with great caution. We have encountered only a few patients whose soft tissue tumors could be so designated. Treatment is local excision.

MALIGNANT

Malignant Granular Cell Myoblastoma

The malignant variant of granular cell myoblastoma is indeed rare.[34] Some authors consider the organoid type to be similar to an alveolar

TABLE 19.2. TWENTY-THREE CASES OF MALIGNANT GRANULAR CELL MYOBLASTOMA

Case No.	Author (s)	Year of Publication	Age/Sex	Site of Lesion	Metastases	End Results
1	Ravich et al[25]	1945	31 M	Urinary bladder	Lymph nodes, bones, liver spleen, lungs, pericardium, peritoneum, prostate	17 mo (dead)
2	Powell[6]	1946	26 F	Subcutaneous nodules	Ovaries, retroperitoneum	240 mo
3	Dunnington[38]	1948	40 M	Eyelid	Generalized	24 mo
4	Ceelen[39]	1949	45 F	Left arm	Axillary lymph nodes, breast, and lungs	54 mo
5	Schwidde[40]	1951	21 F	Right thigh	Brain and humerus	37 mo
6	Ross et al[35]	1952	60 M	Lumbosacral area	Inguinal lymph nodes and lungs	36 mo
7	Ibid[35]	1952	58 F	Skin of left ankle	Inguinal lymph nodes	96 mo (dead)
8	Ibid[35]	1952	33 F	Subcutaneous tumor of left thigh	Local recurrence	8 mo
9	Crawford and De Bakey[41]	1953	50 F	Breast	Left lung, liver and celiac axis	12 mo (dead)
10	Gamboa[36]	1955	30 F	Right thigh	Inguinal lymph nodes and left lung	60 mo
11	Svejda and Horn[42]	1958	48 F	Groin	Small intestine, liver, myocardium, lungs, urinary bladder, and thigh muscle	36 mo (dead)
12	Bussanny et al[43]	1958	40 M	Larynx nodes	Cervical lymph nodes	24 mo (dead)
13	Hunter and Dewar[34]	1960	73 F	Colon	None	15 mo
14	Caby et al[44]	1960	40 F	Thigh	Inguinal lymph nodes	156 mo (dead)
15	Obiditsch-Mayer and Salzer-Kuntschik[45]	1961	23 F	Esophagus	Regional lymph nodes	Died post-operatively
16	Krieg[46]	1962	64 F	Biceps and brachii muscle	Lung, liver vertebral bones, mediastinal, retroperitoneal, and axillary lymph nodes	14 mo (dead)
17	Nitze[47]	1966	66 M	Buccal mucosa	Retro-ocular	18 mo (dead)
18	Mackenzie[48]	1967	82 F	Left loin	Lungs, lymph nodes, and breast	39 mo (dead)
19	McCabe and Harman[49]	1969	69 M	Tongue	Cervical lymph nodes	Dead

(Continued)

TABLE 19.2. *(Continued)*

Case No.	Author(s)	Year of Publication	Age/Sex	Site of Lesion	Metastases	End Results
20	Al-Sarraf et al[50]	1971	35 M	Ischiorectal mass	Inguinal lymph nodes	—
21	Kuchemann[51]	1971	38 F	Right shoulder	Axillary lymph nodes	—
22	Cadotte[37]	1973	60 F	Right thigh	Local invasion, inguinal lymph nodes and lungs	9 mo (dead)
23	Das Gupta	1981	64 M	Back	Local recurrence lymph nodes, lungs and other viscera	6 mo (dead)

Courtesy Cadotte,[37] Cancer 33:1417, 1974.

soft part sarcoma.[29] However, there is a non-organoid type that probably can be classified as a malignant variant of granular cell myoblastoma. In 1952, Ross, Miller, and Foote[35] could find only four unequivocal cases of malignant granular cell myoblastoma, to which they added three of their own. In 1955, Gamboa[36] reviewed the literature and added one case of his own, bringing the total to 11. Cadotte[37] reviewed the literature in 1974 and concluded that there were only 22 documented cases.[6,25,35,37-51] In our surgical oncology service, one additional case has been treated. Table 19.2 summarizes the clinical history of these 23 cases. In our patient, the primary tumor was in the interscapular region, and the ipsilateral axilla contained metastatic tumor. The patient died within six months and autopsy showed diffuse metastatic involvement of the viscera. Based on the scanty information on the 22 earlier patients[6,25,35,37-51] and on observation of our own patient (Table 19.2), it appears that these neoplasms are aggressive. Primary treatment should consist of radical excision and, when indicated, lymph node dissection. Following initial excision, adjuvant systemic chemotherapy is in order. However, the types of agents and the program that might yield the best end result are not yet known.

Alveolar Soft Part Sarcoma

Christopherson, Foote, and Stewart[52] first described this entity in 1952. Costero[53] and Udekwu and Pulvertaft[54] later published specific histopathologic evidence which indicated that alveolar soft part sarcoma was an unusual type of malignant mesenchymal tumor. Although rare,[55] clinically these tumors have a distinct history of slow growth, local infiltration, and delayed visceral metastases.

They occur in all age groups from neonates to adults in their seventh decade, but are most commonly encountered in young adults between the ages of 20 and 35 years; they are far more common in women than in men. The average age of discovery in women is 20 years and in men about 10 years later. There seems to be no racial predilection.

The usual history is of a comparatively slow-growing asymptomatic mass located in one of the extremities. Of the original 12 cases reported by Christopherson et al.,[52] ten were in an extremity. The tumor may also arise from the anterior abdominal wall, the perianal region, the retroperitoneum,[56] and the head and neck region.[52,56A-65] It is always associated with skeletal muscles or musculofascial planes, and it is usually well circumscribed.

Lieberman and co-workers[58] analyzed 53 cases of alveolar soft part sarcoma seen at Memorial Sloan-Kettering Cancer Center and presented survival data on 46 patients. We have treated six patients with this tumor. Five were women and one was a man 69 years old. The clinical histories of these six patients are summarized in Table 19.3. Alveolar soft part sarcomas in the head and neck region are extremely rare. Up to 1979 only eleven cases were recorded (Table 19.4).[52,56A,60-66]

Alveolar soft part sarcoma runs an indolent but inexorable course, with a tendency to me-

TABLE 19.3. CLINICAL SUMMARY OF SIX CASES OF ALVEOLAR SOFT PART SARCOMA (UNIVERSITY OF ILLINOIS PATIENTS)

Patient	Age	Sex	Location	Treatment	Recurrence or Metastases	End Result
1	21	F	Upper lateral arm 4 × 1 cm tumor	Wide soft tissue excision	—	6½ yr N.E.D.*
2	36	F	Medial thigh 5 × 7 tumor	Wide soft tissue excision	Local recurrence after 1 yr; lesion excised	5 yr N.E.D. since treatment of local recurrence
3	69	M	Lateral aspect of thigh 3 × 2 cm	Wide soft tissue excision	—	5½ yr N.E.D.
4	39	F	Lower thigh 3 × 3 cm	Wide soft tissue excision	—	6 yr, 2 mo N.E.D.
5	21	F	Anterior aspect of right thigh 6 × 7 cm. Ovoid mass attached to femoral nerve	Wide soft tissue excision	—	3 yr N.E.D.
6	62	F	Left inguinal region 5 × 4 cm. Initially thought to be a lymph node and biopsied	Wide soft tissue excision. Specimen showed a focal tumor, 1 cm diameter, 8 cm distal from the original primary	—	2 yr N.E.D.

No evidence of disease.

tastasize to lungs, liver, skeleton, and, infrequently, to the lymph nodes. In Lieberman and co-workers'[58] series, three patients had lung metastases 15 years after the onset of illness.

Treatment for alveolar soft part sarcoma is wide soft tissue excision. A major amputation is seldom indicated. The author's personal experience is based only on tumors located in the extremities, and for none of them was amputation required (Table 19.3). Based on a five-year survival analysis it appears that radical excision alone is adequate. However, in larger lesions or lesions located in the head and neck area, a combination of radiation therapy and systemic chemotherapy probably is in order (Table 19.4).

In the series reported by Lieberman et al.,[58] of 43 patients 83 percent survived two years and 47 percent for ten years. Of the six patients treated by the author, four are living at the end of five years and the remaining two are still disease-free two years after primary treatment. It is recognized that these neoplasms have a propensity to recur at a late date and also have the potential to metastasize after a long time. However, based on five-year followup study it appears that an adequate wide excision is sufficient for local control of these tumors, without compromising the functioning of the extremity.

Malignant Mesenchymoma

This diagnosis is rarely encountered today. As described in Chapter 4, if, in an unusual situation, the exact histogenesis of the given tumor cannot be adequately documented, the management of the tumor should depend on the predominant malignant tissue component. For example, a tumor containing different tissue elements with a preponderance of malignant lipoblasts should be treated as an undifferentiated liposarcoma (grade 3 or 4). In most instances, the natural history of this tumor is similar to that of high-grade liposarcoma.

Malignant Mesothelioma

Pleural or peritoneal mesotheliomas are rare malignant neoplasms. Because of the association of pleural mesothelioma with asbestos exposure, this type of malignancy has engendered considerable curiosity; however, the neoplasm is rare and general guidelines for management

TABLE 19.4. ALVEOLAR SOFT PART SARCOMA IN THE HEAD AND NECK REGION

Author(s)	Year of Publication	Age/Sex	Location	Size	Treatment	End Result
Smetana and Scott[60]	1951	27 M	R posterior cervical triangle	Weight 51 gm	Excision	Died 1 yr. Metastases to lungs, heart, brain
Smetana and Scott[60]	1951	28 F	Inferior to angle L mandible	1.5 cm	Radiation (unspec. amt); excision 3 yr thereafter	No recurrence 4 yr after surgery
Christopherson et al[52] (Patient 8 of Lieberman et al[58])	1952	12 F	Base of tongue	5.0 cm	Excision	No recurrence after 5 yr
Caldwell et al[61]	1956	4 M	Base of tongue	4.0 cm	Excision	Unknown
Ushijima and Tamura[62]	1957	26 F	Tongue	5.0 cm	Excision	Unknown
Vakil and Sirsat[63]	1963	45 M	R orbit	Unknown	Excision	Recurrence after few months orbit exenterated. Died
Vakil and Sirsat[63]	1963	10 F	Tongue	Unknown	Excision	Recurrence after 6 mo
Gingrass et al[64]	1967	24 M	L temporal region	3.0 cm	Excision	No recurrence after 6 mo
Varghese et al[65]	1968	13 F	L orbit	Unknown	Orbital exenteration	Recurrence after few months
Buchanan[56A]	1974	17 F	R lower jaw	?	Wide excision including the ramus (rt.)	Lymph node metastases 1 yr later, recurrence in neck, died 4 yr later with metastases
Spector et al[66]	1979	17 F	Tongue	?	Excision	Dead of disease 5 yr after diagnosis. Tumor became apparent after childbirth

are not yet possible. Strictly speaking, these are soft somatic tissue neoplasms, but seldom are they treated as such. In the unusual instance in which the diagnosis can be made early, a pleurectomy might be of some value. However, in most instances the diagnosis is made after the patient has massive pleural effusion, and the treatment becomes palliative, with judicious thoracentesis, radiation therapy, and chemotherapy. Long-term cures are rare.

A clinical diagnosis of peritoneal or pelvic mesothelioma is based on abdominal or pelvic symptoms. These tumors can be operated upon by removing the gross tumor along with the adjacent viscera, but the incidence of local recurrence is extremely high (Fig. 19.2).

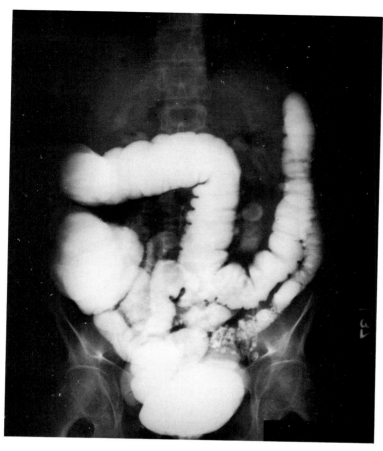

Figure 19.2. Peritoneal mesothelioma in 55-year-old woman. Note the impingement of the sigmoid due to serosal implants and pressure. She was first seen because of changing bowel habits. The diagnosis was established by exploratory celiotomy. Treatment consisted of removal of peritoneal implants and segmental resection of the sigmoid colon.

REFERENCES

1. Strong EW, McDivitt RW, Brasfield RD: Granular cell myoblastoma. Cancer 25:415, 1970
2. Vance SF III, Hudson RP Jr: Granular cell myoblastoma: Clinicopathologic study of forty-two patients. Am J Clin Path 52:208, 1969
3. Horn RC Jr, Stout AP: Granular cell myoblastoma. Surg Gynecol Obstet 76:315, 1943
4. Moscovic EA, Azar HA: Multiple granular cell tumors ("myoblastomas"). Cancer 20:2032, 1967
5. Papageorgiou S, Litt JZ, Pomeranz JR: Multiple granular cell myoblastomas in children. Arch Dermat 96:168, 1967
6. Powell EB: Granular cell myoblastoma. Arch Path 42:517, 1946
7. Kirschner H: Uber elnen Fall von maligne entartetem Myoblastenmyon der Mamma. Bruns Beitr Klin Chir 204:87, 1962
8. Hagen JO, Soule EH, Gores JF: Granular cell myoblastoma of the oral cavity. Oral Surg 14:454, 1961
9. Rafel SS: Granular cell myoblastoma. Oral Surg 15:192, 1962
10. Gray SH, Gruenfeld, GE: Myoblastoma. Am J Cancer 30:699, 1937
11. Friedman RM, Hurwitt ES: Granular cell myoblastoma of the breast. Am J Surg 112:75, 1966
12. Pope TA: Laryngeal myoblastoma. Arch Otolaryngol 81:80, 1965
13. Nussbaum M, Haselkorn A: Granular cell myoblastoma in parotid gland. NY State J Med 72:2887, 1972
14. De Gouveici OF, Pereira AA, Netto BM, et al: Granular cell myoblastoma of the esophagus. Gastroenterology 54:805, 1960
15. Keshishian JM, Alford TC: Granular cell myoblastoma of the esophagus. Am Surg 30:263, 1964
16. Archer FL, Harrison RW, Moulder PV: Granular cell myoblastoma of the trachea and carina treated by resection and reconstruction. J Thor Cardiovasc Surg 45:539, 1963
17. Rojer CL: Multicentric endobronchial myoblastoma. Arch Otolaryngol 82:652, 1965
18. Weitzner S, Oser JF: Granular cell myoblastoma of bronchus. Am Rev Resp Dis 97:923, 1968
19. Goldman ML, Gottlieg LS, Zamchek N: Granular cell myoblastoma of the stomach and colon. Am J Dig Dis 7:432, 1962
20. Schwartz DT, Gaetz HP: Multiple granular cell myoblastomas of the stomach. Am J Clin Path 44:453, 1965

21. Winne BE, Bacon HE: Myoblastoma of the anal canal. Dis Colon Rectum 4:206, 1961
22. Wellmann KF, Tsai CY, Reyes FB: Granular cell myoblastoma in pancreas. NY State J Med 78:1270, 1975
23. LiVolsi VA, Perzin KH, Badder EM et al: Granular cell tumor of the bilary tract. Arch Path 95:13, 1973
24. Reul GH, Rubio PA, Berkman NL: Granular cell myoblastoma of the cystic duct: A case associated with hydrops of the gallbladder. Am J Surg 129:583, 1975
25. Ravich A, Stout AP, Ravich RA: Malignant granular cell myoblastoma involving the urinary bladder. Ann Surg 121:361, 1945
26. Svesko VS: Granular cell myoblastoma of the vulva. Am J Obstet Gynecol 87:143, 1963
27. Wolfe DS, Mackles A: Uncommon myogenic tumors of the female genital tract. Obstet Gynecol 22:199, 1963
28. Doyle WF, Hutchinson JR: Granular cell myoblastoma of the clitoris. Am J Obstet Gynecol 100:589, 1968
29. Stout AP, Lattes R: Tumors of the Soft Tissues, fasc 3, series 2. Washington DC, AFIP, 1967
30. Tauber EB, Goldman L, Bassett C: Mesenchymoma, a new type of turban tumor. Arch Dermat Syph 37:444, 1938
31. Stout AP: Mesenchymoma, the mixed tumor of mesenchymal derivatives. Ann Surg 127:278, 1948
32. LeBer MS, Stout AP: Benign mesenchymomas in children. Cancer 15:598, 1962
33. Bugg ET, Mathews RS: Benign mesenchymoma. South Med J 63:268, 1970
34. Hunter DT Jr, Dewar JP: Malignant granular cell myoblastoma: report of a case and review of the literature. Am Surg 26:554, 1960
35. Ross RC, Miller TR, Foote FW Jr: Malignant granular cell myoblastoma. Cancer 5:112, 1952
36. Gamboa LG: Malignant granular cell myoblastoma. Arch Path 60:663, 1955
37. Cadotte M: Malignant granular cell myoblastoma. Cancer 33:1417, 1974
38. Dunnington JH: Granular cell myoblastoma of the orbit. Arch Ophthalmol 40:1422, 1948
39. Ceelen W: Uber die Natur der sog. Myoblastome (zugleich ein Bericht uber eine maligne Myoblastengeschwulst). Zentralbl f allg Path U path Anat 85:289, 1949
40. Schwidde, JT: Meyers R, Sweeney DB: Intracerebral metastatic granular cell myoblastoma. J Neuropath Exper Neurol 10:303, 1951
41. Crawford ES, De Bakey ME: Granular cell myoblastoma: Two unusual cases. Cancer 6:786, 1953
42. Svejda J, Horn V: Disseminated granular cell pseudotumor, so-called metastasizing granular cell myoblastoma. J Path Bacteriol 75:343, 1958
43. Busanny-Caspari W, Hammer CH: Zur Malignitat der sogenanntem Myoblastenmyome. Zentralbl Allg Pathol 98:401, 1958
44. Caby F, Duperrat B, Eoochard JC: Un cas de tumeur dAbrikoffof a evolution maligne. Mem Acad Chir 86:585, 1960
45. Obiditsch-Mayer I, Salzer-Kuntschik M: Malignant granular cell neuroma, so-called "myoblastoma" of the esophagus. Beitr Path Anat 125:357, 1961

46. Krieg AF: Malignant granular cell myoblastoma: Case report. Arch Path 74:251, 1962
47. Nitze von H: Das sogenannte Myoblastenmyom und weine maligne Verlaufsform. Z Laryngol Rhinol Otol 45:740, 1966
48. Mackenzie DH: Malignant granular cell myoblastoma. J Clin Path 20:739, 1967
49. McCabe MM, Harman JW: Malignant myoblastoma: A case report. J Irish Med Assoc 62:284, 1969
50. Al-Sarraf M, Loud AV, Vaitkevicius VM: Malignant granular cell tumor. Arch Path 91:550, 1971
51. Kuchemann von K: Malignes granulares Neurom (Granularzell-myoblastom) Fallbericht und Literaturubersicht. Zentralbl Allg Pathol 114:426, 1971
52. Christopherson WM, Foote JW Jr, Stewart FW: Alveolar soft part sarcomas: Structurally characteristic tumors of uncertain histogenesis. Cancer 5:100, 1952
53. Costero I: Recent advances in the knowledge concerning chemodectomas. Lab Invest 12:270, 1963
54. Udekwu FA, Pulvertaft FJ: Studies of an alveolar soft tissue sarcoma. Br J Cancer 19:744, 1965
55. Ekfors TO, Kalimo H, Rantakokko V, Latvala M, Parviner M: Alveolar soft part sarcoma. A report of two cases with some histochemical and ultrastructural observations. Cancer 43:1672, 1979
56. Mathew T: Evidence supporting neural crest origin of an alveolar soft part sarcoma: An ultrastructural study. Cancer 50:507, 1982
56A. Buchanan G: Two rare tumors involving the infratemporal fossa: Alveolar soft part sarcoma and haemangiopericytoma. J Laryngol Otol (London): 89:375, 1975
57. Balfour RS: The alveolar soft-part sarcoma: Review of the literature and report of case. J Oral Surg 32:214, 1974
58. Lieberman PH, Foote FW Jr, Stewart FW, et al: Alveolar soft part sarcoma. JAMA 198:1047, 1966
59. Olson RAJ, Perkins KD: Alveolar soft-part sarcoma in the oral cavity: Report of a case. J Oral Surg 34:73, 1976
60. Smetana HF, Scott WF Jr: Malignant tumors of nonchromaffin paraganglia. Milit Surg 190:330, Oct 1951
61. Caldwell JB, Hughes KW, Fadell EJ: Alveolar soft-part sarcoma of the tongue: Report of a case. J Oral Surg 14:342, 1956
62. Ushijima H, Tamura Z: A report of two cases of alveolar soft-part sarcoma and their histological variations. Acta Pathologica Japonica (Suppl) 7:851, 1957
63. Vakil VV, Sirsat MV: The natural history of alveolar soft-part sarcomas. Indian J Path Bacteriol 6:19, 1963
64. Gingrass R, Mladick R, Pickrell L, Punyahotra V: Malignant nonchromaffin paraganglioma or alveolar soft-part sarcoma in the temporal region. Plast Reconstr Surg 40:463, 1967
65. Varghese S, Nair G, Joseph TA: Orbital malignant non-chromaffin paraganglioma: Alveolar soft tissue sarcoma. Br J Ophthalmol 52:713, 1968
66. Spector RA, Travis LW, Smith J: Alveolar soft part sarcoma of the head and neck. Laryngoscope 89:1301, 1979

20

Childhood Sarcoma

Tapas K. Das Gupta

Pessimism regarding childhood cancers was at one time so rampant that, as late as 1941, Ladd and Gross,[1] in their textbook *Surgery of Infancy and Childhood*, were exhorting physicians to develop a more positive attitude, since 25 percent of all children with renal embryomas could be permanently cured. They urged their colleagues to make an attempt at cure rather than adopt a nihilistic attitude as soon as the diagnosis of a pediatric neoplasm was established. In the last 40 years the outlook for childhood cancer has become increasingly hopeful.

It is now generally agreed that a large number of pediatric solid tumors are indeed curable, and that they constitute one of the important areas in which the combination of three therapeutic modalities—surgery, radiation therapy, and chemotherapy—has produced exciting end results in recent years. The first neoplasm to fall before this combined attack was Wilms' tumor. The survival rate in children in the most successful arm of the national Wilms' tumor study is now well above 85 percent, and in certain of tbe early stages of that disease, it is approaching 100 percent.[2-4] It seems likely that other types will soon be successfully treated, and pediatric solid tumors, especially soft tissue sarcomas, will come to be considered a curable entity.

INCIDENCE OF SOFT TISSUE SARCOMAS

Fraumeni and Miller[5] reviewed the death certificates of all children under 15 years of age who died of cancer in the United States during the five-year period 1960 to 1964. They found that 12 (0.6 percent) died before the age of 28 days, the death rate in these infants being 6.25 per one million live births. Table 20.1 summarizes the mortality data on the various forms of cancer (including leukemia) in children under 5 years of age and infants under 28 days. Table 20.2 shows the death rate from sarcoma in children under the age of 15 years, the highest being 5.08 for neuroblastoma and the lowest, 0.02 for malignant schwannoma.[6] The cancer mortality in children under 15 years points to the overall rarity of pediatric soft tissue sarcomas, although all histogenetic types are encountered.

The relationship between soft tissue sarcomas and congenital anomalies has been studied off and on by several authors.[7-10] The association of aniridia, hemihypertrophy, and Wilms' tumor appears to be a consistent observation.[10] Similarly, in diseases such as von Recklinghausen's neurofibromatosis, children are seen with a variety of different soft tissue tu-

TABLE 20.1. COMPARISON OF MORTALITY FROM MALIGNANCY IN CHILDREN IN THE UNITED STATES UNDER FIVE YEARS OF AGE AND INFANTS UNDER 28 DAYS OF AGE 1960–1964*

	Under 5 Yr	Under 28 Days		
Neoplasms	No. Deaths	No. Deaths	(Rate per 10^6 Live Births)	Percent†
Leukemia	4,592	44	2.11	1.0
Neuroblastoma	1,049	27	1.30	2.6
Brain tumor	1,035	7	0.34	0.7
Wilms' tumor	696	9	0.43	1.3
Liver cancer, primary	196	10	0.48	5.1
Teratoma	111	9	0.43	8.1
Sarcoma	1,940	12	0.58	1.2
Other	—	12	0.58	—
Total	9,619	130	6.25	1.4

*Adapted from Fraumeni and Miller.[5]
†Percent of neonatal deaths among type-specific cancers in children under five years of age, eg, for leukemia (44 × 100/4,592 = 1.0).

mors.[11] Sloane and Hubbell[7] described four children with congenital anomalies in a small series of 20 soft tissue sarcomas. In the series from the University of Illinois reported by Wood and Das Gupta,[12] however, and in the more updated ma-

TABLE 20.2. DEATH RATE FROM DIFFERENT TYPES OF SARCOMA IN CHILDREN UNDER 15 YEARS OF AGE IN THE UNITED STATES 1960–1966*

Neoplasm	No. Deaths	Death Rate (per million/yr)
Neuroblastoma	2,093	5.08
Wilms' tumor	1,585	3.85
Osteosarcoma	647	1.57
Ewing's sarcoma	384	.93
Chondrosarcoma	20	0.05
Rhabdomyosarcoma	644	1.56
Retinoblastoma	243	0.59
Blood vessel tumor	85	0.21
Fibrosarcoma	81	0.20
Neurofibrosarcoma	46	0.11
Liposarcoma	35	0.08
Meningiosarcoma	27	0.07
Synovial sarcoma	24	0.06
Leiomyosarcoma	24	0.06
Ganglioneuroblastoma	23	0.06
Malignant schwannoma	7	0.02

*The difference in time intervals does not affect comparisons, since there were only minor variations in annual rates of specific neoplasms in the periods studied. Modified from RW Miller, 1969.[6]

terial reported here, no concomitant congenital anomalies were observed.

Recognition of soft tissue sarcomas in children is relatively recent. In 1876, Duzan[13] described 183 tumors of infancy and childhood, and Picot,[14] in 1883, reviewed 424. Neither of these early authors mentioned sarcomas of the soft somatic tissues. In contrast, in 1952 Arey[15] described 62 pediatric neoplasms, of which 18 percent were soft tissue sarcomas. Since then, several large series have been reported.[12,16-20]

A more detailed discussion of the clinicopathologic features and methods of management of the various histologic types of soft tumors can be found in the appropriate chapters elsewhere in this book. This chapter deals only with features unique to malignant soft tissue tumors in children.

Soft tissue sarcomas are seen in all anatomic areas and appear to have no sexual or racial predilection. Wood and Das Gupta[12] reported a series of 31 pediatric cases from the University of Illinois. Since then, 41 new cases have been added. In this combined series of 72 patients, 34 tumors (47 percent) were located in the head and neck region and 6 (8 percent) in the genitourinary tract. A similar anatomic distribution in the head and neck region was noted in Mayo Clinic material (Table 20.3). Although we have not treated any case of intrathoracic soft tissue sarcoma, recently Crist et al.[17] found

TABLE 20.3. ANATOMIC DISTRIBUTION OF SOFT TISSUE SARCOMAS IN CHILDREN IN TWO SERIES

Major Anatomic Location	U of I Series (1981)	Mayo Clinic Series (1968)[16]
Head and neck	34	51
Upper extremities	6	18
Trunk	6	10
Lower extremities	12	23
Retroperitoneum	2	5
Pelvis and perineum	6	28
Gastrourinary tract	6	0
Totals	72	135

this to be the primary tumor in 17 (2.6 percent) of the 646 children registered in the Intergroup Rhabdomyosarcoma Study. The tumor appeared to arise from the mediastinum in ten patients, the pleura in four, and the lung in three.

HISTOLOGIC TYPE

Although all types of soft tissue sarcoma have been reported in children,[21-34] the three most common are rhabdomyosarcoma, fibrosarcoma,

and malignant peripheral nerve tumors. Table 20.4 shows the histologic types encountered in three series. In the past, a large number of these tumors were placed in the category of unclassified sarcomas. Probably this accounts for such a large number of this group in Pack and Ariel's[20] series, as well as in the series reported from the Mayo Clinic by Soule and associates.[16] Recently, electron microscopy has shown that the majority of so-called undetermined histogenetic types are in reality rhabdomyosarcomas. In our own group of 72 patients, three sarcomas were deemed unclassifiable. However, from a therapeutic standpoint they were classified as rhabdomyosarcomas and treated accordingly.

Table 20.5 shows the incidence of various histologic types in different anatomic locations encountered in our series. It is apparent that a preponderance occurred in the head and neck region. This observation is in keeping with other published reports.[12,16,18,20,35]

CLINICAL FEATURES

The major presenting complaint is usually of a painless, slow-growing mass. Occasionally pain is present, and two of the children in our series

TABLE 20.4. SOFT TISSUE SARCOMAS IN CHILDREN: HISTOLOGIC TYPES IN THREE SERIES

Histologic Type	U of I (1981)	Pack and Ariel[20]* (1958)	Soule et al.[16]† (1968)
Rhabdomyosarcoma	44	4	75
Sarcoma of undetermined histogenesis	3	23	27
Fibrosarcoma	15	4	6
Malignant solitary schwannoma	2	7	0
Neurofibrosarcoma with von Recklinghausen's disease	1	0	5
Liposarcoma	2	7	2
Synovial cell sarcoma	3	3	10
Leiomyosarcoma	1	0	3
Dermatofibrosarcoma protuberans	0	1	2
Malignant hemangiopericytoma	0	0	3
Malignant mixed mesenchymoma	0	0	1
Extraosseous osteogenic sarcoma	0	0	1
Angiosarcoma	0	2	0
Epithelioid sarcoma	1	0	0
Totals	72	51	135

*Memorial Sloan-Kettering Cancer Center.
†Mayo Clinic.

TABLE 20.5. ANATOMIC SITES AND HISTOLOGIC TYPES OF SOFT TISSUE SARCOMAS IN CHILDREN (UNIVERSITY OF ILLINOIS SERIES OF 72 PATIENTS)

Histologic Type	Head and Neck	Upper Extremity	Trunk	Perineum and Pelvis	Lower Extremity	Retroperitoneum	GU Tract and Misc.	Total
Rhabdomyosarcoma	24	2	4	3 (perianal)	5	0	6	44
Fibrosarcoma	7	1	1	3	2	1	0	15
Solitary malignant schwannoma	0	0	1	0	1	0	0	2
Malignant schwannoma with von Recklinghausen's disease	1	0	0	0	0	0	0	1
Liposarcoma	0	1	0	0	1	0	0	2
Synovial cell sarcoma	0	0	0	0	3	0	0	3
Leiomyosarcoma	0	1	0	0	0	0	0	1
Epithelioid sarcoma	0	1	0	0	0	0	0	1
Unclassified	2	0	0	0	0	1	0	3
Total	34	6	6	6	12	2	6	72

were first seen because of vocal changes or tonsillitis. The diagnostic methods required are similar to those used for adults and are discussed in Chapter 5.

Head and Neck Region

It should be assumed, a priori, that all childhood solid tumors in the head and neck region, with the exception of enlarged lymph nodes, are malignant unless proved otherwise by histologic examination. All too often, children have been sent to us after inadequate excision of a supposedly innocuous tumor in the head and neck region, which at a later date was found to be a sarcoma.

Although all types of sarcoma occur in this region, rhabdomyosarcoma and fibrosarcoma are the most common. Table 20.6 shows the relative frequency of specific histologic types of tumors in the head and neck region in four rel-

TABLE 20.6. INCIDENCE OF MALIGNANT HEAD AND NECK TUMORS IN FOUR LARGE SERIES

Histologic Type	M.D. Anderson Hospital[35] (1965)	J.J. Conley[37] (1970)	Children's Hosp. Boston[36] (10-year study— 1973)	U of I Series (1981)
Rhabdomyosarcoma	30	24	20	24
Fibrosarcoma	6*	22*	11*	7
Solitary malignant schwannoma	0	0	2	0
Malignant schwannoma with von Recklinghausen's disease	0	0	0	1
Malignant histiocytoma	0	0	2	0
Malignant hemangiopericytoma	0	0	2	0
Malignant hemangioendothelioma	2	2	2	0
Malignant mesenchymoma	0	4	2	0
Leiomyosarcoma	0	1	0	0
Unclassified	0	0	0	2
Total	38	53	41	34

*Includes neurofibrosarcomas.

atively large series. It is obvious that, after rhabdomyosarcoma and fibrosarcoma are excluded,
the incidence of other types is rare and purely
random. The occurrence of hemangiopericytoma in one series and the absence of leiomyosarcoma in others is purely coincidental. In our
series of 34 head and neck tumors, 24 were
rhabdomyosarcomas, 7 were fibrosarcomas, 1
was a malignant schwannoma associated with
von Recklinghausen's disease, and 2 were unclassified. The orbital region showed the highest incidence of tumor (Fig. 20.1), the majority
being rhabdomyosarcomas. The predilection of
embryonal rhabdomyosarcomas for the orbital
region has been observed by many other authors.[35-42] Recently Sutow and associates[42A] found
that in 202 children with rhabdomyosarcoma in
the head and neck region, the primary site was
the eye and orbit in 52 instances, the parameningeal region in 93 (18 in the middle ear and
mastoid, 23 in the nasal cavity and paranasal
sinuses, 39 in the nasopharynx, 13 in the infratemporal fossa), and miscellaneous head and
neck locations, including the scalp and face, in
57 instances.

In tumors of the head and neck region, the
location of the primary correlates with the physical findings. Tumors near the orbit result in
ptosis or proptosis. Large tumors in the mandibular region limit mobility of the jaw. If the
lesion is primarily located in the laryngopha-
ryngeal region, there frequently is a change in
the voice. One such case of laryngeal rhabdomyosarcoma was treated at the University of
Illinois Hospital (Table 7.4, Chapter 7). In tumors located in the nasopharynx the principal
complaint is nasal stuffiness or epistaxis. In recent years, computerized axial tomography has
been found to be extremely useful as a noninvasive means of assessing the extent of the tumor and the results of treatment.[43]

Soft Tissue Sarcoma of the Extremities
Eighteen instances (25 percent) of childhood soft
tissue sarcoma of the extremities were encountered in our series, compared with 41 cases (30
percent) in the Mayo Clinic material (Table 20.3).
The extremities are the next most common site
after the head and neck region. Diagnosis is
sometimes missed because of a low index of
suspicion (Fig. 20.2).

Soft Tissue Sarcomas of the Trunk
As in all other locations, in the majority of patients these tumors are subcutaneous. In the six

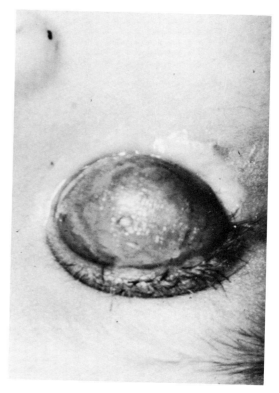

Figure 20.1. Two-and-one-half-year-old boy with embryonal rhabdomyosarcoma of right eyelid. *(Courtesy of
EJ Liebner, M.D., Radiation Therapy Section, University
of Illinois Hospital)*

patients (8.3 percent) in our series, all tumors
were subcutaneous, and in one patient there
was evidence of destruction of the ribs. Raney
and colleagues[43A] found that of the 407 evaluable
patients registered with the Intergroup Rhabdomyosarcoma Study, 30 (7.4 percent) had a
primary sarcoma of the trunk. The chest wall
was the commonest anatomic site. Forty percent
of the 30 patients had alveolar rhabdomyosarcoma, 20 percent had the embryonal type, 20
percent had extraskeletal Ewing's sarcoma, 17
percent had undifferentiated sarcoma, and 3
percent had the pleomorphic type.

Sarcomas of the Pelvis and Perineum
The pelvic sarcomas in general represent tumors arising from the urogenital tract, usually
rhabdomyosarcomas (Table 13.13, Chapter 13).

In female children these tumors usually arise
in the vagina, but occasionally in the urethra or
urinary bladder. When the tumor arises in the
vagina, the most common symptom is a blood-

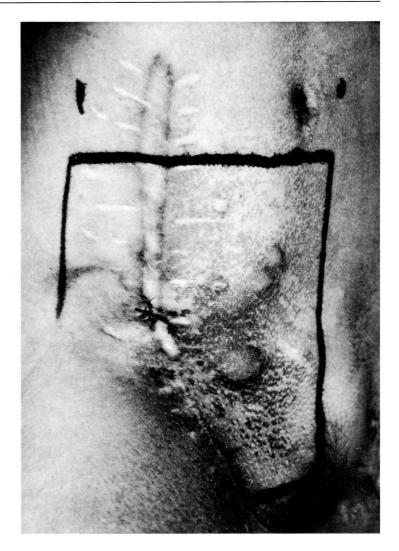

Figure 20.2. Local recurrence at the site of an excision and groin dissection in an 11-year-old girl. The original tumor, 2 × 2 cm, was on the medial thigh. The tumor was disregarded for one year. She was sent to us after the inguinal node had enlarged. A monobloc excision of the primary, along with node dissection, showed extensive involvement of the inguinofemoral nodes by metastatic rhabdomyosarcoma. She was treated with radiation therapy and the VAC regimen. However, within one-and-one-half years after treatment of the primary, metastatic skin nodules, along with bone metastases, were noted. She died within four months of the appearance of the metastatic nodules shown here.

tinged vaginal discharge. If the diagnosis is missed at this stage, the tumor enlarges and becomes visible through the outlet. It resembles a cluster of grapes, leading to the descriptive term of sarcoma botryoides (Fig. 20.3A and 20.3B). Similarly, sarcoma botryoides can occur in the urinary bladder (Fig. 4.48, Chapter 4).

In male children a pelvic tumor frequently represents a sarcoma of the prostate. A male infant with a palpable pelvic tumor and an enlarged prostate should be assumed to have a rhabdomyosarcoma of the prostate unless proved otherwise.

Tumors can also arise in the paratesticular tissues and scrotum. A number of such instances have been encountered by us and by other authors.[44-48] Rhabdomyosarcomas of these unusual sites are so rare that general guidelines for management cannot be developed. Recently, Penchansky and Gallo[49] brought to our attention a group of renal tumors that they considered rhabdomyosarcomas and suggested that these tumors be separated from conventional Wilms' tumors. However, further corroborative evidence is required before subclassifying a group of renal tumors in children as renal rhabdomyosarcomas.

Fibrosarcomas of the pelvis are rare (Fig. 20.4A to 20.4C). In our series of 72 childhood sarcomas, only three such cases were encountered; and in the Mayo Clinc material, only one. These tumors are usually diagnosed because of a large pelvic mass. The number of children with this tumor is so small that no comments can be forwarded regarding its natural history.

Retroperitoneal Sarcomas

Retroperitoneal sarcomas occur rarely in children,[34,50-55] and there were only two cases in our series. One of these was a fibrosarcoma; in the other, an exact histologic diagnosis could not be ascertained and the child was treated as for an embryonal rhabdomyosarcoma. The child with fibrosarcoma was a 15-month-old girl referred because of a large abdominal tumor. The mass was regular and firm. An exploratory procedure revealed a large retroperitoneal tumor, which was resected. The specimen showed this to be a fibrosarcoma, which we were unable to remove completely. Postoperative irradiation and systemic chemotherapy were given without any effect, and the infant died of bladder invasion and ureteral obstruction 11 months after the exploratory celiotomy.

The management principles of retroperitoneal malignant mesenchymal tumors are in general the same for children as for adults. A review of published case reports[34,49-54] and evaluation of our own clinical material[55] lead us to conclude that individual tumor types behave identically in children and adults, with the probability that when encountered in childhood there probably is a better chance of control with the use of multimodality therapy.

TREATMENT OF CHILDHOOD SOFT TISSUE SARCOMAS

The attitude toward treatment of childhood sarcomas has evolved through several stages. The early literature is replete with anecdotal case reports indicating that treatment was futile. However, Pack and Ariel[20] pointed out that in their experience most infants and children tolerated a radical procedure well and therefore should not be deprived of a curative operation. Today it is well established that children can not only withstand an indicated operative procedure, but that pediatric soft tissue sarcomas in general carry a better prognosis than do their counterparts in adults.

The indications and technique for the operations are described in Chapter 6, and with the realization that multiple modalities can be used with excellent end results, extreme radical procedures are becoming unnecessary. The de-

tails of radiotherapy and chemotherapy methods are discussed in Chapters 7 and 8. The types of treatment offered to the 72 patients in the University of Illinois series are shown in Table 20.7. The use of multimodality therapy has recently become more common. As indicated, 37 of 44 patients with rhabdomyosarcoma, plus those with unclassified sarcoma, were treated by means of operation, radiation therapy, and chemotherapy.

NATURAL HISTORY OF SPECIFIC HISTOLOGIC TYPES

Rhabdomyosarcoma

This constitutes the most common form of soft tissue sarcomas in children.[16-19,23,38-44,55A,55B] Sixty-one percent of the patients in our series had this type of sarcoma. Soule et al.[16] reported a 55.5 percent incidence in their series at the Mayo Clinic. The tumor is seen with equal frequency in both sexes and the most common anatomic site is the head and neck region (Fig. 20.1). Table 20.8 shows the distribtion of embryonal rhabdomyosarcoma in different anatomic sites in both children and adults. A detailed discussion of the management of various histologic types of rhabdomyosarcoma can be found in Chapter 13. In this section only the features applicable to rhabdomyosarcomas in infancy and childhood are discussed.

End Results in Rhabdomyosarcoma. Rhabdomyosarcomas, for the sake of reporting end results, have been classified into three stages. Stage I represents only localized tumor, stage II represnts localized tumor infiltrating the surrounding tissues or with regional node metastases, and stage III represents widespread metastases. The clinical system currently in use by the Intergroup Rhabdomyosarcoma Study (IRS)[56] is described in Chapter 13. In this method the patients are classified into four groups after resection of the primary tumor. Group 1 consists of patients in whom all the tumor could be resected. Group 2 includes those in whom all the gross tumor is resected but microscopic residua are found, or those with extensive regional disease and metastases to the regional lymph nodes. Group 3 are those in whom resection was incomplete, and group 4, those with distant metastases present at the time of initial treatment.

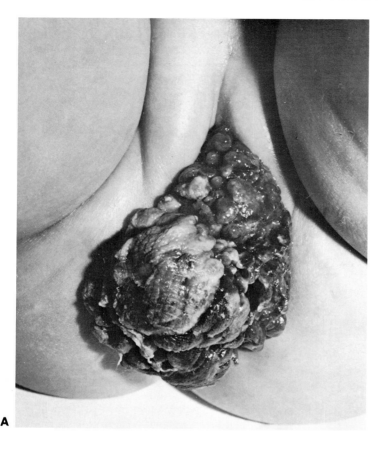

Figure 20.3. (A) Botryoid sarcoma of the vagina in a 13-month-old infant. **(B)** Following preoperative course of actinomycin D and radiation therapy, the protruding tumor dramatically subsided. *(Courtesy of H. Firor, M.D. Cleveland, Ohio)*

A

Pratt and co-workers,[57] who classified rhabdomyosarcomas into the conventional three stages (Chapter 13), subclassified stage III into two groups, A and B. In stage III-A, the bone marrow is free of disease, whereas in stage III-B there is marrow involvement. This subclassification is probably a better method for assessing patients with generalized rhabdomyosarcoma. Although occasional instances of control of advanced cases are recorded, generally the treatment of stage III (Group 4) patients is considered as only palliative. Table 20.9 shows the types of treatment and the end results in 24 patients with stages I and II embryonal rhabdomyosarcoma whom we treated. (This table excludes the data on orbital and genitourinary tract rhabdomyosarcomas. For a review of the end results in these two anatomic sites, the reader is referred to Tables 13.9 and 13.13, Chapter 13.) The best results were achieved when all three treatment modalities were combined. Fifteen of the 17 patients (88 percent) lived disease-free for two years, and 14 (82 per-

cent) were disease-free at five years. It is our opinion that, if an initial aggressive approach is undertaken and a multimodal method of management is used, stage I rhabdomyosarcomas are controllable and a large number of stage IIs can also be salvaged. Our optimism is shared by most other authors[3,4,39-44,56,57]

Primary rhabdomyosarcomas of the head and neck region represent 35 percent of all rhabdomyosarcomas in children and young adults. Excluding the orbit, this site has always carried the poorest prognosis for the patient. In 1965, Masson and Soule[58] found that only 9 percent of their 88 patients with rhabdomyosarcomas of the head and neck were known to be alive, and that 49 percent had died within one year of diagnosis. Although node involvement is not uncommon, the usual lethal spread is hematogenous or directly into the central nervous system. The results of the early combined therapy programs were impressive, and survival rates of 13 percent prior to 1967 were increased to 55 percent in patients treated between 1967 and

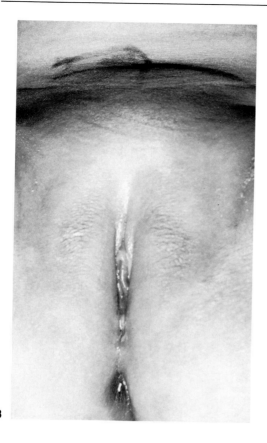

B

1973 in one series.[59] Among the 123 children with primary head and neck lesions (excluding the orbit) in the Intergroup Rhabdomyosarcoma Study (IRS), 60 percent were male; 74 percent had lesions of the embryonal cell type. Among these children, 63 percent were in clinical group 3 and an additional 19 percent were in clinical group 2. Only 15 percent were in clinical group 4, and 4 percent were in clinical group 1. Thus, both complete excision of the tumor or the presence of metastatic disease at the time of diagnosis were relatively uncommon. Of those patients admitted to the study between 1972 and 1976, 56 percent had survived, the mean duration of survival being two years. Sutow et al.[42A] recently updated the end result data from the Intergroup Rhabdomyosarcoma Study. These authors calculated the three-year disease-free survival in 103 patients with rhabdomyosarcoma of the head and neck region. The relapse-free survival rate was 91 percent (21/23) for those with primary tumor of the eye or orbit, 46 percent (20/44) for those with parameningeal pri-

maries, and 75 percent (27/36) for those with tumors located in other sites in the head and neck region. Eight percent of the children relapsed after two years. This improvement in end results in the last decade speaks well for the multimodal treatment program being used by the study group. Initial recurrence of head and neck rhabdomyosarcoma in the IRS has been predominantly local or regional (76 percent), but ultimately has been distant. The predominant regional spread was into the central nervous system via a meningeal route adjacent to the parameningeal primary tumor, and this form of extension was uniformly lethal.[60]

Patients with primary rhabdomyosarcoma of the orbit have a more favorable prognosis than do those with rhabdomyosarcoma in any other site.[39,61,62] These tumors are well controlled by radiation therapy.[36,62,63] Orbital exenteration should be kept in reserve for recurrent tumors.

Raney et al.[43A] analyzed the end result data on 30 patients with rhabdomyosarcoma of the trunk. They concluded that the prognosis was most favorable for patients with paraspinal tumors: seven (70 percent) of ten were disease-free at a median of 4.7 years. The next most favorable results were in patients with abdominal wall tumors: three of five with localized tumor were disease-free at a median of five years. The patients with chest wall tumors had the least favorable prognosis: five of ten (50 percent) with localized tumor were disease-free at a median of 4.7 years. Hays[64] summarized the experience of the Intergroup Rhabdomyosarcoma Study with extremity tumors, which comprised 23 percent of all tumors. Of 83 completely evaluated patients with rhabdomyosarcoma who were admitted to the IRS between 1972 and 1976 and therefore have had a minimum of two years' surveillance, there has been a notable difference in survival related to the clinical groups. Of 21 patients in clinical group 1 (complete local excision), the relapse rate has been 14 percent and mortality 10 percent two years after diagnosis. In clinical group 2 (grossly excised tumors, with microscopic residual tumor, positive nodes, or local extension), the relapse rate has been 19 percent, and mortality 9 percent among 32 patients two years after diagnosis. However, among the 14 patients in clinical group 3, nine have had relapses and four have died.

Hays et al.[57A] recently updated the Intergroup Rhabdomyosarcoma Study end result data on extremity tumors. Of the 102 evaluable pa-

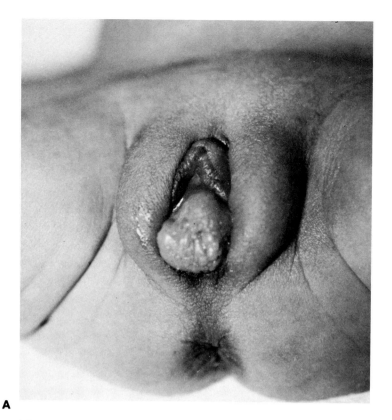

A

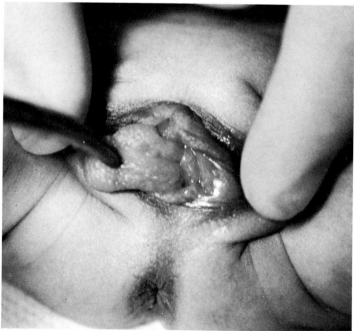

B

Figure 20.4. **(A)** An unusual instance of a benign fibrous polyp protruding from the vagina. **(B)** Polyp pulled out to show the entire extent. **(C)** Micrograph of the polyp. Note polypoid structure covered by mature squamous epithelieum, with occasional downfoldings; composed of fibrovascular stroma with scattered foci of chronic inflammatory cells (H&E. Original magnification × 5.) *(Courtesy of H. Firor, M.D. Cleveland, Ohio)*

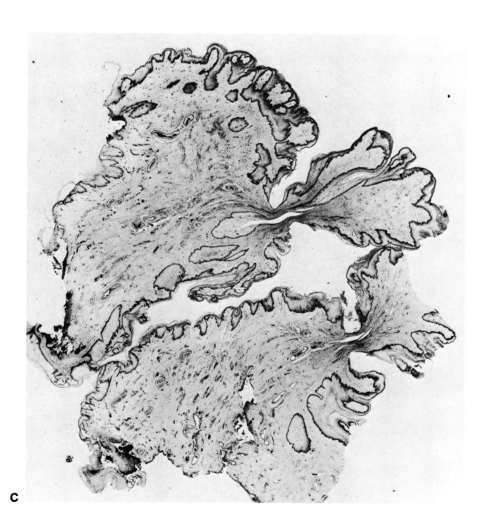

C

TABLE 20.7. TREATMENT OF 72 CASES OF SOFT TISSUE SARCOMAS IN CHILDREN (UNIVERSITY OF ILLINOIS SERIES)*

Histologic Type	No. of Patients	Wide Excision and RT	Wide Excision, RT, CT	Wide Excision and CT	Wide Excision	Excision Biopsy CT and RT
Rhabdomyosarcoma	44	3†	32	4	0	5
Fibrosarcoma	15	4	3	0	8	0
Unclassified sarcoma	3	0	3	0	0	0
Solitary malignant schwannoma	2	1	0	0	1	0
Malignant schwannoma with von Recklinghausen's disease	1	0	1	0	0	0
Liposarcoma	2	0	0	0	2	0
Synovial cell sarcoma	3	0	1	2	0	0
Leiomyosarcoma	1	0	0	1	0	0
Epithelioid sarcoma	1	0	1	0	0	0
Total	72	8	41	7	11	5

*RT = Radiation therapy; CT = Chemotherapy.
†Parents refused chemotherapy.

TABLE 20.8. ANATOMIC DISTRIBUTION OF EMBRYONAL RHABDOMYOSARCOMA IN CHILDREN AND ADULTS (UNIVERSITY OF ILLINOIS SERIES OF 59 PATIENTS)

Site	Children	Adults	Total
Orbital region	7	1	8
Other head and neck sites	17/15*	6/4	23/19
Trunk and peritoneum	4/2	4/2	8/4
Perineum and pelvis	3/1		3/1
Lower extremity	5/4	1/1	6/5
Upper extremity	2/2	2/1	4/3
Gastrourinary tract	6	1	7
Total	44 (74.5%)	15 (25.4%)	59

*Number in numerator represents total number of patients, and in the denominator, patients with stage I or stage II disease.

TABLE 20.9. END RESULTS OF THERAPY IN 24 PATIENTS WITH STAGES I AND II EMBRYONAL RHABDOMYOSARCOMA (UNIVERSITY OF ILLINOIS SERIES)*

Treatment	No. Patients	Disease-free at 2 Yr	Disease-free at 5 Yr
Wide excision, radiation therapy, and chemotherapy	17	15	14
Wide excision and radiation therapy	2	1	1
Wide excision and chemotherapy	3	2	2
Chemotherapy and radiation therapy	2	0	0

*Exclusive of orbital and genitourinary tract sarcomas.

tients followed up for 2.5 to 7.5 years, five of the six treated by amputation had relapses. Seven (35 percent) of the 21 in clinical group 1, and nine (33 percent) of the 27 in clinical group 2, also had relapses. Thirteen (72 percent) of the 18 in clinical group 3, although responsive to the chemotherapy and radiation therapy regimen, died of the disease. Of the 30 patients in clinical group 4, 25 were dead at the time of the report. These authors found that the relapse rate could be correlated with the histologic subtype. In their series, patients with the alveolar type of rhabdomyosarcoma had the highest incidence of relapse, and 44 percent of the primary tumors in the extremities were of the alveolar variety. In contrast, in the orbital locations, in which the best end results were achieved, only 10 percent were alveolar. Hays and coworkers concluded that the poor end results associated with the extremity rhabdomyosarcomas were directly attributable to the high incidence of the alveolar subtype. However our data on the alveolar subtype do not lead us to this conclusion. In our experience the alveolar type reponds to multimodal treatment in the same manner as the embryonal type, and our data, albeit in a much smaller group of patients, are comparable in all the histologic subgroups of rhabdomyosarcomas.

Embryonal rhabdomyosarcoma of the urogenital tract in children of both sexes poses a major therapeutic challenge. Too often, too much is done too late, with attendant bad end results. Our experience with urogenital tract rhabdomyosarcomas is discussed in detail in Chapter 13 and data are given in Table 13.13. Suffice it to reemphasize in this section that only early diagnosis and the immediate application of multimodal therapy will improve the end result.[40-48,64-76]

Crist and co-workers[17] recently summarized prognosis by primary site as has been done by the investigators of the Intergroup Rhabdomyosarcoma Study. These authors collected a total of 345 cases of rhabdomyosarcoma. The anatomic distribution and the two-year disease-free survival rates were as follows: orbit 34 (77 percent), head and neck 127 (51 percent), trunk 30 (50 percent), extremities 72 (42 percent), retroperitoneum 24 (42 percent), bladder and prostate 41 (68 percent), and intrathoracic 17 (24 percent).

The history of the management of rhabdomyosarcoma was rather uneventful until about 1965. Prior to the use of effective radiotherapy,[63] surgical approaches were the only form of therapy, and more than 85 percent of children and young adults with this disease died.[77] Development of radical surgical procedures only slightly improved the results. The general effect on long-range survival was not dramatic, and survival rates appeared to reach a plateau of approximately 25 percent.[18,78-83] The combined effect of dactinomycin and radiation on rhabdomyosarcoma was demonstrated in 1959 by D'Angio, Farber, and Maddock.[85] In 1961, Pinkel and Pickren[85] suggested that a surgery, radiotherapy, and chemotherapy regimen be employed as prophylactic therapy in patients both with and without known residual or metastatic tumors. The use of chemotherapy in all pediatric patients with rhabdomyosarcoma, irrespective of site or extent of disease, was advocated by Sutow et al. in 1970.[86] The terms "combined therapy" or "combination therapy" then came into use and implied that surgery should be followed routinely by radiotherapy and a long-range chemotherapy program.

A major advance in the evaluation of this form of management was a prospective study in 1967 carried out by the Childrens Cancer Study Group (CCSG), which randomized chemotherapy and nonchemotherapy.[87,88] In this series it appeared that patients with microscopic residual tumor had survival rates comparable to those of patients in whom an apparent complete excision had been achieved. Previously and concurrently (1968–1974), similar studies were carried out in a number of institutions caring for childhood rhabdomyosarcoma, and surgery followed by local radiation therapy and a prolonged course of multiple-agent chemotherapy soon became standard in the United States.[39,76,89,90] For the first time, the results of the overall treatment of rhabdomyosarcoma were dramatically improved. Even in the initial series[39,91] the percentage of long-range survivors among patients without tumor dissemination was doubled in chemotherapy-treated groups.

Subsequent trends in the treatment of rhabdomyosarcoma included the following: (1) development of more intensive chemotherapy (or chemotherapy-radiotherapy) regimens for patients with unresectable rhabdomyosarcomas, in an attempt to increase the rate of resectability or provide long-range control.[92] This was the origin of the concept of initial elective tumor suppression by a primary chemotherapy (or chemotherapy-radiotherapy) regimen followed by a secondary, and sometimes limited, surgical procedure to remove residual tumor[93,94]; (2) attempts to control disseminated rhabdomyosarcoma by resection of metastatic lesions; (3) an attempt to minimize or eliminate the use of radiotherapy in patients with rhabdomyosarcoma, in some instances by using longer or more intensive chemotherapeutic regimens[96]; (4) intensive therapy programs, including more radical surgery, intensive radiotherapy, and prolonged periods of chemotherapy with multiple agents[44,89] in children with more advanced stages of the disease, with at times encouraging results; and (5) an attempt to avoid major therapeutic surgery entirely by the more intensive use of chemotherapeutic agents, or chemotherapy-radiotherapy regimens, in rhabdomyosarcomas in the orbit and pelvic organs.[59,93]

Hays[64] recently summarized the pertinent findings of cancer study groups in the United States concerned with pediatric oncology. These groups accrued a total of 750 patients from 75 qualifying institutions during the years 1972–1978. Patients were divided into four clinical groups on the basis of (1) extent of disease at the time of diagnosis and (2) the surgical procedure performed. Each patient was then randomly assigned to one of two therapy arms (Table 20.10). A total of 474 patients was analyzed. Among the 67 children in clinical group 1, the use of local radiotherapy did not result in any significant difference in the survival rate. Between 92 and 96 percent of the children were alive, with local recurrence rates of 3.7 percent and 5.5 percent, respectively, at the time of Hays's[64] report.

In clinical group 2, the clinical trial concerned the evaluation of two chemotherapy regimens, namely, VAC for two years or a regimen

TABLE 20.10. THE INTERGROUP RHABDOMYOSARCOMA STUDY (IRS)
THE CLINICAL GROUPS ARE DEFINED AND THE CHEMOTHERAPY-RADIOTHERAPY REGIMENS THAT ARE EMPLOYED FOLLOWING RANDOMIZATION ARE INDICATED

Group I.	Localized disease, completely resected (regional nodes not involved) a. Confined to muscle or organ of origin b. Contiguous involvement—Infiltration outside the muscle or organ of origin, as through fascial planes	RANDOMIZE	A. Vincristine dactinomycin cyclophosphamide B. Radiotherapy + vincristine dactinomycin cyclophosphamide
Group II.	a. Grossly resected tumor with microscopic residual disease (nodes negative) b. Regional disease, completely resected (nodes positive or negative) c. Regional disease with involved nodes, grossly resected, but with evidence of microscopic residual disease.	RANDOMIZE	C. Radiotherapy + vincristine dactinomycin D. Radiotherapy + vincristine dactinomycin cyclophosphamide
Group III. Group IV.	Incomplete resection or biopsy with gross residual disease Metastatic disease present at onset	RANDOMIZE	E. Radiotherapy + vincristine dactinomycin cyclophosphamide F. Radiotherapy + vincristine dactinomycin cyclophosphamide adriamycin

Courtesy DM Hays, World J Surgery 4:15, 1980.

of intensive vincristine and dactinomycin for one year. All patients received local radiation therapy. There were no significant differences between the results of these two regimens after two years of therapy. Of the 110 patients evaluated, 73 percent had no evidence of disease and 82 percent were alive in 1978.

Patients in clinical group 3, with an incomplete local surgical resection or simple biopsy of a localized tumor, and those in clinical group 4, with metastasis at the time of diagnosis, were randomized between two more intensive chemotherapy regimens. These patients had surgical procedures as indicated (and as frequently as necessary) and received radiotherapy (when possible) six weeks following the initiation of therapy. They were randomized between regimens of pulse VAC alone and pulse VAC plus adriamycin. The results of the use of these two chemotherapy regimens in clinical groups 3 and 4 were not significantly different. More than 72 percent of the 199 patients in clinical group 3 and 65 to 73 percent of the 102 patients in clinical group 4 responded to chemotherapy with varying degrees of regression of these advanced tumors. In approximately 25 percent, a state of complete response (no demonstrable tumor) was achieved prior to the course of radiation therapy at six weeks. The use of clinical grouping in the Intergroup Rhabdomyosarcoma Study (IRS), as opposed to conventional staging, proved effective in distinguishing the prognostic categories.

The recommended basic radiation dosage in the IRS was (1) 5,000 rads in five weeks for patients with possible (or known) microscopic residual disease and (2) 6,000 rads in six weeks for bulk disease (clinical groups 2 and 4). Dosage was graduated downward as patient age decreased, and for specific sites.

These clinical studies are still in progress and the Intergroup Rhabdomyosarcoma Study participants are addressing themselves to the more subtle questions of how children with localized resectable diseases can be cured with less therapy, thereby minimizing therapy-related complications; and how in locally advanced disease the duration of remission can be prolonged with modification and alteration of various chemotherapeutic regimens.

Sarcomas of Undetermined Histogenesis

One of our three patients in whom the histogenesis of the tumor could not be determined is still living. From a histologic standpoint, the differential diagnosis of these round cell anaplastic tumors still remains extremely difficult.[96] Recently, childhood extraskeletal Ewing's sarcoma has been recognized, and the therapeutic and prognostic criteria for this tumor are becoming increasingly clear.[97,98]

There still remains the problem of rhabdoid sarcoma[99] and other highly anaplastic round cell sarcomas of infancy and childhood.[100] The morphogenesis of these tumors requires further clarification. From an operational standpoint, however, until these tumors are properly catalogued the treatment should be along the same lines as for rhabdomyosarcoma, that is, a combination of all three modalities.

Fibrosarcoma

In most respects fibrous tissue proliferations in older children are comparable to those in adults. But those occurring in infants and young children commonly exhibit features that suggest a more aggressive behavior. Stout[101] was the first to call attention to this group of tumors. He reported a series of 44 fibrous tumors in children that he designated "juvenile fibromatosis." In these lesions he noted that the degree of cellular differentiation was not a reliable criterion for predicting clinical behavior. Some innocent-appearing fibrous tumors recurred repeatedly, and occasionally even necessitated amputation of an extremity. Only rarely were tumors of this type observed to invade vital structures and cause death. These tumors did not metastasize.

In 1962, Stout[102] described 23 tumors in children that he distinguished from juvenile fibromatosis and considered to be fibrosarcomas. In a collective review of 61 cases of fibrosarcoma in children, he found 31 patients who had been followed up for at least five years and who could, with reasonable assurance, be said to have juvenile fibrosarcoma. Metastasis occurred in two. Two of his own patients also had metastasis, making a total of 4 (7.4 percent) of 54 children who had metastatic disease. The difficulties encountered in separating the cellular fibromatoses from fibrosarcomas have been stressed by Stout.[101,102]

The histologic dividing line between fibromatosis and fibrosarcoma is usually exceedingly fine, and the pathologist may be faced with an almost impossible situation. Enzinger[103] summarized the problem well in discussing aggressive fibromatosis in 12 infants and young children. He stated that, although the histologic features of these tumors indicated a diagnosis of fibrosarcoma, the clinical course of the tumor was more in keeping with the concept of juvenile fibromatosis, in which the tumor is regionally aggressive, tends to recur locally, but rarely if ever metastasizes. Since the clinical course of the tumor, at least in infants and young children, would appear to be less aggressive than a similar-appearing tumor in adults, Soule and co-workers[16] elected to classify a group of active fibroblastic tumors in infants and children as juvenile fibrosarcomas. We agree with the pathologic concept proposed by Stout,[101,102] Enzinger,[103] and Soule et al.[16] In the case of a poorly differentiated fibrous tissue tumor, particularly in older children, that has a solid cellular pattern, pleomorphism of the tumor cells, tumor necrosis, and a rapid clinical course, it would appear justifiable to diagnose fibrosarcoma, with the probability of a malignant clinical course similar to that seen in adults. One should not routinely resort to major excision as the primary form of treatment in these cases, but should evaluate each case carefully before planning treatment.

End Results in Fibrosarcoma. The results of treatment in our series of 15 fibrosarcomas are summarized in Table 20.11. All 15 patients were eligible for five-year end result study: 13 (87 percent) lived disease-free for two years and 10 (66 percent) for five years. In all these 15 patients the resected margins were microscopically free of tumor. In 11, the size of the primary tumor was less than 5 cm. Although fibrosarcoma has not been staged as comprehensively as rhabdomyosarcoma, a similar staging method should be used in reporting the end results. A modified form of the American Joint Commission staging system (Chapter 5) would prove useful in all future end result reporting.

In our series of 15 children with fibrosarcoma, five (33 percent) died of the tumor. Three of these five showed widespread metastases at autopsy, and the sites of involvement were about the same as in adult fibrosarcoma. In the fourth, autopsy was not performed but there was clinical evidence of pulmonary metastases. The case history of the fifth patient is somewhat puzzling. This girl, at age 10 years, had had a mid-thigh amputation elsewhere for a fibrosarcoma of the popliteal space. At age 11, pulmonary metastases developed and she was seen by another group who elected not to treat her. She continued to remain asymptomatic and the pulmonary nodules remained stationary for one year. At this time she was referred to the University of Illinois Hospital, but the parents refused any form of treatment. She was observed at periodic intervals and the pulmonary tumors continued to remain stationary. However, four and one half years after amputation they suddenly started to enlarge and she was placed on a VAC regimen without much benefit. She died at age 15.

Chung and Enzinger[104] reviewed the files of the Armed Forces Institute of Pathology and found 53 cases of fibrosarcoma in children five years of age or younger. Of the 48 children about whom adequate data were available, four (8.3 percent) had died of metastatic tumor. From the files of the Mayo Clinic, Soule and Pritchard[101] reviewed 40 cases of fibrosarcoma in infants and children and accepted an additional 70 reported cases as satisfying the criteria for infantile fibrosarcoma.[12,101] These authors used the same histologic criteria used for adults. In the 110 cases reviewed, 68 of the patients were in the first quinquennium of life, 13 in the second, and 29 in the third. Eleven patients (10 percent) died of the tumor. Both Chung and Enzinger[104] and Soule and Pritchard[105] reported a lower mortality than seen in our small group of patients. Soule and Pritchard[101] concluded that children younger than five years have a 7.3 percent chance of metastatic spread, even though the local recurrence rate is 43 percent. They found that children who were 10 years of age or older had

TABLE 20.11. END RESULTS OF TREATMENT OF FIBROSARCOMA IN 15 PATIENTS AT THE UNIVERSITY OF ILLINOIS

Treatment	No. Patients	Alive at 2 Yr	Disease-free at 5 Yr
Wide excision	8	7	6
Wide excision, radiation therapy	4	3	3
Wide excision, radiation therapy, chemotherapy	3	3	1

a metastatic rate of 50 percent at five-year fol-lowup.

Enzinger[103] has splendidly summarized the problem of diagnosis, management, and prog-nosis of fibrous tissue tumors in children. The most common form is the aggressive type of fibromatoses. These tumors usually infiltrate the surrounding structures, occasionally killing by local invasion. In this respect, the natural his-tory of the majority of juvenile fibromatoses is comparable to aggressive fibromatoses in adults.[12,106] Therefore, in the majority of younger children, an initial conservative excision should be adequate for control of the primary tumors. In contrast, we think that in older children, if the histologic examination shows a solid cellular pattern, a high degree of pleomorphism, and tumor necrosis, then the treatment should be similar to that of adult fibrosarcoma.

Solitary Malignant Schwannoma

The incidence of peripheral nerve tumors in children is indeed low. These tumors, strictly speaking, are not soft tissue sarcomas but tra-ditionally have been included with mesenchy-mal benign or malignant tumors.[107-109] Das Gupta and Brasfield[107] found only 12 (5 percent) soli-tary malignant schwannomas in children out of a total of 232 cases. In the present University of Illinois series, only two are in children. For lack of adequate information, these young patients should be viewed for the present as having a tumor with the same biologic behavior as that in adults.

Neurofibrosarcoma Associated with von Recklinghausen's Disease

Although the incidence of neurofibrosarcomas in children with von Recklinghausen's disease is higher than for solitary malignant schwan-nomas, it is still rare to see such a tumor in a child with multiple neurofibromatosis. One such patient was encountered in our group. A more detailed discussion of this entity will be found in the section on von Recklinghausen's disease (Chapter 14).

End Results in Malignant Schwannoma. Ma-lignant schwannomas are rare at all ages, par-ticularly in children.[107-109] In our present material we have come across three patients with neu-rogenic tumors. Two were solitary malignant schwannomas and the other was associated with von Recklinghausen's disease. Of the two pa-tients with solitary malignant schwannoma in our group, one is living disease-free after five years. The second, a 15-year-old boy, died within two years of initial treatment. This boy pre-sented with a mass on the left side of the neck. Biopsy showed it to be a solitary malignant schwannoma. He was subjected to a left radical neck dissection, postoperative radiation ther-apy, and cyclical chemotherapy. During the pe-riod of chemotherapy the lesion recurred and all attempts at local control with further oper-ation and radiation therapy failed. The disease progressed and the boy died of metastases within six months of development of local recurrence. We have treated only one patient, a 15-year-old girl, with von Recklinghausen's disease in whom a malignant schwannoma (buttock) was found. She died within one year of diagnosis.

Liposarcoma

This is one of the most commonly encountered-soft tissue sarcomas in adults, but it is unusual in children. In 1959, Kauffman and Stout[110] re-viewed their experience with lipoblastic tumors in children and also critically reviewed other published cases. They found 15 acceptable cases and added 13 patients of their own. In this group of 28, very young or adolescent children har-bored the majority of these tumors. Most of the tumors studied by Kauffman and Stout[110] were well differentiated and occurred in young chil-dren. Only four were followed up for five years or more, one of whom died five years after ini-tial treatment. Two patients had not been fol-lowed up and the remainder were followed for periods of seven months to three years. Two patients had local recurrence. In our present group, only two patients had liposarcoma (Ta-bles 20.4 and 20.5). Both were girls, aged five and seven years, respectively. The primary tu-mors were located in the upper and lower ex-tremities. Both were treated with wide local ex-cision and are living disease-free after five years.

Lipoblastomatosis

This is a rare benign condition that usually oc-curs in infants less than 1 year old.[110-114] The tumors are usually located in the lower extrem-ities. The growth is lobulated and is composed of benign embryonal lipoblasts. Its microscopic pattern may easily be confused with that of a well-differentiated myxoid liposarcoma (Fig. 4.8, Chapter 4). Vellios and associates,[111] Kauffman and Stout,[110] and Enterline and associates[112] de-

scribed six cases of this condition. Chung and
Enzinger[113] described 35 collected cases, 88 percent of which occurred before the age of three
years. The oldest child in this series was 7 years
of age. We have treated one such case in a girl
of 13 years (Chapter 4). Three years after conservative local excision of the tumor the child
is doing well without any local recurrence.

Synovial Cell Sarcoma

Three cases of this tumor were encountered in
our series of 72 childhood sarcomas. Soule et
al.[16] described a cluster of ten such patients seen
at the Mayo Clinic. Crocker and Stout[25] reported
that this sarcoma accounted for only 1.8 percent
of malignant mesenchymal tumors in children.
These authors collected 33 patients from the literature and added ten of their own. This appears to be an aggressive tumor (six of their ten
patients died). Of our three patients (Tables 20.4
and 20.5), two are living, one for five years and
the other for four years. The third case is too
recent to evaluate. We routinely use adjuvant
chemotherapy in children with synovial cell sarcoma, and in our experience the prognosis appears to have improved.

Leiomyosarcoma

Only rarely does this tumor occur during childhood. In 1962, Yannopoulos and Stout[38] found
31 acceptable cases from the many published
reports. In addition, they reviewed ten of their
own cases believed to represent malignant
smooth muscle tumors. Botting and associates[115]
reviewed the Mayo Clinic experience and found
the same difficulty in histologic diagnosis that
Yannopoulos and Stout[38] encountered. In our
own group, only one patient could be classified
as having leiomyosarcoma. Yannopoulos and
Stout[38] concluded that leiomyosarcomas of the
soft tissues show a less aggressive behavior in
children than in adults. In contrast, Botting and
co-workers[115] concluded that the tumor is aggressive in children. Our patient with a leiomyosarcoma of the upper arm has been disease-
free for eight years after a forequarter amputation.

Neuroblastoma
(Malignant Ganglioneuroma)

These tumors and all other types of malignant
tumors arising from the sympathochromaffin
system (Table 3.1, Chapter 3) are frequently encountered in children. Neuroblastomas and their
biologic behavior are discussed in Chapter 14

and will not be repeated here. Suffice it to emphasize that today the natural history of these
tumors is now better understood, with resultant
improvement in management and prognosis in
children.[116–118]

Several other types of soft tissue sarcoma
have been encountered, both in our own series
and other large series (Tables 20.4 and 20.5).
These are rare, and a detailed discussion of all
the individual types will be found in sections
dealing with these entities in general.

On the basis of our experience and all the
evidence cited herein, it appears that a significant advance has been made in the management of common pediatric mesenchymal neoplasms. In rhabdomyosarcoma the role of
multimodal therapy has been established, and
in others, successful treatment programs are
being developed.[119]

REFERENCES

1. Ladd WE, Gross RE: Abdominal Surgery of Infancy and Childhood. Philadelphia, Saunders,
   1941
2. Maurer HM: Solid tumors in children. N Engl J
   Med 299:1345, 1978
3. Pinkel D: Curability of childhood cancer. JAMA
   235:1049, 1976
4. D'Angio G: Pediatric cancer in perspective: Cure
   is not enough. Cancer 35:866, 1975
5. Fraumeni JF Jr, Miller RW: Cancer deaths in the
   newborn. Am J Dis Child 117:186, 1969
6. Miller RW: Fifty-two forms of childhood cancer:
   United States mortality experience 1960–1966. J
   Pediat 75:685, 1969
7. Sloane JA, Hubbell MM: Soft tissue sarcomas in
   children associated with congenital anomalies.
   Cancer 23:175, 1969
8. Bjorklund SL: Hemihypertrophy and Wilms' tumor. Acta Paediat Scand 44:287, 1955
9. Ishak KG, Glunz PR: Hepatoblastoma and he-
   patocarcinoma in infancy and childhood. Cancer
   20:396, 1967
10. Miller RW, Fraumeni JF Jr, Manning MD: As-
    sociation of Wilms' tumor and aniridia, hemi-
    hypertrophy and other congenital malforma-
    tions. N Engl J Med 270, 1964
11. Wander JW, Das Gupta TK: Neurofibromatosis.
    In Current Problems in Surgery, vol XIV, no. 2,
    Feb. 1977
12. Wood DK, Das Gupta TK: Soft tissue sarcomas
    in infancy and childhood. J Surg Oncol 5:387,
    1973
13. Duzan CJ: Du Cancer Chez les Enfants. Paris,
    Ponsot, 1876
14. Picot C: Des tumerus malignes Chez les enfants.
    Rev Med de La Suisse Rom., 1883
15. Arey JB: Cancer in infancy and childhood. Penn
    Med J 55:553, 1952

16. Soule EH, Mahour GH, Mills SD, Lynn HB: Soft-tissue sarcomas of infants and children: A clinicopathologic study of 135 cases. Mayo Clin Proc 43:313, 1968

17. Crist WM, Raney RB Jr, Newton W, Lawrence W, Jr, Tefft M, Foulkes MA: Intrathoracic soft tissue sarcomas. Cancer 50:598, 1982

18. Pack GT, Ariel IM: Sarcomas of the soft somatic tissues in infants and children: A clinicopathologic study of 75 cases. J Pediat Surg 2:402, 1967

19. Ariel IM, Pack GT: Cancer and Allied Diseases of Infancy and Childhood. Boston, Little Brown, 1960

20. Pack GT, Ariel IM: Sarcomas of the soft somatic tissues in infants and children. In Tumors of the Soft Somatic Tissues; A Clinical Treatise. New York, Hoeber-Harper, 1958, pp 281, 543

21. Stout AP: Hemangiopericytoma: A study of twenty-five cases. Cancer 2:1027, 1949

22. Fisher JH: Hemangiopericytoma: A review of twenty cases. Canad Med Assoc J 83:1136, 1960

23. Nash A, Stout AP: Malignant mesenchymomas in children. Cancer 14:524, 1961

24. Kauffman SL, Stout AP: Extraskeletal osteogenic sarcomas and chondrosarcomas in children. Cancer 16:432, 1963

25. Crocker DW, Stout AP: Synovial sarcomas in children. Cancer 12:1123, 1959

26. Das Gupta TK: Tumors and tumor-like conditions of the adipose tissue. In Current Problems in Surgery. Chicago, Year Book Medical Publishers, 1970

27. Dutz W, Stout AP: Kaposi's sarcoma in infants and children. Cancer 13:684, 1960

28. Kauffman SL, Stout AP: Hemangiopericytoma in children. Cancer 13:695, 1960

29. Kauffman SL, Stout AP: Histocytic tumors (fibrous xanthoma and histiocytoma) in children. Cancer 14:469, 1961

30. Perez CA, Vietti T, Ackerman LV, Eagleton MD, Powers WE: Tumors of the sympathetic nervous system in children: An appraisal of treatment and results. Radiology 88:750, 1967

31. Kauffman SL, Stout AP: Congenital mesenchymal tumors. Cancer 18:460, 1965

32. Heimburger IL, Battersby JS: Primary mediastinal tumors of childhood. J Thor Cardiovasc Surg 50:92, 1965

33. Woods JE, Murray JE, Vawter GF: Hand tumors in children. Plast Reconstr Surg 46:130, 1970

34. Cozzutto C, De Bernardi B, Guarino M, Comelli A, Soave F: Retroperitoneal fibrohistiocytic tumors in children (report of 5 cases). Cancer 42:1350, 1978

35. MacComb WS, Fletcher GH: Pediatric tumors. In Cancer of the Head and Neck. Baltimore, Williams and Wilkins, 1967, p 428

36. Jaffe BF: Pediatric head and neck tumors: A study of 178 cases. Laryngoscope 83:1644, 1973

37. Conley JJ: Tumors of the Head and Neck in children. In Concepts in Head and Neck Surgery. Grune and Stratton, New York, 1970, p 181

38. Yannopoulos K, Stout AP: Smooth muscle tumors in children. Cancer 15:958, 1962

39. Jaffe N, Filler RM, Farber S, et al: Rhabdomyosarcoma in children: Improved outlook with a multidisciplinary approach. Am J Surg 125:482, 1973

40. Ragab AH, Vietti TJ, Perez CA, Daisilee HB: Malignant tumors of the soft tissues. In Sutow WW, Vietti TJ, Fernbach W (eds): Clinical Pediatric Oncology. St. Louis, Mosby, 1973

41. D'Angio GH, Evans A: Soft tissue sarcomas. In Bloom GJ, et al (eds): Cancer in Children. Berlin, Springer-Verlag, 1975

42. Jenkin RDT: Rhabdomyosarcoma in childhood. In Godden OJ (ed): Cancer in Childhood. Toronto, Ontario Cancer Treatment and Research Foundation, 1972

42A. Sutow WW, Lindberg RD, Gehan EA, Ragab AH, Raney RB Jr, Ruymann F, Soule EH: Three-year relapse-free survival rates in childhood rhabdomyosarcoma of the head and neck. Cancer 49:2217, 1982

43. Raney RB Jr, Zimmerman RA, Bilaniuk LT et al: Management of craniofacial sarcoma in childhood assisted by computed tomography. Int J Radiat Oncol Biol Phys 5(4):529, 1977

43A. Raney RB Jr, Ragab AH, Ruymann F, Lindberg RD, Hays DM, Gehan EA, Soule EH: Soft-tissue sarcoma of the trunk in childhood. Cancer 49:2612, 1982

44. Ghavimi F, Exelby PR, D'Angio GJ, et al: Combination therapy of urogenital embryonal rhabdomyosarcoma in children. Cancer 32:1178, 1973

45. Littman R, Tessler AN, Valensi Q: Paratesticular rhabdomyosarcoma: A case presentation and review of the literature. J Urol 108:290, 1972

46. Markland C, Kedia K, Fraley EE: Inadequate orchiectomy for patients with testicular tumors. JAMA 224:1025, 1975

47. Arlen M, Grabstald H, Witemore WF Jr: Malignant tumors of the spermatic cord. Cancer 23:525, 1969

48. Olney LE, Narayana A, Loening S, Culp DA: Intrascrotal rhabdomyosarcoma. Urology 14:113, 1979

49. Penchansky L, Gallo G: Rhabodmyosarcoma of the kidney in children. Cancer 44:285, 1979

50. Pack GT, Tahah EJ: Primary retroperitoneal tumors. A study of 120 cases. Int Abst Surg 99:209, 1954

51. Sandberg DH, Edwards WM: Report of a case of xanthogranuloma of the retroperitoneal space. Br J Urol 34:47, 1962

52. Kurgly M, Emanuel B, Smallberg W, Veiga S: Retroperitoneal xanthogranuloma. Pediatrics 30:608, 1962

53. Bissada NK, Fried FA: Retroperitoneal xanthogranuloma: Case report and review of the literature. J Urol 110:354, 1973

54. Kahn LB: Retroperitoneal xanthogranuloma and xanthosarcoma (malignant fibrous xanthoma). Cancer 31:411, 1973

55. Felix E, Wood DW, Das Gupta TK: Retroperitoneal soft tissue sarcomas. In Current Problems in Cancer. Chicago, Year Book Medical Publishers, July, 1981

55A. Hays DM, Soule EH, Lawrence W Jr, Gehan EA, Maurer HM, Donaldson M, Raney RB Jr, Tefft M: Extremity lesions in the Intergroup Rhabdomyosarcoma (IRS-I): A preliminary report. Cancer 49:1, 1982

55B. Lawrence W Jr, Hays DM, Moon TE: Lymphatic metastasis with childhood rhabdomyosarcoma. Cancer 39:556, 1977

56. Johnson DG: Trends in surgery for childhood rhabdomyosarcoma. Cancer 35(6):916, 1975

57. Pratt CB, Husto HO, Fleming ID, Pinkel D: Coordinated treatment of childhood rhabdomyosarcoma with surgery, radiotherapy, and combination chemotherapy. Cancer Res 32:606, 1972

58. Masson JK, Soule EH: Embryonal rhabdomyosarcoma of the head and neck: Report on 88 cases. Am J Surg 110:585, 1965

59. Kilman JW, Clatworthy HW Jr, Newton WA Jr, Grosfeld JL: Reasonable surgery for rhabdomyosarcoma: A study of 67 cases. Ann Surg 178:346, 1973

60. Tefft M, Fernandez C, Donaldson M, Newton W, Moon TE: Incidence of meningeal involvement by rhabdomyosarcoma of the head and neck in children: A report of the Intergroup Rhabdomyosarcoma Study (IRS). Cancer 39:665, 1977

61. Donaldson SS, Castro JR, Wilbur JR, Jesse RH Jr: Rhabdomyosarcoma of head and neck in children: Combination treatment by surgery, irradiation, and chemotherapy. Cancer 31:28, 1973

62. Liebner EJ: Embryonal rhabdomyosarcoma of the head and neck in children: Correlation of stage, radiation dose, local control and survival. Cancer 37:2777, 1976

63. Cassady JR, Sagerman RH, Tretter P, Ellsworth RM: Radiation therapy for rhabdomyosarcoma. Radiology 91:116, 1968

64. Hays DM: The management of rhabdomyosarcoma in children and young adults. World J Surg 4:15, 1980

65. Weissman MJ, Gaeta JF, Albert DJ: Childhood urogenital sarcoma. J Surg Oncol 6:109, 1972

66. Russi MF: Rhabdomyosarcoma of the bladder and prostate in children: A study of seven patients. Urol Digest 10:27, 1961

67. Goodwin WG: Rhabdomyosarcoma of the prostate in a child: First 5-year survival. Trans Amer Assoc GU Surgeons 58:186, 1967

68. Marshall VF: A five-year cure of rhabdomyosarcoma of the prostate in childhood. J Ped Surg 4:366, 1969

69. D'Angio GH, Tefft M: Radiation therapy in the management of children with gynecologic cancers. Ann NY Acad Sci 142:675, 1967

70. Ghazali S: Embryonic rhabdomyosarcoma of the urogenital tract. Br J Surg 60:124, 1973

71. Grosfeld JL, Smith JP, Clatworthy HW: Pelvic rhabdomyosarcoma in infants and children. J Urol 107:673, 1972

72. Hilgers RD, Malkasian GD, Soule EH: Embryonal rhabdomyosarcoma (botryoid type) of the vagina—A clinicopathologic review. Am J Obstet Gynecol 107:484, 1970

73. Tank ES, Fellman SL, Wheeler ES, et al: Treatment of urogenital tract rhabdomyosarcoma in infants and children. J Urol 107:324, 1972

74. Bartholomew TH, Gonzales ET, Starling KA, Harberg FJ: Changing concepts in management of pelvic rhabdomyosarcoma in children. Urology 13:613, 1979

75. Rutledge F, Sullivan MP: Sarcoma botryoides. Ann NY Acad Sci 142:694, 1967

76. Clatworthy HW Jr, Braren V, Smith JP: Surgery of bladder and prostatic neoplasms in children. Cancer 32:1157, 1973

77. Mackenzie AR, Whitmore WF Jr, Melamed MR: Myosarcomas of the bladder and prostate. Cancer 22:833, 1968

78. Pack GT, Eberhart WF: Rhabdomyosarcoma of skeletal muscle—Report of 100 cases. Surgery 32:1023, 1952

79. Jones IS, Reese AB, Kraut J: Orbital rhabdomyosarcoma: An analysis of 62 cases. Am J Ophthalmol 61:721, 1966

80. Linscheid RL, Soule EH, Henderson ED: Pleomorphic rhabdomyosarcomata of the extremities and limb girdles. A clinicopathological study. J Bone Joint Surg 47-A:715, 1965

81. Keyhani A, Booher RJ: Pleomorphic rhabdomyosarcoma. Cancer 22:956, 1968

82. Hardin CA: Radical amputation for sarcoma of the extremities including postoperative resection of pulmonary metastasis. Ann Surg 167:359, 1968

83. Hilgers RD, Malkasian GD, Soile EH: Embryonal rhabdomyosarcoma (botryoid type) of the vagina. Am J Obstet Gynecol 107:484, 1970

84. D'Angio GJ, Farber S, Maddock CL: Potentiation of x-ray effects by actinomycin D. Radiology 73:175, 1959

85. Pinkel D, Pickren J: Rhabdomyosarcoma in children. JAMA 175:293, 1961

86. Sutow WW, Sullivan MP, Ried HL, et al: Prognosis in childhood rhabdomyosarcoma. Cancer 25:1384, 1970

87. Heyn RM, Holland R, Newton WA Jr, et al: The role of combined chemotherapy in the treatment of rhabdomyosarcoma in children. Cancer 34:2828, 1974

88. Heyn R, Holland R, Joo P, et al: Treatment of rhabdomyosarcoma in children with surgery, radiotherapy and chemotherapy. Med Pediatr Oncol 3:21, 1977

89. Ghavimi F, Exelby PR, D'Angio GJ, et al: Multidisciplinary treatment of embryonal rhabdomyosarcoma in children. Cancer 35:677, 1975

90. Razek AA, Perez CA, Lee FA, et al.: Combined treatment modalities of rhabdomyosarcoma in children. Cancer 39:2415, 1977

91. Erlich FE, Haas JE, Kiesewetter WB: Rhabdomyosarcoma in infants and children. J Pediatr Surg 6:571, 1971

92. Wilbur JR: Combination chemotherapy for embryonal rhabdomyosarcoma. Cancer Chemother Rep 58:281, 1974

93. Rivard G, Ortega J, Hittle R, Nitschke R, Karon M: Intensive chemotherapy as primary treatment for rhabdomyosarcoma of the pelvis. Cancer 36:1593, 1975

94. Kumar APM, Wrenn EL Jr, Fleming ID, Hustu HO, Pratt CB: Combined therapy to prevent complete pelvic exenteration for rhabdomyosarcoma of the vagina or uterus. Cancer 37:118, 1976

95. Talley RW: Chemotherapy of soft tissue sarcomas. Proc Nat Cancer Conf 7:889, 1973

96. Gonzalez-Crussi F, Black-Schaeffer S: Rhabdomyosarcoma of infancy and childhood: Problems

of morphologic classification. Am J Surg Path 3:151, 1979

97. Tefft M, Fernandez C, Newton W, Soule EH, Moon T: Round cell tumors: Ewing's vs. rhabdomyosarcoma. Int J Radiat Oncol Biol Phys (suppl 2) 2:26, 1977

98. Gillespie JJ, Roth LM, Wills ER, Einhorn LH, Willman J: Extraskeletal Ewing's sarcoma: Histologic and ultrastructural observations in three cases. Am J Surg Path 3:99, 1979

99. Beckwith JB, Palmer NG: Histopathology and prognosis of Wilms' tumor. Cancer 41:1937, 1978

100. Gonzalez-Crussi F, Goldschmidt RA, Hseuh W, Trujillo YP: Infantile sarcoma with intracytoplasmic filamentous inclusions, distinctive tumor of possible histiocytic origin. Cancer 49:2365, 1982

101. Stout AP: Juvenile fibromatosis. Cancer 7:953, 1954

102. Stout AP: Fibrosarcoma in infants and children. Cancer 15:1028, 1962

103. Enzinger FM: Fibrous tumors of infancy. In Tumors of Bone and Soft Tissue: A Collection of Papers Presented at the 8tb Annual Clinical Confrence on Cancer, 1963, at the University of Texas, MD Anderson Hospital and Tumor Institute, Houston, Texas. Chicago, Year Book Medical Publishers, 1965, p 375

104. Chung EB, Enzinger FM: Infantile fibrosarcoma. Cancer 38:729, 1976

105. Soule EH, Pritchard DJ: Fibrosarcoma in infants and children: A review of 110 cases. Cancer 40:1711, 1977

106. Das Gupta TK, Brasfield RD, O'Hara J: Extraabdominal desmoids. A clinicopathological study. Ann Surg 170:109, 1969

107. Das Gupta TK, Brasfield RD: Solitary malignant schwannoma. Ann Surg 171:419, 1970

108. Brasfield RD, Gas Gupta TK: Von Recklinghausen's disease: A clinicopathologic study. Ann Surg 175:86, 1972

109. Hawkins DB, Luxford WM: Schwannomas of the head and neck in children. Laryngoscope 90:1921, 1980

110. Kauffman SL, Stout AP: Lipoblastic tumors of children. Cancer 12:912, 1959

111. Vellios F, Baez J, Schumacker HB: Lipoblastomatosis: A tumor of fetal fat different from hibernoma: Report of case, with observations on embryogenesis of human adipose tissue. Am J Path 34:1149, 1958

112. Enterline HT, Culberson JD, Rochlin DB, Brady LW: Liposarcoma: A clinical and pathological study of 53 cases. Cancer 13:932, 1960

113. Chung EB, Enzinger FM: Benign lipoblastomatosis. An analysis of 35 cases. Cancer 32:482, 1973

114. Shear M: Lipoblastomatosis of the cheek. Br J Oral Surg 5:173, 1967

115. Botting AJ, Soule EH, Brown AL: Smooth muscle tumors in children. Cancer 18:711, 1965

116. Evans AE, Albo V, D'Angio GJ, Finklestein JZ, Keiken S, Santulli T, et al: Cyclophosphamide therapy for localized neuroblastoma. Cancer 38:655, 1976

117. Filler RM, Traggis DG, Jaffe N, et al: Favorable outlook for children with mediastinal neuroblastoma. J Pediatr Surg 7:136, 1972

118. Evans AE, Albo V, D'Angio GH et al: Factors influencing survival of children with nonmetastatic neuroblastoma. Cancer 38:661, 1976

119. Dritschilo A, Weichselbaum R, Cassady JR, et al: The role of radiation therapy in the treatment of soft tissue sarcomas of childhood. Cancer 42:1192, 1978

Index

Page numbers in italics refer to an illustration; page numbers followed by (t) refer to a table.